MEDICINES

MEDICINES

The Comprehensive Guide

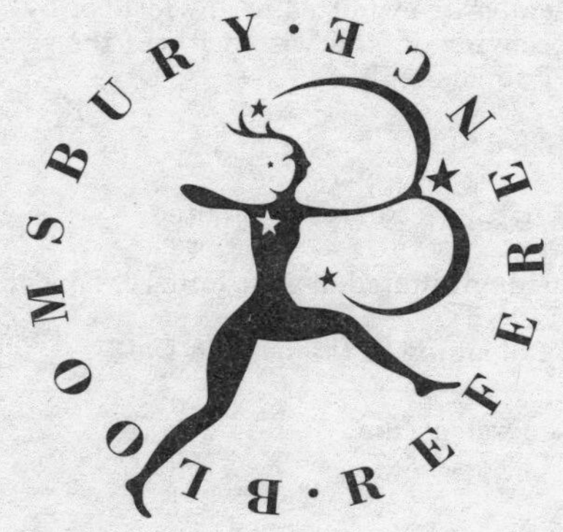

BLOOMSBURY

ACKNOWLEDGEMENTS

CONSULTANTS AND CONTRIBUTORS

Dr Ian Morton BSc, PhD (Technical Consultant)
Judith Hall BSc (Consultant Editor)

Tom Carter BSc
Deborah Carter BSc
Alyson Fox BSc
Rachel Gilbert BSc
Dr Richard Goble MB, BS
Dr Hilary Graham BSc, MB, BS
Zosia Kmietowicz BSc
Harry Shapiro BA, Dip.Lib.
Ayaz Sheikh BSc

Clark Robinson Limited acknowledge the help and advice in the creation of this book received from Dr John Bunyan, Ann and Michael Darton, Dr Andrew Herxheimer and Professor Malcolm Lader.

While the creators of this work have made every effort to be as accurate and up-to-date as possible, medical and pharmaceutical knowledge is constantly changing and the application of it to particular circumstances depends on many factors. Therefore readers are urged always to consult a qualified medical specialist for individual advice. The contributors, editors, consultants and publishers of this book can not be held liable for any errors and omissions, or actions that may be taken as a consequence of using it.

First published 1988

Bloomsbury Publishing Limited, 2 Soho Square, London W1V 5DE

British Library Cataloguing in Publication Data

Medicines.
1. Drugs – For encyclopaedias
615'.1'0321

ISBN 0 7475 0226 9

10 9 8 7 6 5 4 3 2

Designed by Malcolm Smythe
Typeset by Action Typesetting Limited, Gloucester
Printed in Great Britain by
Richard Clay Ltd, Bungay, Suffolk

CONTENTS

Preface vii

Introduction viii

Prescribing Drugs xv

The Drug Industry xxi

The Misuse of Drugs xxvii

Medicines: A to Z 1

Glossary 607

Chart of Common Disorders 614

Home Medicine Cabinet 616

PREFACE

This dictionary is a comprehensive guide to the range of medicines that are available in the United Kingdom today. It is not intended to be a guide to the prescription or administration of drugs; a qualified practitioner should always be consulted before any medicine is taken.

How to use this book

The book is divided into three sections. It begins with an introduction to medicinal drugs in general. This is accompanied by articles on the prescription of drugs, the pharmaceutical industry, and the non-medicinal abuse of drugs. Second, the A to Z forms the major part of the book. Third, there is a glossary of medical and technical terms not defined in the A to Z, a chart of common disorders (giving access to the main A to Z), and a guide to the practical preparation of a home medicine cabinet.

The articles in the A to Z describe the medicinal drugs currently available, listed under their generic and proprietary names. There are also articles describing major drug types (indicated by *), substances such as vitamins and minerals (although these are not strictly drugs) that are administered therapeutically, and various preparations (such as "cough sweets" or medicated bandages) that contain drugs.

The A to Z is cross-referenced so that further information may be found quickly. Cross-references are indicated by SMALL CAPITALS. Many of the articles list warnings (indicated by ✚) about the use of a particular drug, and a description of the possible side-effects (indicated by ▲).

W.H. – Clark Robinson Limited, London 1988

INTRODUCTION

This dictionary is concerned with the wide range of medicines available in Britain that are used in the prevention, diagnosis and treatment of disease. Although vitamins are included in this definition, there is less emphasis in the main part of the book on dietary supplements in general, or on "social" drugs (such as alcohol, caffeine, nicotine, and so on), except where they are of direct medical relevance. There is, additionally, coverage of some related medical items such as special bandages.

he book may be of interest and use to various groups of people, especially medical and paramedical workers at the training stage of their careers. These might include nurses, pharmacists, doctors and students of biomedical subjects such as pharmacology. However, it will also be of undoubted interest and use to non-specialists with a general or personal interest in medicines.

The dictionary is cross-referenced in a way that allows identification of the main active components of medicines under their generic names (the approved chemical name, such as paracetamol) or under the proprietary name (the trade name of that particular formulation, such as Panadol). There is also cross-referencing that relates a drug to a major pharmacological class of drugs.

Although this book is in no sense a medical dictionary, it should make it possible, starting from an interest in a certain type of drug, to obtain some idea of the purpose behind its use in disease, and also some of the difficulties (such as side-effects) that might be encountered.

To provide the reader with some background in this area, the following account describes the roles of both prescription and "over-the-counter" drugs, and in particular points to the benefits, risks and complexities of drug action that make these risks difficult to calculate.

Drug safety

The safety of the chemicals we refer to as "medicines" or "drugs" is an issue that needs to be confronted whenever they are prescribed or used, and here this dictionary should prove helpful. No drug is "safe" in the sense that it can never harm any individual, and this applies equally to those chemicals not always thought of as drugs (for instance vitamins, food additives or nicotine). The dose may be critical; vitamins are important for good health but, if taken in excess, the same chemicals can cause toxic effects. Unfortunately, this has often been shown to occur. Pharmacology (the study of how drugs work) and toxicology (the study of the adverse effects of chemicals) have always been closely related. The comment on early 19th-century practice – 'patients may have died, but they died cured' – is still relevant today. In the 20th century dramatic improvements in the remedies for a host of common, or not so common, complaints have been made, although treatments available at the present time for AIDS and cancer tend to exemplify the 19th-century dilemma.

Prescription of drugs

In spite of advances resulting from the outstanding success of medicinal chemists and pharmacologists in producing new drugs for both humans and animals, there is still some uncertainty as to how we are to use them wisely and responsibly. Clearly the medical profession, whether in general or hospital practice, must shoulder this task and the training of doctors in this area is of steadily increasing complexity. This dictionary indicates medicines that are available in Britain only on medical prescription; these require unambiguous instructions and advice from physicians and pharmacists as to their proper use. These instructions may include the size and frequency of dose, possible interactions with other drugs, and likely side-effects.

However desirable clear instructions may be in an ideal world, in practice difficulties may arise for various reasons, and here the dictionary may help people to take a co-operative and responsible part in their own treatment. In the case of side-effects or contra-indications, the patient needs to know of the possibility of adverse reactions in advance so that the doctor can be informed if these occur, and intervene or offer alternative treatment.

Non-prescription or "over-the-counter" drugs

Many potentially dangerous drugs can be obtained on prescription only, but some of those more commonly available are neither easy to use correctly nor entirely free from side-effects. The risks inherent in self-medication are happily minimized in Britain, where well-trained pharmacists (present for most of the time in chemists' shops) are qualified to give advice when approached with clear queries.

It is common knowledge that the nation's medicine cabinets, bedside drawers and kitchen shelves overflow with part-used or outdated prescriptions, and invitingly-named proprietary medicines acquired for complaints of which perhaps little recollection remains. The temptation to indulge in self-medication is often greatest at just those times when professional help is unavailable. Moreover, in an age of mass travel, sufferers may find themselves in a country where proprietary drugs, including, for example, antibiotics or steroids, are available "over-the- counter". Often, they have only the generic name to guide them in their purchase. In these circumstances this dictionary may prove invaluable. Other readers will be helped in choosing a sensible collection of basic medicines for their everyday needs.

Why do drugs have side-effects?

Side-effects may be of two basic kinds. First, some may be inherent in the way a drug acts pharmacologically and these may prove very difficult or impossible to circumvent. The side-effect of drowsiness and sedation, for example, is so common with the antihistamines used in the treatment of hay fever that it is accepted by most sufferers as inevitable; with more recent preparations of these drugs, however, this inconvenience is minimized by chemical alterations that restrict the drug's access to the brain. Similarly, conventional "sleeping pills" naturally tend to reduce alertness in the morning, and shorter-acting benzodiazepine drugs of this class are now available. In cases like these, co-operation between patient and physician may result in finding a more individually acceptable preparation.

Other side-effects may be less predictable and are often referred to as "idiosyncratic" (when there is a true allergic response by the

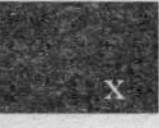

body's immune system). These adverse reactions can present a very real risk and are difficult to predict other than by asking the patient about any previous reactions to particular classes of drugs, for example, antibiotics. However, this depends on the patient being able to recall drug names and classes over long periods of time. Even a little knowledge of this sort is very desirable.

Why is there variability in drug response?

Drug therapy would be very much simplified if we were all exactly alike, but the very differences that make us the individuals we are also cause changes in sensitivities and responses to chemicals, including drugs. With an obvious difference such as body size, it follows that it would be unrealistic to expect a normal recommended dose to be as effective in a large man as it would be in a small woman of half the weight. Similarly, a drug dose may be less well absorbed when taken after a meal than it would be on an empty stomach.

It is less obvious why some drugs have different, even opposite, effects in young children, and among people of different social groups or sexes. We are, however, products of our environment and our genes, and we are becoming increasingly aware that it is the genes in particular that may effect our metabolism and hence our sensitivity to drugs. Because our genetic make-up varies with family, race and sex, it may soon become possible to make an informed guess as to the outcome of a given therapy when a patient's full family history is known.

Problems inherent in treating the very young or elderly, pregnant women and other special cases, are so great that it is almost certainly better to take no medication unless advised by a physician. In view of all these complicating factors, no doses have been recommended in this dictionary.

What are drug interactions?

Uncertainties in predicting the outcome of treatment by a single drug become considerably more complicated when two or more drugs are taken at the same time, because interactions between them are quite likely. Thus, for example, a "social" drug such as alcohol may markedly aggravate the eroding effect of aspirin on the stomach lining, or enhance the sedative effect of antihistamine or other depressant drugs. In this way, two commonly available chemicals, each with an acceptable risk factor, may become potentially dangerous in unorthodox combination. Some of these risks may be avoided by sufficient knowledge about certain products. But conversely, ignorance of the composition of medicines may lead to accidental overdose. An example may be seen in the uses of cold cures: many of these contain a full dose of paracetamol and, if taken together with headache treatment also containing paracetamol, would cause some overdosage.

What is drug dependence or addiction?

Drug dependence is a term that describes the overall situation in which, after using a drug continuously, the individual suffers in some way if the treatment is suddenly stopped. The body has become tolerant to the drug and an increased dosage may then be required over a period of time to elicit the same effect. Withdrawal symptoms may be seen; these are commonly the reverse of the expected effect of the drug (for example, anxiety following the use of a tranquillizer, or a rise in blood pressure when the treatment to lower it is stopped). These symptoms, whether psychological or physical in manifestation, are the principal reason why a treatment is only gradually withdrawn or replaced by another. It has been recognized only recently that some quite common medicines (for example, tranquillizers of the benzodiazepine class) produce marked habituation over an extended period of time.

It is generally known that some "social" drugs (chemicals taken non-medically or illicitly) cause habituation or addiction. Examples such as heroin and, of course, alcohol come readily to mind. That these problems exist also with prescription drugs is disturbing, and further highlights the need for useful dialogue between patient and doctor.

The versatile aspirin tablet

It should be clear from the points raised already that ingestion of any chemical has its risks. To some extent these risks are dose-related, and this can be illustrated by the use of aspirin at different dose levels for different purposes.

At doses much lower than are commonly used at present, aspirin may, in the future, become standard continuous therapy as a prophylactic, to prevent disease and prolong life. Clinical trials still in progress suggest it may, in middle life, give some protection from arterial thrombotic disease, with a consequent lower risk of clot formation in the blood vessels of the heart and brain. This would, in turn, reduce the risk of heart attacks and strokes.

At perhaps five or ten times this dose the standard aspirin tablet (300 mg), for use against minor aches and pains and fevers, does its job quite effectively, although many people find the accompanying dyspepsia (a stomach pain like indigestion) a problem. There is commonly also a variable but usually small blood loss from minor haemorrhages in the intestine. These normally pass unnoticed, except when some anaemia results after long-term use. Some patients suffer asthma-like symptoms, the origin of which may not be fully recognized; aspirin commonly produces an allergic response in those who are susceptible. Rarely, an individual may even die from an idiosyncratic adverse response to perhaps a single aspirin tablet.

At even higher dosages, the sufferer from rheumatoid arthritis may find that the beneficial effects of aspirin on joint pain and movement often outweigh the gastrointestinal upsets and other adverse effects of the drug.

Is paracetamol better than aspirin?

Given these worrying aspects of aspirin's action it is disturbing to learn how many tons of it are consumed annually, and to discover that perhaps one person in three takes a preparation containing salicylates on any given day. For this reason, paracetamol has been actively promoted as an alternative medication. But paracetamol has only weak anti-inflammatory action and is not so effective against pain resulting from tissue injury (although it is an effective antipyretic in the treatment of fevers).

Moreover, drugs of this class are frequently used for attempted suicide, or "parasuicide" ("mock" suicide, used as a cry for help). Aspirin in overdose is commonly used in suicide attempts. It is most disturbing that paracetamol overdose, unless treated very promptly, results in death some days later from irreversible liver failure, whereas aspirin overdose is easier to deal with.

Are the benefits of drug therapy worth the risks involved?

The answer to this question must be 'yes', but with reservations. This brief account of some of the problems associated with drug therapy is intended to help the reader to understand why no drug should be taken casually or carelessly. However, there are enormous benefits to be gained from the considerable range of drugs available when a medical condition warrants their use. Examples of drugs – many quite recently developed – that may be used to alleviate suffering and prolong life are known to all, yet there are always new steps to be taken and much is still little understood. At all stages the contribution that this dictionary may make towards effective communication between patient, physician and pharmacist can only be of value.

Dr Ian Morton
Senior Lecturer in Pharmacology
King's College London

PRESCRIBING DRUGS

The prescribing of a drug or other medication by a family doctor can be a difficult decision in the face of what are sometimes conflicting pressures. These pressures take on relative strengths according to the circumstances. Some of them might be as follows:

- Pressure from the patient/client to be given at least some sort of prescription, and not to leave the surgery "empty-handed", without a tangible outcome of the consultation.
- Pressure from the pharmaceutical industry to recognize the patient as a clinical "problem" requiring treatment (for example, sleeplessness requiring sleeping tablets), rather than as a more complex whole-person problem.
- Pressure against taking into account economic considerations. The Department of Health circulates doctors with literature reminding them of the cost of medication.
- Pressure to maintain rational prescribing considerations, attempting to match the clinical problem with an appropriate therapeutic pharmacological response.

There are subtle variations on these themes, and there are also subconscious or subliminal pressures on doctors when they are prescribing. The final act of prescribing may therefore be entirely rational or in some cases somewhat irrational. The doctor's intentions may be open and shared by the patient, or concealed as in the prescription of a placebo. Prescribing may therefore be done as a result of client demand, mutual understanding or even the doctor's desperation.

Good prescribing demands a therapeutic intention, and doctors must therefore bear certain factors in mind. For instance, a prescribed drug should be effective, cheap where possible, as free as possible from side-effects, and easily administered. Other considerations are lack of toxicity in overdose, and length of effective shelf-life or efficacy after opening. It is to be hoped that these considerations are increasingly taken into account during the development of new drugs, but nevertheless the strong influence of advertising and fashion often seems to override progress in these areas.

A doctor's choice

A family doctor has a bewildering array of drugs to choose from. He or she receives a barrage of advertising from the drug industry, a sort of "peer review" from medical colleagues, professional guidance from organizations such as Which? (Drug and Therapeutics Bulletin), as well as insistent but variable suggestions from a relatively well-informed lay public.

The doctor also has reference books produced by the drug industry and by the state as guides to prescribing. These invaluable manuals, such as the Monthly Index of Medical Specialities (MIMS) and the British National Formulary (BNF), indicate conditions, drugs, treatment regimes, dosages, contra-indications, side-effects, and so on, as well as the cost of drugs. It is one of a doctor's responsibilities to assimilate as much of this information a possible.

Drugs are called by their chemical names, by agreed and approved generic names (as in the British Pharmacopoeia – BP) and by commercial, trade or proprietary names. Such a system is necessary to enable the doctor and pharmacist to be absolutely sure that they are prescribing the correct preparation.

There is very sensible pressure on doctors to prescribe generically, but this is of course countered energetically by drug company advertising.

Hospitals generally construct their own prescribing formulary and tend to stick to generic prescribing. This is much less the case in general practice, although some family doctors have adopted formularies or constructed their own. If all doctors were to prescribe generically there would be a considerable saving to the National Health Service budget.

How drugs are prescribed

Prescribing by doctors within the British National Health Service is done using a prescription pad or Form FP10, on which the

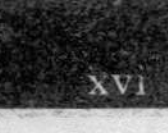

doctor writes the name of the drug, dosage information and total to be dispensed. This is taken by the patient to a pharmacist (commonly called a chemist in Britain) who dispenses the drug according to the prescription. Prescribed drugs are free for children and the elderly, as well as for full-time students, people on low incomes and those with exemption certificates (such as pregnant and lactating women). Doctors may also prescribe drugs privately, and in such cases the patient then pays the chemist at the retail price. Some doctors do their own dispensing.

Many medicines are taken without being prescribed by doctors because the patients know or are advised by friends, relatives, pharmacists or the media to take drugs such as simple analgesics (for example aspirin or paracetamol), antihistamines for conditions such as hay fever, or mixtures to treat coughs, diarrhoea or indigestion. The doctors' help is sought only when the patient is not confident about the problem or does not know of a cheap and readily available effective remedy. About 99 per cent of all homes contain some medication, and about one-third of this is self-prescribed and bought at a chemist's shop.

Drugs and disease

A doctor meets a vast array of conditions, some of which require very powerful or potentially dangerous drugs needing skilled management – for example, in the treatment of heart failure or cancer. At other times prescribing may be very simple, such as choosing an antifungal cream to treat athlete's foot. It is through the study of pharmacology (the science of the action of drugs) and therapeutics (the use of drugs clinically), together with competence in diagnosis, that the doctor is able to match a patient's clinical condition with a particular treatment.

The drugs chosen should be as "friendly" to the patient as possible. For example, doctors tend to select systemic drugs that are easily taken by mouth and which reliably produce effective treatment levels in the body with a minimum of side-effects. The doctor needs to know whether the drug should be taken with, before or after food, if it reacts with alcohol, or if it is made inactive by certain foods (as some antibiotics are by milk). The doctor should be aware, if a woman is pregnant, whether the drug would harm the unborn baby. The doctor also needs to know whether a patient is taking any other form of medication – for example, a traveller taking prophylactic antimalarial tablets or a woman taking the oral contraceptive pill – because there could be serious pharmacological interactions between these and other prescribed drugs.

Retail phramacists in Britain are now required to use a micro-computer when printing their labels for bottles or packets of drugs. Information stored on the computer relates to side-effects, drug interactions, and so on, and is a valuable safety precaution.

Some compromises clearly have to be made. For example, eye drops and certain lotions have a very short life after opening, as has glyceryl trinitrate (commonly used to treat angina), which is ineffective after about a month.

The balance between therapeutic effect and dangerous or unwanted side-effects is a constant consideration. It is widely known, for example, that steroids can control such serious disorders as asthma, rheumatoid arthritis and polymyalgia, but the prolonged systemic use of steroids is hazardous and has serious disadvantages. Similarly anti-cancer treatment, which aims at killing cancer cells, constantly falls just short of killing the patient too, and doctors have to monitor the patient's overall condition carefully and be prepared to stop the drugs or adjust the dose as the patient's condition dictates.

Many drugs are prescribed for short episodes, such as antibiotics for tonsillitis or a course of anti-inflammatory drugs for the neuromuscular condition known as "frozen shoulder". Others may have to be taken on a permanent basis, as in the treatment of hypertension, thyroid disease, epilepsy, diabetes or gout. Patients on long-term medication require carefully planned repeat prescribing, with a built-in review according to the particular properties of the drug concerned. For example, depressed or manic patients taking the fairly frequently prescribed lithium carbonate need regular blood tests to check thyroid function.

Prescribing in general practice

Two-thirds of general practice prescribing is for repeat prescriptions; 95 per cent of such requests are immediately granted without discussion, and 55 per cent of patients over 75 years of age are on regular repeat prescriptions.

Certain drugs, such as powerful painkillers and some hypnotics, cause "tolerance", which means that they become progressively less effective in a given dose, and therefore have to be given in increasingly large amounts. This is a comparable situation to drug addiction or alcoholism, and can be a serious prescribing problem.

A common difficulty in general practice concerns the patients' compliance. Many patients receive a doctors' prescription but never take the medicine, although the doctor believes they are doing so according to instructions. Similarly, patients may take only a small amount of a particular course – typically stopping as soon as the symptoms improve or seem to disappear, even though the disease itself has not been cured. Very commonly tablets are muddled up in the wrong bottles, and this can lead, for example, to patients taking sleeping pills believing they are their early morning diuretic tablets.

These problems may sound unlikely, but they are in fact very common. A doctor's home visit – particularly to an elderly or confused patient – often reveals horrifying inconsistencies between what the doctor believes the patient is taking and what is actually happening.

Because of the high cost of medication, many patients do not collect all the items on their prescription but only the ones that *they* consider the most important. Furthermore, some studies have shown that young men commonly fail to present their prescriptions to a chemist, because their primary intention in visiting the doctor is to collect a medical certificate to justify absence from work and to claim sick pay.

Clearly these sorts of problems apply to general practice rather than to hospital medicine. Administering drugs through intravenous drips and injections is normally only appropriate where nursing staff are available.

Thus prescribing drugs in general practice requires, for safety, another dimension which ensures patient compliance – that is, *explanation*. It is imperative for a doctor to give the patient a chance to understand the purpose for which the drug is being given, and to explain which possible side-effects may be expected and how to deal with them, as well as to give reasons why a course of a particular duration is required.

Doctors prescribe for infants, children, adults and the elderly. Many paediatric preparations are liquid and are administered by the child's parents, but it is also a good idea for a doctor to be aware of the taste of children's medicines. Tablets for the elderly should be easy to swallow and supplied in containers that can be opened by weak or arthritic hands. Pharmacists are particularly helpful in this last respect.

General practice prescribing is a co-operative exercise between the patient/client, doctor and pharmacist. Good communications between all three leads to a successful outcome. The doctor often requires the pharmacist to "back up" and explain the prescription, however, and studies show that pharmacists spend more time explaining drug treatments to patients than doctors do. Similarly, a patient's first request for help may be to a pharmacist, who may suggest that a doctor's advice or prescription is needed.

The doctor and pharmacist thus work together, with the pharmacist sometimes providing a safety net for errors arising out of a doctor's haste or inexperience. Naturally if a patient already has a clear idea of the medical condition and prescribing rationale, a successful outcome is much more likely to be assured.

Dr Hilary Graham
General Practitioner

THE DRUG INDUSTRY

The pharmaceutical industry, or drug industry as it is commonly called, is one of the most buoyant and expanding areas of commerce of the 20th century. This is because it fills an essential need and yet still has many tasks to fulfil. There are several aspects of the industry which should be distinguished.

First, there is research and development (R & D). This is the activity that, in the long run, produces new medicines, and for this reason will be discussed at greatest length here. It is a highly labour-intensive and expanding field, involving chemical, biological and clinical investigations, and has tended to concentrate in Western countries, where there are scientists and doctors with the necessary specialist skills. As in many industrial endeavours, the United States is the major participant, but Britain also plays an active role in this area. About half of Britain's 2,000 or more research pharmacologists are employed in the industry, with the other half in university and research institutions. This sort of mix seems quite fertile for the growth of new ideas. Other countries with a major involvement include West Germany, France, Switzerland and Italy – all countries with successful chemical industries.

Second, there is toxicological evaluation of the proposed drug, in which studies are carried out according to guidelines set up (in Britain) by the Committee on Safety of Medicines. Experiments are performed by qualified toxicologists trained to identify and predict possible toxic actions that a chemical might have in human patients. These studies are both time-consuming (commonly taking several years to complete) and costly, but are nevertheless essential before use of the chemical people can be considered.

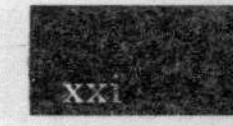

Third, there are pre- and post-marketing clinical trials. These are essential for the all-important confirmation that a drug is effective in humans and for the equally important licensing of drugs. Licensing takes place in countries with statutory bodies entrusted with the job of ensuring new drugs are at least as effective as existing remedies and that they are as safe as possible. These bodies usually also monitor adverse reactions after a drug has been licensed.

Fourth, there is manufacturing and formulation, in which active ingredients (pure drugs) are frequently imported from a parent or manufacturing company located elsewhere, and then incorporated into the often quite complex formulations that are the responsibility of the pharmaceutical chemists. These represent the actual "medicines" (for example, tablets, syrups, ointments or ampoules) that are used in practice.

Fifth, there is marketing, which is targeted throughout the world and differs little from marketing of other products except that, in Britain for example, the target group (doctors) is neither the final consumer nor the person who is financially liable. There is also a critical distinction between proprietary (trade name) and generic (active drug) products which is tied into local licensing and legal arrangements in much the same way as the use of trade marks.

Of course, this 20th-century industrial approach to drug development is by no means the only one. Many of the drugs in use today in the West are of plant or natural origin, and have been listed, often as impure extracts, in our pharmacopoeias for many centuries. In the East, especially in China, such listings cover thousands of remedies and often date back to several centuries BC.

Relationship of industrial activities to academic research

In the past, and probably in the future, the development of new drugs has often been the result of a judicious mix of academic and applied research, in such a way that the various stages leading up to the development of a successful drug are difficult to disentangle. For instance, although many people have a general idea about the story of the discovery and development of insulin or penicillin, or the structure of DNA, to those involved the events were not particularly simple (as recent dramatized accounts have illustrated). Perhaps the truth is that it is often impossible to tell accurately where ideas come from. On the other hand, manpower and effort are generally directed towards a certain useful application.

Given these uncertainties, it seems wise for a country to create an environment where there is proper training of scientists at undergraduate and postgraduate levels, adequate research funds for fundamental academic ("blue skies") research, and a firm industrial base for the exploitation of resultant ideas. Sadly in Britain, direct or indirect government funding for most aspects of scientific research is falling behind in real terms at a time when such research is growing in cost due to improvements in technology. The result is, of necessity, a growing emphasis in academic research on short term (and therefore less costly) projects which are consequently less likely to result in fundamental breakthroughs. This paucity of funding has to be balanced increasingly by charity-sponsored research, commonly directed towards a named disease (such as cancer, diabetes or asthma), and to industry itself funding longer-term projects in co-operation with universities or within its own structure. Just how effective this piecemeal approach will be remains to be seen.

How does industry find a new drug?

There is no simple answer to this question, but the following account deals with the main avenues of exploration.

Natural products have been used since the beginnings of civilization. The main search for these has been directed towards their use in medical remedies or as agents to modify the state of mind. On this latter use it is certainly difficult to find today a hallucinogenic or euphoric plant drug that has not already been tried. Poppy heads have been found in the earliest sites of civilization, and there seems no race that does not know how to produce alcohol. Because man was a 'pharmacologist before he was a farmer' (as one eminent pharmacologist put it), it is not surprising that we have a rich storehouse of products to draw on.

'Natural' does not necessarily mean 'safe', however, in spite of the views of many herbalists old and new. In fact, during the earlier part of this century, much effort in pharmacology was devoted to developing reliable biological tests that allowed potentially lethal natural substances to be used as therapeutic agents at lower dosage. For many such natural substances, the margin between the useful therapeutic dose and the lethal dose is terrifyingly small. Such agents include digitalis, an extract of foxglove leaves used for heart failure (cardiac glycosides); extract of bovine pancreas used to control blood glucose in severe diabetes (insulin); and many plant alkaloids such as atropine (from deadly nightshade) and strychnine (from nux vomica), which have been almost as popular with poisoners as with doctors!

Nevertheless, substances of this sort, to which we must certainly add opium, have proved the starting point for the development of new medicines. These agents have been purified to the stage of knowing the exact chemical composition of the active constituents, followed by systematic modifications of their chemical structure and testing of the resultant compounds. In spite of the spectacular advances, progress has sometimes been slow. It was, for instance, only quite recently that from among the many thousands of morphine-like compounds (from opium) that have been tested, scientists have discovered possible powerful pain-relieving analgesics that are not addictive and do not have other serious side-effects (such as depression of respiration and stimulation of vomiting).

Serendipity is a word popular with experimental scientists – meaning the happy art of making useful discoveries by accident; pharmacology in particular has benefited from this process, and it should always be considered whether some unexpected action of a drug may be usefully harnessed. In fact, many drugs we use today, such as penicillin, have uses deriving from essentially chance observations. This awareness that drug actions are often not predictable has also led to the formal process known as random screening.

In random biological screening, new compounds are investigated in a series of biological tests designed to identify certain actions that might be useful therapeutically. Only very few compounds are thought worthy enough to be passed on to more complicated tests, and eventually to tests on humans. Such screening is very wasteful from many points of view, but has certainly yielded many useful drugs.

Rational drug design is now becoming a practical method of advance. Not only is it likely to be much less wasteful and chancy than some of the approaches already outlined, but it offers hope of discovering drugs of a genuinely new type to treat hitherto untreatable diseases. If we have a sound understanding of the workings of the body and how it goes wrong in disease, then in principle a suitable type of drug can be designed in the pharmacologist's mind. Then, with the determined help of the medicinal chemist, this can be translated into a drug for testing first in animals and later in human patients.

One man (Sir James Black) has the distinction of doing this particular trick twice, to originate two of the most widely prescribed classes of drugs in history. First, working with colleagues at ICI in the late 1950s, he recognized the importance of the observation that a small change in the chemical structure of a compound similar to adrenaline produced a drug that, in contrast to adrenaline, reduced the heart rate and consequently blood pressure. Today, these so-called beta-blockers are used daily in millions of patients with high blood pressure, angina or abnormal heart rhythms.

Not content with this triumph, Black again exploited some earlier academic findings that suggested that the local hormone histamine acted in the stomach to cause gastric acid secretion by a different mechanism to its action elsewhere, such as causing hay fever (for which antihistamines were already available). After a prolonged and exhaustive search, a different type of antihistamine which was active in the stomach (called an H_2 antagonist) was finally developed by making chemical modifications to the histamine molecule itself. Today this type of drug is the only really effective treatment for peptic ulcers. It should be pointed out, though, that such advances are not accomplished every day, and the examples given also had elements of all the other approaches described.

'Me-too' drugs is the derogatory term for agents developed, often with little extra initiative, out of the fundamental and costly advances of others. The costs of an original investigative programme are huge (perhaps some tens of millions of pounds) and the success rate so low (perhaps one chemical in 100,000 proves to be of real value and sufficiently low in toxicity), that the 'me-too approach' is much favoured, particularly by small companies and unsuccessful competitors. The method is to seek chemically similar compounds with similar pharmacological activity but which do not have effective patent cover, and to promote them actively as alternatives to the parent compound, often in some novel combination with another drug also of value in that application. This approach is understandable on commercial grounds, but does result in many alternative remedies of very similar properties, and this tends to confuse effective therapy and lead to a disinclination by the authorities to license such drugs.

Drugs testing and marketing

When a compound with a promising drug action has been found, there follows an extensive programme of testing to explore and define the new drug's pharmacological actions, often using animals in order to predict what is likely to happen in humans. By law in most countries, the potential drug must then undergo what is described as toxicity testing (in Britain according to regulations laid down by the Committee on Safety of Medicines). Although the usefulness of some of the tests is open to debate, the necessity for toxicological evaluation is unquestionable before exposure of the compound to the public is even considered. Nowadays testing involves extensive studies to evaluate the mutagenic and likely carcinogenic properties of a compound, and studies involving several generations of animals to examine possible effects on the foetus. This is imperative if disasters such as that caused by thalidomide are to be avoided in future.

The clinical pharmacologist can then proceed with testing in humans, termed clinical trials. Initially, healthy male volunteers are exposed to the drug under carefully controlled conditions, with groups taking either the substance being tested or a 'dummy' compound (placebo). Once the pharmacologist is satisfied that the drug is safe and has no undesirable or unexpected side-effects, testing is begun using real patients, again under very controlled conditions. For certain drugs that are known to be toxic, but offer hope for treatment of incurable conditions such as cancer, testing is carried out in patients only. This is mainly because of ethical reasons not only with regard to endangering healthy volunteers, but also with regard to patients who may benefit from taking such drugs when no alternative treatment is effective.

If the final phase of the clinical trial is successful, the drug may be granted a product licence, and the drug is then allowed to be marketed for general use. The clinical trial has not, however, ended – and in a sense it never does because doctors have to file reports on adverse reactions to any drug, and particularly to new ones.

Judith Hall
Research Associate
King's College London

The Misuse Of Drugs

The major personal problems associated with the misuse of mood-altering, or psychoactive, drugs relate to health. But using drugs -- particularly if they are illegal – can bring with it all kinds of other difficulties: damaged personal relationships and job prospects, as well as legal problems, either through the possession of illegal substances or from a need to commit crimes to pay for them.

Most of the drugs discussed here are controlled in Britain under the Misuse of Drugs Act, which aims to prevent the non-medical use of certain drugs. Some of them, such as cannabis and LSD, have no currently recognized medical uses. Others, like amphetamines and heroin, still have a restricted medical use, but are deemed to be drugs that can cause the wider social problem of dependency and are thus more strictly controlled than most of the drugs available to doctors for prescribing.

Some drugs are banned and others (like alcohol and tobacco) are not. Historically this has more to do with the expediencies of politics, economics and international diplomacy than with public health. Legality or otherwise often bears little relation to the potential for physical or psychological damage inherent in a particular drug. However, this article has less to say about familiar legal drugs – such as alcohol, caffeine and tobacco than about those that are "controlled".

Definitions

Several terms can be employed to describe the non-medical use of drugs: drug dependence, drug addiction, drug abuse, recreational drug use, and so on. Some of these terms have unhelpfully pejorative connotations – "drug addict", for example, conjures up images of somebody who will do anything for a fix – and for many people the very fact that a drug is illegal makes its use, however moderate, "abuse". For the sake of simplicity, all references to drug dependence, chronic drug use, and so on denote circumstances in which drug abuse has become the dominant feature of an individual's life, to the detriment of relationships, work and health.

Significant medical terms include tolerance, withdrawal and dependence. Tolerance occurs when the body becomes tolerant to the effects of a drug, so that increasingly higher doses are needed to achieve the same effect. Withdrawal is the reaction of the body to the sudden absence of a drug to which it has adapted. Symptoms of withdrawal can range from the headaches some people experience if they miss their morning cup of coffee to the influenza-like effects of heroin withdrawal and the possibly fatal convulsions or seizures that can accompany the sudden cessation of alcohol or barbiturates. Physical dependence occurs when somebody continues to take drugs in order to avoid the physical discomfort of withdrawal. A person can suffer withdrawal symptoms and be physically dependent on a drug without any lasting desire to carry on taking it. For example, this can happen when somebody who has been given morphine in hospital for chronic pain over a period of time is suddenly taken off the drug before going home.

Drug misuse – the risks

Drug effects are strongly influenced by the amount taken, how much has been taken before, what the user wants and expects to happen, the surroundings in which it is taken, and the reactions of other people. All these influences are themselves tied up with social and cultural attitudes to, and beliefs about drugs, as well as more general social conditions. Even the same person may react differently at different times. So it is usually misleading to make simple cause-and-effect statements such as "drug X always causes condition Y".

Many people who use drugs come to no harm and may feel they have benefited from the effects of drugs in improving their social, intellectual or physical performance or helping them to relax. And they may well be right. But there are very serious risks, and some of the most significant aspects of the risks of drug taking relate to all or most drugs, whether they are illegal or not.

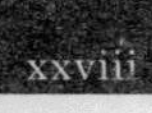

Taking a drug carries with it the risks specific to that drug or drug type. What follows is a guide to the general dangers of taking *any* drug.

Too much

In the short term, taking too much of a drug at once risks accidents, because the person may be out of control, may suffocate (by choking on vomit if he or she is unconscious) or may even overdose. The greatest potential for overdosing exists with drugs such as alcohol, barbiturates or heroin, because they depress the nervous system and in sufficient quantity can cause, for example, respiratory collapse. Overdosing is also a risk when drugs are used together or within a short time of each other. This "doubling up" can cause a fatal overdose that might not have occured if only one of the drugs had been used. Alcohol, for instance, is often implicated in what may initially be regarded as a heroin or tranquillizer overdose.

Over a longer time period, too much drug use can have multiple adverse effects on somebody's life. There can be problems with relationships with family and friends, finding or keeping a job, and keeping healthy – partly because the normal desire for food is diminished. Spare money is diverted into buying drugs and energy is used in finding the money for drugs (which may lead to crime).

Wrong time, wrong place

Even in moderate doses, most of the drugs described here (except stimulants such as amphetamines and cocaine) impair bodily control, reaction time and attention span. This means that no matter how people feel, they will be less able to drive a vehicle or operate machinery and so will become a danger to themselves and others. Low doses of stimulants can enhance performance – which is the main reason why people take them – but performance rapidly deteriorates as the dose is increased.

No two people are the same

Drugs affect different people in different ways – much depends on individual physical and psychological make-up, as the following examples show. A person with a latent mental condition can suffer long-term damage through taking LSD just once. Any drug that increases heart-rate by even a small degree, such as cannabis, can be painful for somebody suffering from angina. One person might still be standing after ten pints of lager, whereas another is on the floor after only two glasses of wine. The lighter your body weight, the greater will be the effects of drugs and so the risks are greater for a small person than for somebody who is heavier.

Injecting

For various reasons, injecting is the most dangerous way of taking a drug. Users who share their injecting equipment put themselves in the high-risk category for contracting the AIDS virus, because blood is one of the ways in which the virus is transmitted. Where needles, syringes and so on are being shared, injecting into the muscle or just under the skin is just as dangerous as injecting into a vein. Furthermore, AIDS is not the only disease associated with injecting. In fact, users are more at risk from contracting hepatitis, which is also a life-threatening, blood-borne disease.

With an injection, all the drug is taken at once. As a result, an overdose is more likely than if the drug is smoked or sniffed, when it is taken a little at a time and allows the user to stop if he or she wants to.

Some users try to inject drugs such as barbiturates, tranquillizers and painkillers, which are not meant to be injected because they are in pill form and do not dissolve properly when crushed. The filler used to make up the tablets can be highly irritant to the skin tissues. Similarly, illicit drugs in powder form, such as heroin, amphetamine and cocaine, are often adulterated with other material that does not dissolve for injecting. In all these cases, users may suffer from abscesses, abnormal swelling of the limbs or serious inflammation of the veins. Abscesses can also occur through using unsterilized or dirty equipment for injecting.

What is it?

Drugs offered on the illicit market are not always what they are claimed to be, and a wide range of impurities or contaminants can get into drugs sold on the street. This may result from the unsterile environment of illegal drug manufacture, or because drugs are mixed (or "cut") with a number of substances to increase their weight and therefore the seller's profit. A sample of street heroin, for example, could contain any combination of talc, glucose powder, flour, chalk dust or another drug substance such as barbiturate powder. An added danger is that even if users know what they are getting, they cannot tell how strong it is in relation to what they are used to taking. An unusually pure sample could easily cause an overdose.

DRUGS THAT DEPRESS THE NERVOUS SYSTEM

Alcohol

The most commonly available and misused depressant drug is alcohol. It is the drug most often used to enhance the effects of other depressants and, when taken with barbiturates, tranquillizers or heroin, can precipitate an overdose that might not otherwise have happened. And as with barbiturates, sudden withdrawal from alcohol can be fatal.

Barbiturates

These are the best-known of the drugs classified as hypnosedatives – that is, drugs which calm people down (sedatives) and in higher doses act as sleeping pills (hypnotics).

Short-acting barbiturates used as sleeping pills are the ones most often taken for their intoxicating effects. They include Tuinal, Seconal and Nembutal, and there is little doubt that they are the most inherently dangerous of the drugs misused in Britain. Partly because of these dangers, their only recommended medical use is for the treatment of severe intractable insomnia.

Barbiturates come in the form of tablets, ampoules, suppositories, solutions or commonly as coloured capsules. They are usually taken by mouth; misusers also generally take them by mouth, occasionally with alcohol, but may also prepare the powders for injection.

Barbiturates depress the central nervous system in the same way alcohol does. They produce similar effects lasting from three to six hours, depending on dose. A small dose usually makes people feel relaxed, as if they have had one or two drinks, and it is possible for the user to control the effects to some extent. With larger doses this becomes difficult, and the sedative effects take over.

Somebody trying to keep awake after a moderate to large dose (several pills) is often clumsy, with poor control of speech and body movements, which can result in accidental injury. Somebody in this state can be extremely happy, very miserable or just confused.

Large doses can produce unconsciousness and eventually respiratory failure and death. Death from overdose is an ever-present danger because the fatal amount is very near the normal dose. These effects and dangers are worse if alcohol has also been taken.

Tolerance and dependence are likely to develop with barbiturates. The dependence has a strong physical (as well as psychological) basis. So after high doses the withdrawal effects can include irritability, nervousness, sleeplessness, faintness and sickness, twitching and delirium. If convulsions occur, there may also be lasting brain damage. Sudden withdrawal from high doses of barbiturates can kill.

Heavy users are also vulnerable to bronchitis and pneumonia (because the cough reflex is depressed), hypothermia (because the drug blocks normal responses to cold) and repeated accidental overdose. Most of these risks are increased if the drug is injected. Injecting barbiturates is possibly the most dangerous form of drug abuse.

Benzodiazepine tranquillizers

Benzodiazepines are the most commonly prescribed minor tranquillizers (for daytime anxiety relief) and hypnotics (to promote sleep). They include products such as Valium, Librium and Ativan. Because of a relative absence of undesirable side-effects (such as drowsiness and poor co-ordination) and their relative safety in overdose, the benzodiazepines have come to replace barbiturates as prescribed sedatives and sleeping pills.

Most benzodiazepine treatments involve long-term repeat prescriptions, and up to half of these are issued without the doctor seeing the patient. Twice as many women as men use these drugs.

Prescribed or stolen benzodiazepines are available on the illicit market. They are often taken to help users through periods when their main choice of drug is unavailable, or to augment the effects of other depressant-type drugs, such as alcohol or opiates, and to offset the effect of amphetamine sulphate. It has been reported, however, that benzodiazepines – particularly temazepam – are the street drugs of choice in some areas, and may be prepared for injection.

Benzodiazepines depress mental activity and alertness, but do not generally make people as drowsy or clumsy as the

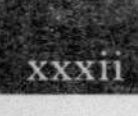

barbiturates. But they do affect driving and similar skills. Like alcohol, tranquillizers can sometimes release aggression by lowering inhibitions. Any benzodiazepine in a high enough dose can cause sleep. These effects usually last three to six hours. Many more benzodiazepines than barbiturates have to be taken to give a lethal dose. Like the other effects described, this could happen at a lower dosage level if alcohol has also been taken.

On their own, benzodiazepines rarely produce the feeling of happiness that comes with barbiturates or alcohol. After up to two weeks' continuous use, benzodiazepines may become ineffective as sleeping pills, and after four months ineffective against anxiety. Dependence is probably mainly psychological. The "pills" are relied upon to help cope with pressures or problems, and there may be severe anxiety and panic if the drug is temporarily unavailable.

Sometimes severe withdrawal symptoms occur if tolerance effects or stressful life events have led the user to increase the dose. Generally mild withdrawal symptoms can occur in a substantial minority of patients after a few years' treatment with normal therapeutic doses, and in the majority after six to eight years. Withdrawal effects after suddenly stopping benzodiazepines often take several days to appear and then last for two to three weeks or longer. They can include insomnia, anxiety, perceptual hypersensitivity, tremor, irritability, nausea and vomiting, and after unusually high doses may include convulsions and mental confusion. These are not life-threatening, and not as common as with the barbiturates, but can be extremely distressing. Withdrawal symptoms seem particularly noticeable with shorter- acting benzodiazepines such as lorazepam and temazepam.

DRUGS THAT REDUCE PAIN

Opiates

These are a group of drugs derived from the opium poppy which have generally similar effects, notably analgesia. As well as being prescribed as painkillers, opiates have medical uses as cough suppressants and anti-diarrhoea agents. Opium is the dried 'milk' of the opium poppy. It contains morphine and codeine, both effective painkillers, and from morphine it is not difficult to produce heroin, which is more than twice as potent as morphine.

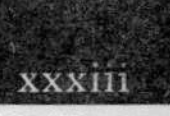

When misused, opiates can be smoked, swallowed or dissolved in water and injected. Heroin is rarely swallowed (because this is relatively ineffective), but it can be smoked or sniffed like cocaine. When smoked, heroin powder is heated and the fumes inhaled, commonly through a small tube – a practice known as 'chasing the dragon'. Some opiate mixtures are effectively rendered non-injectable by the substance used to dilute or dissolve the powder. This is the case with methadone mixture, which is one reason why it is frequently prescribed to opiate addicts.

Other opiates include pethidine (often used as a painkiller in childbirth), dipipanone (Diconal), dihydrocodeine (DF 118) and buprenorphine (Temgesic). Illicit users often crush tablets such as Diconal or Temgesic for injecting. They are not meant for this purpose and using them in this way may cause abscesses, blood clots, gangrene or inflammation of a vein.

In Britain, illicit heroin is usually around 20 to 30 per cent pure, adulterated with anything from glucose powder and chalk dust to barbiturate powder.

Pure opiates in moderate doses produce a range of mild effects in addition to killing pain. Like sedatives they depress brain activity, including reflexes such as coughing, breathing and heart-rate. They also widen blood vessels (giving a feeling of warmth) and cause constipation by reducing bowel activity.

Even with doses high enough to create feelings of great happiness, there is little interference with sensation, muscle co-ordination or intellect, although at higher doses lethargy takes over. Overdose results in unconsciousness and coma, and (very rarely) death from respiratory failure. Overdose is more likely if other depressant drugs such as alcohol or barbiturates are used at the same time.

Opiates cause a relaxed detachment from pain, desires and anxiety. They make people feel drowsy, warm and content, and relieve stress and discomfort. In people who have developed physical dependence and tolerance to opiates, however, pleasure is replaced by the relief of getting the drugs. They need it just to stay "normal".

Along with or instead of these reactions, a first-time user often feels sick and vomits, especially after injecting. Sniffing heroin gives a slower and weaker effect than injection. When heroin is smoked, its effects can be expected to come on as quickly as after injection, but to be less strong.

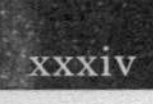

Overdoses can occur when people take what was their usual dose after coming off drugs for a time and tolerance has faded. After several weeks on high doses, sudden withdrawal causes discomfort similar to influenza. The effects start eight to twenty-four hours after the last dose of heroin and include aches, tremor, sweating and chills, sneezing and yawning, and muscular spasms. They gradually fade in seven to ten days, but a feeling of weakness and loss of well-being may last for several months. Physical dependence is not as important as the strong psychological dependence developed by some long-term users. Dependence of any kind is not inevitable, however.

Damage to the body is common among opiate users, although not usually from the drugs themselves. Damage is caused by repeated injections, often with dirty needles, and by the substances mixed with the drugs. Also apathy and reduced appetite can contribute to disease because of poor diet, self-neglect and living conditions associated with bad housing. As tolerance/dependence develops, money problems exacerbate self-neglect and a poor quality of life.

DRUGS THAT STIMULATE THE NERVOUS SYSTEM

Amphetamines

These drugs were commonly prescribed in pill form during World War II to combat physical fatigue, and in the 1950s and 1960s they were used as anti-depressants and slimming pills. Most amphetamines available on the streets today is in the form of illicitly produced amphetamine sulphate powder. Mainly it is sniffed, but increasingly in some parts of Britain it is injected.

Amphetamine sulphate has a purity of only about 15 per cent or less and is heavily adulterated. Because it is of such low purity, heavy users can consume several grams a day.

Amphetamines arouse and activate the user in much the same way as the body's natural adrenaline. Breathing and heart-rate speed up, the pupils widen and appetite decreases. The user feels more energetic, confident and cheerful. Because of these effects, there is a risk of psychological dependence. As the body's energy lessens, the main feelings may become anxiety, irritability and restlessness. High doses (especially if repeated over several days) can produce delirium, panic, hallucinations and feelings of persecution.

The effects of a single dose last about three to four hours, and leave the user feeling tired. The body may need a couple of days to recover fully. To maintain the desired effects, regular users have to take increasing doses, often many times the prescribed medical dose. When they eventually stop, they are likely to feel depressed, dull and very hungry, because amphetamines merely postpone tiredness and hunger and do not satisfy the body's need for rest and food. Heavy use also carries the risk of damaged blood vessels and heart failure, especially among people with already high blood pressure or heart-rate, or among people (such as athletes) who take strenuous exercise while using the drug.

Regular users of high doses may develop delusions, hallucinations and feelings of persecution. Sometimes these develop into mental disorder from which it can take several months to recover. High doses also weaken the user because of lack of sleep and food, and lower resistance to disease. All of these factors can have serious effects on health.

Caffeine

This is the most commonly used stimulant drug, found in small quantities in coffee, tea, chocolate and cola drinks. Consumption of 500 to 600 mg of caffeine a day (around 8 cups of instant coffee or tea) can cause anxiety and restlessness. At 15 cups a day, effects such as light flashes and ringing in the ears may be experienced, together with insomnia, faster heart-rate and breathing, muscle tremor and nausea, vomiting and diarrhoea. Regular drinkers often feel tired and irritable if they miss their usual morning coffee; psychological dependence can develop to such an extent that people find it hard to stop drinking coffee even for medical reasons – such as high blood pressure or anxiety.

Cocaine

Cocaine is a white powder, derived from the leaves of the South American coca shrub, with powerful stimulant properties similar to amphetamine. It is occasionally injected, sometimes mixed with heroin, but more commonly a small amount is sniffed through a tube and absorbed into the blood supply via the nasal membranes. Cocaine can also be smoked through a process known as "freebasing", in which the cocaine base is "freed" from the acid hydrochloride. The drug known as "Crack" is simply freebased cocaine produced by a simpler method.

Cocaine is harder to obtain and more expensive than amphetamine sulphate powder, but people already involved in drug taking circles can currently obtain 60 to 70 per cent pure cocaine for about six or seven times the price of a gram of amphetamine. In fact, it is even more expensive compared to amphetamine than the price difference suggests, because an average "dose" of amphetamine sulphate can last hours, whereas a line of cocaine normally lasts for only about 20 to 30 minutes, and freebase or crack for much less than that. The typical 'weekend' user might sniff ¼ gram or so over the weekend; regular users with sufficient resources might consume one to two grams a day. Some freebase cocaine is available in Britain, but there is so far no evidence of a significant commercial market in "crack".

Like amphetamines, cocaine causes excitement and mental exhilaration, producing feelings of well-being, reduced hunger, indifference to pain and tiredness, and great physical strength and mental capacity. Sometimes these effects are replaced by anxiety or panic, however. When sniffed, the mental effects peak after about 15 to 30 minutes and then are reduced. To maintain the effect the drug may have to be taken more frequently.

Large doses or a number of quickly repeated doses over a period of hours can give the person feelings of anxiety, agitation and persecution, and can produce hallucinations. These effects generally fade as the drug disappears from the body. The after-effects of cocaine include tiredness and depression. High doses can cause death from respiratory failure or heart attack, but this is a rare occurrence.

Users are often tempted to step up the dose because of the feelings of physical and mental well-being produced by cocaine. Users who stop taking the drug feel tired, sleepy and depressed, which reinforces the temptation to repeat the dose. With regular use, increasingly unpleasant effects develop and these generally persuade people to stop using it for a while. Happiness is replaced by an uncomfortable state of restlessness, excitability, sickness, sleeplessness and weight loss. With continued use this may change into a persecuted state of mind. Regular users may seem nervous, excitable and suspicious. Confused exhaustion caused by lack of sleep is also common. All these effects generally clear up once the use is stopped. Repeated sniffing damages the nasal membranes and may damage the structure separating the nostrils.

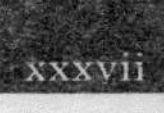

Tobacco

More people are regular users of tobacco than of any other drug, and some drug users have reported that it was harder to give up cigarettes than heroin. Even so, nicotine is the cause of many chronic health conditions, including coronary heart disease and lung cancer. More people in Britain die from tobacco-related diseases than from the effects of all the other drugs put together, including alcohol – at least 100,000 every year.

DRUGS THAT ALTER PERCEPTION

Cannabis

Cannabis – also called hash, pot or grass – does not fit easily into any drug group. In low doses, it can be a sedative: in high doses, a hallucinogenic. It is by far the most widely used illegal drug in Britain – several million people have tried it at least once. It is most commonly smoked, often mixed with tobacco, but it can also be swallowed, usually mixed with food.

The results of taking cannabis (by smoking a "joint") depend largely on the expectations, motivations and mood of the user, the amount used, and the situation. Most people do not experience much at first, and "learn" which effects to look out for. The most common, and also most sought-after, effects are talkativeness, cheerfulness, relaxation and greater appreciation of sound and colour. Cannabis reduces people's ability to do complicated tasks and can affect short-term memory. Because people cannot concentrate as well, it is dangerous to drive or work machinery after taking cannabis.

With higher doses, vision may be distorted. Inexperienced people using high doses, and others using the drug when anxious or depressed, may find their unpleasant feelings strengthened. Sometimes they experience short-term panic. There is virtually no danger of a fatal overdose. The effects generally start a few minutes after smoking. They may last up to one hour with low doses, and for several hours with high ones. Normally there is no hangover.

There is no proof that cannabis use over a long time causes lasting damage to physical or mental health. This may be because the kinds of study needed to detect slow-to-develop and uncommon results have not been done. However, like tobacco smoke, frequently inhaled cannabis probably causes bronchitis and other breathing disorders, and may cause lung cancer.

People who use cannabis are more likely to try other drugs. Likewise people who smoke tobacco or drink are more likely to try cannabis. In neither case is there any evidence that using one drug actually causes people to use another. Cannabis does not seem to produce physical dependence, although regular users can come to feel a psychological need for the drug's effects.

As with other calming drugs, people who often get "high" on cannabis may appear apathetic, dull and neglect their appearance, but there is no evidence that cannabis destroys people's motivation to work. But, while intoxicated, users do less well on tasks requiring concentration. The effects of cannabis may cause special risks for people with existing respiratory or heart disorders. Heavy use by people with disturbed personalities can bring on a temporary mental disorder.

LSD and other psychedelics

In Britain, the main psychedelic drugs are LSD and hallucinogenic 'magic' mushrooms. Lysergic acid diethylamide – LSD – is a white powder, but the minute amounts sufficient for a 'trip' are generally mixed with other substances and formed into tablets or capsules to be taken by mouth. In solution, the drug may also be taken absorbed on paper, gelatine sheets or sugar cubes. The strength of the preparations is uncertain, and often substances offered as LSD contain no LSD at all. Nevertheless three or four "tabs" of LSD would induce a full-blown hallucinogenic experience.

A trip begins about 30 minutes or an hour after taking LSD. It peaks after two to six hours and fades after about 12 hours, depending on the dose. It usually goes through several stages. Experiences are hard to describe, partly because they vary, and partly because they can be very different from our normal ways of seeing the world. Effects depend on the user's mood and situation, as well as the dose. They often include an awareness of strong colours and distortion of vision and hearing. But true hallucinations – believing something is there when it is not – are rare. Reactions may include heightened self-awareness and mystical or ecstatic experiences. A feeling of being outside one's body is commonly reported. Brief but vivid re-experiences of a part of a previous trip ("flashbacks") have also been described, especially after frequent use. These can leave the person feeling disorientated, and can be distressing, but are only rarely dangerous.

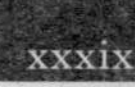

Unpleasant reactions ("bad trips") may include depression, dizziness, disorientation and sometimes panic. These are more likely if the user is unstable, anxious or depressed, or in hostile or unfamiliar surroundings. Deaths because of suicide or hallucinations, although much publicized, are rare.

LSD is not always used as an aid to insight. Smaller doses may be taken in a more casual, recreational fashion, but because such tiny amounts are sufficient to induce quite marked effects it can be difficult to control fully the amount used. There is no proof of physical damage from repeated use of LSD: the main hazards are psychological. Acute anxiety or brief mental disorders may occur, but can usually be dealt with by reassurance from a friend. Prolonged serious disorders are also rare; they are most likely in people with already existing mental problems.

It is difficult to combine a trip with a task requiring concentration. The ability to drive, for instance, is seriously reduced. People who do drive while under the influence of the drug could endanger themselves and others. There is no physical dependence. Frequent use is discouraged by the fact that, for several days after taking LSD, further doses are less effective.

Magic mushrooms

The main varieties of hallucinogenic mushrooms found in Britain are Fly Agaric (Amanita muscaria) and Liberty Cap.

Magic mushrooms have very similar effects to LSD. The biggest danger lies in picking the wrong mushrooms, which may turn out to be highly poisonous rather than "mind blowing". Magic mushrooms are usually eaten, either alone or with food.

Harry Shapiro
Drugs Information Officer

The author wishes to acknowledge
the Institute for the Study of Drug
Dependence in preparing this article.

AAA Spray (*Armour*) is a proprietary, non-prescription, ANTISEPTIC mouth and throat spray, used to treat a sore throat, irritation caused by post-nasal drip, or minor infections. Apart from its antiseptic constituent, AAA Spray also contains a very small proportion of the local ANAESTHETIC BENZOCAINE.

Abicol (*Boots*) is a proprietary ANTIHYPERTENSIVE drug, available only on prescription, used to treat high blood pressure (hypertension) and to slow the heart rate. Produced in the form of tablets, Abicol's active constituents are the RAUWOLFIA ALKALOID reserpine and the DIURETIC bendrofluazide. It is not recommended for administration to children.
✚/▲ warning/side-effects: *see* BENDROFLUAZIDE; RESERPINE.

Abidec (*Parke, Davis*) is a proprietary non-prescription MULTIVITAMIN compound that is not available from the National Health Service. Produced in the form of capsules and drops, Abidec contains RETINOL (vitamin A), several forms of vitamin B (THIAMINE, RIBOFLAVINE, PYRIDOXINE and NICOTINAMIDE), ASCORBIC ACID (vitamin C) and ERGOCALCIFEROL (vitamin D).

acebutolol is a BETA-BLOCKER, a drug used in the treatment of angina (heart pain) and cardiac arrhythmias (heartbeat irregularities). It is also used to treat high blood pressure (*see* ANTIHYPERTENSIVE) usually in conjunction with a THIAZIDE DIURETIC. Acebutolol is also used to decrease the heart rate and to control other symptoms that occur in hyperthyroidism. Administration is oral in the form of capsules, or in the case of emergency treatment of cardiac arrhythmias it may be given by slow intravenous injection.
✚ warning: acebutolol should not be given to patients with asthma or bronchospasm, excessive acidity in the metabolism, partial heart block or slowness of the heartbeat. It should be administered with great care to patients with heart failure (failure of the heart to contract effectively).
▲ side-effects: the most common are nausea, vomiting, diarrhoea, fatigue and dizziness, although slow heartbeat, hypotension (low blood pressure) and cold toes and fingers may also occur.
Related articles: SECADREX; SECTRAL.

Acepril (*Duncan, Flockhart*) is a proprietary ANTIHYPERTENSIVE drug, available only on prescription, used to treat high blood pressure and cardiac failure, particularly when THIAZIDES or BETA-BLOCKERS have failed or are not tolerated. Produced in the form of tablets (in three strengths), Acepril is a preparation of the powerful enzyme inhibitor captopril.
✚/▲ warning/side-effects: *see* CAPTOPRIL.

acetazolamide is a mildly DIURETIC drug used to treat pressure in the eyeball (glaucoma) by reducing the formation of the aqueous humour. Secondary uses include the treatment of grand mal and focal epilepsy, the accumulation of fluid in the tissues (oedema), and premenstrual tension. Administration is oral in the form of tablets or capsules, or by injection or infusion; some forms are not recommended for children. Sodium and/or potassium supplements may be

A

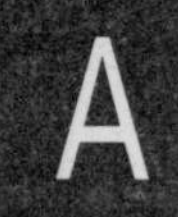

required during treatment.
✚ warning: acetazolamide should not be administered to patients with sodium or potassium deficiency, or with malfunction of the adrenal glands, and should be administered with caution to patients who are pregnant or lactating, diabetic, or who have gout. Monitoring of the blood count and of electrolyte levels is essential.
▲ side-effects: there may be drowsiness, numbness and tingling of the hands and feet, flushes and headache, thirst, and frequency of urination.
Related article: DIAMOX.

acetohexamide is a drug used to treat (adult-onset) diabetes mellitus, one of the SULPHONYLUREAS which work by augmenting insulin secretion (as opposed to compensating for its absence). Administration is oral in the form of tablets.
✚ warning: acetohexamide should not be administered to patients who suffer from liver or kidney disease, from endocrine disorders or from stress; who are pregnant or lactating.
▲ side-effects: there may be some sensitivity reaction (such as a rash).
Related article: DIMELOR

Acetoxyl (*Stiefel*) is a proprietary, non-prescription, topical preparation for the treatment of acne. Produced in the form of a gel (in two strengths – 2.5% and 5%), its active constituent is benzoyl peroxide, which has both KERATOLYTIC and ANTIMICROBIAL properties.
✚/▲ warning/side-effects: *see* BENZOYL PEROXIDE.

acetylcholine chloride is a PARASYMPATHOMIMETIC drug which, in very mild solution and in combination with a mild solution of MANNITOL, is used to irrigate the eye during eye surgery. By itself it has the effect of rapidly contracting the pupil (miosis). Acetylcholine is the natural neurotransmitter released from cholinergic nerves (see ANTICHOLINERGIC).

acetylcysteine is a MUCOLYTIC drug, used to reduce the viscosity of sputum and thus facilitate expectoration (the coughing up of sputum) in patients with disorders of the upper respiratory tract, such as asthma and bronchitis. It may also be used to treat abdominal complications associated with cystic fibrosis; to increase lachrymation (the production of tears); or as an antidote to overdosage of PARACETAMOL. Administration is oral in the form of a solution of dissolved granules, as eye-drops, by injection or infusion, or by nebulisation through a face-mask or mouthpiece.
✚ warning: acetylcysteine should be administered with caution to patients who are elderly or those with severe respiratory insufficiency.
▲ side-effects: there may be nausea and vomiting, and stomatis (inflammation of the mouth).
Related articles: FABROL; ILUBE; PARVOLEX.

Achromycin (*Lederle*) is a proprietary form of the tetracycline ANTIBIOTIC tetracycline hydrochloride, available only on prescription. Used to treat many types of microbial and fungal infection all over the body – particularly on the skin, on the face, and around and in the ears and eyes – Achromycin is produced in many forms: as tablets (in two types), as

a syrup, as an ointment (in two strengths), as an ophthalmic oil suspension (for use as drops), and powdered in vials for reconstitution and injection. Some forms are not recommended for children.
✚/▲ warning/side-effects: *see* TETRACYCLINE.

Achromycin V (*Lederle*) is a form of the proprietary tetracycline antibiotic ACHROMYCIN that also contains a buffer – a substance that does not change its acid-alkali balance (pH) if it is diluted. Produced in the form of capsules and as a syrup, it is not recommended for children.
✚/▲ warning/side-effects: *see* TETRACYCLINE.

Acidol-Pepsin (*Sterling Research*) is a proprietary non-prescription compound used to make up a deficiency of hydrochloric acid and other digestive juices in the stomach. Produced in the form of tablets, Acidol-Pepsin contains betaine hydrochloride together with the gastric enzyme pepsin.
✚/▲ warning/side-effects: *see* BETAINE HYDROCHLORIDE.

Aci-Jel (*Ortho-Cilag*) is a proprietary, non-prescription, ANTISEPTIC preparation used to treat non-specific vaginal infections and restore acidity to the vagina. Produced in the form of a jelly (accompanied by a special applicator), Aci-Jel's active constituent is acetic acid, which has an antibacterial activity.
▲ side-effects: there may be local irritation and/or inflammation.

Acnegel (*Kirby-Warrick*) is a proprietary, non-prescription, topical preparation for the treatment of acne. Produced in the form of a gel (in two strengths – 5% and 10% – the latter under the trade name Acnegel Forte), its active constituent is benzoyl peroxide, which has both KERATOLYTIC and ANTIMICROBIAL properties.
✚/▲ warning/side-effects: *see* BENZOYL PEROXIDE.

Acnidazil (*Janssen*) is a proprietary, non-prescription, topical preparation for the treatment of acne. Produced in the form of a cream, its active constituents are benzoyl peroxide, which has both KERATOLYTIC and ANTIBACTERIAL properties, and the ANTIFUNGAL agent miconazole nitrate.
✚/▲ warning/side-effects: *see* BENZOYL PEROXIDE; MICONAZOLE.

acrosoxacin is an unusual ANTIBACTERIAL agent used to treat the sexually-transmitted disease gonorrhoea in patients who are allergic to penicillin, or whose strain of gonorrhoea is resistant to penicillin-type antibiotics. Administration is oral in the form of capsules. It is not recommended for children.
✚ warning: acrosoxacin should be administered with caution to patients who have impaired kidney or liver function, or who are pregnant.
▲ side-effects: there may be dizziness, drowsiness and headache such as to interrupt concentration or intricacy of movement or thought; there may also be gastrointestinal disturbances.
Related article: ERADACIN.

Actal (*WinPharm*) is a proprietary, non-prescription, compound ANTACID that is available also from the National Health Service. Used to treat acid stomach and indigestion, and produced in the form of tablets for chewing, and as a

A

suspension, Actal's active constituent is ALEXITOL SODIUM.

Acthar Gel (*Armour*) is a proprietary preparation of adrenocorticotrophic HORMONE (ACTH, or corticotrophin), available only on prescription. The hormone controls the secretions of corticosteroids by the adrenal glands. In the form of injections of the hormone in a hydrolysed gelatin base, Acthar Gel replaces hormonal deficiency and treats rheumatic diseases, skin and nerve disorders, asthma and hay fever, and gastrointestinal disturbances. It may also be administered to test adrenal function.

ACTH/CMC (*Ferring*) is a proprietary preparation of adrenocorticotrophic HORMONE (ACTH, or corticotrophin), available only on prescription. The hormone controls the secretions of corticosteroids by the adrenal glands. In the form of injections of the hormone in a carmellose base, ACTH/CMC replaces hormonal deficiency and treats rheumatic diseases, skin and nerve disorders, asthma and hay fever, and gastrointestinal disturbances. It may also be administered to test adrenal function.

Actidil (*Wellcome*) is a proprietary non-prescription ANTIHISTAMINE drug used to treat various allergic conditions, particularly conditions of the nose (allergic rhinitis) and skin (urticaria). It may also be used to assist sedation or as a premedication before surgery. Produced in the form of tablets and as a syrup for dilution (the syrup once dilute retains potency for 14 days), Actidil is a preparation of triprolidine hydrochloride.

✚/▲ warning/side-effects: *see* TRIPROLIDINE.

Actifed (*Wellcome*) is a proprietary, non-prescription, compound nasal and respiratory DECONGESTANT that is not available from the National Health Service. Produced in the form of tablets and as a syrup for dilution (the syrup once dilute retains potency for 14 days), Actifed contains the SYMPATHOMIMETIC VASOCONSTRICTOR ephedrine and the ANTIHISTAMINE triprolidine.
✚/▲ warning/side-effects: *see* EPHEDRINE; TRIPROLIDINE.

Actifed Compound Linctus (*Wellcome*) is a proprietary, non-prescription, compound cough preparation that is not available from the National Health Service. Produced in the form of an elixir for dilution (the elixir once dilute retains potency for 14 days), the Compound Linctus contains the SYMPATHOMIMETIC VASOCONSTRICTOR ephedrine, the ANTIHISTAMINE triprolidine, and the NARCOTIC ANTITUSSIVE dextromethorphan.
✚/▲ warning/side-effects: *see* DEXTROMETHORPHAN; EPHEDRINE; TRIPROLIDINE.

Actifed Expectorant (*Wellcome*) is a proprietary, non-prescription, compound EXPECTORANT that is not available from the National Health Service. Produced in the form of an elixir for dilution (the elixir once dilute retains potency for 14 days), the preparation contains the VASOCONSTRICTOR ephedrine, the ANTIHISTAMINE triprolidine, and the expectorant guaiphenesin.
✚/▲ warning/side-effects: *see* EPHEDRINE; TRIPROLIDINE.

Actinac (*Roussel*) is a proprietary

lotion, to be made up from powder and a diluent solvent, representing a topical treatment for acne. Available only on prescription, Actinac's active constituents include the broad-spectrum ANTIBIOTIC CHLORAMPHENICOL and the STEROID HYDROCORTISONE.

actinomycin D is an ANTIBIOTIC drug that is also CYTOTOXIC, and therefore used to treat cancer (particularly cancer of the kidney, the womb or the testes). In addition it has immunosuppressive properties and may be used in combination with other similar drugs during transplant surgery to prevent tissue rejection. Dosage is critical to each individual patient. Administration is by injection of a bolus of the drug into a vein.

✚ warning: suppression of the bone-marrow's function of producing red blood cells is inevitable, and regular blood counts are essential.

▲ side-effects: hair loss is common, even to total baldness; there may be inflammation of the mucous lining of the mouth (stomatitis), nausea and vomiting. There may also be increased sensitivity to radiotherapy.
Related article: COSMEGEN LYOVAC.

Actonorm (*Wallace*) is a proprietary non-prescription ANTACID that is not available from the National Health Service. In its basic form it is produced as a gel containing no more than the long-lasting antacid ALUMINIUM HYDROXIDE together with the antifoaming agent dimethicone and the mildly laxative MAGNESIUM HYDROXIDE. But in the form of tablets or as powder for solution, Actonorm contains many more constituents intended to impart ANTISPASMODIC properties (that relax the muscular walls of the intestines), including such powerful drugs as the SMOOTH MUSCLE RELAXANT papaverine and the ANTICHOLINERGIC atropine. In any form, Actonorm is not recommended for children.

✚/▲ warning/side-effects: *see* ATROPINE; PAPAVERINE.

Actraphane (*Novo*) is a proprietary intermediate-duration combination of mixed INSULINS (isophane insulin 70%, neutral insulin 30%) used to treat patients with diabetes mellitus.

Actrapid (*Novo*) is a proprietary quick-acting preparation of neutral INSULIN, used to treat patients with diabetes mellitus.

Acupan (*Carnegie*) is a proprietary non-narcotic ANALGESIC, available only on prescription, used to treat severe pain (such as that following surgery, or in cancer or toothache). Produced in the form of tablets and in ampoules for injection, Acupan is a preparation of nefopam hydrochloride.

✚/▲ warning/side-effects: *see* NEFOPAM.

acyclovir is a powerful ANTIVIRAL agent that also has some ANALGESIC properties, used specifically to treat viral infection by herpes viruses (such as shingles, chickenpox, cold sores including genital sores, and herpes infections of the eye). It works by inhibiting the action of one of the enzymes in cells used by the virus to replicate itself. To be effective, however, treatment of an infection must begin early. The drug may also be used to prevent others at risk from contracting a herpes disease. Administration is oral, topical or by infusion.

✚ warning: acyclovir should be administered with caution to patients who are pregnant or who have impaired kidney function. To be effective, treatment of an infection must begin as early as possible. Adequate fluid intake must be maintained.

▲ side-effects: applied topically, there may be a temporary burning or stinging sensation; some patients experience a localized drying of the skin. Taken orally, acyclovir may give rise to gastrointestinal disturbance and various changes in the composition of the blood; there may also be fatigue and a rash.
Related article: ZOVIRAX.

Adalat is a proprietary CALCIUM-ANTAGONIST VASODILATOR, available only on prescription, used to treat angina pectoris, coldness and numbness of the fingers (Raynaud's phenomenon) and (under the trade name Adalat Retard) high blood pressure (hypertension). Produced in the form of a liquid (in capsules) and as sustained-release tablets, the active constituent in both preparations is nifedipine. Neither preparation is recommended for children.

✚/▲ warning/side-effects: *see* NIFEDIPINE.

Adcortyl (*Squibb*) is a proprietary form of the ANTI-INFLAMMATORY glucocorticoid (CORTICOSTEROID) drug triamcinolone acetonide, available only on prescription. Produced in the form of ointment or cream, Adcortyl is used to treat skin infections (such as dermatitis), psoriasis, insect bites and sunburn; a version is available that includes the ANTIBIOTIC NEOMYCIN and the antimicrobial agent gramicidin known as Adcortyl with Graneodin. In ORABASE paste, Adcortyl is used to treat oral and dental inflammations. Produced as injections, Adcortyl is used in two different ways in order to achieve either of two distinct purposes: intradermal injection relieves some scaly skin diseases (such as lichen planus); injection directly into a joint relieves pain, swelling and stiffness (such as with rheumatoid arthritis, bursitis and tenosynovitis).

✚/▲ warning/side-effects: *see* GRAMICIDIN; TRIAMCINOLONE ACETONIDE.

Addamel (*KabiVitrum*) contains additional electrolytes and trace elements for use in association with Vamin (proprietary) infusion fluids, for the intravenous nutrition of a patient in whom feeding via the alimentary tract is not possible.

Addiphos (*KabiVitrum*) contains additional phosphate for use in association with Vamin (proprietary) infusion fluids, for the intravenous nutrition of a patient in whom feeding via the alimentary tract is not possible.

adrenaline is a hormone (a catecholamine) produced and secreted by the central core (medulla) of the adrenal glands. Like the closely-related NORADRENALINE, it represents one contributory element of the sympathetic nervous system in that, as a neurotransmitter (transmitting neural impulses between nerves, and between nerves and muscles), it relays a response to stress. In the face of stress, the body thus uses adrenaline (and noradrenaline) to organize constriction of the small blood vessels (vasoconstriction, so

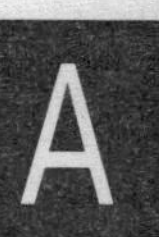

increasing blood pressure), increased blood flow through the heart while the heart rate is raised, increased rate and depth of respiration, and relaxation of the muscles of the intestinal walls and bronchioles. And it is to effect one or more of these responses that adrenaline, as a SYMPATHOMIMETIC, may be administered therapeutically. In an emergency, for example, adrenaline may be injected to restart the heart, or to treat for anaphylactic shock. Because adrenaline relaxes bronchial muscles it is used to relieve bronchial spasm in acute attacks of bronchial asthma, in which case it is injected subcutaneously. Intramuscular injections are given for control of prolonged asthma attacks. In addition, adrenaline administered simultaneously with a local ANAESTHETIC considerably lengthens the duration of effect of the anaesthetic. More commonly, adrenaline is administered in solution in eye-drops to treat glaucoma. Administration is by injection or inhalation; one proprietary solution is in the form of a cream.

✚ warning: adrenaline should be administered with caution to patients who suffer from insufficient blood supply to the heart, from high blood pressure (hypertension), from diabetes, or from overactivity of the thyroid gland (hyperthyroidism), or who are already taking drugs that affect the heart or mood.

▲ side-effects: there is an increase in heart rate; there may also be headache, anxiety, and coldness in the fingertips and toes. High dosage may lead to tremor and the accumulation of fluid in the lungs. Adrenaline in eye-drops may cause redness of the eye.

Related articles: BROVON; EPIFRIN; EPPY; GANDA; ISOPTO EPINAL; MARCAIN; MIN-I-JET ADRENALINE; RYBARVIN; SIMPLENE; XYLOCAINE; XYLOTOX.

Adriamycin (*Farmitalia Carlo Erba*) is a proprietary ANTIBIOTIC drug that is also CYTOTOXIC, and therefore used to treat cancer (particularly leukaemia, lymphoma and certain solid tumours). Available only on prescription, it is produced in the form of powder for reconstitution as a medium for fast-running infusion (generally at three-week intervals). Its active constituent is doxorubicin hydrochloride.

✚/▲ warning/side-effects: *see* DOXORUBICIN HYDROCHLORIDE.

adsorbed diphtheria and tetanus vaccine is diphtheria and tetanus vaccine adsorbed on to a mineral carrier.
see DIPHTHERIA AND TETANUS VACCINE.

adsorbed diphtheria, tetanus and pertussis vaccine is diphtheria, pertussis and tetanus (DPT) VACCINE adsorbed on to a mineral carrier.
see DIPHTHERIA, PERTUSSIS AND TETANUS (DPT) VACCINE.

adsorbed tetanus vaccine is tetanus VACCINE adsorbed on to a mineral carrier.
see TETANUS VACCINE.

Aerosporin (*Calmic*) is a proprietary form of the ANTIBIOTIC drug polymyxin B sulphate, available only on prescription, which is used to treat many infective organisms (particularly in the urinary tract), but which is also fairly toxic. It is produced in the form

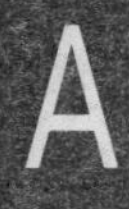

of powder for reconstitution as a medium for injections.

✚/▲ warning/side-effects: *see* POLYMYXIN B SULPHATE.

Afrazine (*Kirby-Warrick*) is a proprietary non-prescription preparation of the nasal DECONGESTANT oxymetazoline hydrochloride, a SYMPATHOMIMETIC, that is not available from the National Health Service. It is produced in the form of nose-drops (in two strengths) and as a nasal spray.

✚/▲ warning/side-effects: *see* OXYMETAZOLINE HYDROCHLORIDE.

Agarol (*Warner-Lambert*) is a proprietary, non-prescription, compound LAXATIVE that is not available from the National Health Service. Produced in the form of a liquid (mixture) for dilution (the mixture once dilute retains potency for 28 days), Agarol contains the seaweed extract gel agar, together with phenolphthalein and liquid paraffin.

▲ side-effects: laxative effects may continue for several days; there may be dysfunction of the kidneys, leading possibly to discoloration of the urine. A mild skin rash may appear.

Agiolax (*Radiol*) is a proprietary non-prescription form of the stimulant LAXATIVE senna together with the bulking-agent laxative ispaghula; it is not available from the National Health Service. Produced in the form of granules for solution in water, Agiolax is not recommended for children aged under 5 years.

✚/▲ warning/side-effects: *see* ISPAGHULA HUSK; SENNA.

Aglutella Azeta (*G F Dietary Supplies*) is a proprietary (non-prescription) brand of gluten-free cream-filled wafers which are also low in protein, sodium and potassium. They are intended for consumption by patients with gluten sensitivity (as with coeliac disease), amino-acid abnormalities (such as phenylketonuria), or kidney or liver failure.

Aglutella Gentili (*G F Dietary Supplies*) is a proprietary (non-prescription) brand of gluten-, sucrose- and lactose-free pasta – spaghetti, spaghetti rings, macaroni, macaroni spirals, and tagliatelle – intended for consumption by patients with gluten sensitivity (as with coeliac disease), amino-acid abnormalities (such as phenylketonuria), or kidney or liver failure.

Akineton (*Abbott*) is a proprietary preparation of the anticholinergic drug biperiden, available only on prescription, used to relieve some of the symptoms of parkinsonism (*see* ANTIPARKINSONISM), specifically tremor of the hands, overall rigidity of posture, and the tendency to produce an excess of saliva. It is thought to work by compensating for the lack of dopamine in the brain that is the major cause of such parkinsonian symptoms, and is produced in the form of tablets and in ampoules for injection.

✚/▲ warning/side-effects: *see* BIPERIDEN.

Akrotherm (*Napp*) is a proprietary non-prescription cream for topical application, designed to act as a local VASODILATOR to improve the blood circulation in conditions such as bruising and inflammation of the veins. Active constituents include histamine oxycholesterol and acetylcholine chloride.

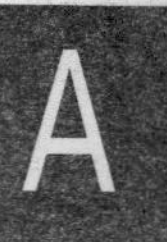

Alavac-P (*Bencard*) is a set of proprietary DESENSITIZING VACCINES prepared from 12 varieties of common grass pollens for the prevention and treatment of hay fever and pollen asthma. Available only on prescription and administered by injection, Alavac-P pollen preparations are of carefully-annotated different allergenic effect, so that the process of desensitisation, as regulated by a doctor, can be progressive.

✚ warning: injections should be administered under close medical supervision, and following a comprehensive case history of the patient.

Alavac-S (*Bencard*) is a proprietary set of up to 6 preparations of common allergens (including the house dust mite) prepared to the patient's requirements for use in desensitising patients who are allergic to them. Available only on prescription and administered by injection, Alavac-S allergen preparations are of carefully-annotated different allergenic effect, so that the process of desensitisation, as regulated by a doctor, can be progressive.

✚ warning: injections should be administered under close medical supervision, and following a comprehensive case history of the patient.

Albay (*Dome/Hollister-Stier*) is either of two preparations – of bee venom and of wasp venom – for use in diagnosing and desensitising patients who are allergic to them. Available only on prescription, solutions of one or the other venom are administered as injections in increasingly less dilute form so that treatment is progressive.

✚ warning: injections should be administered under close medical supervision and in locations where emergency facilities for full cardio-respiratory resuscitation are immediately available. Albay preparations should not be given to patients who are pregnant, or who suffer from asthma.

Albucid (*Nicholas*) is a proprietary ANTIBACTERIAL, available only on prescription, used to treat eye infections. Produced in the form of eye-drops and (under the trade name Albucid Ointment) as an ointment (in either a water-miscible base or an oily base), Albucid's active constituent is the SULPHONAMIDE sulphacetamide sodium.
see SULPHACETAMIDE.

Albumaid (*Scientific Hospital Supplies*) is the brand name of a series of proprietary foods for special diets, as required mostly in hospitals and clinics. They are produced as powders for reconstitution. Albumaid Complete contains protein, amino acids, vitamins, minerals and trace elements, and has no carbohydrate or fat. Albumaid XP contains protein, carbohydrate, vitamins and minerals, amino acids but less than 0.01% phenylalanine, and no fat. Albumaid XP Concentrate contains protein, vitamins, minerals and trace elements, amino acids but less than 0.025% phenylalanine, and no carbohydrate or fat. Other Albumaid preparations generally follow the pattern of Albumaid XP but instead of a minimum content of phenylalanine contain minimum quantities of (respectively) the amino acids cystine, histidine, methionine or tyrosine.

alclometasone dipropionate is a

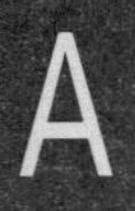

CORTICOSTEROID drug used for topical application to treat inflammatory skin disorders in which the cause of inflammation is deemed not to be infection – in particular to treat eczema. Administration is as a cream or an ointment. Dosage should be the minimum to achieve the required response.

✚ warning: as with all corticosteroids, alclometasone diproprionate treats the symptoms and does not treat any underlying disorder. An undetected infection may thus become worse although its symptoms may be suppressed by the drug.

▲ side-effects: side-effects are rare, but may include skin sensitivity and hair growth.
Related article: MODRASONE

Alcobon (*Roche*) is a powerful proprietary ANTIFUNGAL drug, available only on prescription, used to treat systemic infections by yeasts (such as candidiasis, or thrush). Produced for hospital use only in the form of tablets and in infusion flasks, Alcobon is a preparation of flucytosine.

✚/▲ warning/side-effects: *see* FLUCYTOSINE.

Alcoderm (*Alcon*) is a proprietary non-prescription skin EMOLLIENT (softener and soother), used to treat dry or itchy skin. Produced in the form of a cream and a lotion, Alcoderm's major constituents are liquid paraffin and a moisturizer.

alcohol is the name of a class of compounds derived from hydrocarbons. The alcohol in alcoholic drinks is ethyl alcohol (or ethanol) and is produced by the fermentation of sugar by yeast. Alcohol is ultimately a depressant, at high doses producing sleep (HYPNOTIC), general anaesthesia (ANAESTHETIC), and eventually coma and death. At low doses (consumption) it reduces social inhibitions, so can be effectively a stimulant. It has marked diuretic actions, and produces vasodilatations, particularly in the skin. As a food, alcohol has calorific values between carbohydrates and fats, and as a nutritional substitute in alcoholics may lead to vitamin deficiencies.

For medical purposes, a strong solution of ethyl alcohol can be used as an ANTISEPTIC (particularly to prepare skin before injection) or as a preservative. Another form of alcohol, methyl alcohol (or methanol) is perhaps better known as wood alcohol. In the body it is oxidized more slowly than ethyl alcohol, forming poisonous products that may cause blindness and/or death. Methylated spirits is a mixture of ethanol with a little methanol and other petroleum hydrocarbons; one form is alternatively called surgical spirit or rubbing alcohol.

Alcopar (*Wellcome*) is a proprietary non-prescription ANTHELMINTIC drug, used to treat infections by roundworms, specifically by hookworms. Produced in the form of granules in sachets for solution in water, Alcopar is a preparation of bephenium hydroxynaphthoate.

▲ side-effects: see BEPHENIUM.

Alcos-Anal (*Norgine*) is a proprietary non-prescription preparation combining a soothing agent and an ANTISEPTIC, used to treat and soothe piles (haemorrhoids) and itching around the anus. It is produced in the form of suppositories and

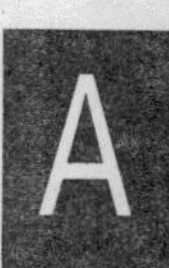

(under the trade name Alcos-Anal Ointment) as an ointment.

alcuronium chloride is a SKELETAL MUSCLE RELAXANT, of the type known as competitive or non-depolarizing. It is used during surgical operations to achieve long-duration paralysis. Administration is by injection, but only after the patient has been rendered unconscious – the muscle spasm it causes might be painful to a conscious patient. *Related article:* ALLOFERIN.

Aldactide 50 (*Gold Cross*) is a proprietary potassium-sparing DIURETIC drug, available only on prescription, used to treat congestive heart failure and high blood pressure (*see* ANTIHYPERTENSIVE). Produced in the form of tablets, Aldactide 50 is a compound of the weak but catalytic diuretic spironolactone together with the THIAZIDE hydroflumethiazide. A half-strength version of the compound is also available (under the trade name Aldactide 25).
✚/▲ warning/side-effects: *see* HYDROFLUMETHIAZIDE; SPIRONOLACTONE.

Aldactone (*Searle*) is a proprietary potassium-sparing DIURETIC drug, available only on prescription, used to treat congestive heart failure, high blood pressure (*see* ANTIHYPERTENSIVE), cirrhosis of the liver, and the accumulation of fluids within the tissues (oedema). Produced in the form of tablets, Aldactone is a preparation of the comparatively weak diuretic spironolactone.
✚/▲ warning/side-effects: *see* SPIRONOLACTONE.

Aldomet (*Merck, Sharp & Dohme*) is a proprietary form of the powerful drug methyldopa, which is thought to act on the central nervous system (the brain). Available only on prescription, Aldomet is used – usually in combination with a diuretic drug – to treat moderate to very high blood pressure (*see* ANTIHYPERTENSIVE), and is produced in the form of tablets (in three strengths) and in ampoules for injection (as methyldopate hydrochloride).
✚/▲ warning/side-effects: *see* METHYLDOPA.

Alembicol D (*Alembic*) is a proprietary preparation of fatty acids derived from coconut oil, used as a dietary supplement in patients who suffer from impaired absorption of fats. In the form of a liquid, it is available either without prescription or on prescription, at the discretion of the doctor.

Aleudrin (*Lewis*) is a proprietary BETA-RECEPTOR STIMULANT BRONCHODILATOR, available only on prescription, used to treat asthma and bronchitis. Produced in the form of tablets and as a solution for spraying, Aleudrin is a preparation of the SYMPATHOMIMETIC isoprenaline sulphate.
✚/▲ warning/side-effects: *see* ISOPRENALINE.

Alevaire (*Winthrop*) is a proprietary non-prescription MUCOLYTIC, used to reduce the viscosity of sputum and thus facilitate expectoration (coughing up phlegm). It is produced in the form of a liquid for spraying or nebulization, representing a mild solution of TYLOXAPOL.

Alexan (*Pfizer*) is a proprietary preparation of the CYTOTOXIC drug cytarabine used to treat cancer, particularly acute forms of leukaemia. Available only on

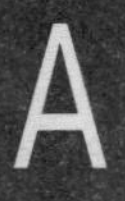

prescription, it is produced in ampoules for injection.
✚/▲ warning/side-effects: *see* CYTARABINE.

Alexan 100 (*Pfizer*) is a proprietary preparation of the CYTOTOXIC drug cytarabine used to treat cancer, particularly acute forms of leukaemia. Available only on prescription, it is produced in ampoules for intravenous infusion, and is five times as strong as Alexan.
✚/▲ warning/side-effects: *see* CYTARABINE.

alexitol sodium is a non-proprietary (non-prescription) ANTACID, used to treat indigestion and acid stomach. It is produced in the form of tablets, and is not recommended for children.

alfacalcidol is a synthesized form of CALCIFEROL (vitamin D), used to make up body deficiencies, particularly in the treatment of types of hypoparathyroidism and rickets. Calcium levels in the body should be regularly monitored during treatment. Administration is oral in the form of capsules or drops.
✚ warning: overdosage may cause kidney damage. Although an increased amount of vitamin D is necessary during pregnancy, high body levels while lactating may cause corresponding high blood levels of calcium in the breast-fed infant.
Related article: ONE-ALPHA

alfentanil is a narcotic ANALGESIC, used for short surgical operations, for outpatient surgery, or in combination to enhance the effect of general ANAESTHETICS (particularly barbiturate) drugs. Administration is by intravenous infusion, and may be continuous during prolonged surgical procedures. Its proprietary form is on the controlled drugs list.
✚ warning: respiration may become depressed during and following treatment; the use of alfentanil to assist with childbirth may lead to respiratory depression in the newborn. Alfentanil should therefore be administered with caution to patients who already suffer from respiratory disorders. Dosage should be reduced for the elderly and for patients who suffer from chronic liver disease.
▲ side-effects: there may be respiratory depression (severely shallow breathing), worsened by nausea and vomiting; the heart rate may slow and blood pressure fall.
Related article: RAPIFEN.

Algesal (*Duphar*) is a proprietary non-prescription COUNTER-IRRITANT preparation which, in the form of a cream applied to the skin, produces an irritation of sensory nerve endings that offsets the pain of underlying muscle or joint ailments. It is not recommended for children aged under 6 years.
✚ warning: Algesal should not be used on inflamed or broken skin, or on mucous membranes.

Algicon (*Rorer*) is a proprietary non-prescription ANTACID compound that has an additional suppressant effect on the muscles controlling the flow of food along the alimentary canal, so discouraging any reflux backwards. Produced in the form of tablets and as a suspension, Algicon contains ALUMINIUM HYDROXIDE and several magnesium and potassium salts. It is not recommended for children.

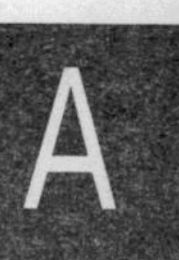

✚ warning: Algicon should not be administered to patients with kidney failure, or who are very weak. Diabetics should be wary of taking it because it contains sucrose.

Algipan (*Wyeth*) is a proprietary non-prescription COUNTER-IRRITANT compound which, in the form of a cream or a spray applied to the skin, produces an irritation of sensory nerve endings that offsets the pain of underlying muscle or joint ailments. The spray also has a chilling effect.
✚ warning: Algipan should not be used on inflamed or broken skin, or on mucous membranes.

Alka-Donna (*Carlton*) is a proprietary, non-prescription, ANTICHOLINERGIC compound that is not available from the National Health Service. It is used to treat muscle spasm of the intestinal walls, and the resulting gastrointestinal discomfort. Produced in the form of tablets (to be sucked) and as a suspension, Alka-Donna's active constituents are belladonna alkaloids, aluminium hydroxide and magnesium trisilicate.
✚/▲ warning/side-effects: *see* ALUMINIUM HYDROXIDE; BELLADONNA; MAGNESIUM TRISILICATE.

Alka-Donna-P (*Carlton*) is a form of the proprietary ANTICHOLINERGIC compound ALKA-DONNA that is not available from the National Health Service, and is on the cotrolled drugs list because it additionally contains the BARBITURATE phenobarbitone.
✚/▲ warning/side-effects: *see* PHENOBARBITONE.

Alkeran (*Wellcome*) is a proprietary CYTOTOXIC drug, available only on prescription, used to treat multiple myeloma, breast cancer and cancer of the ovary. Produced in the form of tablets (in two strengths) and (under the trade name Alkeran Injection) as powder for reconstitution with a solvent for injection, Alkeran is a preparation of melphalan.
✚/▲ warning/side-effects: *see* MELPHALAN.

Allbee with C (*Robins*) is a proprietary, non-prescription MULTIVITAMIN preparation that is not available from the National Health Service. Used to treat vitamin deficiencies and produced in the form of capsules, Allbee with C – as its name indicates – consists of several forms of vitamin B (THIAMINE, RIBOFLAVINE, PYRIDOXINE, NICOTINAMIDE and PANTOTHENIC ACID) together with ASCORBIC ACID (vitamin C).

Allegron (*Dista*) is a proprietary ANTIDEPRESSANT, available only on prescription, used to treat depressive illness. It is also used for children to stop bed-wetting at night. Produced in the form of tablets (in two strengths), Allegron is a preparation of the TRICYCLIC drug nortriptyline hydrochloride.
✚/▲ warning/side-effects: *see* NORTRIPTYLINE.

Aller-eze is a proprietary non-prescription ANTIHISTAMINE, in which the active constituent is clemastine hydrogen fumarate.
✚/▲ warning/side-effects: *see* CLEMASTINE.

Alloferin (*Roche*) is a proprietary SKELETAL MUSCLE RELAXANT, available only on prescription, of the type known as competitive or non-depolarizing. It is used during surgical operations, but

A

only after the patient has been rendered unconscious. Produced in ampoules for injection, Alloferin is a preparation of alcuronium chloride.

✚/▲ warning/side-effects: *see* ALCURONIUM CHLORIDE.

allopurinol is a XANTHINE-OXIDASE INHIBITOR, a drug used to combat an excess of uric acid in the blood, and thus to try to prevent gout. Once begun – provided that there are no acute gout attacks – treatment should be continued indefinitely. Administration is oral in the form of tablets, but before beginning treatment an inflammatory analgesic should be administered for about 4 weeks.

✚ warning: if an acute gout attack or a rash with high temperature occurs, treatment should cease at once, and continue only after the attack has subsided. Allopurinol should be administered with caution to patients who suffer from liver or kidney disease.

▲ side-effects: there may be gastrointestinal disturbances. Rarely, there may be headache, dizziness and high blood pressure (hypertension), hair loss, and/or problems with the sense of taste.

Related articles: ALORAL; ALULINE; CAPLENAL; COSURIC; HAMARIN; ZYLORIC.

Allpyral-G (*Dome/Hollister-Stier*) is a proprietary set of 5 grass pollen preparations for use in desensitizing patients who are allergic to such pollen (and so suffer from hay fever). Available only on prescription and administered by injection, Alavac-P pollen preparations are of carefully annotated different allergenic effect, so that the process of desensitization, as regulated by a doctor, can be progressive.

✚ warning: injections should be administered under close medical supervision and in locations where emergency facilities for full cardio-respiratory resuscitation are immediately available.

Allpyral Specific (*Dome/Hollister-Stier*) is a proprietary set of preparations of common allergens, including (under the separate trade name Allpyral Mite Fortified House Dust) the house dust mite, for use in desensitizing patients who are allergic to them. Available only on prescription and administered by injection, Allpyral preparations are of carefully annotated different allergenic effect, so that the process of desensitization, as regulated by a doctor, can be progressive.

✚ warning: injections should be administered under close medical supervision and in locations where emergency facilities for full cardio-respiratory resuscitation are immediately available.

allyloestrenol is a PROGESTOGEN, an analogue of the natural female sex HORMONE progesterone, responsible for the changing state of the lining of the womb preparatory to, or during, pregnancy. It is used to treat recurrent miscarriage or failure of a blastocyst to implant following conception; it may also be used to treat premenstrual tension. Administration is oral in the form of tablets.

✚ warning: allyloestrenol should not be administered to patients with undiagnosed vaginal bleeding, incomplete abortion, or any form of thrombosis; and should be administered with caution to

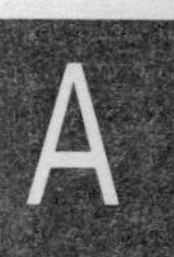

patients who are diabetic, who suffer from high blood pressure (hypertension), from heart, liver or kidney disease, or who are lactating.

▲ side-effects: there may be skin disorders (such as acne), accumulation of fluid in the tissues (oedema) and associated weight gain, breast tenderness, and/or gastrointestinal disturbances. *Related article:* GESTANIN.

almasilate suspension is a non-proprietary non-prescription ANTACID preparation that has an additional suppressant effect on the muscles controlling the flow of food along the alimentary canal, so discouraging any reflux backwards. It is also used to treat the symptoms of peptic ulcer or acidity in the stomach. Produced in the form of a liquid, almasilate suspension is not recommended for children.

Almazine (*Steinhard*) is a proprietary ANXIOLYTIC, used as a tranquillizer especially in relieving attacks of phobia. Produced in the form of tablets (in two strengths), Almazine is a preparation of the BENZODIAZEPINE lorazepam.

✚/▲ warning/side-effects: *see* LORAZEPAM.

Almevax (*Wellcome*) is a proprietary VACCINE against German measles (rubella) in the form of a solution containing live but attenuated viruses of the Wistar RA27/3 strain. Available only on prescription, and administered in the form of injection, it is intended specifically for the immunization of non-pregnant women.

Alophen is a powerful proprietary, non-prescription, compound LAXATIVE containing several strong, natural ingredients. Produced in the form of pills, Alophen contains essence of aloes, belladonna extract, phenolphthalein and ipecacuanha – all effective in their own right.

▲ side-effects: laxative effects may continue for several days; there may be dysfunction of the kidneys, leading possibly to discoloration of the urine. A mild skin rash may appear.

Aloral (*Lagap*) is a proprietary form of the XANTHINE-OXIDASE INHIBITOR allopurinol, used to treat high levels of uric acid in the bloodstream (which may otherwise cause gout). Available only on prescription, Aloral is produced in the form of tablets (in two strengths).

✚/▲ warning/side-effects: *see* ALLOPURINOL.

aloxipirin is a non-narcotic ANALGESIC. It is a form of ASPIRIN that additionally contains a buffer (a substance that does not change its acid-alkali balance) that counters acidity. This means that aspirin's detrimental effect on the lining of the stomach is considerably reduced.

✚/▲ warning/side-effects: *see* ASPIRIN.
Related article: PALAPRIN FORTE.

alpha-blockers (alpha-adrenoceptor antagonists) are drugs that inhibit the action of the hormones ADRENALINE, NORADRENALINE and related substances (known at the catecholamines) at sites in the body where the recognition site for these substances is known as an alpha type. The main effect of alpha-blockers is to lower the blood pressure and they are therefore used to treat some types of hypertension. They are also used to treat poor

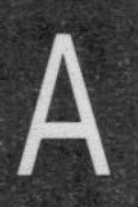

circulation in the extremities of the body and an excess of catecholamines in the body. Examples include PHENTOLAMINE and PRAZOSIN.

Alphaderm (*Norwich Eaton*) is a proprietary cream preparation containing urea (10%) with the corticosteroid hydrocortisone (1%) dispersed in a slightly oily base. Available only on prescription, the cream is used as a topical application for the treatment of ichthyosis (dry and horny epidermis) and other mild inflammations of the skin.
✚/▲ warning/side-effects: *see* HYDROCORTISONE.

Alpha Keri (*Bristol-Myers*) is a proprietary non-prescription skin emollient (softener and soother) for use in the bath. Containing mineral and lanolin oils, it can also be massaged into the skin to treat dry or itchy areas.

alpha tocopheryl acetate is a form of VITAMIN E (tocopherol), used to treat body deficiency and generally as a vitamin supplement. Administration is oral in the form of tablets for chewing, capsules and in suspension, or as a paraffin-based ointment.
Related articles: EPHYNAL; VITA-E.

Alphosyl (*Stafford-Miller*) is a proprietary non-prescription preparation used to treat eczema and psoriasis. Produced in the form of a water-based cream and as a lotion, Alphosyl's major active constituent is COAL TAR extract.

Alphosyl HC (*Stafford-Miller*) is a proprietary COAL TAR and corticosteroid preparation, available only on prescription, used to treat psoriasis. Produced in the form of a water-based cream, Alphosyl HC's steroid constituent is hydrocortisone.
✚/▲ warning/side-effects: *see* HYDROCORTISONE.

alprazolam is an ANXIOLYTIC drug, one of the BENZODIAZEPINES used to treat anxiety in either the short or the long term. Administration is oral in the form of tablets. It is not recommended for children.
✚ warning: alprazolam may reduce a patient's concentration and intricacy of movement or thought; it may also enhance the effects of alcohol consumption. Prolonged use or abrupt withdrawal should be avoided. It should be administered with caution to patients who suffer from respiratory difficulties, glaucoma, or kidney or liver disorders; who are in the last stages of pregnancy; or who are elderly or debilitated.
▲ side-effects: there may be drowsiness, dizziness, headache, dry mouth and shallow breathing; hypersensitive reactions may occur.
Related article: XANAX.

alprostadil is a hormonal drug (a prostaglandin) used to maintain he status quo in babies born with the congenital heart defect ductus arteriosus, while emergency preparations are made for corrective surgery and intensive care. Administration is by infusion in dilute solution.
✚ warning: monitoring of arterial pressure is essential; a close watch must also be kept for haemorrhage.
▲ side-effects: in addition to the symptoms of the congenital defect, administration of the drug may cause breathing difficulties, low blood pressure

(hypotension) and slow OR fast heart rate, high temperature and flushing. Prolonged use may cause bone deformity and damage to the pulmonary artery.
Related article: PROSTIN VR.

Alrheumat (*Bayer*) is a proprietary, non-steroid, ANTI-INFLAMMATORY, non-narcotic ANALGESIC drug, available only on prescription, used to relieve pain – particularly arthritic and rheumatic pain – and to treat other musculo-skeletal disorders. Its active constituent is ketoprofen, and it is produced in the form of capsules and anal suppositories. Not recommended for children, Alrheumat should be administered with care to patients with a peptic ulcer, gastrointestinal haemorrhage or asthma, or who are pregnant or lactating.
✚/▲ warning/side-effects: *see* KETOPROFEN.

Altacaps (*Roussel*) is a proprietary non-prescription ANTACID preparation that is not available from the National Health Service, used to soothe heartburn, infection of the oesophagus, hiatus hernia and peptic ulcer. Produced in the form of a suspension within gelatin capsules, Altacaps contain the antacid-deflatulent HYDROTALCITE together with the antifoaming agent DIMETHICONE. It is not recommended for children.

Altacite (*Roussel*) is a proprietary non-prescription ANTACID that is not available from the National Health Service. Produced in the form of tablets for chewing and as a sugar-free suspension, Altacite's active constituent is HYDROTALCITE, a readily-dissociated compound that also has deflatulent properties.

Altacite Plus (*Roussel*) is a proprietary non-prescription ANTACID preparation used to soothe acid stomach, indigestion, flatulence and peptic ulcer. Produced in the form of a suspension, Altacite Plus contains the antacid-deflatulent HYDROTALCITE together with the antifoaming agent DIMETHICONE, and is not recommended for children aged under 8 years. A version of Altacite Plus is produced in the form of tablets, but is not available from the National Health Service.

Alu-cap (*Riker*) is a proprietary non-prescription ANTACID preparation used to soothe an acid stomach. It is produced in the form of capsules containing aluminium hydroxide, and is not recommended for children.
✚/▲ warning/side-effects: *see* ALUMINIUM HYDROXIDE.

Aludrox (*Wyeth*) is a proprietary non-prescription ANTACID preparation used to soothe acid stomach, indigestion and peptic ulcer. It is produced in the form of a gel containing aluminium hydroxide, and is not recommended for children aged under 2 years. Versions of Aludrox available only on prescription are produced in the form of tablets under the trade name Aludrox Tablets; and as a gel or a suspension (incorporating AMBUTONIUM BROMIDE and magnesium salts) under the trade name Aludrox SA. Aludrox SA suspension is not recommended for children.
✚/▲ warning/side-effects: *see* ALUMINIUM HYDROXIDE.

Aluhyde (*Sinclair*) is a proprietary non-prescription ANTACID compound that is not available from the National Health Service. It is used to treat

A

acidity of the stomach resulting from spasm of the muscular stomach wall. Produced in the form of tablets containing aluminium hydroxide, MAGNESIUM TRISILICATE and an anticholinergic extract of belladonna, Aluhyde is not recommended for children.
✚/▲ warning/side-effects: *see* ALUMINIUM HYDROXIDE; BELLADONNA.

Aluline (*Steinhard*) is a proprietary form of the XANTHINE-OXIDASE INHIBITOR allopurinol, used to treat high levels of uric acid in the bloodstream (which may otherwise cause gout). Available only on prescription, Aluline is produced in the form of tablets (in two strengths).
✚/▲ warning/side-effects: *see* ALLOPURINOL.

alum is used therapeutically as an astringent, particularly to treat mouth pain and in mouth-washes.
✚ warning: treatment with alum may in fact cause tissue damage and actually defer healing.

aluminium acetate is an astringent DISINFECTANT, used primarily to clean sites of infection and inflammation, particularly in the case of weeping or suppurating wounds or sores, eczema, and infections of the outer ear. Administration is in the form of a lotion (containing aluminium acetate in dilute solution) or as drops.
Related article: XYLOPROCT.

aluminium chloride is a powerful antiperspirant. Administration is topical in the form of a lotion or aerosol comprising a 20% solution. It also acts as an astringent.
✚ warning: Keep away from the eyes; do not shave armpit within 12 hours of application there.
▲ side-effects: there may be skin irritation (which may require treatment with a corticosteroid).
Related articles: ANHYDROL FORTE; DRICLOR.

aluminium glycinate is an ANTACID which, because it is relatively insoluble in water, is long-acting when retained in the stomach.
Related article: PRODEXIN.

aluminium hydroxide is an ANTACID which, because it is relatively insoluble in water, is long-acting when retained in the stomach. Used to treat digestive problems from acid stomach to peptic ulcers or oesophageal reflux. Administration is oral in the form of tablets for chewing or sucking, as a gel, or in a compound liquid mixture. Some proprietary preparations are not recommended for children.
Related articles: ACTONORM; ALGICON; ALKA-DONNA; ALU-CAP; ALUDROX; ALUHYDE; ANDURSIL; ANTASIL; ASILONE; DIJEX; DIOVOL; GASTROCOTE; GASTRON; GAVISCON; GELUSIL; KOLANTICON; KOLANTYL; LOASID; MAALOX; MUCAINE; MUCOGEL; POLYALK REVISED FORMULA; POLYCROL; PYROGASTRONE; SILOXYL; SIMECO; TOPAL; UNIGEST.

Alunex (*Steinhard*) is a proprietary non-prescription ANTIHISTAMINE, used to treat allergic conditions such as hay fever and urticaria. Produced in the form of tablets, Alunex is a preparation of chlorpheniramine maleate. It may cause drowsiness.
✚/▲ warning/side-effects: *see* CHLORPHENIRAMINE.

Alupent (*Boehringer Ingelheim*) is

a proprietary compound BRONCHODILATOR, available only on prescription, which works as a selective SMOOTH MUSCLE RELAXANT. Administered orally in the form of tablets, as an aerosol spray (under the trade name Alupent Aerosol) or as a sugar-free syrup (under the trade name Alupent Syrup) to treat bronchospasm, it thus relieves the effects of asthma, emphysema and chronic bronchitis. A dilute solution is also produced in ampoules for injection (under the trade name Alupent Injection). A much stronger form, however, may be used in injection or infusion (under the trade name Alupent Obstetric) to prevent premature labour in pregnant women by causing relaxation of the uterine muscles. In every form of Alupent, the active constituent is the BETA-RECEPTOR STIMULANT orciprenaline sulphate.
✚/▲ warning/side-effects: *see* ORCIPRENALINE.

Alupram (*Steinhard*) is a proprietary ANXIOLYTIC and SKELETAL MUSCLE RELAXANT, available only on prescription. Produced for both purposes in the form of tablets (in three strengths), Alupram is a preparation of the BENZODIAZEPINE diazepam.
✚/▲ warning/side-effects: *see* DIAZEPAM.

Aluzine (*Steinhard*) is a proprietary DIURETIC drug, available only on prescription, used to treat the accumulation of fluids in the tissues (oedema), particularly caused by kidney failure. Produced in the form of tablets (in three strengths), Aluzine is a preparation of frusemide.
✚/▲ warning/side-effects: *see* FRUSEMIDE.

Aluzyme (*Phillips Yeast*) is a proprietary non-prescription MULTIVITAMIN compound that is not available from the National Health Service. Produced in the form of tablets, it is used as a vitamin supplement and tonic. In addition to the vitamin B substances THIAMINE, RIBOFLAVINE, NICOTINIC ACID and FOLIC ACID, Aluzyme contains dried yeast.

alverine citrate is an ANTISPASMODIC drug used to treat muscle spasm in both the gastrointestinal tract (leading to abdominal pain and constipation) and the uterus or vagina (leading to menstrual discomfort). Administration is oral in the form of capsules and soluble granules. It is not recommended for children.
✚ warning: alverine citrate should not be administered to patients who suffer from paralytic ileus.
Related articles: NORMACOL; SPASMONAL.

amantadine hydrochloride is an ANTIVIRAL agent used to prevent infection with the influenza A2 virus (but not other types of influenza virus) and in the treatment of shingles. It is also used to treat parkinsonism, although it truly benefits only a relatively small proportion of patients. Nevertheless, it improves such symptoms as tremor or rigidity, and there are few side-effects. Administration is oral in the form of capsules or as a dilute syrup.
✚ warning: amantadine should not be administered to patients who suffer from gastric ulcers or from epilepsy. It should be administered with caution to patients who suffer from heart, liver or kidney disease, psychosis, or long-term eczema; who are

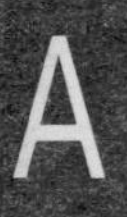

pregnant or lactating; who are in a state of confusion; or who are elderly. Withdrawal of treatment must be gradual.

▲ side-effects: there is commonly restlessness and inability to concentrate; there may also be dizziness and insomnia, gastrointestinal disturbances, swelling resulting from fluid retention in the tissues, and skin discoloration. A regular blood count is advisable.
Related article: SYMMETREL.

Ambaxin (*Upjohn*) is a proprietary ANTIBIOTIC, available only on prescription, used to treat systemic bacterial infections and infections of the upper respiratory tract, the ear, nose and throat, and the urogenital tracts. Produced in the form of tablets, Ambaxin is a preparation of the broad-spectrum penicillin bacampicillin hydrochloride.
✚/▲ warning/side-effects: *see* BACAMPICILLIN HYDROCHLORIDE.

ambutonium bromide is an ANTISPASMODIC drug used to assist in treating a peptic ulcer. Mildly ANTICHOLINERGIC too, it is administered orally in the form of a dilute suspension containing other antispasmodics.

✚ warning: ambutonium bromide, like all anticholinergics, inhibits the secretions of the stomach, thus slowing the process of digestion, leading possibly to constipation. It should be administered with caution to patients who suffer from retention of urine, heart disease, or muscular disorders of the intestines.

▲ side-effects: there may be thirst and a constantly dry mouth, visual disturbances with sensitivity to light, pressure within the eyeballs (glaucoma), an oscillating or irregular heartbeat, and/or difficulty in urinating.
Related article: ALUDROX.

amethocaine hydrochloride is a local ANAESTHETIC used in creams and in solution for topical application or instillation into the bladder, and in eye-drops for ophthalmic treatment. It is absorbed rapidly from mucous membrane surfaces.

✚ warning: topical administration may cause initial stinging. It should be given with caution to patients with epilepsy, impaired cardiac conduction or respiratory damage, or with liver damage.

▲ side-effects: rarely, there are hypersensitive reactions.
Related article: MINIMS AMETHOCAINE HYDROCHLORIDE; NOXYFLEX.

Amfipen (*Brocades*) is a proprietary ANTIBIOTIC, available only on prescription, used to treat systemic bacterial infections and infections of the upper respiratory tract, the ear, nose and throat, and the urogenital tracts. Produced in the form of capsules (in two strengths), as a powder for reconstitution, as a syrup (in two strengths, under the trade name Amfipen Syrup), and in vials for injection (in two strengths, under the name Amfipen Injection), Amfipen represents a preparation of the broad-spectrum penicillin ampicillin.
✚/▲ warning/side-effects: *see* AMPICILLIN.

amikacin is an ANTIBIOTIC drug (a semisynthetic aminoglycoside), used to treat several serious bacterial infections, particularly those that prove to be resistant to

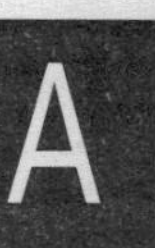

the more generally-used aminoglycosides GENTAMICIN and TOBRAMYCIN. Administration is by intramuscular or intravenous injection.

✚ warning: amikacin should not be administered to patients who are pregnant (because the drug can cross the placenta), and should be administered with caution to patients with impaired function of the kidney. Careful monitoring for toxicity is advisable during treatment.

▲ side-effects: there may be deafness; temporary kidney malfunction may occur.

Amikin (*Bristol-Myers*) is a proprietary preparation of the aminoglycoside ANTIBIOTIC amikacin, available only on prescription, used to treat several serious bacterial infections, particularly those that prove to be resistant to the more generally used aminoglycoside GENTAMICIN. Amikin is produced in vials for injection or infusion (as amikacin sulphate) in two strengths.

✚/▲ warning/side-effects: *see* AMIKACIN.

Amilco (*Norton*) is a proprietary potassium-sparing DIURETIC drug, available only on prescription, used to treat oedema associated with congestive heart failure, high blood pressure (*see* ANTIHYPERTENSIVE) and cirrhosis of the liver. Produced in the form of tablets, it represents a compound of the weak but catalytic diuretic AMILORIDE hydrochloride together with the THIAZIDE hydrochlorothiazide.

✚/▲ warning/side-effects: *see* HYDROCHLOROTHIAZIDE.

amiloride is a mild DIURETIC drug that causes the retention of potassium (it is potassium-sparing) and is thus commonly used in combination with other diuretics – such as the THIAZIDES – that normally cause a loss of potassium from the body. It is then used particularly to treat the accumulation of fluids in the tissues (oedema).

✚ warning: amiloride should not be administered to patients who have high blood potassium levels or who are taking potassium supplements; it should be administered with caution to patients who suffer from cirrhosis of the liver or impaired kidney function, are diabetic, or are pregnant.

▲ side-effects: there may be skin rashes. Some patients become confused.

Related articles: AMILCO; FRUMIL; KALTEN; MIDAMOR; MODURET 25; MODURETIC; NORMETIC; SYNURETIC.

Aminex (*Cow & Gate*) is a brand of non-prescription lactose- and sucrose-free biscuits intended for consumption by patients suffering from lactose or sucrose intolerance, amino-acid abnormalities (such as phenylketonuria), kidney failure, or cirrhosis of the liver. Mostly carbohydrate, the biscuits contain a small proportion of fat, and less than 1% of protein.

aminobenzoic acid is an unusual drug, sometimes classed as one of the VITAMIN B complex, that helps to protect the skin from ultraviolet radiation. For this reason, aminobenzoic acid is a constituent in many suntan lotions, but also in some barrier preparations to ward off the effects of repeated radiotherapy. Administration is topical, in the form of creams and lotions.

✚ warning: protection is temporary, and creams and lotions must be reapplied

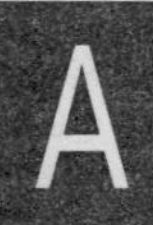

every so often. Some patients are in any case more sensitive to ultraviolet radiation than others.
Related articles: COPPERTONE SUPERSHADE 15; DELIAL 10; PIZ BUIN; RoC TOTAL SUNBLOCK; SPECTRABAN.

Aminofusin L600 (*Merck*) is a proprietary form of nutrition for intravenous infusion into patients who are unable to take in food via the alimentary canal. Available only on prescription, it contains amino acids, the sugar-substitute sorbitol, vitamins and electrolytes.

Aminofusin L1000 (*Merck*) is the same as AMINOFUSIN L600 with the addition of ethanol (ethyl alcohol).

Aminofusin L Forte (*Merck*) is much like AMINOFUSIN L600 but contains more amino acids, vitamins and electrolytes, but no sorbitol.

aminoglutethimide is a drug used to treat advanced breast cancer in women who have passed the menopause or had both ovaries removed. It may also be used to palliate the effects of advanced cancer of the prostate gland in men. Administration is oral in the form of tablets.
✚ warning: simultaneous corticosteroid treatment is essential to replace hormones absent. Despite initial symptoms of toxicity, dosage must be progressively increased over 2 to 4 weeks.
▲ side-effects: commonly there is drowsiness; there may even be a rash resembling measles.
Related article: ORIMETEN.

Aminogran (*Allen & Hanburys*) is a proprietary non-prescription form of nutritional supplement for patients with amino-acid abnormalities (such as phenylketonuria). It comprises a food supplement containing all essential amino acids except for phenylalanine. There is in addition a mineral mixture – intended to be combined with the food supplement, or for use with independent synthetic diets – containing all necessary minerals.

aminophylline is a BRONCHODILATOR used mostly in sustained-release forms of administration, generally to treat moderate but chronic asthma over periods of around 12 hours at a time. It can alternatively be used to treat cardiac, pulmonary or renal oedema, and angina pectoris. Administration is usually oral in the form of tablets, but may be by injection or suppositories. It is not recommended for children.
✚ warning: treatment should initially be gradually progressive in quantity administered. Aminophylline should be administered with caution to patients who suffer from heart or liver disease, or from peptic ulcer; or who are pregnant or lactating.
▲ side-effects: there may be nausea and gastrointestinal disturbances, an increase or irregularity in the heartbeat, and/or insomnia. Treatment in the form of suppositories may cause proctitis.
Related articles: PHYLLOCONTIN CONTINUS; THEODROX.

Aminoplasmal (*Braun*) is a proprietary form of nutrition for intravenous infusion into patients who are unable to take in food via the alimentary canal. Available only on prescription, it contains amino acids and electrolytes. Various strengths

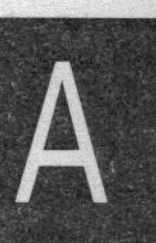

are produced, differentiated by suffixes to the trade name: Ped, L3, L5 and L10.

Aminoplex 12 (*Geistlich*) is a proprietary form of nutrition for intravenous infusion into patients who are unable to take in food via the alimentary canal. Available only on prescription, it contains amino acids, malic acid and electrolytes. Another version, Aminoplex 5, additionally contains the sugar-substitute sorbitol and ethanol (ethyl alcohol); a third version, Aminoplex 14, additionally contains vitamins.

Aminoven 12 (*MCP Pharmaceuticals*) is a proprietary form of nutrition for intravenous infusion into patients who are unable to take in food via the alimentary canal. Available only on prescription, it contains synthesized amino acids and electrolytes.

amiodarone is a potentially toxic drug used to treat severe irregularity of the heartbeat, especially in cases where for one reason or another alternative drugs cannot be used. It is also used in the treatment of angina pectoris. Administration is oral in the form of tablets, or by injection.

✚ warning: amiodarone should not be administered to patients who suffer from very slow heartbeat, thyroid dysfunction, or shock; or who are pregnant or lactating. Dosage in each individual case should be the minimum to achieve the desired results. There should be regular testing of thyroid, liver and pulmonary function.

▲ side-effects: deposits on the cornea of the eyes and associated sensitivity to light are inevitable, but reversible on withdrawal of treatment. There may be other neurological effects.

Related article: CORDARONE X.

amitriptyline is an ANTIDEPRESSANT drug that also has sedative properties. The sedation may be a benefit to agitated or violent patients, or to those who care for them. In contrast to the treatment of depressive illness, however, the drug may be used to prevent bed-wetting at night in youngsters. Administration is oral in the form of tablets, capsules or a dilute mixture. It is not recommended for young children.

✚ warning: amitriptyline should not be administered to patients who suffer from heart disease or psychosis; it should be administered with caution to patients who suffer from diabetes, epilepsy, liver or thyroid disease, glaucoma or urinary retention; or who are pregnant or lactating. Withdrawal of treatment must be gradual.

▲ side-effects: common effects include loss of intricacy in movement or thought, dry mouth and blurred vision; there may also be difficulty in urinating, sweating and irregular heartbeat, behavioural disturbances, a rash, a state of confusion, and/or a loss of libido. Rarely, there are also blood deficiencies.

Related articles: DOMICAL; ELAVIL; LENTIZOL; TRYPTIZOL.

ammonia and ipecacuanha is a non-proprietary formulation intended as an EXPECTORANT to promote the expulsion of excess bronchial secretions. It is not available as a mixture from the National Health Service. In effect, the mixture is a dilute solution of two potential EMETICS.

ammonium chloride is an EMETIC that in dilute solution may be used instead as a constituent of expectorant mixtures (sometimes in combination with opiates as cough suppressants). But it is more often for its acidifying properties that ammonium chloride is used: either to rectify the body's acid/alkali balance in a patient who is dehydrated, or for the therapeutic acidification of the urine.
Related articles: BENILYN EXPECTORANT; HISTALIX.

amodiaquine is an ANTIMALARIAL drug used as one of the major weapons against tertian malaria; it is sometimes also used to treat leprosy or rheumatoid arthritis. Administration is oral in the form of tablets.
✚ warning: amodiaquine should be administered with caution to patients who suffer from impaired liver or kidney function, porphyria, or psoriasis. Regular ophthalmic examination is recommended.
▲ side-effects: there may be nausea, vomiting and headache; some patients enter a state of lethargy. Blood disorders may occur. Prolonged treatment may lead to deposits on the cornea of the eyes and a greyish discoloration of the skin, fingernails and palate.
Related article: CAMOQUIN.

***amoebicidal** drugs prevent or treat infection by the microscopic protozoan organisms known as amoebae. Best known and most used are chloroquine and metronidazole – metronidazole particularly to counter the intestinal forms of infection (amoebic dysentery) and chloroquine to treat infection of the liver. Both subject their patients to some potentially unpleasant side-effects. In cases in which amoebic cysts are being passed on defecation but there are no further symptoms, the drug of choice is diloxanide furoate.
✚/▲ warning/side-effects: *see* CHLOROQUINE; DILOXANIDE FUROATE; METRONIDAZOLE.
Related articles: AVLOCLOR; FLAGYL; FLAGYL S; FURAMIDE; METROLYL; ZADSTAT.

Amoxidin (*Lagab*) is a proprietary ANTIBIOTIC, available only on prescription, used to treat systemic bacterial infections and infections of the upper respiratory tract, of the ear, nose and throat, and of the urogenital tracts; it is sometimes also used to treat typhoid fever and to treat dental infections. Produced in the form of capsules (in two strengths), Amoxidin is a preparation of the broad-spectrum PENICILLIN amoxycillin.
✚/▲ warning/side-effects: *see* AMOXYCILLIN.

Amoxil (*Bencard*) is a proprietary ANTIBIOTIC, available only on prescription, used to treat systemic bacterial infections and infections of the upper respiratory tract, of the ear, nose and throat, and of the urogenital tracts; it is sometimes used also to treat typhoid fever. Produced in the form of capsules (in two strengths), as sugar-free soluble (dispersible) tablets, as a syrup for dilution (the potency of the syrup once diluted is retained for 14 days), as a sugar-free syrup for dilution (in two strengths; the potency of the syrup once diluted is retained for 14 days), as a suspension for children, in the form of powder in sachets, as a sugar-free powder in sachets, and

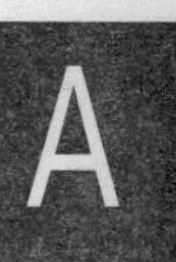

as a powder in vials for reconstitution as a medium for injection, Amoxil is a preparation of the broad-spectrum PENICILLIN amoxycillin.
✚/▲ warning/side-effects: *see* AMOXYCILLIN.

amoxycillin is a broad-spectrum penicillin-type ANTIBIOTIC, closely related to AMPICILLIN. Easily absorbed, it is used to treat many infections and especially infections of the urogenital tracts, the upper respiratory tract, or the middle ear. It is also sometimes used to treat typhoid fever or to prevent infection following dental surgery. Administration is oral in the form of capsules or liquids, or by injection.
✚ warning: amoxycillin should not be administered to patients who are known to be allergic to penicillin-type antibiotics; it should be administered with caution to those with impaired kidney function.
▲ side-effects: there may be sensitivity reactions such as rashes, high temperature and joint pain. Allergic patients may suffer anaphylactic shock. The most common side-effect, however, is diarrhoea.
Related articles: AMOXIDIN; AMOXIL; AUGMENTIN.

amphotericin is an ANTIBIOTIC used particularly to treat infection by fungal organisms. Unlike similar antibiotics it can be given by infusion, and is extremely important in the treatment of systemic fungal infections and is active against almost all fungi and yeasts. It is a toxic drug and side-effects are common. Administration is oral in the form of tablets, lozenges or liquids, or by infusion.
✚ warning: amphotericin should not be administered to patients who are already undergoing drug treatment that may affect kidney function. During treatment by infusion, tests on kidney function are essential; the site of injection must be changed frequently.
▲ side-effects: treatment by infusion may cause nausea, vomiting, severe weight loss and ringing in the ears (tinnitus); some patients experience a marked reduction in blood potassium. Prolonged or high dosage may cause kidney damage.
Related articles: FUNGILIN; FUNGIZONE.

ampicillin is a broad spectrum penicillin-type ANTIBIOTIC much like TETRACYCLINE in its effect. Easily absorbed – although absorption is reduced by the presence of food in the stomach or intestines – it is used to treat many infections and especially infections of the urogenital tracts, of the upper respiratory tract, or of the middle ear. Many bacteria have over the past two decades, however, become resistant to ampicillin. Administration is oral in the form of capsules or liquids, or by injection.
✚ warning: ampicillin should not be administered to patients who are known to be allergic to penicillin-type antibiotics; it should be administered with caution to those with impaired kidney function.
▲ side-effects: there may be sensitivity reactions such as minor rashes, high temperature and joint pain. Allergic patients may suffer anaphylactic shock. The most common side-effect, however, is simply diarrhoea.
Related articles: AMPICLOX;

A

AMPIFEN; AMPILAR; BRITCIN; FLU-AMP; MAGNAPEN; PENBRITIN; VIDOPEN.

Ampiclox (*Beecham*) is a proprietary ANTIBIOTIC, available only on prescription, used to treat systemic bacterial infections and infections of the upper respiratory tract, of the ear, nose and throat, and of the urogenital tracts. Produced in vials for injection, Ampiclox is a compound preparation of the broad-spectrum PENICILLIN ampicillin and the penicillin cloxacillin. A weaker version (under the trade name Ampiclox Neonatal) is produced in the form of a sugar-free suspension and as a powder for reconstitution as a medium for injection, and is used to treat or prevent infections in newborn or premature babies.
✚/▲ warning/side-effects: *see* AMPICILLIN; CLOXACILLIN.

Ampilar (*Lagab*) is a proprietary ANTIBIOTIC, available only on prescription, used to treat systemic bacterial infections and infections of the upper respiratory tract, of the ear, nose and throat, and of the urogenital tracts. Produced in the form of capsules (in two strengths), and as a syrup (in two strengths, the stronger labelled forte), Ampilar is a preparation of the broad-spectrum PENICILLIN ampicillin.
✚/▲ warning/side-effects: *see* AMPICILLIN.

amsacrine is a synthetic ANTICANCER agent that has the effect of halting the production of new, potentially cancerous cells. It is used specifically in the treatment of acute leukaemia in adults. Administration is by infusion.
✚ warning: amsacrine should be administered with caution to patients with heart disease, liver or kidney damage, or who are pregnant or elderly. Blood monitoring, particularly in relation to potassium levels, is essential. The capacity of the bone-marrow to produce blood cells is depressed.
▲ side-effects: nausea and vomiting, with hair loss, is common. The drug is a skin irritant. Rarely, patients have suffered convulsions.
Related article: AMSIDINE

Amsidine (*Parke-Davis*) is a proprietary ANTICANCER drug, available only on prescription, used to treat certain forms of leukaemia. It works by preventing the production of new, potentially cancerous cells. Produced in the form of a concentrate for intravenous infusion, generally for hospital use only, Amsidine is a preparation of amsacrine.
✚/▲ warning/side-effects: *see* AMSACRINE.

amylobarbitone is a BARBITURATE, used only when absolutely necessary as a HYPNOTIC to treat severe and intractable insomnia. Administration is oral in the form of tablets and capsules, or (as amylobarbitone sodium) by injection. Proprietary forms are all on the controlled drugs list.
✚ warning: amylobarbitone should not be administered to patients whose insomnia is caused by pain, who have porphyria, who are pregnant or lactating, who are elderly or debilitated, or who have a history of drug (including alcohol) abuse. It should be administered with caution to those with kidney, liver or lung disease. Use of the drug should be avoided as far as possible. Repeated doses are cumulative in effect, and may lead to real sedation; abrupt

withdrawal of treatment, on the other hand, may cause serious withdrawal symptoms. Tolerance and dependence (addiction) occur readily.
▲ side-effects: concentration and the speed of movement and thought are affected. There may be drowsiness, dizziness and shallow breathing, with headache. Some patients experience hypersensitivity reactions. (The drug enhances the effects of alcohol consumption.)
Related articles: AMYTAL; SODIUM AMYTAL; TUINAL.

Amytal (*Lilly*) is a proprietary HYPNOTIC drug, a BARBITURATE, and on the controlled drugs list; it is used to treat persistent and intractable insomnia. A dangerous and potentially addictive drug, it is produced in the form of tablets (in five strengths) and is a preparation of amylobarbitone. It is not recommended for children.
✚/▲ warning/side-effects: *see* AMYLOBARBITONE.

Anacal (*Panpharma*) is a proprietary compound CORTICOSTEROID preparation, available only on prescription, used in topical application to treat inflammation of the colon and rectum, piles (haemorrhoids) and related conditions. Produced in the form of rectal ointment and as anal suppositories, Anacal is a preparation that includes the steroid prednisolone and the antiseptic hexachlorophane. It is not recommended for children aged under 7 years.
✚/▲ warning/side-effects: *see* HEXACHLOROPHANE; PREDNISOLONE.

Anadin (*Whitehall Laboratories*) is a proprietary, non-prescription compound non-narcotic ANALGESIC produced in the form of tablets and as capsules. Anadin is a preparation of aspirin, caffeine and quinine sulphate.
✚/▲ warning/side-effects: *see* ASPIRIN; CAFFEINE; QUININE.

Anadin Extra (*Whitehall Laboratories*) is a proprietary, non-prescription compound non-narcotic ANALGESIC produced in the form of tablets and as capsules. Anadin is a preparation of aspirin, caffeine and paracetamol.
✚/▲ warning/side-effects: *see* ASPIRIN; CAFFEINE; PARACETOMOL.

***anaesthetic** is a drug that reduces sensation; such drugs affect either a specific local area – a local anaesthetic – or the whole body with loss of conciousness – a general anaesthetic.

The drug used to induce general anaesthesia is generally different from the drug or drugs used to continue it. Frequently used drugs for the induction of anaesthesia include THIOPENTONE SODIUM and ETOMIDATE. For the continuance of anaesthesia, common drugs include oxygen-nitrous oxide mixtures and HALOTHANE. Prior to induction, a patient is usually given a premedication, a drug to calm the nerves and to promote diuresis (passing of water), an hour or so before an operation is due. Such premedications include OPIATES and BENZODIAZEPINES. Other drugs in addition to general anaesthetics are used during surgery; for most internal surgery a SKELETAL MUSCLE RELAXANT, or perhaps a narcotic ANALGESIC, is also required.

Local anaesthetics are injected or absorbed in the area of the body where they are intended to take effect; they work by temporarily impairing the functioning of local nerves. Frequently used local anaesthetics include LIGNOCAINE, which is often used in dental surgery. One form of local anaesthesia, known as epidural anaesthesia, is produced by injection of anaesthetic into the membranes surrounding the spinal cord, which causes numbness from the abdomen down. Epidurals are used mainly during childbirth. Common epidural anaesthetics are LIGNOCAINE and BUPIVACAINE HYDROCHLORIDE.

Anaflex (*Geistlich*) is a proprietary non-prescription antibacterial and ANTIFUNGAL ANTIBIOTIC used to treat fungal infections of the mouth and the throat, and also applied topically to treat many skin infections. Produced in the form of an aerosol spray, as a water-miscible cream, as a dusting-powder (with talc), as a paste, and in the form of lozenges (which are not recommended for children aged under 6 years); the aerosol, paste and powder should only be used externally. Anaflex is a preparation of the drug POLYNOXYLIN.

Anafranil (*Geigy*) is a proprietary ANTIDEPRESSANT, available only on prescription, used to relieve the symptoms of depressive illness and as an additional treatment in phobic and obsessional states. It is also used to treat attacks of muscular weakness that occur in narcolepsy. Produced in the form of capsules (in three strengths), as sustained-release tablets (under the name Afranil SR), as a syrup (the potency of the dilute syrup lasts for 7 days), and in ampoules for injection, Anafranil is a preparation of the tricyclic antidepressant clomipramine hydrochloride. None of these preparations is recommended for children.

✚/▲ warning/side-effects: *see* CLOMIPRAMINE HYDROCHLORIDE.

***analgesic** is a drug that relieves pain. Because pain is a subjective experience that can arise from many causes, there are many ways that drugs can be used to relieve it. However, the term analgesic is best restricted to two main classes of drug.

First, NARCOTIC analgesics are drugs such as MORPHINE that have powerful actions on the central nervous system and alter the perception of pain. Because of the numerous possible side- effects, the most important of which is drug dependence (habituation), this class is usually used under medical supervision, and normally the drugs are only available on prescription. Other notable side-effects commonly include depression of respiration, nausea and sometimes hypotension, constipation, inhibition of coughing, and constriction of the pupils. Other members of this class include HEROIN, PENTAZOCINE, methadone, PETHIDINE and CODEINE, in descending order of potency with respect to their ability to deal with severe pain.

Second, non-narcotic analgesics are drugs such as ASPIRIN that have no serious tendency to produce dependence, but are by no means free of side-effects. This class is referred to by many names, including weak analgesics and, in medical circles, NSAIDs (non-steroidal anti-inflammatory drugs). The latter term refers to the valuable ANTI-INFLAMMATORY action of some members of the class (a property shared with the CORTICOSTEROIDS). This class of drug is used for a variety of purposes, ranging from

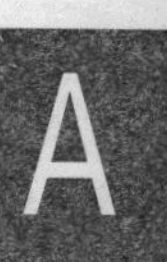

mild aches and pains (at normal dosage) to the treatment of rheumatoid arthritis (at higher dosage). PARACETAMOL does not have strong anti-inflammatory actions, but, as with other drugs in this class, has the valuable ability to lower raised body temperature (ANTIPYRETIC action). In spite of these important actions and uses, all members of the class have side-effects of concern, which for ASPIRIN-like drugs include gastrointestinal upsets ranging from dyspepsia to serious haemorrhage. Other examples of drugs of this class include IBUPROFEN and INDOMETHACIN. Often drugs in this class are used in combination with each other (e.g. paracetamol and codeine) or with drugs of other classes (e.g. caffeine).

Apart from these two main classes, there are other drugs that are sometimes referred to as analgesics because of their ability to relieve pain (e.g. local anaesthetics in the USA). To achieve the degree of pain relief necessary for major surgical operations general ANAESTHETICS are used, but often in conjunction with narcotic analgesics.

Ananase Forte (*Fisons*) is a proprietary non-prescription preparation of the enzyme bromelains, used to treat inflammation (particularly of the veins, or in and around the eye), bruising or swelling; it may also be used to treat skin conditions, skin ulceration and damaged tissue as in burns or sprains. Ananase Forte has also been used to treat bronchitis. Its actions result from the effect of breaking down complex molecules into simpler ones (much like a digestive enzyme); it is thought thus to dissolve dead tissue, cellular debris and congealed blood for rapid transportation away from the site of inflammation. It is produced in the form of tablets.

✚/▲ warning/side-effects: *see* BROMELAINS.

Anapolon 50 (*Syntex*) is a proprietary form of the anabolic STEROID oxymetholone, available only on prescription, used to build up the body following major surgery or long-term debilitating disease, or to treat osteoporosis (brittle bones). Sometimes administered also to treat sex-hormone-linked cancers, it is additionally used in the treatment of certain forms of anaemia, although how it works in this respect – and even whether it works – remains the subject of some debate: variations in patient response are wide. It is produced in the form of tablets.

✚/▲ warning/side-effects: *see* OXYMETHOLONE.

Ancoloxin (*Duncan, Flockhart*) is a proprietary ANTI-EMETIC, available only on prescription, used to prevent nausea and vomiting. Produced in the form of tablets, Ancoloxin is a preparation of the ANTIHISTAMINE meclozine hydrochloride together with pyridoxine hydrochloride (vitamin B_6) and is not recommended for children.

✚/▲ warning/side-effects: *see* MECLOZINE; PYRIDOXINE.

ancrod is an effective ANTICOAGULANT derived from an enzyme that is a constituent of the venom of the Malaysian pit-viper. It works by breaking down the protein fibrinogen which is necessary for the formation of blood clots. The effects may be experienced for between 12 and 24 hours (and in some cases an antidote may have to be administered too – although that

A

may also cause sensitivity problems). Its therapeutic use is in the treatment of deep-vein thrombosis (blood clots), especially the sort that occur following surgery, and it is occasionally used to prevent thrombosis. Administration is by injection.

✚ warning: ancrod should not be administered to patients who are pregnant; it should be administered with extreme caution to those with haemophilia or other bleeding disorders (such as ulcers), high blood pressure (hypertension), severe liver disease, or who have had recent surgery (especially of the eye or nervous system). The antidote should be on hand in case of emergency, preferably with fresh (frozen) plasma as back-up. Initial infusion must be administered slowly, and during treatment there must be constant blood monitoring.

▲ side-effects: the major side-effects are bleeding and sensitivity/allergic reactions. Brittle bones and hair loss may result from prolonged use. *Related article:* ARVIN.

Andrews (*Sterling Health*) is a proprietary, non-prescription ANTACID, produced in the form of a powder. By disolving various amounts in water, the solution may also be used as a laxative or simply a refreshing drink. Andrews contains sodium bicarbonate and magnesium sulphate.

✚/▲ warning/side-effects: *see* MAGNESIUM SULPHATE; SODIUM BICARBONATE.

Androcur (*Schering*) is a proprietary hormonal drug that acts as a male sex HORMONE antagonist. Available only on prescription, it is used to treat severe hypersexuality and sexual deviation in men. Produced in the form of tablets, Androcur is a preparation of the anti-androgen cyproterone acetate.

✚/▲ warning/side-effects: *see* CYPROTERONE ACETATE.

androgens are male sex HORMONES that stimulate the development of male sex organs and male secondary sexual characteristics. In men they are produced primarily by the testes in the form of testosterone and androsterone. However in both men and women, androgens are also produced by the adrenal glands, and in women small quantities are also secreted by the ovaries. An excessive amount in women causes masculinization. There are also synthetic androgens. Therapeutically, androgens are administered to make up hormonal deficiency, and may also be used to treat sex-hormone-linked cancers, such as breast cancer in women.

✚ warning: androgens should not be administered to patients who suffer from male-sex-hormone-linked cancers, such as cancer of the prostate gland, or who are pregnant.

▲ side-effects: there is salt and water retention, with increased bone growth. In women there is masculinization. *see* TESTOSTERONE.

Andursil (*Geigy*) is a proprietary non-prescription compound ANTACID that is not available from the National Health Service. Used to treat severe indigestion, heartburn, gastric and peptic ulcers, and hiatus hernia, it is produced in the form of a sugar-free suspension representing a preparation of ALUMINIUM HYDROXIDE, MAGNESIUM

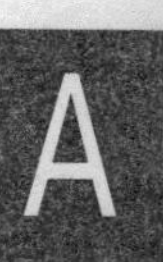

HYDROXIDE, MAGNESIUM CARBONATE and the antifoaming agent DIMETHICONE. Tablets containing the same constituents but without magnesium hydroxide are also available. Neither of these preparations is recommended for children.

Anectine (*Calmic*) is a proprietary MUSCLE RELAXANT, available only on prescription, that has an effect for only 5 minutes. It is used to relax muscles during surgical anaesthesia and this facilitates some surgical procedures (e.g. inserting a ventilator into the windpipe). Produced in ampoules for injection, Anectine is a preparation of suxamethonium chloride.
✚/▲ warning/side-effects: *see* SUXAMETHONIUM CHLORIDE.

Anethaine (*Evans*) is a proprietary non-prescription local ANAESTHETIC, used to treat painful skin conditions and itching. Produced in the form of a water-miscible cream for topical application, Anethaine is a preparation of amethocaine hydrochloride.
✚/▲ warning/side-effects: *see* AMETHOCAINE.

Aneurone (*Philip Harris*) is a proprietary mixture prescribed principally to stimulate the appetite. Available on prescription only to private patients, it is a syrup preparation of STRYCHNINE hydrochloride, THIAMINE hydrochloride (vitamin B_1), CAFFEINE, compound GENTIAN infusion and SODIUM ACID PHOSPHATE for dilution (the potency of the syrup once diluted is retained for 14 days).

Angilol (*DDSA Pharmaceuticals*) is a proprietary ANTIHYPERTENSIVE BETA-BLOCKER, available only on prescription, used not only to treat high blood pressure (hypertension), but also to relieve angina pectoris (heart pain) and to slow and/or regularize the heartbeat in order to prevent a recurrent heart attack. The drug may also be used to treat an excess of thyroid hormones in the bloodstream (thyrotoxicosis) or to try to prevent migraine attacks. Produced in the form of tablets (in four strengths), Angilol is a preparation of the beta-blocker propranolol hydrochloride.
✚/▲ warning/side-effects: *see* PROPRANOLOL.

Anhydrol Forte (*Dermal*) is a proprietary medicated antiperspirant, available only on prescription, used to treat abnormally heavy sweating (hyperhydrosis) of the armpits, hands and feet. Produced in a roll-on bottle, Anhydrol Forte is a 20% solution of aluminium chloride hexahydrate. The solution is inflammable so care should be taken when it is used.
✚/▲ warning/side-effects: *see* ALUMINIUM CHLORIDE.

Anodesyn (*Crookes Products*) is a proprietary non-prescription ointment used to soothe and treat piles (haemorrhoids) and anal itching. Also available in the form of anal suppositories, Anodesyn is a compound preparation that includes the SYMPATHOMIMETIC ephedrine hydrochloride and the local ANAESTHETIC lignocaine hydrochloride. Prolonged use should be avoided.
✚/▲ warning/side-effects: *see* EPHEDRINE HYDROCHLORIDE; LIGNOCAINE.

Anquil (*Janssen*) is a proprietary ANTIPSYCHOTIC drug, available only on prescription, used to treat psychosis (especially schizophrenia) and as a major

A

TRANQUILLIZER in patients undergoing behavioural disturbance. It is used to treat deviant and antisocial sexual behaviour, and it may also be used in the short term to treat severe anxiety (especially in the case of terminal disease) or to treat an intractable hiccup. Produced in the form of tablets, Anquil is a preparation of the powerful drug benperidol. It is not recommended for children.
✚/▲ warning/side-effects: *see* BENPERIDOL.

Antabuse (*CP Pharmaceuticals*) is a proprietary preparation of the drug disulfiram, available only on prescription. It is used as an adjunct in the treatment of alcoholism because, in combination with the consumption of even small quantities of alcohol, it gives rise to unpleasant reactions – such as flushing, headache, palpitations, nausea and vomiting. Produced in the form of tablets, Antabuse is not recommended for children.
✚/▲ warning/side-effects: *see* DISULFIRAM.

***antacid** is a drug that effectively neutralizes the hydrochloric acid that the stomach produces as a means of digestion. Much of indigestion is caused by an excessive quantity of acids in the stomach (particularly after alcohol consumption), and simple indigestion can be complicated by the effects of stomach acids on peptic ulcers or hernias. Antacids thus reduce acidity, but may themselves cause flatulence or diarrhoea as side-effects. Antacids may also impair the absorption of other drugs. Most used and best known antacids include ALUMINIUM HYDROXIDE, SODIUM BICARBONATE, MAGNESIUM HYDROXIDE and CALCIUM CARBONATE.

Antasil (*Stuart*) is a proprietary non-prescription compound ANTACID that is not available from the National Health Service. Used to treat severe indigestion, heartburn, gastric and peptic ulcers, and flatulence, it is produced in the form of tablets and as a liquid, both being a preparation of ALUMINIUM HYDROXIDE and magnesium hydroxide with the antifoaming agent DIMETHICONE. Neither form is recommended for children.

antazoline is an ANTIHISTAMINE used to treat topical allergic conditions. It is thus used in combination with other drugs to treat allergic skin irritations, stings and bites, and in combination with other antihistamines to relieve the symptoms of allergic conjunctivitis. Administration is in the form of a cream or as eye-drops.
Related articles: OTRIVINE-ANTISTIN; R.B.C.; VASOCON A.

Antepar (*Wellcome*) is a proprietary non-prescription ANTHELMINTIC drug used to treat infestation by threadworms or roundworms. A laxative administered simultaneously is often expedient. Produced in the form of tablets and as an elixir for dilution (the potency of the elixir once diluted is retained for 14 days), Antepar is a preparation of piperazine hydrate.
✚/▲ warning/side-effects: *see* PIPERAZINE.

Antepsin (*Ayerst*) is a proprietary drug used to promote the healing of peptic ulcers in the stomach and duodenum. Available only on prescription, it is thought to work by forming a protective coating over an ulcer under which the ulcer is then able to heal. It is

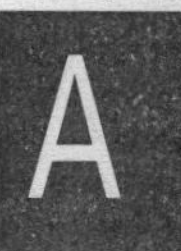

also used in the treatment of acid stomach. Produced in the form of tablets, Antepsin is a preparation of the aluminium sucrose sulphate sucralfate.
✚/▲ warning/side-effects: *see* SUCRALFATE.

***anthelmintic** drugs destroy or rid the body of parasitic worms (such as flukes, roundworms or tapeworms). Most worms infest the intestines; diagnosis often corresponds to evidence of their presence as shown in the faeces. Drugs can then be administered, and the worms are killed or anaesthetized and excreted in the normal way. Complications arise if the worms migrate within the body, in which case in order to make the environment in the body untenable for the worms, the treatment becomes severely unpleasant for the patient. Most used and best known anthelmintics include PIPERAZINE, MEBENDAZOLE and MEPACRINE.

Anthical (*May & Baker*) is a proprietary non-prescription ANTIHISTAMINE, used to treat allergic symptoms of itching and rashes. Produced in the form of a cream, Anthical is a preparation of mepyramine maleate and ZINC OXIDE.
✚/▲ warning/side-effects: *see* MEPYRAMINE.

Anthisan (*May & Baker*) is a proprietary non-prescription ANTIHISTAMINE, used to treat allergic conditions (such as hay fever) and symptoms of itching and rashes. Produced in the form of tablets and as a cream, Anthisan is a preparation of mepyramine maleate.
✚/▲ warning/side-effects: *see* MEPYRAMINE.

Anthranol (*Stiefel*) is a proprietary antipsoriatic, available only on prescription, used to treat serious non-infective skin inflammation, in particular psoriasis. Produced in the form of an ointment (in three strengths), Anthranol is a preparation of the powerful drug dithranol with salicylic acid.
✚/▲ warning/side-effects: *see* DITHRANOL; SALICYLIC ACID.

anthrax vaccine is generally required only by patients who are exposed to anthrax-infected hides and carcases, or who handle imported bonemeal, fishmeal and feedstuffs. Available only on prescription, this vaccine consists of a suspension administered by injection in three doses over 9 weeks followed by another shot after 6 months; thereafter there may be an annual booster if necessary.

***anti-allergic** drugs relieve the symptoms of allergic sensitivity to specific substances. These substances may be endogenous (in the patients body), or they may be exogenous (present in the environment). Because allergic reactions generally cause the internal release of histamine, the most effective drugs for the purpose are the ANTIHISTAMINES. However, some allergic reactions include inflammatory symptoms, and in such cases the CORTICOSTEROIDS may afford useful relief. How certain corticosteroids may relieve asthmatic symptoms is not fully understood, but the effect may be due to the reduction of inflammatory responses in the lining of the airways. There are many other types of drugs that also treat the symptoms of asthma, including the SYMPATHOMIMETICS and the ANTICHOLINERGIC or xanthine BRONCHODILATORS. In allergic emergencies – anaphylactic

A

shock – blood pressure is severely lowered and initial treatment is generally an injection of ADRENALINE (which may have to be repeated), followed by intravenous infusion of an antihistamine (such as CHLORPHENIRAMINE). SODIUM CHROMOGLYCATE is an anti-allergic drug that prevents the release of histamine from cells, unlike antihistamines which antagonize histamine.

***antiarrhythmic** drugs strengthen and regularize a heartbeat that has become unsteady and is not showing its usual patter of activity. But because there are many ways in which the heartbeat can falter – atrial tachycardia, ventricular tachycardia, atrial flutter or fibrillation, and the severe heartbeat irregularity that may follow a heart attack (myocardial infarction), for example – there is a variety of drugs available, each for a fairly specific use. Best known and most used antiarrhythmic drugs include DIGOXIN (a CARDIAC GLYCOSIDE), VERAPAMIL (a CALCIUM ANTAGONIST) and LIGNOCAINE (a local ANAESTHETIC, especially used for ventricular arrhythmia); also extremely effective are the BETA-BLOCKERS (which also treat high blood pressure and angina pectoris).

***anti-asthmatic** drugs relieve the symptoms of bronchial asthma or prevent recurrent attacks. The symptoms of asthma include spasm of the muscles in the bronchial passages and make breathing difficult, so some anti-asthmatic drugs are BRONCHODILATORS and some are also SMOOTH MUSCLE RELAXANTS. The SYMPATHOMIMETICS are drugs in common use, notable examples being SALBUTAMOL and TERBUTALINE. In an emergency situation, CORTICOSTEROIDS may also be required to limit inflammatory responses in the mucous membranes of the air passages, and are being increasingly used by inhalation in the prevention of asthmatic attacks. But there are many other types of drugs used in the treatment of asthma. In the prevention of asthmatic attacks, regular dosage of SODIUM CHROMOGLYCATE is the preferred therapy, although some patients use KETOTIFEN instead. ANTIHISTAMINES may also be used, although they are perhaps more useful in treating other allergic symptoms (such as hay fever or rashes).
see ANTI-ALLERGIC.

***antibacterial** drugs include ANTIBIOTICS that destroy bacteria (and may have less effect on other micro-organisms). The major group is that of the PENICILLINS (including penicillin, CLOXACILLIN, FLUCLOXACILLIN, AMPICILLIN, AMOXYCILLIN and BACAMPICILLIN); others are CEPHALOSPORINS, TETRACYCLINES. Other antibacterials include GENTAMICIN and KANAMYCIN, and ERYTHROMYCIN. Some, such as the SULPHONAMIDES (which are not technically antibiotics), are most commonly administered in combination because antibiotic-resistant strains of bacteria have now become troublesome. ANTISEPTICS and DISINFECTANTS all have antibacterial properties.

***antibiotics** are drugs that destroy infective organisms or that prevent them from reproducing. Most commonly, such drugs are themselves derived from other organisms. Antibiotics treat infections caused mostly by bacteria or fungal agents; some are effective

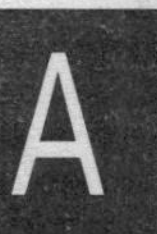

against other microbes or against worms. The use of antibiotics has revolutionized medical therapy in the twentieth century. However, over-use of some has led to the emergence of a number of resistant infective organisms. Individual patients may experience allergic reactions to certain antibiotics. High dosage may cause an imbalance in the body's normal content of harmless or useful bacteria, which may in turn lead to severe symptoms or further infection. *see* ANTIBACTERIAL; ANTIFUNGAL; ANTIVIRAL.

***anticancer** drugs are mostly CYTOTOXIC: they work by interfering one way or another with cell replication or production, so preventing the growth of new tissue. Inevitably, this means that normal cell production is also affected and thus there may be some severe side-effects. They are generally administered in combination in a series of treatments known collectively as chemotherapy. But there are other forms of anticancer therapy. In cases where the growth of a tumour is linked to the presence of a sex hormone (as with some cases of breast cancer or cancer of the prostate gland), treatment with sex hormones opposite to the patient's own sex can be extremely beneficial, although side-effects may be psychologically stressful. The CORTICOSTEROIDS PREDNISONE and PREDNISOLONE are also used as anticancer drugs in the treatment of the lymphatic cancer Hodgkin's disease and other forms of lymphoma, and may be helpful additionally in halting the progress of hormone-linked breast cancer.

***anticholinergic** drugs inhibit the action, release or production of the substance acetylcholine (a neurotransmitter), which plays an important part in the nervous system, and tends to relax smooth muscle, to reduce the secretion of saliva, digestive juices and sweat, and to dilate the pupil of the eye. They may thus be used as ANTISPASMODICS, in the treatment of parkinsonian symptoms or of peptic ulcers, and in ophthalmic examinations. However, use of such drugs is commonly accompanied by side-effects that include dry mouth, dry skin, blurred vision, an increased heart rate, constipation and difficulty in urinating. ATROPINE is an example of an anticholinergic drug.

***anticoagulants** are agents that prevent the clotting of blood and disolve blood clots that have formed. The blood's own natural anticoagulant is HEPARIN, probably still the most effective anticoagulant known. Synthetic anticoagulants (such as WARFARIN, NICOUMALONE and PHENINDIONE) take longer to act and work by affecting clotting factors within the blood; they are thus less capable than heparin of breaking up clots that have already formed. Therapeutically, anticoagulants are used to prevent the formation of, and to treat blood clots in, conditions such as thrombosis and embolism, especially following surgery. They are also used to prevent blood clots in patients fitted with a heart pacemaker or with arteriosclerosis.

***anticonvulsant** drugs prevent the onset of epileptic seizures or reduce their severity if they do occur. The best known and most used anticonvulsant is SODIUM VALPROATE, which is used to treat all forms of epilepsy; others

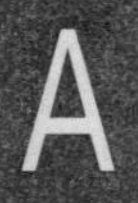

include those used solely to treat grand mal forms of epilepsy (such as CARBEMAZEPINE and PHENYTOIN) and those used solely to treat petit mal forms (such as ETHOSUXIMIDE). In every case, dosage must be adjusted to the requirements of each individual patient.

***antidepressants** are drugs that relieve the symptoms of depressive illness. There are two main groups of drugs used for the purpose. One is the group nominally called tricyclic antidepressants, which include AMITRYPTILINE, IMIPRAMINE and DOXEPIN, and are effective in alleviating a number of associated symptoms – although they have anticholinergic side-effects. The other group consists of the monoamine-oxidase inhibitors (MAOIs), including for example ISOCARBOXAZID, TRANYLCYPROMINE and PHENELZINE, which are now used less commonly because they have severe side-effects. A third type of antidepressant consists of the amino acid TRYPTOPHAN. Caution must be taken in prescribing antidepressant drugs.

***antidiarrhoeal** drugs prevent the onset of diarrhoea or assist in treating it if the symptom is already present. Yet the main medical treatment while diarrhoea lasts is always the replacement of fluids and minerals. Because there is a perceived need on the part of the general public, however, antidiarrhoeals are generally available, without prescription. Many are adsorbent mixtures that bind faecal material into solid masses; such mixtures include those containing KAOLIN, CHALK or METHYLCELLULOSE – preparations which may also be useful in controlling faecal consistency for patients who have undergone colostomy or ileostomy. Other antidiarrhoeals work by reducing the movement of the intestines (peristalsis) and this slows down the movement of faecal material: OPIATES such as CODEINE PHOSPHATE and MORPHINE are efficient at this. Diarrhoea caused by inflammatory disorders may be relieved by treatment with CORTICOSTEROIDS.

***anti-emetic**, or antinauseant, drugs prevent vomiting, and are therefore used primarily to prevent travel sickness, to relieve vertigo experienced by patients with infection of the organs of balance in the ears, or to alleviate nausea in patients undergoing chemotherapy for cancer. No specific type of drugs is used for the purpose, although most of the ANTIHISTAMINES are effective. HYOSCINE is also useful, as in many cases are the PHENOTHIAZINE derivatives (such as CHLORPROMAZINE and PROCHLORPERAZINE). In all cases, treatment causes drowsiness and reduces concentration, and enhances the effects of alcohol consumption. Anti-emetic drugs should not be administered to treat vomiting in pregnancy: most can cause harm to a foetus.

***anti-epileptic** drugs are more usually described as anticonvulsant drugs (even though mild forms of epilepsy may not cause convulsions). *see* ANTICONVULSANT.

***antifungal** drugs are ANTIBIOTICS that treat or prevent infection by fungal agents. Many fungal infections are in fact associated with some immune deficiency in the patient, a deficiency that should be corrected if treatment is to succeed. For systemic fungal infections the drug of choice is

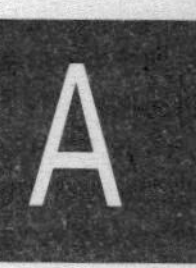

AMPHOTERICIN, which can be administered by infusion, and is active against almost all fungi and yeasts. Side-effects, however, are common. FLUCYTOSINE is an effective antifungal agent, a synthetic drug taken orally; sensitivity reactions occur in some patients. GRISEOFULVIN is primarily used to treat infection in hair or nails; it too is administered orally. For topical treatment, the IMIDAZOLE group of drugs is generally effective (including MICONAZOLE and KETOCONAZOLE), although in the treatment of candidiasis (thrush), NYSTATIN may often be preferred.

***antihistamines** are drugs that inhibit the effects in the body of histamine. Such a release occurs naturally as the result of a patient's coming into contact with a substance to which he or she is allergically sensitive, and the resultant symptoms if not more serious may be those of hay fever, urticaria, itching (pruritus) or even asthma. Many antihistamines also have ANTI-EMETIC properties, and are thus used to prevent travel sickness, vertigo, or the effects of chemotherapy in the treatment of cancer. Side-effects following administration commonly include drowsiness (and a small number of antihistamines are used as sedatives), dizziness, blurred vision, gastrointestinal disturbances and a lack of muscular co-ordination.

Conventially, only the earlier discovered drugs that act on histamine's H_1 receptors are referred to by the general name 'antihistamines'. Somewhat confusingly, however, the recently discovered drugs used in the treatment of peptic ulcers (e.g. CIMETIDINE, RANITIDINE) are also antihistamines, but act on another class of receptor (H_2) that is involved in gastric secretion.

see ASTEMIZOLE; AZATADINE MALEATE; BROMPHENIRAMINE MALEATE; CINNARIZINE; CLEMASTINE; CYCLIZINE; CYPROHEPTADINE HYDROCHLORIDE; DIMENHYDRINATE; DIMETHINDENE MALEATE; DIPHENHYDRAMINE HYDROCHLORIDE; HYDROXYZINE HYDROCHLORIDE; MEBHYDROLIN; MEPYRAMINE MALEATE; MEQUITAZINE; OXATOMIDE; PHENINDAMINE TARTRATE; PHENIRAMINE MALEATE; PROMETHAZINE HYDROCHLORIDE; TERFENADINE; TRIMEPRAZINE TARTRATE; TRIPROLIDINE HYDROCHLORIDE.

***antihypertensive** drugs reduce high blood pressure (hypertension – a group of diseases of different origins) and so reduce a patient's risk of heart attacks, kidney failure or a stroke; many also treat angina pectoris (heart pain). There are several large groups of drugs used for the purpose, each with a specific mode of action, but before any drugs are administered a check should be made on the patient's diet and lifestyle to see if therapy without drugs can be advised. All DIURETIC drugs act as antihypertensives, and often a mild diuretic may be all that is required. If further treatment is necessary, any of the BETA-BLOCKERS may be used, with or without simultaneous administration of a diuretic. Other treatments include the use of a VASODILATOR (such as NIFEDIPINE or HYDRALAZINE). Some antihypertensive drugs act directly on the brain centre responsible for monitoring blood pressure: these include the RAUWOLFIA ALKALOIDS. Other antihypertensives inhibit the factors in the body that respond to stress, so preventing the release of hormones such as

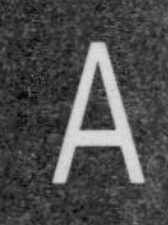

adrenaline and noradrenaline: these include DEBRISOQUINE. All require frequent and regular monitoring.

***anti-inflammatory** drugs are those used to reduce inflammation (the body's defensive reaction when tissue is injured). The way they work depends on the type of drug (e.g. CORTICOSTEROID or NSAID), but may involve actions such as the reduction of blood flow to the inflamed area, or an inhibitory effect on the chemicals released in the tissue that cause the inflammation.

***antimalarial** drugs are used to treat or prevent malaria. The disease is caused by infection of the red blood cells with a small organism called a protozoon (of the genus Plasmodium) which is carried by the Anopheles mosquito. Infection occurs as a result of the mosquito's bite. Two drugs frequently used to treat malaria are CHLOROQUINE and AMODIAQUINE. However, in some parts of the world, some forms of the protozoon that causes malaria are resistant to chloroquine; in such cases, the traditional remedy for malaria, QUININE, is used. Quinine may also be used in patients who cannot tolerate chloroquine. The prevention of malaria by drugs cannot be guaranteed. However, adminsitration of chloroquine, PROGUANIL or PYRIMETHAMINE before, and for a period after, travelling to a tropical place is thought to provide reasonable protection.

***antimicrobials** are drugs used in the treatment of infection by micro-organisms (such as bacteria, viruses and fungi).

***antinauseants** are usually described as anti-emetics, although theoretically they remedy nausea (the sensation that makes people feel as if they are about to vomit) rather than prevent vomiting. The term is used occasionally to make this distinction.
see ANTI-EMETIC.

***antiparkinsonism** drugs are used to treat parkinsonism, which is the symptoms of a number of disorders of the central nervous system, including muscle tremor and rigidity (extrapyramidal symptoms), especially in the limbs, and results from an imbalance of the actions of the neurotransmitters acetylcholine and dopamine. In classic Parkinson's disease this is due to the degeneration of dopamine-containing nerves; however, parkinsonian extrapyramidal side-effects may be caused by treatment with several types of drugs, especially ANTIPSYCHOTICS (e.g. HALOPERIDOL). Treatment of parkinsonism may be by ANTI-CHOLINERGIC drugs (e.g. BENZHEXOL), or by drugs that increase dopamine release (e.g. LEVODOPA). The former class is more useful for controlling fine tremor – including that induced by drugs – and the latter class for overcoming difficulty in commencing movement and slowness brought about by degenerative disease. Overcompensation is common and a good balance difficult to achieve.

***antiperspirants** are substances that help to prevent sweating. Medically they are needed only in cases of severe hyperhydrosis – when some disorder of the sweat glands causes constant and streaming perspiration. In such cases, aluminium chloride in mild solution is an effective

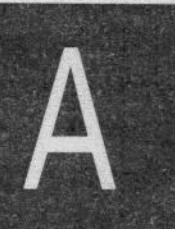

treatment. Dusting powders may also be useful to dry the skin. But in all other cases there should be no need for antiperspirants, and indeed they may be harmful in preventing the body's normal means of cooling from functioning adequately.
✚/▲ warning/side-effects: *see* ALUMINIUM CHLORIDE.

***antiprotozoal** drugs are used to treat infections by a type of organism called a protozoon. There are a number of different kinds of protozoa. There is a wide range of drugs used to treat protozoal infections. Most of the drugs specifically affect only one type of protozoon. For example, antimalarial drugs are used to treat and prevent disease caused by a protozoon of the genus Plasmodium. Other protozoa that cause disease in humans are Leishmania, which cause black fever (kala-azar); Trypanosoma which cause sleeping sickness and Chagas' disease; Trichomona which are common throughout the world and cause the sexually transmitted infection trichomoniasis; and Giardia which are also found throughout the world and cause intestinal problems. The drugs most commonly used against Trichomona are METRONIDAZOLE and NIMORAZOLE, against Giardia are METRONIDAZOLE or MEPACRINE, and against Leishmania is SODIUM STIBOGLUCONATE. A number of different drugs are used against Trypanosoma.

***antipsychotic**, or neuroleptic, drugs calm and soothe patients without impairing consciousness. They are used mainly to treat psychologically disturbed patients, particularly those who manifest the complex behavioural patterns of schizophrenia, but in the short term they may also be used to treat severe anxiety. Affecting mood, they may also worsen or help to alleviate depression. Antipsychotics exert their effect by acting in the brain. They exibit many side-effects, including abnormal face and body movements, and restlessness; these may resemble the symptoms of the condition being treated. The use of other drugs may be required to control these side-effects. Antipsychotic drugs include HALOPERIDOL, FLUPENTHIXOL DECANOATE and the PHENOTHIAZINE derivatives, especially CHLORPROMAZINE and THIORIDAZINE; SULPIRIDE demands careful adjustment of dosage depending on effect; BENPERIDOL is used mostly to control antisocial sexual behaviour or hyperactivity. Those antipsychotics with markedly depressant side-effects are known as major TRANQUILLIZERS.

***antipyretic** drugs reduce high body temperature. Best known and most used antipyretic drugs include the ANALGESICS ASPIRIN, PARACETAMOL, MEFENAMIC ACID and PHENYLBUTAZONE.

***antirheumatic** drugs are used to relieve the pain and the inflammation of rheumatism and arthritis, and sometimes of other musculo-skeletal disorders. The primary form of treatment is with non-steroidal ANTI-INFLAMMATORY (NSAID) non-narcotic ANALGESICS such as ASPIRIN, SODIUM SALICYLATE, the aspirin-paracetamol ester BENORYLATE, INDOMETHACIN, FENOPROFEN, IBUPROFEN and PHENYLBUTAZONE.
CORTICOSTEROIDS may also be used for their notable anti-inflammatory properties. Suitable steroids include

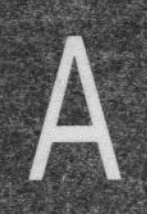

PREDNISOLONE and TRIAMCINOLONE. Finally, there are some drugs that seem to halt the progressive advance of rheumatism; some have unpleasant side-effects, others may take up to 6 months to have any effect. They include gold (in the form of SODIUM AUROTHIOMALATE) and PENICILLAMINE, and some drugs otherwise mostly used as IMMUNOSUPPRESSANTS.

***antiseptics** are agents that destroy micro-organisms, or inhibit their activity to a level such that they are less or no longer harmful to health. Antiseptics are used to treat the skin and living tissue. The term DISINFECTANT is sometimes used synonymously.

***antiserum** is a general term used to describe certain preparations of blood serum. Antiserums are used to provide (passive) immunity to diseases, or to provide some measure of treatment if the disease has already been contracted. The general term used to describe the disease-causing entity is "antigen". If an antigen is injected into an animal, the animal produces antibodies in response to the antigen. An antiserum is a sample of blood serum containing these antibodies. Most antiserums are prepared from blood of antigen-treated horses, and when the purified antiserums are used to immunize humans they may react to the animal preparation to some degree.

***antispasmodic**, or spasmolytic, drugs relieve spasm (rigidity) in smooth muscle (muscle that is not under voluntary control, such as the muscles in the upper respiratory tract and those of the intestinal walls), and form part of the group of drugs known collectively as SMOOTH MUSCLE RELAXANTS. They are therefore most used as BRONCHODILATORS or to relieve abdominal pain due to intestinal colic; however, they may also be used to stimulate the heart in the treatment of angina pectoris (heart pain). Best known antispasmodics include the BELLADONNA alkaloids, PIPERIDOLATE HYDROCHLORIDE and OPIATES such as PAPAVERINE. Many of them give rise to ANTICHOLINERGIC side-effects.

Antistin-Privine (*Ciba*) is a proprietary non-prescription compound solution for use in treating allergic nasal conditions such as hay fever. Not available from the National Health Service, and produced in the form of nose-drops and a nasal spray, it is a combination of the ANTIHISTAMINE antazoline sulphate and the SYMPATHOMIMETIC naphazoline. *see* ANTAZOLINE.

***antitubercular,** or antituberculous, drugs are used in combination to treat tuberculosis. The initial phase of treatment usually employs three drugs (ordinarily a selection between ISONIAZID, RIFAMPICIN, STREPTOMYCIN, and ETHAMBUTOL) in order to tackle the disease as efficiently as possible, while reducing the risk of encountering bacterial resistance. If the first line of treatment was successful, after about 2 or 3 months treatment usually continues with only two of the initial three drugs (one of which is generally isoniazid).

If the first line of treatment was not successful, for example because the patient suffered intolerable side-effects or because the disease was resistant to drugs, then other drugs (e.g.

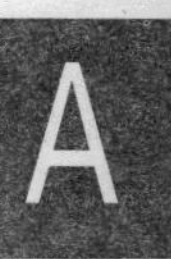

CAPREOMYCIN and CYCLOSERINE) are used to treat the patient. The duration of treatment depends on the combination of drugs used.

*__antitussives__ are drugs that assist in the treatment of coughs. Sometimes the term antitussive is used to describe only those drugs that suppress coughing rather than drugs used to treat the cause of coughing. Cough suppressants include OPIATES such as DEXTROMETHORPHAN, NOSCAPINE, METHADONE and CODEINE. They tend to cause constipation as a side-effect and so should not be used for prolonged periods. Other antitussive preparations are EXPECTORANTS and DEMULCENTS. Expectorants are drugs used to decrease the viscosity of mucus or to increase the secretion of liquid mucus in dry, irritant, unproductive coughs, the idea being that air passages will become lubricated, thereby making the cough more productive. Expectorants include AMMONIUM CHLORIDE and IPECACUANHA. These expectorants are included in many proprietary compound cough medicines. Demulcents also help to reduce the viscosity of mucus and relieve dry, unproductive coughs. All of these drugs are used to soothe coughs rather than treat the underlying cause of the cough, such as an infection.

*__antivenin__ is an antidote to the poison in a snake-bite, a scorpion's sting, or a bite from any other poisonous creature (such as a spider). Normally, it is an ANTISERUM, and is injected into the bloodstream for immediate relief. Identification of the poisonous creature is important so that the right antidote can be selected.

*__antiviral__ drugs mostly treat only the symptoms of virus infections: very few drugs seem to have any effect on the viruses themselves, and in most cases infection has to be left virtually to resolve itself in the course of time. However, there are several drugs that are effective in dealing with viruses of the herpes family, and particularly in combating herpes simplex (which infects the skin, mucous membranes and eyes). They include ACYCLOVIR, IDOXURIDINE, VIDARABINE and INOSINE PRANOBEX. AMANTADINE may also be used to treat herpes zoster (shingles), and is sometimes also used to prevent some types of flu in patients at risk (although many types of flu can be prevented alternatively by vaccination).

Antoin (*Cox*) is a proprietary non-prescription compound ANALGESIC that is not available from the National Health Service. Used to relieve mild to moderate pain anywhere in the body, and produced in the form of soluble (dispersible) tablets, Antoin is a preparation of aspirin with the OPIATE codeine phosphate and the mild stimulant caffeine citrate. It is not recommended for children.
✚/▲ warning/side-effects: *see* ASPIRIN; CAFFEINE; CODEINE PHOSPHATE.

Antraderm (*Brocades*) is a proprietary form of the powerful drug dithranol, available on prescription, used to treat serious non-infective skin inflammations, particularly psoriasis. It is produced in the form of a wax stick for topical application. In three strengths, the strongest under the trade name Antraderm Forte, the weakest under the name Antraderm Mild, it is available only on prescription, except for Antraderm Mild.

A

✚/▲ warning/side-effects: *see* DITHRANOL.

Anturan (*Geigy*) is a proprietary preparation of the drug sulphinpyrazone, available only on prescription, used to treat and prevent gout, and especially recurrent attacks of arthritic gout. It works by reducing blood levels of uric acid by increasing its excretion in the urine. It is produced in the form of tablets (in two strengths). The effectiveness of Anturan in children has not been established.
✚/▲ warning/side-effects: *see* SULPHINPYRAZONE.

Anugesic-HC (*Parke-Davis*) is a proprietary CORTICOSTEROID preparation, available only on prescription, used to treat piles (haemorrhoids) and itching, swelling and inflammation in the anal region. Produced in the form of a cream (for application with a rectal nozzle), and as anal suppositories, it is a preparation that includes the steroid hydrocortisone acetate, the anti-parasitic benzyl benzoate, and the local anaesthetic pramoxine hydrochloride, together with mild astringents and antiseptics. It is not recommended for children.
✚/▲ warning/side-effects: *see* BENZYL BENZOATE; HYDROCORTISONE.

Anusol (*Warner*) is a proprietary, non-prescription, soothing preparation used to treat piles (haemorrhoids) and itching and discomfort in the anal region. Produced in the form of a cream (for application with a rectal nozzle), as an ointment (for similar application), and as anal suppositories, it is a preparation of the mild astringent ZINC OXIDE with other astringents and an antiseptic. It is not recommended for children.

Anusol-HC (*Warner*) is a proprietary CORTICOSTEROID preparation, used to treat piles (haemorrhoids) and inflammation in the anal region. Produced in the form of an ointment (for application with a rectal nozzle) and as anal suppositories, it is a preparation of the corticosteroid hydrocortisone acetate, the anti-parasitic benzyl benzoate, and the mild astringent ZINC OXIDE, with other astringents and antiseptics. It is not recommended for children.
✚/▲ warning/side-effects: *see* BENZYL BENZOATE; HYDROCORTISONE.

***anxiolytic** drugs relieve medically diagnosed anxiety states and should be prescribed only for patients whose anxiety in the face of stress is actually hindering the prospect of its resolution. Treatment should be at the lowest dosage effective, and must not be prolonged: psychological dependence (if not physical addiction) readily occurs and may make withdrawal difficult. Best known and most used anxiolytic drugs are the BENZODIAZEPINES, such as DIAZEPAM, CHLORDIAZEPOXIDE, LORAZEPAM and CLOBAZAM; others include MEPROBAMATE and some of the ANTIPSYCHOTIC drugs used in low dosage. The benzodiazepines are sometimes used in the relief of withdrawal symptoms caused by addiction to other drugs (such as alcohol). Drugs of this class may also be referred to as minor TRANQUILLIZERS.

Anxon (*Beecham*) is a proprietary ANXIOLYTIC drug, available on prescription only to private patients, used to treat anxiety, stress, irritability and insomnia, or to assist in the treatment of acute alcohol withdrawal symptoms; it is sometimes also

used as a SKELETAL MUSCLE RELAXANT, for example in the treatment of multiple sclerosis. Produced in the form of capsules (in two strengths), Anxon is a preparation of the long-acting benzodiazepine ketazolam, and is not recommended for children.
✚/▲ warning/side-effects: *see* KETAZOLAM.

Apisate (*Wyeth*) is a proprietary APPETITE SUPPRESSANT that is on the controlled drugs list. Produced in the form of sustained-release tablets, Apisate is a preparation of the amphetamine-related drug diethylpropion hydrochloride together with a vitamin supplement of THIAMINE (vitamin B_1), RIBOFLAVINE (vitamin B_2), PYRIDOXINE (vitamin B_6), and the B vitamin derivative NICOTINAMIDE. Treatment must be in the short term and under strict medical supervision; the drug is not recommended for children.
✚/▲ warning/side-effects: *see* DIETHYLPROPION HYDROCHLORIDE.

APP (*Consolidated*) is a proprietary compound ANTISPASMODIC drug, available on prescription only to private patients. It is used in the treatment of gastrointestinal muscle spasm, travel sickness, peptic ulcers or other gastrointestinal disturbances. Produced in the form of tablets and as a powder, APP is a preparation of the OPIATE papaverine, together with the ANTI-CHOLINERGIC homatropine methylbromide, and the ANTACIDS aluminium hydroxide, calcium carbonate, magnesium carbonate and magnesium trisilicate. It is not recommended for children.
✚/▲ warning/side-effects: *see* CALCIUM CARBONATE; MAGNESIUM CARBONATE; PAPAVERINE.

***appetite suppressants** are intended to assist in the medical treatment of obesity – in which the primary therapy has to be in the form of diet. They work either by acting on the brain or by bulking out the food eaten so that the body feels it has actually taken more than it has. Appetite suppressants that act on the brain include DIETHYLPROPION HYDROCHLORIDE, FENFLURAMINE HYDROCHLORIDE and PHENTERMINE; bulking agents include STERCULIA and METHYLCELLULOSE. Treatment should be in the short term only: psychological dependence readily occurs.

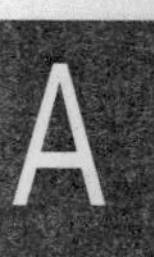

Apresoline (*Ciba*) is a proprietary VASODILATOR, available only on prescription, used to treat moderate to severe high blood pressure (hypertension). It can also be used to treat heart failure. It is a useful adjunct to diuretic and beta-blocker therapy. Produced in the form of tablets (in two strengths) and as a powder for reconstitution as a medium for injection, Apresoline is a preparation of hydralazine hydrochloride.
✚/▲ warning/side-effects: *see* HYDRALAZINE.

Aprinox (*Boots*) is a proprietary DIURETIC, available only on prescription, used to treat high blood pressure (*see* ANTIHYPERTENSIVE) and the accumulation of fluid within the tissues (oedema). Produced in the form of tablets (in two strengths), Aprinox is a preparation of the THIAZIDE bendrofluazide.
✚/▲ warning/side-effects: *see* BENDROFLUAZIDE.

Aproten (*Ultrapharm*) is a proprietary non-prescription brand of gluten-free, low protein food preparations, for the use of patients with phenylketonuria

A

and similar amino acid abnormalities, kidney or liver failure, cirrhosis of the liver, coeliac disease, or gluten sensitivity. It is produced in the form of various types of pasta, as biscuits, as crispbread and as flour.

aprotinin is a drug that has the effect of inhibiting certain digestive enzymes secreted by the pancreas. It is thus primarily used to assist in the treatment of pancreatitis, particularly after surgery on or around the pancreas. As well as affecting the digestive enzymes it is thought to affect enzymes involved in forming blood clots. It is thus also thought to have ANTICOAGULANT properties and may also be used to prevent thrombosis following surgery elsewhere in the body.
▲ side-effects: some patients experience serious sensitivity reactions (that may require emergency treatment).
Related article: TRASYLOL.

Apsifen (*Approved Prescription Services*) is a proprietary non-narcotic ANALGESIC, available only on prescription, used to relieve pain, particularly the pain of rheumatic disease and other musculo-skeletal disorders. It is produced in the form of tablets, which can be film- or sugar-coated; the film-coated are available in 3 strengths and the sugar-coated in 2 strengths. Apsifen is a preparation of the ANTI-INFLAMMATORY drug IBUPROFEN.
✚/▲ warning/side-effects: *see* IBUPROFEN.

Apsin V.K. (*Approved Prescription Services*) is a proprietary ANTIBIOTIC, available only on prescription, used to treat bacterial infections of the skin and of the ear, nose and throat, and especially staphylococcal infections that prove to be resistant to penicillin. Produced in the form of tablets and as a syrup (in two strengths) for dilution (the potency of the syrup once dilute is retained for 7 days if stored at a temperature below 15 degrees centigrade), Apsin V.K. is a preparation of the PENICILLIN phenoxymethyl-penicillin.
✚/▲ warning/side-effects: *see* PHENOXYMETHYLPENICILLIN.

Apsolol (*Approved Prescription Services*) is a proprietary ANTIHYPERTENSIVE drug, available only on prescription, used not only to treat high blood pressure (hypertension), but also to relieve angina pectoris (heart pain) and to slow and/or regularize the heartbeat in order to prevent a recurrent heart attack or to relieve anxiety. The drug may also be used to treat the effects of an excess of thyroid hormones in the bloodstream (thyrotoxicosis) or to try to prevent migraine attacks. Produced in the form of tablets (in four strengths), Apsolol is a preparation of the BETA-BLOCKER propranolol hydrochloride.
✚/▲ warning/side-effects: *see* PROPRANOLOL.

Apsolox (*Approved Prescription Services*) is a proprietary ANTIHYPERTENSIVE drug, available only on prescription, used not only to treat high blood pressure (hypertension), but also to relieve angina pectoris (heart pain) and to slow and/or regularize the heartbeat in order to prevent a recurrent heart attack. The drug may also be used to treat the effects of an excess of thyroid hormones in the bloodstream (thyrotoxicosis). Produced in the form of tablets (in four strengths), Apsolox is a preparation of the

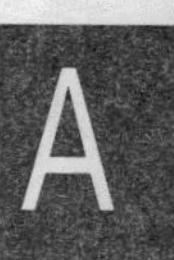

BETA-BLOCKER oxprenolol hydrochloride.
✚/▲ warning/side-effects: *see* OXPRENOLOL.

Aquadrate (*Norwich Eaton*) is a proprietary non-prescription preparation, used to treat conditions in which the skin becomes scaly and hardens in layers. It is used to treat certain eczemas and chronic dry skin conditions. Produced in the form of a cream, Aquadrate is a preparation of the natural DIURETIC urea.

Aquadry (*Thackraycare*) is a proprietary non-prescription medical adhesive (with a brush) used in the maintenance of a stoma (a surgically produced outlet in the skin surface following the surgical curtailment of the intestines).

aqueous iodine solution is a non-proprietary solution of iodine and potassium iodide in water (and is known also as Lugol's solution). It is used as an iodine supplement for patients suffering from an excess of thyroid HORMONES in the bloodstream (thyrotoxicosis), especially prior to thyroid surgery.
✚/▲ warning/side-effects: *see* IODINE.

arachis oil is peanut oil, used primarily as an EMOLLIENT in treating crusts on skin surfaces in such conditions as psoriasis, cradle cap, dandruff and eczema (often in combination with calamine). It is also a constituent in many anal suppositories.

Aradolene (*Rorer*) is a proprietary non-prescription COUNTER-IRRITANT cream which, applied topically, causes irritation. This irritation in turn offsets the pain of underlying muscle and joint ailments. It is thus used to treat rheumatic pains, and is a preparation of diethylamine salicylate together with natural oils.

Aramine (*Merck, Sharp & Dohme*) is a proprietary SYMPATHOMIMETIC VASOCONSTRICTOR, available only on prescription, most often used to raise blood pressure in a patient under general anaesthesia or in conditions of severe shock. It is a preparation of metaraminol in ampoules for injection or infusion.
✚/▲ warning/side-effects: *see* METARAMINOL.

Arelix (*Hoechst*) is a proprietary DIURETIC, available only on prescription, used to treat mild to moderate high blood pressure (*see* ANTIHYPERTENSIVE). Produced in the form of sustained- release capsules, Arelix is a preparation of piretanide. There has been insufficient experience of the use of this drug in children and therefore dosage recommendations for children have not been made.
✚/▲ warning/side-effects: *see* PIRETANIDE.

Arfonad (*Roche*) is a proprietary preparation of the GANGLION BLOCKER drug trimetaphan camsylate, available only on prescription, used to reduce blood pressure to a low level (hypotension) during surgery. It is produced in ampoules for injection; it may also be administered by intravenous infusion.
✚/▲ warning/side-effects: *see* TRIMETAPHAN CAMSYLATE.

Arilvax (*Wellcome*) is a proprietary form of VACCINE against yellow fever. It consists of a suspension containing live

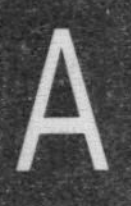

but attenuated viruses, which are cultured in chick embryos. Available only on prescription, it is produced in vials with a diluent. It is not recommended for children under the age of 9 months.
✚ warning: see YELLOW FEVER VACCINE.

Arobon (*Nestlé*) is a proprietary non-prescription preparation used to treat diarrhoea. Produced in the form of a sugar-free powder (to be taken orally in liquid), Arobon is a preparation of the adsorbent substance CERATONIA in a mixture of starch and cocoa.

Arpicolin (*RP Drugs*) is a proprietary preparation of the ANTICHOLINERGIC drug procyclidine hydrochloride, available only on prescription, used in the treatment of parkinsonism and to control tremors induced by drugs (*see* ANTIPARKINSONISM). Produced in the form of a syrup (in two strengths), Arpicolin is not recommended for children.
✚/▲ warning/side-effects: *see* PROCYCLIDINE.

Arpimycin (*RP Drugs*) is a proprietary ANTIBIOTIC, available only on prescription, used both to treat many forms of infection (particularly pneumonia and legionnaires' disease) and to prevent others (particularly sinusitis, diphtheria and whooping cough); it is also used as an alternative to penicillin-type antibiotics in patients who are allergic or whose infections are resistant to penicillins. Produced in the form of a mixture (in three strengths) for dilution (the potency of the syrup once diluted is retained for 7 days), Arpimycin is a preparation of the macrolide antibiotic erythromycin.
✚/▲ warning/side-effects: *see* ERYTHROMYCIN.

Arret (*Janssen*) is a proprietary ANTIDIARRHOEAL drug, which works by reducing the speed at which material travels along the intestines. Produced in the form of capsules and as a syrup (for adults), Arret is a preparation of the OPIATE loperamide hydrochloride. It is not recommended for children aged under 4 years.
✚/▲ warning/side-effects: *see* LOPERAMIDE.

Artane (*Lederle*) is a proprietary preparation of the ANTICHOLINERGIC drug benzhexol hydrochloride, available only on prescription, used in the treatment of parkinsonism and to control tremors and involuntary movement. Produced in the form of tablets (in two strengths), as a powder (for oral use), and as sustained-release capsules ("Sustets"), Artane is not recommended for children.
✚/▲ warning/side-effects: *see* BENZHEXOL HYDROCHLORIDE.

Artracin (*DDSA Pharmaceuticals*) is a proprietary non-steroidal ANTI-INFLAMMATORY non-narocotic ANALGESIC, available only on prescription, used to treat the pain of rheumatic and other musculo-skeletal disorders (including gout). Produced in the form of capsules (in two strengths), Artracin is a preparation of indomethacin. It is not recommended for children.
✚/▲ warning/side-effects: *see* INDOMETHACIN.

Arvin (*Armour*) is a proprietary preparation of the ANTICOAGULANT ancrod, available only on prescription (and

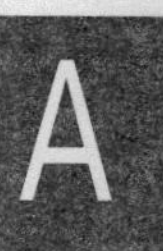

generally only for hospital use), used to treat or prevent thrombosis (blood clots). Administration is by injection. Arvin Antidote is also available for emergencies.

✚/▲ warning/side-effects: *see* ANCROD.

Asacol (*Tillotts*) is a proprietary form of the drug mesalazine, used to treat patients who suffer from ulcerative colitis but who are unable to tolerate the more commonly used drug sulphasalazine. Available only on prescription, Asacol is produced in the form of resin-coated tablets; it is not recommended for children.

✚/▲ warning/side-effects: *see* MESALAZINE.

Ascabiol (*May & Baker*) is a proprietary non-prescription preparation of BENZYL BENZOATE in suspension, used to treat infestation of the skin of the trunk and limbs by itch-mites (scabies) or sometimes to treat infestation by lice. A skin irritant, it is not suitable for use on the head, face and neck; for children it should be in diluted form (or another preparation should be used).

✚ warning: keep Ascabiol away from the eyes, and avoid taking it in by the mouth.

▲ side-effects: there is commonly skin irritation; there may also be a temporary burning sensation. Sensitivity may cause a rash.

Ascalix (*Wallace*) is a proprietary non-prescription ANTHELMINTIC drug used to treat infestation by threadworms or roundworms. Produced in the form of a syrup (in bottles and in sachets), Ascalix is a preparation of piperazine hydrate.

✚/▲ warning/side-effects: *see* PIPERAZINE.

ascorbic acid is the chemical name of the water-soluble VITAMIN C. Essential in the diet, the vitamin is instrumental in the development and maintenance of cells and tissues. Deficiency leads to scurvy and to certain other disorders associated particularly with the elderly. Good food sources are green vegetables and citrus fruits. Vitamin C supplements are rarely necessary; when they are, it is only in small quantities. Administration is oral in the form of tablets, or by injection.

✚ warning: ascorbic acid in food is lost by over-cooking or through the action of ultraviolet light.

Related article: REDOXON.

Aserbine (*Bencard*) is a proprietary non-prescription cream containing three acids (malic, benzoic and salicylic) and other additives, used to cleanse and remove hard, dry, dead skin from ulcers, burns and bedsores so that natural healing can take place. The same preparation is also available in the form of a solution.

✚ warning: contact with the eyes should be avoided, and Aserbine should only be applied externally.

Asilone (*Berk*) is a proprietary non-prescription ANTACID compound that is not available from the National Health Service. It is used to treat acid stomach, flatulence, heartburn and gastritis, and to soothe peptic ulcers. It is produced in the form of tablets, as a gel for dilution, and as a suspension for children (under the trade name Asilone Infant Suspension) for dilution. The potency of Asilone once dilute is retained for 14 days. Asilone is a combination of the antacids ALUMINIUM

A

HYDROXIDE and MAGNESIUM OXIDE ("magnesia") together with the antifoaming agent DIMETHICONE.

Asmaven (*Approved Prescription Services*) is a proprietary form of the BETA-RECEPTOR STIMULANT BRONCHODILATOR salbutamol, available only on prescription. It is able to relax the muscles of the breathing airways and is thus used in the treatment of asthma and bronchitis. Asmaven is sometimes used in the management of premature labour. It is produced in the form of tablets (in two strengths) and as a solute inhalant. Using the inhalant, patients should not exceed the prescribed dose and should be careful to follow the manufacturer's directions.
✚/▲ warning/side-effects: *see* SALBUTAMOL.

Aspav (*Cox*) is a proprietary compound ANALGESIC, available only on prescription, used to relieve pain, especially pain following surgery or caused by inoperable cancer. Produced in the form of dissolvable tablets, Aspav is a combination of aspirin and the OPIATE papaveretum. It is not recommended for children.
✚/▲ warning/side-effects: *see* ASPIRIN; PAPAVERETUM.

Aspellin (*Rorer*) is a proprietary non-prescription LINIMENT which, applied to the skin, produces an irritation that in turn counteracts rheumatic pain or pains in muscles and joints or tendons. It may also soothe chilblains. Also available in the form of a spray, Aspellin's active constituents include ASPIRIN, menthol and camphor.
✚ warning: Aspellin should not be used on inflamed or broken skin, or on mucous membranes.

Aspergum (*Plough*) is a proprietary non-prescription preparation of aspirin in the form of chewing-gum. It is not available from the National Health Service.
✚/▲ warning/side-effects: *see* ASPIRIN.

aspirin, or acetylsalicylic acid, is a well known and widely used non-narcotic ANALGESIC that also has ANTI-INFLAMMATORY properties and is useful in reducing high body temperature (ANTIPYRETIC). As an analgesic it relieves mild to moderate pain, particularly headache, toothache, menstrual pain and the aches of rheumatic disease. Its temperature-reducing capacity helps in the treatment of the common cold, fevers or influenza. Aspirin is also used as an ANTICOAGULANT. In tablet form, aspirin may irritate the stomach lining and many forms of soluble aspirin, in trying to avoid this drawback, include chalk. Other proprietary forms combine aspirin with such drugs as codeine or paracetamol. Administration is oral or, rarely, by injection. It is advised that aspirin should not be administered to children aged under 12 years. Some people are allergic to aspirin.
✚ warning: irritation of the stomach lining may, in susceptible patients, cause nausea, vomiting, pain and bleeding (which may lead to anaemia if prolonged). Overdosage may cause ringing in the ears (tinnitus), dizziness, nausea, vomiting, headache, hyperventilation, and sometimes a state of confusion or delirium followed by coma. Aspirin may also dispose a patient to bronchospasm, which in asthmatic patients may prove problematic. Repeated

overdosage may result in kidney damage.

▲ side-effects: gastric irritation with or without haemorrhage is common, although such effects may be neutralized to some extent by taking the drug after food. Aspirin may enhance the effect of some hypoglycaemic and anticoagulant drugs.
Related articles: ANTOIN; ASPAV; ASPELLIN; ASPERGUM; CAPRIN; CLARADIN; CODIS; DOLOXENE COMPOUND; EQUAGESIC; HYPON; LABOPRIN; LEVIUS; MIGRAVESS; MYOLGIN; NU-SEALS ASPIRIN; PALAPRIN FORTE; PAYNOCIL; ROBAXISAL FORTE; SAFAPRYN; SOLPRIN; TRANCOPRIN; VEGANIN.

astemizole is an ANTIHISTAMINE drug used primarily to treat allergic symptoms such as hay fever, conjunctivitis and skin rashes. Administration is oral in the form of tablets, or as a suspension.

✚ warning: astemizole should not be administered to patients who are pregnant, and should be administered with caution to those with epilepsy, glaucoma, liver disease or enlargement of the prostate gland.

▲ side-effects: sedation is minimal for an antihistamine, although there may be headaches and/or weight gain.
Related article: HISMANAL.

A.T. 10 (*Sterling Research*) is a proprietary non-prescription preparation of CALCIFEROL (vitamin D) in the form of its analogue dihydrotachysterol. Used to increase the absorption and improve the use of calcium in the body, A.T. 10 is produced as a solution in a dropper bottle; administration is oral only.

✚ warning: see DIHYDROTACHYSTEROL.

Atarax (*Pfizer*) is a proprietary ANTIHISTAMINE, available only on prescription. It is used to treat emotional disturbances and anxiety (*see* ANXIOLYTIC) which may manifest as physical symptoms. It is also used to treat physical conditions caused by allergy (such as itching and mild rashes). Atarax may also be used as a sedative (e.g. before or after surgery), and as an ANTI-EMETIC. Produced in the form of tablets (in two strengths) and as a syrup (under the trade name Atarax Syrup), Atarax is a preparation of hydroxyzine hydrochloride.

✚/▲ warning/side-effects: *see* HYDROXYZINE HYDROCHLORIDE.

atenolol is a BETA-BLOCKER drug which is capable of reducing the heart rate and the heart's force of contraction. It is used to treat high blood pressure (*see* ANTIHYPERTENSIVE), angina, changes in heart rhythm and heart attacks. It is not recommended for children.

✚ warning: atenolol should be administered with caution to those who are pregnant or lactating, to patients undergoing anaesthesia, and to those with asthma. The dose of atenolol should be reduced in the event of kidney failure. Special attention should be paid to signs of heart failure; atenolol should be administered with caution to patients who may be susceptible to heart failure. As with other beta-blockers, treatment with atenolol should not be discontinued abruptly.

▲ side-effects: the heartbeat may slow more than intended; there may be some gastrointestinal or respiratory disturbance, and tiredness of muscles. Fingers and toes may

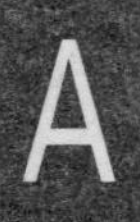

turn cold. Rarely, there are rashes.
Related article: TENORMIN.

Atensine (*Berk*) is a proprietary ANXIOLYTIC, available on prescription only to private patients, used both as an anxiolytic or minor TRANQUILIZER (to treat states of anxiety, insomnia and nervous tension) and to relieve muscle spasm and cerebral palsy. It may also be used as a premedication for dental operations. Produced in the form of tablets (in three strengths), Atensine is a preparation of the BENZODIAZEPINE diazepam.
✚/▲ warning/side-effects: *see* DIAZEPAM.

Ativan (*Wyeth*) is a proprietary ANXIOLYTIC, available only on prescription, used as an anxiolytic or minor TRANQUILLIZER (to treat anxiety, phobias, and as a HYPNOTIC in insomnia), as a sedative or premedication before surgery, and – as an emergency treatment – to control status epilepticus (in which epileptic fits succeed each other so closely that the patient does not recover consciousness and is gradually deprived of oxygen). Produced in the form of tablets (in two strengths) and in ampoules for injection, Ativan represents a preparation of the BENZODIAZEPINE lorazepam.
✚/▲ warning/side-effects: *see* LORAZEPAM.

Atkinson and Barkers (*Strenol*) is a proprietary, non-prescription preparation of infant's gripe mixture. It contains the ANTACIDS sodium bicarbonate and magnesium carbonate.
✚/▲ warning/side-effects: *see* SODIUM BICARBONATE; MAGNESIUM CARBONATE.

Atlas Dermalex is a proprietary non-prescription ANTIBACTERIAL in the form of a water-miscible cream, used primarily to prevent bedsores and to moisturize dry skin. Active constituents include TRICLOSAN.

Atmocol (*Thackray*) is a proprietary non-prescription aerosol deodorant, used to freshen and sanitize a stoma (an outlet from the intestines to the surface of the skin).

atracurium besylate is a SKELETAL MUSCLE RELAXANT, the effects of which can be reversed by other drugs. Administration is by injection, usually under general anaesthetic during surgery – effects on the muscles of a conscious patient may be painful.
✚ warning: patients treated with atracurium besylate must have their respiration controlled and monitored until the drug's effects have worn off or been antagonized. The effect of repeated dosage, unlike that of most competitive muscle relaxants, is not cumulative. Some patients may be sensitive to this drug, and its safety during pregnancy or caesarean section is not known.
▲ side-effects: rarely, atracurium may cause transient hypotension (lowered blood pressure).
Related article: TRACRIUM.

Atromid-S (*ICI*) is a proprietary form of the drug clofibrate, available only on prescription, used to treat high levels of cholesterol or other lipids (fats) in the blood. Atromid-S is produced as gelatin capsules, and is not recommended for children.
✚/▲ warning/side-effects: *see* CLOFIBRATE.

atropine is a powerful ANTICHOLINERGIC drug obtained from plants including belladonna (deadly nightshade). It is able to depress certain functions of the autonomic nervous system, and is a useful ANTISPASMODIC. In combination with morphine it may be used as a premedication to relax the muscles prior to surgery. It is also used to dilate the pupil of the eye for ophthalmic surgery (although this requires care in order not to trigger off latent glaucoma). Atropine is able to decrease gastric acid secretion and is therefore sometimes used to treat peptic ulcers. Administration is oral, as eye-drops, or by injection.

✚ warning: atropine should not be administered to patients with enlargement of the prostate gland.

▲ side-effects: there is commonly dry mouth and thirst; there may also be visual disturbances, and constipation.

atropine methonitrate is a less toxic salt of the ANTICHOLINERGIC ATROPINE, used as an ANTISPASMODIC, particularly in the treatment of pyloric stenosis (obstruction of the stomach exit) when surgery is not possible. It is also used as a BRONCHODILATOR in the treatment of asthma and whooping cough in children. Administration is oral in the form of a solution, or by means of an inhaler. In general, however, the use of the drug is not recommended.

✚ warning: atropine methonitrate should not be administered to patients with glaucoma; it should be administered with caution to those with heart problems and rapid heart rate, ulcerative colitis, urinary retention or enlargement of the prostate gland; who are elderly; or who are lactating. Some people may be allergic to this drug.

▲ side-effects: there is commonly dry mouth and thirst; there may also be visual disturbances (including sensitivity to light), flushing, irregular heartbeat, dry skin, rashes, difficulty in urinating and constipation. Rarely, there may be high temperature accompanied by delirium.

Related article: EUMYDRIN; ISO-BROVON.

atropine sulphate is used as a secondary drug in the treatment of gastrointestinal disorders that involve muscle spasm of the intestinal wall. Administration is oral in the form of tablets, by injection or as eye-drops.

✚ warning: atropine sulphate should not be administered to patients who suffer from glaucoma; it should be administered with caution to those who suffer from heart problems and rapid heart rate, ulcerative colitis, urinary retention or enlargement of the prostate gland; who are elderly; or who are pregnant or lactating.

▲ side-effects: there is commonly dry mouth and thirst; there may also be visual disturbances, flushing, irregular heartbeat, sensitivity to light and constipation. Rarely, there may be high temperature accompanied by delirium or hallucinations.

Related article: ISOPTO ATROPINE.

Atrovent (*Boehringer Ingelheim*) is a proprietary preparation of the ANTICHOLINERGIC BRONCHODILATOR ipratropium bromide, available only on prescription, used to treat chronic bronchitis and other disorders of the upper respiratory tract. It is

A

produced in the form of an aerosol spray (in two strengths, the stronger under the name Atrovent Forte) and as a solution for use in a nebulizer. Using either method, patients should not exceed the prescribed dose and should be careful to follow the manufacturer's directions; treatment should be initiated under hospital supervision.

✚/▲ warning/side-effects: *see* IPRATROPIUM.

Attenuvax (*Morson*) is a proprietary VACCINE against measles (rubeola), available only on prescription. It is a powdered preparation of live but attenuated measles viruses for administration by injection. Attenuvax is not usually recommended for children aged under 12 months.

✚ warning: attenuvax should not be administered to patients who suffer from any infection, particularly tuberculosis; who are allergic to chicken, chicken feathers or eggs (the viruses are cultured in chick-embryo tissue); who have known immune-system abnormalities; who are pregnant; or who are already taking corticosteroid drugs (except for replacement therapy), cytotoxic drugs or undergoing radiation treatment. It should be administered with caution to those who suffer from epilepsy or any other condition potentially involving convulsive fits. The vaccine contains NEOMYCIN, so should not be administered to those who are allergic to this drug.

▲ side-effects: there may be inflammation at the site of injection. Rarely, there may be high temperature, a rash, swelling of the lymph glands and/or pain in the joints.

Audax (*Napp*) is a proprietary non-prescription non-narcotic ANALGESIC in the form of ear-drops, used to soothe pain associated with infection of the outer or middle ear. Its active constituent is choline salicylate.

✚ warning: see CHOLINE SALICYLATE.

Audicort (*Lederle*) is a proprietary ANTI-INFLAMMATORY, ANTI-BACTERIAL and ANTIFUNGAL, available only on prescription, used in the treatment of bacterial and/or fungal infections of the outer ear. It contains the CORTICOSTEROID triamcinolone acetonide, the local ANAESTHETIC benzocaine, the ANTIBIOTIC neomycin, and the antifungal drug undecenoic acid.

✚/▲ warning/side-effects: *see* BENZOCAINE; NEOMYCIN; TRIAMCINOLONE ACETONIDE.

Augmentin (*Beecham*) is a proprietary preparation of the penicillin-like ANTIBIOTIC amoxycillin together with an "extending agent", clavulanic acid, which extends amoxycillin's action and power. It is used primarily to treat infections of the skin, ear, nose and throat, and urinary tract, and is produced in a number of forms: as tablets, as a solution (under the name Augmentin Dispersible), in milder versions as a powder for solution (under the names Augmentin Paediatric and Augmentin Junior), and in vials for injection or infusion (under the trade name Augmentin Intravenous).

✚/▲ warning/side-effects: *see* AMOXYCILLIN.

Auralgicin (*Fisons*) are proprietary non-prescription ear-drops used to soothe pain and treat bacterial infections of the middle ear. In a glycerol base, its

A

active constituents include the local ANAESTHETIC benzocaine, the VASOCONSTRICTOR ephedrine hydrochloride, the ANTIBACTERIAL CHLORBUTOL, and the ANALGESIC phenazone.
✚/▲ warning/side-effects: *see* BENZOCAINE; EPHEDRINE HYDROCHLORIDE.

Auraltone (*Radiol*) are proprietary non-prescription ear-drops used to soothe the pain of an inflamed eardrum or of an infection of the middle ear. In a glycerol base, it contains the analgesic phenazone and local ANAESTHETIC benzocaine.
✚/▲ warning/side-effects: *see* BENZOCAINE.

Aureocort (*Lederle*) is a proprietary ANTIBIOTIC preparation for topical application, available only on prescription, used to treat inflammations of the skin where infection is also present. Produced as a water-miscible cream, an anhydrous ointment, and an aerosol spray, Aureocort contains the CORTICOSTEROID triamcinolone acetonide and the TETRACYCLINE chlortetracycline hydrochloride.
✚/▲ warning/side-effects: *see* CHLORTETRACYCLINE; TRIAMCINOLONE ACETONIDE.

Aureomycin (*Lederle*) is a proprietary broad-spectrum ANTIBIOTIC, available only on prescription, used to treat a wide range of bacterial infections. It is produced in the form of capsules (in which form it is not recommended for women who are pregnant or for children), as a cream and as an ointment. In every form it is a preparation of the TETRACYCLINE chlortetracycline hydrochloride.
✚/▲ warning/side-effects: *see* CHLORTETRACYCLINE.

Aveeno Regular (*Dendron*) is a proprietary non-prescription bath additive for soothing and softening the skin, and to relieve itching in conditions such as prickly heat and eczema. Produced in the form of powder in sachets, it is a preparation of oat protein.

Aveeno Oilated (*Dendron*) is a proprietary non-prescription bath additive for soothing and softening the skin, and to relieve itching in conditions such as prickly heat and eczema. Produced in the form of powder in sachets, it is a preparation of oat protein and liquid paraffin.

Aventyl (*Lilly*) is a proprietary ANTIDEPRESSANT drug, available only on prescription, used to treat depressive illness – but also used to treat nocturnal bedwetting in children (although not recommended for children aged under 6 years or for treatment periods of longer than three months). Produced in the form of capsules (in two strengths) and as a liquid (under the trade name Aventyl Liquid), Aventyl represents a preparation of nortriptyline hydrochloride.
✚/▲ warning/side-effects: *see* NORTRIPTYLINE.

Avloclor (*ICI*) is a proprietary ANTIMALARIAL drug, available only on prescription, used primarily to prevent or treat certain forms of malaria, but also used as an AMOEBICIDAL drug to treat amoebic hepatitis, and to treat rheumatoid arthritis. Produced in the form of tablets, Avloclor is a preparation of chloroquine phosphate. In children under 12 Avloclor is used only to prevent or to supress malaria.
✚/▲ warning/side-effects: *see* CHLOROQUINE.

A

Avomine (*May & Baker*) is a proprietary non-prescription ANTINAUSEANT drug used to treat symptoms of nausea, vomiting and/or vertigo caused by certain diseases, motion sickness, or some forms of drug therapy. Produced in the form of tablets, Avomine is a preparation of promethazine theoclate.
✚/▲ warning/side-effects: *see* PROMETHAZINE THEOCLATE.

Azactam (*Squibb*) is a proprietary ANTIBACTERIAL, available only on prescription, used to treat severe bacterial infections. Produced in the form of powder for reconstitution as a medium for injection or infusion, Azactam is a preparation of aztreonam. It is not recommended for children.
✚/▲ warning/side-effects: *see* AZTREONAM.

Azamune (*Penn*) is a proprietary IMMUNOSUPPRESSANT drug, available only on prescription, used to reduce the possibility of tissue rejection in patients who undergo donor skin grafts or organ transplants. It may also be used to treat other conditions where the more usual corticosteroid therapies have failed. Produced in the form of tablets, Azamune is a preparation of the CYTOTOXIC drug azathioprine.
✚/▲ warning/side-effects: *see* AZATHIOPRINE.

azapropazone is a non-steroidal ANTI-INFLAMMATORY non-narcotic ANALGESIC, used primarily to treat rheumatic and arthritic complaints, gout, and musculo-skeletal pain. Administration is oral in the form of capsules and tablets. It is not recommended for children.
✚ warning: azapropazone should not be administered to patients with peptic ulcer or impairment of kidney function, or who are taking sulphonamides; it should be administered with caution to those with impaired liver function or with allergic disorders, who are elderly, or who are pregnant. It should not be given to patients who are taking phenytoin, drugs that lower the blood sugar level, or anticoagulants.
▲ side-effects: there is commonly a rash; there may also be a sensitivity to light. Sometimes there is accumulation of fluid within the tissues (oedema) and consequent weight gain. There may be gastrointestinal upsets.
Related article: RHEUMOX.

azatadine maleate is an ANTIHISTAMINE drug, used primarily to treat allergic symptoms such as hay fever and urticaria, and those arising from insect bites and stings. Administration is oral in the form of tablets, or as a syrup. Its proprietary form is not recommended for children aged under 12 months.
✚ warning: patients taking azatadine maleate should avoid alcohol. It should be administered with caution to patients who are pregnant, or with glaucoma, urinary retention, intestinal obstruction, enlargement of the prostate gland, peptic ulcer, epilepsy or liver disease.
▲ side-effects: sedation may affect patients' capacity for speed of thought and movement; there may be nausea, headaches and/or weight gain, dry mouth, gastrointestinal disturbances and visual problems.
Related article: OPTIMINE.

azathioprine is a powerful IMMUNOSUPPRESSANT drug used

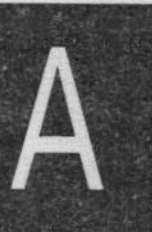

mostly to reduce the possibility of tissue rejection in patients who undergo donor grafts or transplants. It may also be used to treat autoimmune diseases, some collagen disorders, and other conditions where the more usual steroid therapies have failed. Administration is oral in the form of tablets, or by injection.

✚ warning: as with all CYTOTOXIC drugs, patients receiving azathioprine are prone to infections. Constant checking of blood counts is essential to monitor and adjust dosage for any bone-marrow toxicity.

▲ side-effects: there may be suppression of the bone-marrow's function, rashes and liver damage.

Related articles: AZAMUNE; IMURAN.

azlocillin is a penicillin-type ANTIBIOTIC used primarily to treat infections by a type of bacteria called Pseudomonas, and particularly in serious infections of the urinary tract and respiratory tract, and for septicaemia. Administration is by injection or infusion.

✚ warning: azlocillin should not be administered to patients who are known to be allergic to penicillins; it should be administered with caution to those who have impaired kidney function, or who are pregnant.

▲ side-effects: there may be some allergic reactions – such as a rash – and high temperature; some patients experience pain in the joints. Diarrhoea may occur.

Related article: SECUROPEN.

aztreonam is an ANTIMICROBIAL used to treat severe bacterial infections. Administration is by injection or infusion. A relatively recent addition to the pharmacopoeia, aztreonam is thought to arouse fewer sensitivity reactions than are caused by many other antimicrobials. It is not recommended for children.

✚ warning: aztreonam should not be administered to patients who are pregnant; it should be administered with caution to those who are known to be sensitive to penicillin or cephalosporin, who have impaired kidney or liver function, or who are lactating.

▲ side-effects: there may be diarrhoea and vomiting; skin rashes may occur, with pain or inflammation at the site of injection or infusion. Rarely, the composition of the blood changes.

Related article: AZACTAM.

B

bacampicillin hydrochloride is a broad-spectrum penicillin-type ANTIBIOTIC, a derivative of AMPICILLIN that is converted to ampicillin in the bloodstream. Used to treat many infections, especially those of the urogenital areas, upper respiratory tract and middle ear, it is administered orally in the form of tablets.

✚ warning: bacampicillin hydrochloride should not be administered to patients who are known to be allergic to penicillin-type antibiotics; it should be administered with caution to those with impaired kidney function.

▲ side-effects: there may be sensitivity reactions, ranging from a minor rash to urticaria, high temperature and joint pain, or even to anaphylactic shock. The most common side-effect, however, is simply diarrhoea.

Related article: AMBAXIN.

baclofen is a drug used as a SKELETAL MUSCLE RELAXANT that relaxes muscles which are in spasm, especially muscles in the limbs, and particularly when caused by injury or disease in the central nervous system. Although it is chemically unrelated to any other ANTISPASMODIC drug, it has similar clinical uses to certain of the benzodiazepine group of drugs. Administration is oral in the form of tablets or a dilute sugar-free liquid.

✚ warning: baclofen should be administered with caution to patients with impaired cerebrovascular system, epilepsy, or psychiatric conditions, or who are elderly. Initial dosage should be gradually increased (to avoid sedation); withdrawal of treatment should be equally gradual.

▲ side-effects: there may be drowsiness and fatigue, weakness and low blood pressure (hypotension); elderly or debilitated patients may enter a state of confusion. Nausea and vomiting may occur.

Related article: LIORESAL.

Bacticlens (*Smith & Nephew*) is a proprietary non-prescription DISINFECTANT, used to treat minor wounds and burns on the skin. Produced in the form of a solution in sachets, Bacticlens is a preparation of chlorhexidine gluconate.

✚/▲ warning/side-effects: *see* CHLORHEXIDINE.

Bactigras (*Smith & Nephew*) is a proprietary non-prescription dressing in the form of gauze impregnated with chlorhexidine acetate. It is used to treat wounds and ulcers.

✚/▲ warning/side-effects: *see* CHLORHEXIDINE.

Bactrian (*Loveridge*) is a proprietary non-prescription ANTISEPTIC cream used in the treatment of minor burns and abrasions. It contains the antiseptic CETRIMIDE in very dilute solution.

Bactrim (*Roche*) is a proprietary ANTIBACTERIAL available only on prescription, used to treat bacterial infections, especially infections of the urinary tract, sinusitis and bronchitis, and infections of bones and joints. Produced in the form of tablets (in three strengths), as soluble (dispersible) tablets, as a suspension for dilution (the potency of the suspension once dilute is retained for 14 days), as a sugar-free syrup for dilution (the potency of the syrup once dilute is retained for 14 days), in ampoules for injection, and in ampoules for intravenous infusion (following dilution), Bactrim represents a preparation of the SULPHONAMIDE compound co-trimoxazole.

✚/▲ warning/side-effects: *see* CO-TRIMOXAZOLE.

Bactroban (*Beecham*) is a proprietary ANTIBIOTIC, available only on prescription, used in topical application to treat bacterial infections of the skin. Produced in the form of a water-miscible ointment, Bactroban is a preparation of MUPIROCIN in dilute solution.

✚ warning: the ointment may sting on application.

Balanced Salt Solution (*Alcon; CooperVision Optics*) is a proprietary non-prescription sterile solution, used as an eye-wash. It is a preparation of SODIUM CHLORIDE, SODIUM CITRATE, SODIUM ACETATE, MAGNESIUM CHLORIDE and POTASSIUM CHLORIDE.

Balmosa (*Pharmax*) is a proprietary non-prescription COUNTER-IRRITANT cream which, applied topically, causes an irritation of the sensory nerve endings that has the effect of beneficially offsetting the pain of underlying muscle and joint ailments. It is thus used to treat rheumatic pains, lumbago and sciatica. It is a preparation that contains methyl salicylate, camphor, menthol and capsicum resin.

Balneum (*Merck*) is a proprietary non-prescription skin emollient (softener and soother) for use in the bath; it is a preparation of soya oil in a fragrant solution.

Balspray (*Bullen*) is a proprietary skin cleanser and protective spray used to sanitize a stoma (an outlet in the skin surface representing the surgical curtailment of the intestines). A powder for the same purpose is produced under the same name.

bamethan sulphate is a VASODILATOR used to improve blood circulation in the forearms and hands, and calves and feet, during exercise. Administration is oral in the form of tablets.

✚ warning: bamethan sulphate should not be administered to patients who have recently suffered a heart attack; it should be administered with caution to those with angina pectoris. The drug cannot treat the symptoms of poor peripheral circulation that occur while the body is at rest.

▲ side-effects: there may be an increase in the heart rate, and flushing. Low blood pressure may cause dizziness on the patient's rising from a sitting or lying position.
Related article: VASCULIT.

Banocide (*Wellcome*) is a proprietary preparation of the drug diethylcarbamazine, used to treat infestations by filarial worm-parasites (such as those that cause elephantiasis, lymphangitis, loiasis and onchocerciasis). Side-effects are inevitable, and may be severe (but should be treated with other drugs); close monitoring is essential throughout treatment, but particularly at first. Several courses of treatment may be necessary, but the drug is almost always successful. It is produced in the form of tablets.

✚/▲ warning/side-effects: *see* DIETHYLCARBAMAZINE.

Baratol (*Wyeth*) is a proprietary ANTIHYPERTENSIVE drug, available only on prescription, and often used in combination with other

antihypertensives. Produced in the form of tablets (in two strengths), Baratol represents a preparation of (the alpha-blocker) indoramin hydrochloride.
✚/▲ warning/side-effects: *see* INDORAMIN.

barbiturates are a group of drugs derived from barbituric acid, with a wide range of essentially depressent actions. They are used mostly as SEDATIVES and ANAESTHETICS. They work by direct action on the brain, depressing specific centres, and may be slow- or fast-acting; all are extremely effective. However, all also quite rapidly produce tolerance and then both psychological and physical dependence, and for that reason are used as sparingly as possible. Moreover, prolonged use even in small dosage can have serious toxic side-effects, potentially leading to death. Best known and most used barbiturates include the minor tranquillizers amylobarbitone and pentobarbitone, the sedative and anticonvulsant phenobarbitone, and the anaesthetic thiopentone. Administration is oral in the form of tablets, or by injection.
✚ warning: barbiturates should be avoided wherever possible. They should not in any case be administered to patients who suffer from insomnia caused by pain or from porphyria, who are pregnant or lactating, who are elderly, debilitated or very young, or who have a history of drug or alcohol abuse (barbiturates greatly enhance the effects of alcohol). Barbiturates should be administered with caution to those with kidney or liver disease, or impaired lung function. Prolonged use should be avoided, as should abrupt withdrawal of treatment (which might lead to withdrawal symptoms). Tolerance develops when barbiturates are taken repeatedly, an increasingly larger dose being necessary to produce the same effect; continued use leads to psychological and physical dependence.
▲ side-effects: there is drowsiness and dizziness within a hangover effect; there may be shallow breathing and headache. Some patients experience sensitivity reactions that may be serious.
see AMYLOBARBITONE; BUTOBARBITONE; CYCLOBARBITONE CALCIUM; METHYLPHENOBARBITONE; PHENOBARBITONE; QUINALBARBITONE SODIUM; THIOPENTONE SODIUM.

Barquinol HC (*Fisons*) is a proprietary non-prescription CORTICOSTEROID cream used to treat mild inflammations of the skin. Apart from its ANTI-INFLAMMATORY properties it also has some ANTIBACTERIAL and ANTIFUNGAL activity because in addition to the steroid hydrocortisone acetate it also contains the iodine-based antiseptic clioquinol.
✚/▲ warning/side-effects: *see* CLIOQUINOL; HYDROCORTISONE.

Baxan (*Bristol-Myers*) is a proprietary ANTIBIOTIC, available only on prescription, used to treat many infections, especially those of the skin and soft tissues, the respiratory and urinary tracts, and the middle ear. Produced in the form of capsules, and as a suspension (in three strengths) for dilution, Baxan is a

preparation of the cephalosporin cefadroxil monohydrate.
✚/▲ warning/side-effects: *see* CEFADROXIL.

Baycaron (*Bayer*) is a proprietary DIURETIC, available only on prescription, used to treat fluid retention in the tissues (oedema) and high blood pressure (*see* ANTIHYPERTENSIVE); it may thus also be used to treat some of the symptoms of premenstrual syndrome. Simultaneous administration of a POTASSIUM supplement is often advised. Produced in the form of tablets, Baycaron is a preparation of the THIAZIDE-like drug mefruside, and is not recommended for children.
✚/▲ warning/side-effects: *see* MEFRUSIDE.

Bayolin (*Bayer*) is a proprietary non-prescription COUNTER-IRRITANT cream which, when applied topically, causes an irritation of the sensory nerve endings that offsets the pain of underlying muscle and joint ailments. It is used particularly to treat rheumatic pain, and contains a derivative of the anticoagulant HEPARIN together with glycol salicylate and benzyl nicotinate.

Baypen (*Bayer*) is a proprietary broad-spectrum penicillin-type ANTIBIOTIC, used to treat many infections and to prevent others following abdominal and/or uterine surgery. Produced in the form of powder in vials for reconstitution as a medium for injection or infusion, Baypen is a preparation of mezlocillin.
✚/▲ warning/side-effects: *see* MEZLOCILLIN.

BC 500 (*Ayerst*) is a proprietary non-prescription multivitamin supplement that is not available from the National Health Service. It is used to treat deficiency of vitamins B and C, particularly in conditions such as convalescence from debilitating illness or chronic alcoholism, and contains THIAMINE (vitamin B_1), RIBOFLAVINE (vitamin B_2), PYRIDOXINE (vitamin B_6), NICOTINAMIDE (of the B complex), PANTOTHENIC ACID (of the B complex), and ASCORBIC ACID (vitamin C).

BC 500 with Iron (*Ayerst*) is a preparation of the proprietary non-prescription multivitamin supplement BC 500 that also includes IRON in the form of ferrous fumarate. It is used especially to treat deficiencies of vitamins B and C, and of iron (as for example may occur during pregnancy).
✚/▲ warning/side-effects: *see* FERROUS FUMARATE.

BCG vaccine (bacillus Calmette-Guérin vaccine) is a strain of the tuberculosis bacillus that no longer causes the disease in humans but does cause the formation in the body of the specific antibodies, and so can be used as the base for an ANTITUBERCULAR vaccine.

beclamide is an ANTICONVULSANT drug for various epileptic disorders (including grand mal and psychomotor epilepsies) and in the management of some behavioural disorders in non-epileptic patients. Administration is oral in the form of tablets.
✚ warning: beclamide is used as a secondary form of therapy: previous antiepileptic drug treatment should be continued in parallel for a month as treatment with beclamide is gradually introduced.
▲ side-effects: there may be gastrointestinal disturbance

B

and impaired kidney function, leading to weight loss; a rash may appear. Some patients experience dizziness. The white blood cell count may be reduced.
Related article: NYDRANE.

Becloforte (*Allen & Hanburys*) is a proprietary preparation of the CORTICOSTEROID drug beclomethasone dipropionate, available only on prescription, used to treat the symptoms of asthma, chronic bronchitis and emphysema. Produced in an aerosol for topical inhalation, it is not recommended for children.
✚/▲ warning/side-effects: *see* BECLOMETHASONE DIPROPIONATE.

beclomethasone dipropionate is a CORTICOSTEROID used primarily to treat the symptoms of asthma, chronic bronchitis and emphysema. It is thought to work by reducing inflammation in the mucous lining of the bronchial passages, and stemming allergic reactions. For many patients the best results are achieved if a BRONCHODILATOR such as salbutamol is inhaled about 10 minutes before administration. (One proprietary preparation combines the two.) The drug is also used in the form of a cream or an ointment for topical application to treat serious non-infective inflammations on the skin, or as a nasal spray to treat conditions such as hay fever. For bronchial treatment, however, it is produced mostly in aerosols for inhalation, although it is available also as powder for insufflation or as a suspension for nebulization.
✚ warning: as with all corticosteroids, beclomethasone treats the symptoms and has no effect on any underlying infection: such an infection, if remaining undetected, may reach potentially serious proportions while its symptoms are masked by the corticosteroid. In any case, prolonged use should be avoided because of side-effects. Prolonged high doses may give adrenal suppression.
▲ side-effects: some patients undergoing bronchial treatment experience hoarseness; large doses increase a risk of fungal infection. The nasal spray may cause initial sneezing.
Related articles: BECLOFORTE; BECOTIDE; VENTIDE.

Beconase (*Allen & Hanburys*) is a proprietary nasal spray, available only on prescription, used to treat conditions such as hay fever. Produced in both an aerosol and a nasal applicator, Beconase is a preparation of the CORTICOSTEROID beclomethasone dipropionate.
✚/▲ warning/side-effects: *see* BECLOMETHASONE DIPROPIONATE.

Becosym is a proprietary non-prescription VITAMIN B supplement that is not available from the National Health Service. Produced in the form of tablets (in two strengths, the stronger under the trade name Becosym Forte), and as a syrup for dilution (the potency of the syrup once dilute is retained for 14 days), Becosym contains several forms of vitamin B, including THIAMINE, RIBOFLAVINE and PYRIDOXINE.

Becotide (*Allen & Hanburys*) is a proprietary preparation of the CORTICOSTEROID drug beclomethasone dipropionate, available only on prescription, used to treat the symptoms of

asthma, chronic bronchitis and emphysema. It is produced in an aerosol for inhalation (in two strengths, the stronger under the name Becotide 100), in inhalation cartridges (using the name Rotacaps), and as a suspension for nebulization.
✚/▲ warning/side-effects: *see* BECLOMETHASONE DIPROPIONATE.

Bedranol (*Lagap*) is a proprietary ANTIHYPERTENSIVE drug of the BETA-BLOCKER class, available only on prescription, used to treat high blood pressure (hypertension), and also to relieve angina pectoris and to slow and/or regularize the heartbeat in order to prevent a recurrent heart attack. The drug may also be used to treat the effect of an excess of thyroid hormones in the bloodstream (thyrotoxicosis) or to try to prevent migraine attacks. Produced in the form of tablets (in four strengths), Bedranol is a preparation of the beta-blocker propranolol hydrochloride.
✚/▲ warning/side-effects: *see* PROPRANOLOL.

Beecham's Powders (*Beecham Health Care*) is a proprietary, non-prescription cold relief preparation. It contains paracetamol, caffeine and ascorbic acid.
✚/▲ warning/side-effects: *see* ASCORBIC ACID, CAFFEINE, PARACETAMOL.

belladonna is the name of both a solanaceous plant (deadly nightshade) and of the ALKALOIDS produced from it and related plants, from which in turn the drugs ATROPINE (hyoscyamine) and HYOSCINE are extracted. Both of those pure drugs have several uses, but the plant alkaloids too are used therapeutically – mostly (in compounds with aluminium or magnesium salts) to assist in the treatment of gastrointestinal disorders caused by smooth muscle spasm in the intestine, because the alkaloids have antispasmodic properties.
✚ warning: belladonna alkaloids should not be administered to patients with enlargement of the prostate gland or with glaucoma; they should be administered with caution to those with heart problems and rapid heart rate, ulcerative colitis, or urinary retention; who are elderly; or who are lactating.
▲ side-effects: there is commonly dry mouth and thirst; there may also be visual disturbances, flushing, irregular heartbeat and constipation.
Related articles: ALKA-DONNA; ALKA-DONNA-P; ALUHYDE; BELLOCARB; CARBELLON; NEUTRADONNA; PEPTARD.

Bellocarb (*Sinclair*) is a proprietary non-prescription ANTICHOLINERGIC compound that is not available from the National Health Service. It is used to treat muscle spasm of the intestine, and other gastrointestinal upsets including stomach acidity. Produced in the form of tablets, Bellocarb's active constituents are belladonna extract, magnesium trisilicate, and magnesium carbonate.
✚/▲ warning/side-effects: *see* BELLADONNA; MAGNESIUM CARBONATE; MAGNESIUM TRISILICATE.

Benadon (*Roche*) is a proprietary non-prescription VITAMIN B supplement that is not available from the National Health Service. Used to treat vitamin deficiency and associated symptoms, Benadon is a

B

preparation of vitamin B_6: PYRIDOXINE hydrochloride. It is produced in the form of tablets (in two strengths).

Benadryl (*Parke-Davis*) is a proprietary non-prescription ANTIHISTAMINE used to treat the symptoms of (allergy-based) conditions such as hay fever and urticaria. It also has ANTINAUSEANT properties and is used to treat or prevent travel sickness, vertigo and infections of the inner or middle ear. Produced in the form of capsules, Benadryl is a preparation of the somewhat sedative antihistamine diphenhydramine hydrochloride. It is not recommended for children.

✚/▲ warning/side-effects: *see* DIPHENHYDRAMINE HYDROCHLORIDE.

Bendogen (*Lagap*) is a proprietary ANTIHYPERTENSIVE drug, available only on prescription, used to treat moderate to severe high blood pressure (hypertension), especially when other forms of treatment have failed. Administered in combination with a DIURETIC or a BETA-BLOCKER, Bendogen works by inhibiting the release in the body of the neurotransmitter NORADRENALINE. It represents a preparation of bethanidine sulphate, and is produced in the form of tablets (in two strengths).

✚/▲ warning/side-effects: *see* BETHANIDINE SULPHATE.

bendrofluazide is a THIAZIDE DIURETIC that may be used to treat hypertension, either alone or in conjunction with other ANTIHYPERTENSIVE agents, because it has a slight lowering effect on blood pressure. Like the other thiazides, bendrofluazide is used in the treatment of oedema associated with congestive heart failure and renal and hepatic disorders. Blood potassium levels should be monitored in patients taking thiazide diuretics because they may deplete body reserves of potassium. However, potassium supplements or potassium-sparing diuretics should be added only when appropriate (hypercalcaemia is particularly hazardous in the elderly). Administration is oral in the form of tablets.

✚ warning: bendrofluazide should not be administered to patients with kidney failure or urinary retention, or who are lactating. It should be administered with caution to those who are pregnant. It may aggravate conditions of diabetes or gout.

▲ side-effects: there may be tiredness and skin rashes, thirst, nausea, dizziness. In men, temporary impotence may occur.

Related articles: APRINOX; BERKOZIDE; CENTYL; NEO-NACLEX; URIZIDE.

Benemid (*Merck, Sharp & Dohme*) is a proprietary preparation of the compound drug probenecid which, because it reduces blood levels of uric acid by promoting its excretion in the urine, is used primarily to treat gout. Available only on prescription, it is produced in the form of tablets, and is not recommended for children.

✚/▲ warning/side-effects: *see* PROBENECID.

Benerva (*Roche*) is a proprietary non-prescription VITAMIN B supplement that is not available from the National Health Service. Used to treat vitamin deficiency and associated symptoms, Benerva is a preparation of vitamin B_1:

THIAMINE hydrochloride. It is produced in the form of tablets (in six strengths) and (available only on prescription) in ampoules for injection (in two strengths).

Benerva Compound (*Roche*) is a proprietary non-prescription VITAMIN B supplement that is not available from the National Health Service. Used to treat vitamin deficiency and associated symptoms, Benerva Compound is a preparation of various forms of vitamin B; it is produced in the form of tablets.

benethamine penicillin is a penicillin-type ANTIBIOTIC that is used to treat and prevent bacterial infection. Administration is by injection.

✚ warning: benethamine penicillin should not be administered to patients who are known to be allergic to penicillins; it should be administered with caution to those who suffer from impaired kidney function.

▲ side-effects: there may be sensitivity reactions ranging from a minor rash to urticaria and joint pains, and (occasionally) to high temperature or anaphylactic shock.

Related article: TRIPLOPEN.

Bengué's Balsam (*Bengué*) is a proprietary non-prescription COUNTER-IRRITANT ointment which, applied topically, causes an irritation of the sensory nerve endings that offsets the pain of underlying muscle and joint ailments. It is thus used to treat rheumatic pains, and contains methyl salicylate and menthol in a lanolin base.

✚ warning: Lanolin causes sensitivity reactions in some patients.

Bengué's Balsam SG (*Bengué*) is a proprietary non-prescription COUNTER-IRRITANT cream which, applied topically, causes an irritation of the sensory nerve endings that offsets the pain of underlying muscle and joint ailments. It is thus used to treat rheumatic pains, and contains methyl salicylate and menthol in a vanishing-cream base.

Benoral (*Sterling Research*) is a proprietary non-prescription non-narcotic ANALGESIC used to treat mild to moderate pain, especially the pain of rheumatic disease and other musculo-skeletal disorders. Produced in the form of tablets, as a powder in sachets for solution, and as a sugar-free suspension for dilution (the potency of the suspension once dilute is retained for 14 days), Benoral is a preparation of an ester derived from both ASPIRIN and PARACETAMOL called benorylate.

✚/▲ warning/side-effects: *see* BENORYLATE.

benorylate is a non-narcotic ANALGESIC, with both anti-inflammatory and antipyretic actions, that is chemically derived from both ASPIRIN and PARACETAMOL, and is used particularly to treat the pain of rheumatic disease and other musculo-skeletal disorders, and to lower a high temperature. The paracetamol constituent is released more slowly into the bloodstream than the aspirin. Administration is oral in the form of tablets, a solution or a dilute suspension.

✚ warning: benorylate should not be administered to patients intolerant of aspirin, with peptic ulcers, who are already taking aspirin or paracetamol in some other form, or who are aged under

B

12 years. It should be administered with caution to those with allergic conditions, who have impaired kidney or liver function, who suffer from alcoholism, or from dehydration; who are elderly; who are pregnant or lactating; or who are already taking anticoagulant drugs.

▲ side-effects: gastrointestinal disturbance is fairly common, but there may also be nausea and bleeding. Some patients experience hearing disturbances and vertigo. A few proceed to hypersensitivity reactions, blood disorders, or a state of confusion. Prolonged use or overdosage may cause liver damage.
Related article: BENORAL.

benoxinate is an alternative name for the local ANAESTHETIC oxybuprocaine, used in eye-drops. *see* OXYBUPROCAINE.

Benoxyl (*Stiefel*) is a proprietary preparation of the drug benzoyl peroxide, which when applied topically in the form of a cream or an ointment removes hardened or dead skin (it is KERATOLYTIC) while simultaneously treating bacterial infection. It is most used in the treatment of acne. In its standard form (under the name Benoxyl 5) it is produced as both a cream and an ointment, and in a version that additionally contains sulphur (under the name Benoxyl 5 with Sulphur). There is also a stronger version of the standard (produced under the trade name Benoxyl 10) that appears as a lotion, and a corresponding cream that includes sulphur (produced under the name Benoxyl 10 with Sulphur). Finally, there is a preparation that is stronger still (produced under the name Benoxyl 20); it too is marketed as a lotion, and removes hard and dead skin from the edges of skin ulcers and lesions.

✚/▲ warning/side-effects: *see* BENZOYL PEROXIDE.

benperidol is a powerful ANTIPSYCHOTIC drug, used to treat and tranquillize psychotics, especially suitable for treating antisocial and deviant forms of sexual behaviour. Administration is oral in the form of tablets. It is not recommended for children.

✚ warning: benperidol should not be administered to patients who have a reduction in the bone-marrow's capacity to produce blood cells, or certain types of glaucoma. It should be administered only with caution to those with heart or vascular disease, kidney or liver disease, parkinsonism, or depression; or who are pregnant or lactating.

▲ side-effects: sedation and extrapyramidal symptoms are likely to occur. There may also be restlessness, insomnia and nightmares; rashes and jaundice may appear; and there may be dry mouth, gastrointestinal disturbance, difficulties in urinating, and blurred vision. Muscles in the neck and back, and sometimes the arms, may undergo spasms. Rarely, there is weight loss and impaired kidney function.
Related article: ANQUIL.

benserazide is an enzyme inhibitor that is administered therapeutically in combination with the powerful drug levodopa to treat parkinsonism, but not the parkinsonian symptoms induced by drugs (*see* ANTIPARKINSONISM). The benserazide prevents too rapid a breakdown in the body of the levodopa (into dopamine), allowing more levodopa to reach the brain to make up the deficiency (of dopamine) that is the major cause of parkinsonian symptoms. Administration of the combination is oral in the form of capsules.

✚/▲ warning/side-effects: complex mode of action makes side-effects and interactions with many other drugs likely, so great care should be taken in its use. Also *see* LEVODOPA. *Related article:* MADOPAR.

Bentex (*Steinhard*) is a proprietary preparation of the drug benzhexol hydrochloride, available only on prescription, used to relieve some of the symptoms of parkinsonism (*see* ANTIPARKINSONISM), specifically overall rigidity of posture, and the tendency to produce an excess of saliva. (The drug also has the capacity to treat these conditions in some cases where they are produced by drugs.) It is thought to work by compensating indirectly for the lack of dopamine in the brain that is the major cause of such parkinsonian symptoms. Bentex is produced in the form of tablets (in two strengths), to be taken before or after food. Counselling of patients is advised.

✚/▲ warning/side-effects: *see* BENZHEXOL HYDROCHLORIDE.

bentonite is an absorbent powder administered therapeutically in emergencies to absorb corrosive substances like paraquat (the toxic horticultural preparation) in cases of accidental poisoning, and to reduce further absorption by the body. The entire alimentary canal has then to be evacuated, bathed, cleaned and soothed.

Benylin Decongestant (*Parke-Davis*) is a proprietary non-prescription DECONGESTANT that is not available from the National Health Service. Produced in the form of a syrup for dilution (the potency of the syrup once dilute is retained for 14 days), it contains the ANTIHISTAMINE diphenhydramine hydrochloride, the SYMPATHOMIMETIC pseudoephedrine hydrochloride, and sodium citrate. It is not recommended for children aged under 12 months.

✚/▲ warning/side-effects: *see* DIPHENHYDRAMINE HYDROCHLORIDE; SODIUM CITRATE.

Benylin Expectorant (*Parke-Davis*) is a proprietary non-prescription EXPECTORANT that is not available from the National Health Service. Intended to promote the coughing up of bronchial secretions that might otherwise clog the air passages, it contains the expectorant AMMONIUM CHLORIDE, the ANTIHISTAMINE diphenhydramine hydrochloride, sodium citrate, and menthol. It is produced in the form of a syrup for dilution (the potency of the syrup once dilute is retained for 14 days), and is not recommended for children aged under 12 months. A version without ammonium chloride is also available (under the name Benylin Paediatric); and there is a version that additionally includes the ANALGESIC codeine phosphate (under the name Benylin with Codeine).

✚/▲ warning/side-effects: *see* CODEINE PHOSPHATE; DIPHENHYDRAMINE HYDROCHLORIDE; SODIUM CITRATE.

Benzagel (*Bioglan*) is a

B

proprietary preparation of the drug benzoyl peroxide, which when applied topically in the form of a gel removes hardened or dead skin (it is KERATOLYTIC) while simultaneously treating bacterial infection. It is most used in the treatment of acne, and is produced in two strengths (under the names Benzagel 5 and Benzagel 10, the figures representing the percentage of solute).

✚/▲ warning/side-effects: *see* BENZOYL PEROXIDE.

benzalkonium chloride is an astringent ANTISEPTIC that also has some KERATOLYTIC properties and may be used in topical application to remove hard, dead skin from around wounds or ulcers, or to dissolve warts. It is also used on minor abrasions and burns, and (in the form of lozenges to be sucked) on mouth ulcers or gum disease, simply as a disinfectant. For other than oral purposes, administration is topical in the form of a cream or, combined with bromine, as a paint.

✚ warning: in topical application, keep benzalkonium chloride off normal skin.

Related articles: CALLUSOLVE; DRAPOLENE; EMULSIDERM.

benzathine penicillin is a penicillin-type ANTIBIOTIC that is used to treat many bacterial infections. In high dosage it is used especially to treat syphilis (although PROCAINE PENICILLIN appears more effective in this) or to prevent patients at risk from contracting rheumatic fever. Administration is oral in the form of a suspension or drops, or by injection.

✚ warning: benzathine penicillin should not be administered to patients who are known to be allergic to penicillins; it should be administered with caution to those with impaired kidney function.

▲ side-effects: there may be sensitivity reactions ranging from a minor rash to urticaria and joint pains, and (occasionally) to high temperature or anaphylactic shock.

Related article: PENIDURAL.

benzhexol hydrochloride is an ANTICHOLINERGIC agent employed in the treatment of some types of parkinsonism (*see* ANTIPARKINSONISM). It increases mobility and decreases rigidity, but it has only a limited effect on tremors. The tendency to produce an excess of saliva is also reduced by benzhexol. (The drug also has the capacity to treat these conditions in some cases where they are produced by drugs.) It is thought to work by compensating for the lack of dopamine in the brain that is the major cause of such parkinsonian symptoms by reducing the cholinergic excess. Administration – which may be in parallel with the administration of other drugs used for the relief of parkinsonism – is oral in the form of tablets or sustained-release capsules, or as a dilute syrup.

✚ warning: benzhexol hydrochloride should not be administered to patients who have not only tremor but distinct involuntary movements; it should be administered with caution to those with impaired kidney or liver function, cardiovascular disease, glaucoma, or urinary retention. Withdrawal of treatment must be gradual.

▲ side-effects: there may be dry mouth, dizziness and blurred vision, and/or gastrointestinal

disturbances. Some patients experience sensitivity reactions and anxiety. Rarely, and in susceptible patients, there may be confusion, agitation and psychological disturbance (at which point treatment must be withdrawn).
Related articles: ARTANE; BENTEX; BROFLEX.

benzocaine is a mild local ANAESTHETIC used in topical application for the relief of pain in the skin surface or mucous membranes, particularly in or around the mouth and throat, or (in combination with other drugs) in the ears. Administration is in various forms: as lozenges, as a cream, as anal suppositories, as an ointment, and as ear-drops.
✚ warning: prolonged use should be avoided; some patients experience sensitivity reactions.
Related articles: AUDICORT; DEQUACAINE; MEDILAVE; SOLARCAINE.

benzodiazepines are a large group of drugs that have a marked effect upon the central nervous system. That effect varies with different members of the group, however, and some are used primarily as SEDATIVES or HYPNOTICS, whereas others are used more as ANXIOLYTICS, MUSCLE RELAXANTS or ANTICONVULSANTS. Those that are used as hypnotics have virtually replaced the barbiturates, for the benzodiazepines are just as effective but are much safer (there is reduced scope for abuse) – although some caution is necessary in treating patients who suffer from respiratory depression. However, it is now realized that dependence may result from continued usage. Best known and most used benzodiazepines include diazepam (used particularly to control the convulsions of epilepsy or drug poisoning), nitrazepam (a widely used hypnotic), lorazepam (an anxiolytic) and loprazolam (a tranquillizer used to treat insomnia).
✚/▲ warning/side-effects: *see* ALPRAZOLAM; BROMAZEPAM; CHLORDIAZEPOXIDE; CLONAZEPAM; DIAZEPAM; FLUNITRAZEPAM; FLURAZEPAM; KETAZOLAM; LOPRAZOLAM; LORAZEPAM; LORMETAZEPAM; MEDAZEPAM; OXAZEPAM; TEMAZEPAM.

benzoic acid ointment is a non-proprietary compound formulation (known also as Whitfield's ointment) used most commonly to treat patches of the fungal infection ringworm. It contains the ANTIFUNGAL substances benzoic acid and SALICYLIC ACID in an emulsifying ointment base.

benzoin tincture is a non-proprietary compound formulation of balsamic resins used both as a base from which vapours may be inhaled (when added to boiling water) in order to clear the nose, and as a disinfectant in the treatment of bedsores or in the sanitary care of a stoma (an outlet in the skin surface that represents the surgical curtailment of the intestines).

benzoyl peroxide is a KERATOLYTIC agent used in combination with other drugs or with sulphur in the treatment of skin conditions such as acne, or skin infections such as athlete's foot (which is a fungal infection). Administration is topical in the form of a cream, lotion or gel.
✚ warning: benzoyl peroxide

should not be used to treat the skin disease of the facial blood vessels rosacea. Topical application must avoid the eyes, mouth, and mucous membranes. (The drug may bleach fabrics.)

▲ side-effects: some patients experience skin irritation.
Related articles: ACETOXYL; ACNEGEL; ACNIDAZIL; BENOXYL; BENZAGEL; NERICUR; PANOXYL; QUINODERM; QUINOPED; THERADERM.

Benztrone (*Paines & Byrne*) is a proprietary OESTROGEN preparation, available only on prescription, used for replacement therapy in deficiency states, including primary amenorrhoea, delayed onset of puberty, and for the management of symptoms associated with the menopause. Produced in the form of ampoules (in two strengths) for injection, Benztrone is a preparation of the HORMONE oestradiol benzoate.

✚/▲ warning/side-effects: *see* OESTRADIOL.

benztropine mesylate is an ANTICHOLINERGIC agent employed in the treatment of some types of parkinsonism (*see* ANTIPARKINSONISM). It increases mobility and decreases rigidity, but it has only a limited effect on tremors. The tendency to produce an excess of saliva is also reduced. (The drug also has the capacity to treat these conditions in some cases where they are produced by drugs.) It is thought to work by compensating for the lack of dopamine in the brain that is the major cause of such parkinsonian symptoms, and because it additionally has some sedative properties it is sometimes used in preference to the similar drug benzhexol hydrochloride. Administration – which may be in parallel with the administration of levodopa – is oral in the form of tablets, or by injection.

✚ warning: benztropine mesylate should not be administered to patients who suffer not merely from tremor but from distinct involuntary movements; it should be administered with caution to those with impaired kidney or liver function, cardiovascular disease, glaucoma, or urinary retention. Withdrawal of treatment must be gradual.

▲ side-effects: there may be drowsiness, dry mouth, dizziness and blurred vision, and/or gastrointestinal disturbances. Some patients experience sensitivity reactions.
Related article: COGENTIN.

benzydamine hydrochloride has ANALGESIC, local ANAESTHETIC and ANTI-INFLAMMATORY actions. It is used in topical application as a cream to relieve muscle or joint pain, or as a liquid mouthwash or spray to relieve the pain of mouth ulcers and other sores or inflammations in the mouth and throat. Some patients prefer to use the liquid in dilute form.

✚ warning: benzydamine is not recommended for continual use over more than 7 days. As a spray it is not suitable for children aged under 6 years; as a mouthwash it is not suitable for those aged under 13 years.

▲ side-effects: some patients experience a stinging sensation or numbness on initial application.
Related article: DIFFLAM.

benzyl benzoate is a transparent liquid with an aromatic smell, used to treat infestation of the skin of the trunk and limbs by

itch-mites (scabies) or by lice (pediculosis). A skin irritant, it is not suitable for use on the head, face and neck, and treatment of children should be in diluted form (or by another preparation altogether). Administration is in the form of a from-the-neck-down application two days consecutively, without washing in the interval.
Related article: ASCABIOL.

benzylpenicillin is the chemical name for the first of the penicillins. It remains an important ANTIBIOTIC widely used to counter bacterial infections, and especially the more serious systemic forms. It is also used to prevent infection, particularly following the amputation of a limb. Since it is inactivated by digestive acids in the stomach, poorly absorbed in the intestine, and rapidly excreted by the kidneys, it is difficult to maintain an effective concentration, so benzylpenicillin is most commonly administered by injection.
✚ warning: benzylpenicillin should not be administered to patients known to be allergic to penicillins; it should be administered with caution to those with impaired kidney function.
▲ side-effects: there may be sensitivity reactions ranging from a minor rash to urticaria and joint pains, and (occasionally) to high temperature or anaphylactic shock. High doses may in any case cause convulsions.
Related article: CRYSTAPEN.

bephenium is an ANTHELMINTIC drug used specifically to treat infestation of the small intestine by hookworms, which draw blood from the point of their attachment to the intestinal wall and may thus cause iron-deficiency anaemia. Administration is oral in the form of a solution.
▲ side-effects: there may be occasional nausea and vomiting; some patients experience diarrhoea, headache and vertigo.
Related article: ALCOPAR.

Berkatens (*Berk*) is a proprietary CALCIUM ANTAGONIST drug, available only on prescription, used to treat high blood pressure (*see* ANTIHYPERTENSIVE), heartbeat irregularities (*see* ANTI-ARRHYTHMIC), and angina pectoris (heart pain). It works primarily by decreasing the excitability of the cells. Produced in the form of tablets (in four strengths), Berkatens is a preparation of verapamil hydrochloride.
✚/▲ warning/side-effects: *see* VERAPAMIL HYDROCHLORIDE.

Berkmycen (*Berk*) is a proprietary ANTIBIOTIC, available only on prescription, used to treat infections of the soft tissues and respiratory tract. Produced in the form of tablets, Berkmycen is a preparation of the TETRACYCLINE oxytetracycline dihydrate. It is not recommended for children aged under 2 years.
✚/▲ warning/side-effects: *see* OXYTETRACYCLINE.

Berkolol (*Berk*) is a proprietary BETA-BLOCKER, available only on prescription, used to treat high blood pressure (*see* ANTIHYPERTENSIVE), usually in combination with a DIURETIC, to relieve angina pectoris (heart pain) and to slow and/or regularize the heartbeat in order to prevent a recurrent heart attack. The drug may also be used to treat symptoms of hyperthroidism or to reduce frequency of migraine attacks.

B

Produced in the form of tablets (in four strengths), Berkolol is a preparation of the BETA-BLOCKER propranolol hydrochloride.
✚/▲ warning/side-effects: *see* PROPRANOLOL.

Berkozide (*Berk*) is a proprietary DIURETIC, available only on prescription, used to treat high blood pressure (*see* ANTIHYPERTENSIVE) and an accumulation of fluid within the tissues (oedema). Produced in the form of tablets (in two strengths), Berkozide is a preparation of the THIAZIDE bendrofluazide. It is not recommended for children.
✚/▲ warning/side-effects: *see* BENDROFLUAZIDE.

Berotec (*Boehringer Ingelheim*) is a proprietary BRONCHODILATOR, available only on prescription, used to treat conditions such as asthma and chronic bronchitis. Produced in the form of an aerosol inhalant (with metered inhalation) and a solution for nebulization, Berotec is a preparation of fenoterol hydrobromide. Inhalation of the nebulized solution is not recommended for children aged under 6 years.
✚/▲ warning/side-effects: *see* FENOTEROL.

***beta-blockers** (beta-adrenoceptor blockers) are drugs that inhibit the action of the hormonal and neurotransmitter substances ADRENALINE and NORADRENALINE (and the other catecholamines) in the body. These catecholamines are involved in bodily response to stress: among other actions they speed the heart and constrict some blood vessels, so increasing blood pressure, suppress digestion and generally prepare the body for emergency action. In patients with heart conditions, with diseases of the blood vessels or with high blood pressure (hypertension), stresses that release catecholamines may quickly lead to angina pectoris (heart pain) and an inability of the heart to pump blood sufficiently. Beta-blockers are administered so that the receptor sites that would normally react to the presence of the catecholamines remain comparatively inactivated. Beta-blockers are thus used in the treatment of cardiac arrhythmias (heartbeat irregularities) and as ANTIHYPERTENSIVES. However, some of them have additional effects on catecholamine-sensitive receptor sites elsewhere in the body, particularly in the bronchial passages, and care must thus be taken in prescribing for patients with disorders of the respiratory tract, because their use may induce asthma attacks. These drugs are also used to treat the symptoms of over-active thyroid glands (hyperthyroidism). Best known and most used beta-blockers include propranolol, sotalol, oxprenolol and acebutolol.
✚/▲ warning/side-effects: *see* ACEBUTOLOL; ATENOLOL; BETAXOLOL HYDROCHLORIDE; LABETALOL HYDROCHLORIDE; METOPROLOL TARTRATE; NADOLOL; OXPRENOLOL; PENBUTOLOL SULPHATE; PINDOLOL; PRACTOLOL; PROPRANOLOL; SOTALOL HYDROCHLORIDE; TIMOLOL MALEATE.

Beta-Cardone (*Duncan, Flockhart*) is a proprietary BETA-BLOCKER, available only on prescription, used to treat high blood pressure (*see* ANTIHYPERTENSIVE), heartbeat irregularities and angina pectoris (heart pain), and to prevent secondary heart attacks. Produced in the form of tablets

(in three strengths), Beta-Cardone is a preparation of sotalol hydrochloride. It is not recommended for children.
✚/▲ warning/side-effects: *see* SOTALOL HYDROCHLORIDE.

Betadine (*Napp*) is a proprietary non-prescription group of preparations of the ANTISEPTIC povidone-iodine, produced in the form of pessaries, a gel and a solution (all together a vaginal cleansing kit) for the treatment of bacterial infections in the vagina and cervix. A more dilute solution may also be used as a mouthwash and gargle for inflammations in the mouth and throat. For the treatment of skin infections it is produced in solutions of differing concentrations as an aerosol spray, an antiseptic paint, an alcoholic lotion, a scalp and skin cleanser, a shampoo, a skin cleanser solution, and a surgical scrub; it is also produced as a dry powder for insufflation. In the form of a water-miscible ointment it is used to dress leg ulcers.
✚/▲ warning/side-effects: *see* POVIDONE-IODINE.

betahistine hydrochloride is an ANTINAUSEANT drug used specifically to treat the vertigo and nausea associated with Ménière's disease (which also causes constant noises in the ears), although as a VASODILATOR it is also used to treat other disorders and infections of the middle and inner ears. Administration is oral in the form of tablets.
✚ warning: betahistine hydrochloride should not be administered to patients who suffer from disorders that cause abnormal secretion from the adrenal glands (phaeochromocytoma); it should be administered with caution to those who suffer from asthma or peptic ulcer.
▲ side-effects: sometimes the drug, while helping to relieve vertigo, actually causes nausea; some patients experience a headache; rarely, there may be a rash.
Related article: SERC.

betaine hydrochloride is an unusual drug used to increase gastric acids in patients whose stomach secretions have for one reason or another been reduced. Administration is oral in the form of a solution made from crushed tablets dissolved in water, taken through a straw after meals. The tablets also contain the stomach enzyme pepsin. The drug is not recommended for children.
✚ warning: the solution should be taken through a straw (or a glass tube) in order to protect the teeth.
▲ side-effects: high dosage may naturally result in acid stomach and the associated symptoms.
Related article: ACIDOL-PEPSIN.

Betaloc (*Astra*) is a proprietary preparation of the BETA-BLOCKER metoprolol tartrate, available only on prescription, used to control and regulate the heart rate and to treat high blood pressure (*see* ANTIHYPERTENSIVE), angina pectoris (heart pain), or in the treatment of hyperthyroidism; it is additionally used in the prevention of migraine attacks. Produced in a standard form of tablets (in two strengths) and in ampoules for injection, a stronger form is also available (under the trade name Betaloc-SA) as sustained-release tablets ("Durules"). None of these is recommended for children.
✚/▲ warning/side-effects: *see* METOPROLOL TARTRATE.

B

betamethasone is a synthetic CORTICOSTEROID, used for its ANTI-INFLAMMATORY effect to treat many kinds of inflammation, and especially those caused by allergic disorders. Unlike most corticosteroids, it does not cause salt or fluid retention in the body, and is thus particularly useful in treating conditions such as cerebral oedema (fluid retention in the brain). Administration is oral in the form of tablets, or by injection.

✚ warning: betamethasone should be administered with great caution to patients with infectious diseases, chronic renal failure, and uraemia; it should be administered with caution to the elderly (in whom overdosage can cause osteoporosis, "brittle bones"). In children, administration of betamethasone may lead to stunting of growth. As with all corticosteroids, betamethasone treats only inflammatory symptoms; an undetected and potentially serious infection may have its effects masked by the drug until it is well established.

▲ side-effects: systemic treatment of susceptible patients may engender a euphoria – or a state of confusion or depression. Rarely, there is peptic ulcer. *Related articles:* BETNELAN; BETNESOL.

betamethasone dipropionate is a synthetic CORTICOSTEROID used in topical application to treat severe non-infective skin inflammations (such as eczema), particularly in cases where less powerful steroids have failed. Administration is in the form of a cream or ointment, or as a lotion for the scalp.

✚ warning: betamethasone dipropionate should not be administered to patients with the skin blood vessel disorder rosacea, or from any form of internal ulcer. Absorption through the skin where dosage is high may result in a reduction of the secretion of natural corticosteroids by the adrenal glands, with consequent symptoms.

▲ side-effects: as with all corticosteroids, betamethasone dipropionate treats only the external symptoms; an undetected and potentially serious infection may have its effects masked by the drug until it has become well established. There may be local thinning of the skin, with increased hair growth. Younger patients, especially girls, may experience a local outbreak of acne. *Related articles:* DIPROSALIC; DIPROSONE.

betamethasone sodium phosphate is a synthetic CORTICOSTEROID used in topical application to treat both mild, local forms of inflammation (particularly of the eyes, ears or nose, and occasionally also to assist in the treatment of more severe non-infective skin inflammations, such as eczema. Administration is in the form of drops (for eye, ear or nose), and as an ointment.

✚ warning: betamethasone sodium phosphate should not be administered to patients with the skin blood vessel disorder rosacea. Prolonged use may lead to absorption through the skin which in turn may result in a reduction of the secretion of natural corticosteroids by the adrenal glands.

▲ side-effects: as with all corticosteroids, betamethasone sodium phosphate treats only

the external symptoms; an undetected and potentially serious infection may have its effects masked by the drug until it has become well established. There may be local thinning of the skin, with increased hair growth. Younger patients, especially girls, may experience a local outbreak of acne.
Related articles: BETNESOL; VISTA-METHASONE.

betamethasone valerate is a synthetic CORTICOSTEROID used in topical application to treat severe non-infective skin inflammations such as eczema, particularly in cases where less powerful steroids have failed. Administration is in the form of a cream or ointment, or as a lotion. It is also sometimes used for its properties as a BRONCHODILATOR in the treatment of asthma.

✚ warning: betamethasone valerate should not be administered to patients who suffer from the skin blood vessel disorder rosacea, or from any form of internal ulcer. Absorption through the skin where dosage is high may result in a reduction of the secretion of natural corticosteroids by the adrenal glands, with consequent symptoms.

▲ side-effects: as with all corticosteroids, betamethasone valerate treats only the external symptoms; an undetected and potentially serious infection may have its effects masked by the drug until it has become well established. There may be local thinning of the skin, with increased hair growth. Younger patients, especially girls, may experience a local outbreak of acne.
Related articles: BETNOVATE; BETNOVATE-C; BETNOVATE-N; BETNOVATE-RD; BEXTASOL; FUCIBET.

***beta-receptor stimulants** (beta-adrenoceptor stimulants; beta-agonists) are a class of drugs that act at sites, called beta-receptors, that "recognise" the natural neurotransmitters or hormones of the sympathetic nervous system. Drugs that act at such sites are regarded as SYMPATHOMIMETICS. Notable actions of beta-receptor stimulants include bronchodilation, speeding and strengthening of the heart beat and inhibition of contraction of the uterus. Importantly, differences in receptors at different sites allow, for example, beta-receptor stimulant drugs that give bronchodilation in asthma sufferers without overstimulation of the heart (in this case known as beta$_2$-receptor stimulants). The BETA-BLOCKERS have roughly the reverse of the actions of beta-receptor stimulants.

betaxolol hydrochloride is a BETA-BLOCKER of fairly recent introduction used orally to treat high blood pressure (*see* ANTIHYPERTENSIVE); for this purpose administration is in the form of tablets. In dilute solution, however, the drug is also used in the form of eye-drops.

✚ warning: as an antihypertensive drug, betaxolol hydrochloride should not be administered to patients who suffer from asthmatic symptoms; it should be administered with great caution to those with impaired kidney function, or who are nearing the end of pregnancy or who are lactating. Withdrawal of treatment should be gradual. Ophthalmic betaxolol should not be

B

B

administered to patients with severe sinus bradycardia, cardiagenic shock or to patients with overt cardiac failure.

▲ side-effects: there may be some gastrointestinal or slight respiratory disturbance following oral administration. Ophthalmic treatment may result in temporarily dry eyes; some patients experience sensitivity reactions; the drug should be used in those with cardiac disease only as appropriate.

Related articles: BETOPTIC; KERLONE.

bethanechol chloride is a PARASYMPATHOMIMETIC drug. It is used to stimulate motility in the intestines, but perhaps its most common use is to treat urinary retention, particularly following surgery. Administration is oral in the form of tablets or by injection.

✚ warning: Bathanechol chloride should not be administered to patients who suffer from medicinal, urinary or intestinal obstruction. It should be administered with caution to those who suffer from epilepsy, parkinsonism or thyroid disorders, or who are elderly. It should not be administered during pregnancy.

▲ side-effects: there may be sweating, blurred vision, nausea and vomiting, and a slow heart rate.

Related article: MYOTONINE CHLORIDE.

bethanidine sulphate is an ANTIHYPERTENSIVE drug used to treat moderate to severe high blood pressure (hypertension), especially when other forms of treatment have failed. It works by inhibiting the release of the neurotransmitter (catecholamine) noradrenaline. Administration is oral in the form of tablets, usually with a DIURETIC (such as a THIAZIDE) or a BETA-BLOCKER.

✚ warning: bethanidine sulphate should not be administered to patients who suffer from disease of the adrenal glands or from kidney failure; it should be administered with caution to those who are pregnant. Resultant low blood pressure, especially on rising from sitting or lying down, may cause falls in the elderly.

▲ side-effects: there may be low blood pressure (hypotension), nasal congestion, and fluid retention leading to weight gain.

Related articles: BENDOGEN; ESBATAL.

Betim (*Burgess*) is a proprietary BETA-BLOCKER, available only on prescription, used to treat high blood pressure (*see* ANTIHYPERTENSIVE), heartbeat irregularities and angina pectoris (heart pain), and to prevent secondary heart attacks and also migraine. Produced in the form of tablets, Betim represents a preparation of timolol maleate. It is not recommended for children.

✚/▲ warning/side-effects: *see* TIMOLOL MALEATE.

Betnelan (*Glaxo*) is a proprietary CORTICOSTEROID preparation, available only on prescription, used to treat inflammation especially in rheumatic or allergic conditions, and particularly in severe asthma. Produced in the form of tablets, Betnelan is a preparation of the glucocorticoid betamethasone. It is not recommended for children aged under 12 months.

✚/▲ warning/side-effects: *see* BETAMETHASONE.

Betnesol (*Glaxo*) is a proprietary

CORTICOSTEROID preparation, available only on prescription, used to treat local inflammations as well as more widespread rheumatic or allergic conditions, particularly severe asthma. Produced in the form of tablets and in ampoules for injection, Betnesol represents a preparation of the glucocorticoid betamethasone. The tablets are not recommended for children aged under 12 months. Betnesol ear-, eye- and nose-drops and eye ointment are used for local inflammations, and are an alternative preparation of betamethasone sodium phosphate. A preparation is also available that additionally contains the antiseptic ANTIBIOTIC neomycin sulphate; it too is produced in the form of ear-, eye- and nose-drops and eye ointment (under the trade name Betnesol-N).
✚/▲ warning/side-effects: *see* BETAMETHASONE; BETAMETHASONE SODIUM PHOSPHATE; NEOMYCIN.

Betnovate (*Glaxo*) is a proprietary group of CORTICOSTEROID preparations, available only on prescription, used to treat severe non-infective skin inflammations such as eczema, especially in patients who are not responding to less powerful corticosteroids. Produced in the form of a water-miscible cream, an ointment in an anhydrous paraffin base, a lotion, and a scalp application in an alcohol base, Betnovate is a preparation of betamethasone valerate. A rectal ointment (applied with an applicator) and anal suppositories are also available, representing a compound preparation of betamethasone valerate together with the local ANAESTHETIC lignocaine hydrochloride and the VASOCONSTRICTOR phenylephrine hydrochloride.
✚/▲ warning/side-effects: *see* BETAMETHASONE VALERATE; LIGNOCAINE; PHENYLEPHRINE.

Betnovate-C (*Glaxo*) is a proprietary CORTICOSTEROID, available only on prescription, used to treat severe non-infective skin inflammations such as eczema. Produced in the form of a water-miscible cream and an ointment in a paraffin base, Betnovate-C is a compound preparation of the steroid betamethasone valerate and the ANTIMICROBIAL clioquinol.
✚/▲ warning/side-effects: *see* BETAMETHASONE VALERATE; CLIOQUINOL.

Betnovate-N (*Glaxo*) is a proprietary CORTICOSTEROID, available only on prescription, used to treat severe non-infective skin inflammations such as eczema. Produced in the form of a water-miscible cream, an ointment in a paraffin base, and as a lotion, Betnovate-N is a compound preparation of the steroid betamethasone valerate and the ANTIBACTERIAL ANTIBIOTIC neomycin sulphate.
✚/▲ warning/side-effects: *see* BETAMETHASONE VALERATE; NEOMYCIN.

Betnovate-RD (*Glaxo*) is a proprietary CORTICOSTEROID, available only on prescription, used as the basis for maintenance therapy in the treatment of severe non-infective skin inflammation (such as eczema) once control has initially been achieved with BETNOVATE. Produced in the form of a water-miscible cream and as an ointment in an anhydrous paraffin base, Betnovate-RD is a

preparation of betamethasone valerate.
✚/▲ warning/side-effects: *see* BETAMETHASONE VALERATE.

Betoptic (*Alcon*) is a proprietary BETA-BLOCKER, available only on prescription, used in the form of eye-drops to treat various forms of glaucoma. It is a preparation of betaxolol hydrochloride and is not recommended for children.
✚/▲ warning/side-effects: *see* BETAXOLOL HYDROCHLORIDE.

Bextasol (*Glaxo*) is a proprietary CORTICOSTEROID, available only on prescription, used to treat asthma. Produced in an aerosol that emits individually metered doses, Bextasol represents a preparation of the CORTICOSTEROID betamethasone valerate.
✚/▲ warning/side-effects: *see* BETAMETHASONE VALERATE.

bezafibrate is used to reduce the level of fats (lipids) such as cholesterol in the bloodstream when these are raised (hyperlipidaemia). It works by inhibiting lipid synthesis. Generally, it is administered only to patients in whom a strict and regular dietary regime is not having the desired effect, although during treatment such a regime should additionally be adhered to. Administration is oral in the form of tablets.
✚ warning: bezafibrate should not be administered to patients with severely impaired kidney or liver function, disease of the gall bladder, or associated blood disorders, or who are pregnant.
▲ side-effects: there may be nausea and abdominal pain; rarely, there may be itching or urticaria. In men, impotence very occasionally occurs.
Related article: BEZALIP.

Bezalip (*MCP Pharmaceuticals*) is a proprietary preparation of the drug bezafibrate, available only on prescription, used to treat high levels of fats (lipids) such as cholesterol in the bloodstream (hyperlipidaemia). It works by inhibiting production of fat. Produced in the form of tablets (in two strengths, the stronger form under the trade name Bezalip-Mono), it is not recommended for children.
✚/▲ warning/side-effects: *see* BEZAFIBRATE.

Bi-Aglut (*Ultrapharm*) represents a brand of non-prescription gluten-free biscuits. Gluten-, lactose-, and milk-protein-free cracker toast is also available for the dietary needs of patients who are unable to tolerate those substances, such as in coeliac disease.

Bicillin (*Brocades*) is a proprietary ANTIBIOTIC, available only on prescription, used to treat serious infections for which long- term treatment is required, such as gonorrhoea and syphilis, and gas gangrene following amputation. Produced in the form of a powder for reconstitution as a medium for depot injection, Bicillin is a compound preparation of the penicillin-type antibiotics procaine penicillin and benzylpenicillin sodium.
✚/▲ warning/side-effects: *see* BENZYLPENICILLIN; PROCAINE PENICILLIN.

BiCNU (*Bristol-Myers*) is a proprietary CYTOTOXIC drug, available only on prescription, used in the treatment of leukaemia, lymphomas and some solid tumours. It works by disrupting DNA production in new-forming cells and so preventing normal cell reproduction. Produced in the

form of a powder for reconstitution as a medium for injection or in vials, BiCNU is a preparation of carmustine.
✚/▲ warning/side-effects: *see* CARMUSTINE.

Bilarcil is a preparation of the organo-phosphorous drug METRIPHONATE, used specifically to treat infections by parasitic Schistosoma haematobium worms (which cause bilharziasis) in various organs. It is not available in the United Kingdom.

BiNovum (*Ortho-Cilag*) is an ORAL CONTRACEPTIVE, available only on prescription, that combines the OESTROGEN ethinyloestradiol with the PROGESTOGEN norethisterone. It is produced in calender packs of 21 tablets which together with 7 tablet-free days represent one complete menstrual cycle.
✚/▲ warning/side-effects: *see* ETHINYLOESTRADIOL; NORETHISTERONE.

Biogasterone (*Winthrop*) is a proprietary gastric ulcer treatment. Available only on prescription, it protects the stomach lining from excess acid and enzymes in a way that is not well understood. Biogasterone is produced in the form of tablets and is a preparation of carbenoxolone sodium. It is not recommended for children.
✚/▲ warning/side-effects: *see* CARBENOXOLONE SODIUM.

Biophylline (*Delandale*) is a proprietary non-prescription BRONCHODILATOR, used to treat severe restrictions in the bronchial passages, as occur in asthma, and bronchitis. Produced in the form of a sugar-free syrup, Biophylline is a preparation of theophylline hydrate. It is not recommended for children aged under 2 years.
✚/▲ warning/side-effects: *see* THEOPHYLLINE.

Bioplex (*Thames*) is a proprietary drug, available only on prescription, used to treat mouth ulcers. Produced in the form of granules to be dissolved in warm water for use as a mouth-wash, Bioplex is a preparation of the drug carbenoxolone sodium.
✚/▲ warning/side-effects: *see* CARBENOXOLONE SODIUM.

Bioral (*Winthrop*) is a proprietary non-prescription preparation, used to treat mouth ulcers and other sores in and around the mouth. Produced in the form of a gel, Bioral is a preparation of the drug carbenoxolone sodium.
✚/▲ warning/side-effects: *see* CARBENOXOLONE SODIUM.

Biorphen (*Bio-Medical*) is a proprietary ANTICHOLINERGIC drug, available only on prescription, used to relieve some of the symptoms of parkinsonism, especially muscle rigidity and the tendency to produce an excess of saliva (*see* ANTIPARKINSONISM). The drug also has the capacity to treat these conditions in some cases where they are produced by drugs. It is thought to work by compensating for the lack of dopamine in the brain that is the major cause of such parkinsonian symptoms. Produced in the form of a sugar-free elixir, Biorphen represents a preparation of orphenadrine hydrochloride. Counselling of patients is advised.
✚/▲ warning/side-effects: *see* ORPHENADRINE HYDROCHLORIDE.

biperiden lactate is an ANTICHOLERGENIC agent employed in the treatment of some types of parkinsonism (*see* ANTIPARKINSONISM). It increases mobility and decreases rigidity, but it has only a limited effect on tremors. The tendency to produce an excess of saliva is also reduced. (The drug also has the capacity to treat these conditions in some cases where they are produced by drugs.) It is thought to work by compensating for the lack of dopamine in the brain that is the major cause of such parkinsonian symptoms, and because it additionally has some sedative properties it is sometimes used in preference to the similar drug benzhexol hydrochloride. Administration – which may be in parallel with the administration of other drugs used to relieve parkinsonism – is oral in the form of tablets, or by injection.

✚ warning: biperiden should be administered only to patients with mild tremor and rigidity; it should be administered with caution to those with impaired kidney or liver function, cardiovascular disease, glaucoma, or urinary retention. Withdrawal of treatment must be gradual.

▲ side-effects: there may be drowsiness, dry mouth, dizziness and blurred vision, and/or gastrointestinal disturbances. Some patients experience sensitivity reactions.

Related article: AKINETON.

bisacodyl is a stimulant LAXATIVE used not only to promote defecation and relieve constipation, but also to evacuate the colon prior to rectal examination or surgery. It probably works by stimulating the walls of the intestine. Administration is either oral in the form of tablets (full effects are achieved after 10 hours), or topical as anal suppositories (effects achieved within 1 hour). It is not recommended for children.

✚ warning: bisacodyl should not be administered to patients with intestinal obstruction.

▲ side-effects: there may be abdominal pain, nausea,or vomiting. Suppositories sometimes cause rectal irritation.

Related articles: DULCODOS; DULCOLAX.

Bismodyne (*Loveridge*) is a proprietary non-prescription ointment used to soothe and treat piles (haemorrhoids) and anal itching. Also available in the form of anal suppositories and an ointment, Bismodyne is a compound preparation of the ANTISEPTIC hexachlorophane, the local anaesthetic LIGNOCAINE and the mild astringents BISMUTH SUBGALLATE and ZINC OXIDE. Prolonged use should be avoided.

bismuth subgallate is a mild astringent used as a dusting powder in some skin disorders, and as suppositories in the treatment of haemorrhoids. It has also been administered by mouth to help control the odour and consistency of stools in patients with a colostomy or ileostomy

✚ warning: prolonged administration by mouth should be avoided.

▲ side-effects: there may be disturbance of the gastrointestinal tract, discolouration of mucous membranes and mild jaundice.

Related articles: ANUSOL; BISMODYNE

Bisodol (*Whitehall Laboratories*) is a proprietary, non-prescription ANTACID produced in the form of tablets and as a powder. It contains sodium bicarbonate and magnesium carbonate.

✚ warning: *see* MAGNESIUM CARBONATE; SODIUM BICARBONATE.

BJ6 (*Macarthys; Thornton & Ross*) is a proprietary non-prescription ophthalmic preparation, used to treat sore eyes caused by chronically reduced tear secretion. Produced in the form of eye-drops, BJ6 is a preparation of the water-soluble cellulose derivative hypromellose.

bleomycin is an ANTIBIOTIC that also has CYTOTOXIC properties. Unlike most ANTICANCER drugs, however, it has virtually no depressant effect on the blood-producing capacity of the bone-marrow. It is used particularly to treat cancer of the upper part of the gut and of the genital tract, and lymphomas. Sensitivity reactions are not uncommon, the symptoms of which are chills and fever a few hours after administration: these can be dealt with by the simultaneous administration of a CORTICOSTEROID (such as hydrocortisone). Bleomycin is administered by injection. The proprietary preparation of the same name is produced by Lundbeck and is available only on prescription.
✚ warning: high dosage increases a risk of pulmonary fibrosis, a lung disease that is potentially very serious. Regular monitoring of lung function is essential.
▲ side-effects: there is generally nausea and vomiting (for which additional medications may be prescribed). Increased pigmentation of the skin and some hair loss is common. Some patients experience inflammation of the mucous membranes.

Blocadren (*Merck, Sharp & Dohme*) is a proprietary BETA-BLOCKER, available only on prescription, used to treat high blood pressure (*see* ANTI-HYPERTENSIVE), angina pectoris (heart pain) and to prevent migraine and heart attack. Produced in the form of tablets, Blocadren represents a preparation of timolol maleate. It is not recommended for children.
✚/▲ warning/side-effects: *see* TIMOLOL MALEATE.

Bocasan (*Cooper*) is a proprietary non-prescription ANTISEPTIC, used to cleanse and disinfect the mouth. Produced in the form of sealed sachets to be emptied into water to produce a mouth-wash, Bocasin is a preparation of sodium perborate.
✚ warning: see SODIUM PERBORATE.

Bolvidon (*Organon*) is a proprietary ANTIDEPRESSANT, available only on prescription, used to treat depressive illness especially where sedation is needed. Produced in the form of tablets (in three strengths), Bolvidon is a preparation of mianserin hydrochloride. It is not recommended for children.
✚/▲ warning/side-effects: *see* MIANSERIN.

Bonjela (*Reckitt & Colman*) is a proprietary non-prescription oral gel, used to treat mouth ulcers and to relieve pain during teething. Bonjela represents a preparation of choline salicylate (and is sugar-free).
✚ warning: see CHOLINE SALICYLATE.

Boots Covering Cream (*Boots*) is a proprietary non-prescription camouflage cream, in four shades, designed for use in masking scars and other skin disfigurements. It may be obtained on prescription if the skin disfigurement is the result of surgery or is giving rise to emotional disturbance.

B

botulism antitoxin is a preparation that neutralizes the toxins produced by the botulism bacteria (rather than acting to counter the presence of the bacteria, as would a vaccine). In this way, it may be administered not only to people at risk from the disease following exposure to an infected patient, but also to the infected patient as a means of treatment. However, there are some strains of botulism in relation to which the antitoxin is not effective. Moreover, hypersensitivity reactions are common (and it is essential that an administering doctor has all relevant details of a patient's medical history, with regard especially to allergies). Administration is by injection or infusion, depending on whether it is for the purpose of prophylaxis or treatment.

Bradilan (*Napp*) is a proprietary non-prescription VASODILATOR, used to treat circulatory disorders of the hands and feet, chilblains, night cramps, and to limit high blood levels of cholesterol or triglycerides (hyperlipidaemia). Produced in the form of tablets, Bradilan is a preparation of the vitamin B derivative nicofuranose, and is not recommended for children.
✚/▲ warning/side-effects: *see* NICOFURANOSE.

Bradosol (*Ciba*) is a proprietary non-prescription DISINFECTANT, used to treat infections in the mouth and throat. Produced in the form of lozenges, Bradosol is a preparation of the detergent antiseptic domiphen bromide.

bran is perhaps the best-known natural bulking agent used to keep people "regular" or, if necessary, as a LAXATIVE to treat constipation. In either case it works by increasing the overall mass of faeces, so stimulating bowel movement (although in fact the full effect may not be achieved for more than 36 hours). As an excellent form of dietary fibre, bran may be said to reduce the risk of diverticular disease while actively assisting digestion.
✚ warning: bran should not be consumed if there is any possibility of intestinal blockage: adequate fluid intake must be maintained to avoid faecal impaction. Calcium and iron absorption may be impaired.
▲ side-effects: some patients cannot tolerate bran (particularly patients sensitive to the compound gluten).
Related articles: FYBRANTA; LEJFIBRE; PROCTOFIBE; TRIFYBA.

Brasivol (*Stiefel*) is a proprietary non-prescription abrasive preparation, used to cleanse skin that suffers from acne. It is produced in the form of a paste containing particles of aluminium oxide in three grades (fine, medium, and coarse) within a soap base. Treatment ordinarily begins with the fine grade and progresses to the medium and the coarse in more severe cases.

Bravit (*Galen*) is a proprietary non-prescription MULTIVITAMIN supplement that is not available from the National Health Service. It is used to treat deficiency of vitamins B and C, particularly in conditions such as convalescence from debilitating illness or chronic alcoholism, and contains THIAMINE hydrochloride (vitamin B_1), RIBOFLAVINE (vitamin B_2), PYRIDOXINE hydrochloride (vitamin B_6), NICOTINAMIDE (of the B complex) and ASCORBIC ACID (vitamin C).

Bretylate (*Wellcome*) is a

proprietary ANTIARRHYTHMIC drug, available only on prescription, used to treat heartbeat irregularities and to prevent a speeding up of the heart rate. Produced in ampoules for injection, Bretylate is a preparation of the ANTIHYPERTENSIVE drug bretylium tosylate.

✚/▲ warning/side-effects: *see* BRETYLIUM TOSYLATE.

bretylium tosylate is an ANTIHYPERTENSIVE and ANTIARRHYTHMIC drug used primarily to treat heartbeat irregularities and to prevent a speeding up of the heart rate. Administered usually following a heart attack, the drug may cause a marked fall in blood pressure; administration is most often by intramuscular injection.

✚ warning: bretylium tosylate should not be administered to patients who are already taking sympathomimetic drugs.

▲ side-effects: the fall in blood pressure on initial administration may be extreme; there may also be nausea and vomiting.

Related article: BRETYLATE.

Brevinor (*Syntex*) is a proprietary ORAL CONTRACEPTIVE, available only on prescription, that combines the OESTROGEN ethinyloestradiol with the PROGESTOGEN norethisterone. It is produced in packs of 21 tablets which together with 7 tablet-free days represent one complete menstrual cycle.

✚/▲ warning/side-effects: *see* ETHINYLOESTRADIOL; NORETHISTERONE.

Bricanyl (*Astra*) is a proprietary form of the BRONCHODILATOR terbutaline sulphate, available only on prescription, which acts as a selective BETA-RECEPTOR STIMULANT and SMOOTH MUSCLE RELAXANT and so relieves the bronchial spasms associated with such conditions as asthma and bronchitis. It is produced in the form of tablets, as a sugar-free syrup for dilution (the potency of the syrup once dilute is retained for 14 days; it is not recommended for children aged under 3 years), in ampoules for injection, as an inhalant within an aerosol that emits metered doses, in a "spacer inhaler" (metered inhalation using a "spacer tube" and a collapsible extended mouthpiece), in "respules" (single-dose units for nebulization; not recommended for children weighing under 25 kg), and as a respirator solution (for use with a nebulizer or a ventilator). Sustained-release tablets are also available (under the trade name Bricanyl SA). Associated compound preparations are also available, though not from the National Health Service, under the trade names Bricanyl Compound (terbutaline sulphate and guaiphenesin tablets) and Bricanyl Expectorant (a sugar-free terbutaline sulphate and guaiphenesin elixir for dilution: the potency of the elixir once dilute is retained for 14 days). Bricanyl injection and tablets may also be used as a means of slowing premature labour.

✚/▲ warning/side-effects: *see* GUAIPHENESIN; TERBUTALINE.

Brietal Sodium (*Lilly*) is a proprietary preparation of the short-acting general ANAESTHETIC methohexitone, in the form of methohexitone sodium. It is used mainly for the initial induction of anaesthesia or for short, minor operations. Available only on prescription, Brietal Sodium is produced in vials for

B

intravenous injection (in three strengths).
✚/▲ warning/side-effects: *see* METHOHEXITONE SODIUM.

brilliant green and crystal violet paint is a non-proprietary antiseptic paint used primarily to prepare skin for surgery. It combines the two dyes brilliant green and gentian violet (also called crystal violet).
see GENTIAN VIOLET.

Brinaldix K (*Sandoz*) is a proprietary DIURETIC, available only on prescription, used to treat an accumulation of fluid within the tissues (oedema) and high blood pressure (*see* ANTI-HYPERTENSIVE). Produced in the form of tablets, Brinaldix K is a compound preparation of the THIAZIDE-like drug clopamide with the potassium supplement POTASSIUM CHLORIDE.
✚/▲ warning/side-effects: *see* CLOPAMIDE.

Britcin (*DDSA Pharmaceuticals*) is a proprietary ANTIBIOTIC, available only on prescription, used to treat systemic bacterial infections and infections of the upper respiratory tract, of the ear, nose and throat, and of the urogenital areas. Produced in the form of capsules (in two strengths), Britcin is a preparation of the broad-spectrum PENICILLIN ampicillin.
✚/▲ warning/side-effects: *see* AMPICILLIN.

Brocadopa (*Brocades*) is a proprietary form of the immensely powerful drug levodopa, used to treat parkinsonism (*see* ANTIPARKINSONIAM). It is particularly good at relieving the rigidity and slowness of movement associated with the disease, although it does not always improve the tremor. Levodopa is converted inside the body to dopamine – and it is the lack of dopamine in the brain that it is thought Brocadopa compensates for. It is produced in the form of capsules (in three strengths).
✚/▲ warning/side-effects: *see* LEVODOPA.

Broflex (*Bio-Medical*) is a proprietary preparation of the drug benzhexol hydrochloride, available only on prescription, used to relieve some of the symptoms of parkinsonism specifically the overall rigidity of the posture, and the tendency to produce an excess of saliva. The drug also has the capacity to treat these conditions in some cases where they are produced by drugs (*see* ANTIPARKINSONISM). It is thought to work by compensating for the lack of dopamine in the brain that is the major cause of such parkinsonian symptoms. Broflex is produced in the form of a syrup for dilution (the potency of the syrup once diluted is retained for 14 days), to be taken before or after food; counselling of patients is advised. Broflex is not recommended for children.
✚/▲ warning/side-effects: *see* BENZHEXOL HYDROCHLORIDE.

Brolene (*May & Baker*) is a proprietary non-prescription preparation with ANTIFUNGAL and ANTIBACTERIAL properties, used to treat bacterial infections in the eyelid and conjunctiva. Produced in the form of eye-drops, Brolene is a preparation of PROPAMIDINE ISETHIONATE.

bromazepam is an ANXIOLYTIC drug, one of the BENZODIAZEPINES used to treat anxiety in either the short or the long term. Administration is oral in the form of tablets. It is not recommended for children.

✚ warning: bromazepam may reduce a patient's concentration and speed of movement or thought; it may also enhance the effects of alcohol consumption. Prolonged use or abrupt withdrawal of treatment should be avoided. It should be administered with caution to patients with respiratory difficulties, glaucoma, or kidney or liver disease; who are in the last stages of pregnancy; or who are elderly or debilitated.

▲ side-effects: there may be drowsiness, dizziness, headache, dry mouth and shallow breathing; hypersensitivity reactions may occur.
Related article: LEXOTAN.

bromelains is a proteolytic enzyme preparation with actions much like the digestive enzymes of the stomach, that breaks down complex molecules into their constituent amino acids for subsequent absorption. It is administered therapeutically – in the form of tablets – to relieve inflammatory swelling caused by an accumulation of fluid (oedema) in soft tissues. This it is thought to do by dissolving dead tissue, cellular debris and congealed blood for rapid transportation from the site of inflammation.

✚ warning: bromelains should not be administered to patients who are already taking oral anticoagulants; it should be administered with caution to those who suffer from blood clotting abnormalities, or impaired liver or kidney function. (Because the drug is derived from pineapples, it should not be administered either to patients who are allergically sensitive to the fruit.)

▲ side-effects: there may be nausea and vomiting; some patients break out in a rash.
Related article: ANANASE FORTE.

bromhexine hydrochloride is a MUCOLYTIC drug that reduces the viscosity of sputum in the air passages, so making it easier to cough up phlegm. It is particularly useful in treating conditions such as chronic bronchitis where the sputum tends to thicken and adhere to the walls of the air passages. Administration is oral in the form of tablets or a dilute elixir, or by injection.

✚ warning: bromhexine hydrochloride should be administered with caution to patients who suffer from gastric ulcers.

▲ side-effects: there may be gastrointestinal irritation.

bromocriptine is a drug used primarily to treat parkinsonism, but not the parkinsonian symptoms caused by certain drug therapies (*see* ANTIPARKINSONISM). It works by stimulating the dopamine receptors in the brain as if dopamine was present in the correct amount. In this it is slightly different from the more commonly used treatment with levodopa, which actually is converted to dopamine in the body. It is thus particularly useful in the treatment of patients who for one reason or another cannot tolerate levodopa. Occasionally, the two drugs are combined. However, bromocriptine is alternatively used to treat delayed puberty caused by hormonal insufficiency, to relieve certain menstrual disorders, or to reduce or halt lactation. Administration of

B

bromocriptine is oral in the form of tablets and capsules.
✚ warning: full, regular monitoring of various body systems is essential during treatment, particularly to check on whether there is pituitary enlargement.
▲ side-effects: there may be nausea, vomiting, headache, dizziness especially on rising from sitting or lying down (because of reduced blood pressure), and drowsiness. High dosage may cause hallucinations, a state of confusion, and leg cramps.
Related article: PARLODEL.

brompheniramine maleate is an ANTIHISTAMINE, used to treat the symptoms of allergic conditions like hay fever and urticaria; it is also used, in combination with other drugs, in expectorants to loosen a dry cough. Administration is oral in the form of tablets, sustained-release tablets, and a dilute elixir.
✚ warning: brompheniramine maleate should not be administered to patients who are pregnant, or who suffer from glaucoma, urinary retention, intestinal obstruction, enlargement of the prostate gland, or peptic ulcer; it should be administered with caution to those who suffer from epilepsy or liver disease.
▲ side-effects: sedation may affect patients' capacity for speed of thought and movement; there may be nausea, headaches and/or weight gain, dry mouth, gastrointestinal disturbances and visual problems.
Related articles: DIMOTANE; DIMOTANE EXPECTORANT; DIMOTANE PLUS; DIMOTANE WITH CODEINE; DIMOTAPP.

Brompton Cocktails are various compound ANALGESIC elixirs containing MORPHINE or its derivatives (such as DIAMORPHINE – better known as heroin – and COCAINE). They were once widely used for the relief of severe pain during the final stages of terminal disease; now, however, preparations simply of one narcotic analgesic or another are preferred.

Bronchilator (*Sterling Research*) is a proprietary BRONCHODILATOR, available only on prescription, used in the form of an inhalant to treat bronchial asthma and chronic bronchitis. Produced in an aerosol, Bronchilator represents a compound preparation of the two SYMPATHOMIMETIC drugs isoetharine mesylate and phenylephrine hydrochloride. It is not recommended for children.
✚/▲ warning/side-effects: *see* ISOETHARINE; PHENYLEPHRINE.

Bronchodil (*Keymer*) is a proprietary BRONCHODILATOR, available only on prescription, used to treat bronchospasm in asthma and chronic bronchitis. Produced in the form of tablets, as a sugar-free elixir for dilution (the potency of the elixir once dilute is retained for 14 days), in a metered-dose aerosol, and as a respirator solution, Bronchodil is a preparation of the sympathomimetic reproterol hydrochloride. None of these products is recommended for children aged under 6 years.
✚/▲ warning/side-effects: *see* REPROTEROL HYDROCHLORIDE.

***bronchodilator** is any agent that relaxes the smooth muscle of the bronchial passages, so allowing more air to flow in or out. There are many conditions that cause spasm in the bronchial muscles (bronchospasm), but the most common are asthma and bronchitis. The type of drug most commonly used to treat bronchospasm is the SYMPATHOMIMETIC or BETA-RECEPTOR STIMULANT. Sympathomimetic drugs work by stimulating receptors on smooth muscle of the airways that respond to adrenal hormones and sympathetic neurotransmitters – i.e. they are in effect the opposite of beta-blockers – and are generally safe and effective though may become less effective on continued usage. Best known and most used sympathomimetic bronchodilators include SALBUTAMOL, TERBUTALINE, ISOPRENALINE, FENOTEROL, RIMITEROL and EPHEDRINE HYDROCHLORIDE. Other forms of bronchodilator therapy include CORTICOSTEROIDS, ANTIHISTAMINES (which inhibit the allergic response that causes the symptoms of asthma) such as SODIUM CROMOGLYCATE, and such drugs as THEOPHYLLINE. Many bronchodilators are available in the form of aerosols, ventilator sprays or nebulizing mists. In high dosage, some can affect the heart rate. There may also be fine muscular tremor, headaches and nervous tension.

bronopol is an ANTIMICROBIAL agent used as a preservative in shampoos, cosmetics and suppositories.

Brovon (*Napp*) is a proprietary non-prescription compound BRONCHODILATOR, produced as an inhalant spray, used to treat asthma and other conditions involving bronchospasm. It contains several powerful constituents, including the ANTISPASMODIC ANTICHOLINERGIC atropine methonitrate, the SMOOTH MUSCLE RELAXANT papaverine hydrochloride and the SYMPATHOMIMETIC adrenaline. A metered-inhalation aerosol is also available, on prescription only, containing just adrenaline and atropine methonitrate (under the name Brovon Pressurised). Neither of these products is recommended for children.

✚/▲ warning/side-effects: *see* ADRENALINE; ATROPINE METHONITRATE; PAPAVERINE.

Broxil (*Beecham*) is a proprietary ANTIBIOTIC, available only on prescription, used to treat many forms of infection. Produced in the form of capsules, and as a syrup for dilution (the potency of the syrup once dilute is retained for 7 days), Broxil is a preparation of the PENICILLIN derivative phenethicillin.

✚/▲ warning/side-effects: *see* PHENETHICILLIN.

Brufen (*Boots*) is a proprietary non-narcotic ANALGESIC that has valuable additional anti-inflammatory properties. Available only on prescription, Brufen is used to relieve pain – particularly the pain of rheumatic disease and other musculo-skeletal disorders – and is produced in the form of tablets (in three strengths) and as a syrup for dilution (the potency of the syrup once dilute is retained for 14 days) as a preparation of ibuprofen.

✚/▲ warning/side-effects: *see* IBUPROFEN.

Brulidine (*May & Baker*) is a proprietary, non-prescription, antiseptic, water-miscible cream, used to treat minor burns and abrasions.

budesonide is a CORTICOSTEROID drug used primarily to treat the symptoms of asthma, chronic bronchitis and emphysema. It is thought to work by reducing inflammation in the mucous lining of the bronchial passages, and stemming allergic reactions. For many patients the best results are achieved if a BRONCHODILATOR such as salbutamol is inhaled about 10 minutes before administration. The drug is also used to treat the symptoms of nasal allergies such as hay fever. In both cases, administration is by inhaler (either from an aerosol or from a nasal spray).

✚ warning: as with all corticosteroids, budesonide treats the symptoms and has no effect on any underlying infection: such an infection, remaining undetected, may reach potentially serious proportions while its symptoms are masked by the corticosteroid. In any case, prolonged use should be avoided.

▲ side-effects: some patients undergoing bronchial treatment experience hoarseness. Large doses may increase the risk of fungal infection.

Related articles: PULMICORT; RHINOCORT.

bufexamac is an anti-inflammatory agent used (in dilute solution) in topical application to treat mild inflammations of the skin. It is produced in the form of a water-miscible cream.
Related article: PARFENAC.

buffer is a solution in which the concentration of hydrogen ions (pH, i.e. the acid-alkali balance) remains pretty well constant despite any further addition of alkali or acid. The body has its own buffering system, maintaining the pH in the blood and extracellular fluids, known as the bicarbonate system.

bumetanide is a quick-acting powerful DIURETIC with relatively short duration of action, which works by inhibiting reabsorption of ions in part of the kidney known as the loop of Henle. It is used to treat fluid retention in the tissues (oedema) and high blood pressure (*see* ANTIHYPERTENSIVE), and to assist a diseased kidney by promoting the excretion of urine.
Administration is oral in the form of tablets or a sugar-free liquid, or by injection.

✚ warning: bumetanide should not be administered to patients who have suffered kidney diseease or who have gout, diabetes, an enlarged prostate gland, or cirrhosis of the liver. Treatment may cause a deficiency of chloride, potassium and sodium in the body.

▲ side-effects: diuretic effect corresponds to dosage; large doses may cause deafness or ringing in the ears (tinnitus). There may be a skin rash.
Related article: BURINEX.

bupivacaine hydrochloride is a long-acting local ANAESTHETIC that is related to lignocaine but is more powerful and has greater duration of action. Because of this, it is often administered by injection epidurally via the spinal membranes (particularly during labour).

✚ warning: bupivacaine hydrochloride should not be administered to patients who suffer from the neural disorder myasthenia gravis or from heart block, or who are suffering from an insufficient supply of blood (as in shock); it should be administered with caution to those with impaired heart or liver function, or epilepsy. Dosage should be reduced for the elderly or debilitated. Facilities for emergency cardio-respiratory resuscitation should be on hand during treatment.

▲ side-effects: there may be slow heart rate and low blood pressure (hypotension) that may in high dosage tend towards cardiac arrest. Some patients enter states of euphoria, agitation or respiratory depression.
Related article: MARCAIN.

buprenorphine is a narcotic ANALGESIC that is long-acting and is used to treat moderate to severe levels of pain. Although it is thought not to be seriously addictive, it may be dangerous to use in combination with other narcotic analgesics. Administration is oral in the form of tablets, or by injection.

✚ warning: buprenorphine should not be administered to patients who suffer from head injury or intracranial pressure; it should be administered with caution to those with impaired kidney or liver function, asthma, depressed respiration, insufficient secretion of thyroid hormones (hypothyroidism) or low blood pressure (hypotension), or who are pregnant or lactating. Dosage should be reduced for the elderly or debilitated.

▲ side-effects: nausea, vomiting, dizziness, sweating and drowsiness are fairly common. Rarely, there may be shallow breathing.
Related article: TEMGESIC.

Burinex (*Leo*) is a proprietary DIURETIC drug, available only on prescription, used to treat the accumulation of fluids in the tissues (oedema) associated with congestive heart failure, and to assist a diseased kidney by promoting the excretion of urine. Produced in the form of tablets (in two strengths), as a sugar-free liquid, and in ampoules for injection, Burinex represents a preparation of bumetanide. A compound preparation of bumetanide together with the potassium supplement POTASSIUM CHLORIDE is also available (under the name Burinex K). Neither of these products is recommended for children.

✚/▲ warning/side-effects: *see* BUMETANIDE.

Buscopan (*Boehringer Ingelheim*) is a proprietary ANTICHOLINERGIC ANTISPASMODIC drug, available only on prescription, used to treat overactivity or spasm of the smooth muscle of the stomach or intestinal walls (causing constipation) or of the muscles of the vagina (causing painful menstruation). Produced in the form of tablets (not recommended for children aged under 6 years) and in ampoules for injection (not recommended for children), Buscopan is a preparation of the SMOOTH MUSCLE RELAXANT hyoscine butylbromide.

✚/▲ warning/side-effects: *see* HYOSCINE.

buserelin acts as a GONADOTROPHIN-RELEASING HORMONE, and is used therapeutically to treat cancer of the prostate gland. Such a cancer is sex-hormone-linked, and the effect of buserelin is – after an initial, brief formation of testosterone – to halt the production of androgens in the testes. Administration (in the form of buserelin acetate) is by injection or as a nasal spray.

✚ warning: treatment is initially by injection; maintenance of treatment is by nasal spray. Some patients experience increased tumour growth for the first fortnight of treatment, to the extent even of compressing the spinal cord. If necessary, therapy to avoid this complication may include the simultaneous administration of an anti-androgen (such as cyproterone acetate).

▲ side-effects: to all intents and purposes, use of buserelin has the effect of castration. There is weight gain with a rounding of the body and a complete lack of facial hair. There is loss of libido and may be hot flushes.
Related article: SUPREFACT.

busulphan is a CYTOTOXIC drug used principally as a factor in chemotherapy to treat certain forms of leukaemia. It works by direct interference with the DNA of new-forming cells, preventing normal cell replication. Administration is oral in the form of tablets.

✚ warning: prolonged treatment may cause sterility in men and an early menopause in women. Regular and frequent blood counts are essential, for irreversible bone-marrow damage may be caused by overdosage even by a small amount.

▲ side-effects: there is commonly nausea and vomiting; there is often also hair loss. An increase in skin pigmentation may cause a change in coloration. Rarely, there is lung damage.
Related article: MYLERAN.

Butacote (*Geigy*) is a proprietary ANTI-INFLAMMATORY non-narcotic ANALGESIC, available only on prescription (and now generally only in hospitals), used to treat rheumatic disease of the type that causes bone fusion or deformity, especially in the backbone. Produced in the form of tablets (in two strengths), Butacote is a preparation of phenylbutazone.

✚/▲ warning/side-effects: *see* PHENYLBUTAZONE.

Butazolidin (*Geigy*) is a proprietary ANTI-INFLAMMATORY non-narcotic ANALGESIC, available only on prescription (and now generally only in hospitals), used to treat rheumatic disease of the type that causes bone fusion or deformity, especially the backbone. Produced in the form of tablets (in two strengths), Butazolidin is a preparation of phenylbutazone.

✚/▲ warning/side-effects: *see* PHENYLBUTAZONE.

Butazone (*DDSA Pharmaceuticals*) is a proprietary ANTI-INFLAMMATORY non-narcotic ANALGESIC drug, available only on prescription in hospitals, used to treat rheumatic disease involving especially the backbone. Produced in the form of tablets (in two strengths), Butazone represents a preparation of phenylbutazone.

✚/▲ warning/side-effects: *see* PHENYLBUTAZONE.

butobarbitone is a BARBITURATE used only when absolutely necessary as a HYPNOTIC, to treat severe and intractable insomnia. Administration is oral in the form of tablets – the proprietary preparation is on the controlled drugs list – to be taken about half an hour before retiring.

✚ warning: butobarbitone should not be administered to patients whose insomnia is caused by pain, who suffer from porphyria, who are pregnant or lactating, who are elderly or debilitated, or who have a history of drug (including alcohol) abuse.

It should be administered with caution to those who suffer from kidney, liver or lung disease. Use of the drug should be avoided as far as possible. Repeated doses are cumulative in effect, and may lead to real sedation; abrupt withdrawal of treatment, on the other hand, may cause serious withdrawal symptoms. Tolerance and dependence occur readily.

▲ side-effects: concentration and the speed of movement and thought are affected. There may be drowsiness, dizziness and shallow breathing, with headache. Some patients experience hypersensitivity reactions. (The drug enhances the effects of alcohol consumption.)
Related article: SONERYL.

butriptyline is an ANTIDEPRESSANT drug that also has some sedative properties, used to treat depressive illness, especially where there is some degree also of anxiety. Administration of butriptyline is oral in the form of tablets.

✚ warning: butriptyline should not be administered to patients who suffer from heart disease or psychosis; it should be administered with caution to those with diabetes, epilepsy, liver or thyroid disease, glaucoma, or urinary retention; or who are pregnant or lactating. Withdrawal of treatment must be gradual.

▲ side-effects: common effects include a loss of intricacy in concentration, movement and thought, dry mouth, and blurred vision; there may also be difficulty in urinating, sweating, and irregular heartbeat, behavioural disturbances, a rash, a state of confusion, and/or a loss of libido. Rarely, there are also blood deficiencies.
Related article: EVADYNE.

B

C

Cafadol (*Typharm*) is a proprietary non-prescription compound ANALGESIC that is not available from the National Health Service. Used for mild pain, it is produced in the form of tablets. Cafadol is a compound of paracetamol and caffeine.
✚/▲ warning/side-effects: *see* CAFFEINE; PARACETAMOL.

Cafergot (*Sandoz*) is a proprietary ANALGESIC, available only on prescription, used to treat migraine. Produced in the form of tablets and suppositories, Cafergot is a compound of caffeine and ergotamine tartrate. Not recommended for pregnant women or nursing mothers, or those with high blood pressure or heart problems.
✚/▲ warning/side-effects: *see* CAFFEINE; ERGOTAMINE TARTRATE.

caffeine is a weak STIMULANT. Present in both tea and coffee, it is included in many ANALGESIC preparations, often to increase absorption. In the form of caffeine sodium benzoate, it is used as a cardiac stimulant.
✚ warning: caffeine should not be taken simultaneously with aspirin, or increased gastric irritation may occur.
▲ side-effects: excessive doses may cause headache either directly or on withdrawal.

Calaband (*Seton*) is a proprietary non-prescription form of impregnated bandaging, impregnated with ZINC OXIDE, CALAMINE, glycerol and other soothing substances. (Further bandaging is required to hold it in place.)

Caladryl (*Warner-Lambert*) is a proprietary non-prescription ANTIHISTAMINE, used to treat skin irritations, stings and bites, and sunburn. Produced in the form of cream or lotion, Caladryl contains CALAMINE, diphenhydramine hydrochloride and camphor in solution.
✚/▲ warning/side-effects: *see* CALAMINE; DIPHENHYDRAMINE HYDROCHLORIDE.

calamine is a preparation that cools and soothes itching skin. Produced in the form of a lotion, cream or ointment, it is actually a suspension of mainly zinc carbonate.

calamine and coal tar ointment is a preparation combining the soothing effects of CALAMINE (zinc carbonate) and the ANTISEPTIC properties of COAL TAR, which also relieves itching and softens hard skin.

calciferol is the chemical name for the fat-soluble VITAMIN D. It occurs in four main forms (D_1 to D_4) which are formed in plants or in human skin by the action of sunlight. Vitamin D promotes the absorption of calcium and, to a lesser extent, phosphorus into the bones; a deficiency of vitamin D therefore results in bone deficiency disorders, e.g. rickets in children. Good food sources in normal diets include eggs, milk and cheese; fish liver oil is particularly rich as a dietary supplement. However, as with other vitamins, large doses are toxic. Nevertheless, therapeutic replacement of vitamin D in cases of severe deficiency requires quantities of the vitamin best provided (despite the cost) by one of the synthetic vitamin D analogues – such as ALFACALCIDOL, DIHYDROTACHYSTEROL or CALCITRIOL.
Related articles: CHOCOVITE; STEROGYL-15.

Calcimax (*Wallace*) is a proprietary non-prescription mineral-and-VITAMIN compound that is not available from the National Health Service. Produced in the form of a syrup, it contains calcium, several forms of vitamin B (THIAMINE, RIBOFLAVINE, PYRIDOXINE, CYANOCOBALAMIN, NICOTINAMIDE and PANTOTHENOL), ASCORBIC ACID (vitamin C) and CALCIFEROL (vitamin D).

Calciparine (*Labaz*) is a proprietary form of the ANTICOAGULANT heparin calcium, available only on prescription, used to treat various forms of thrombosis. It is produced in syringes and in ampoules for injection.
✚/▲ warning/side-effects: *see* HEPARIN.

Calcisorb (*Riker*) is a proprietary non-prescription preparation used to help reduce high calcium levels in the bloodstream. It effects this by inhibiting calcium absorption from food. Produced in the form of powder for solution in water, or to sprinkle over food (here children should be supervised). Calcisorb is a preparation of sodium cellulose phosphate. It may cause diarrhoea in some users.
✚/▲ warning/side-effects: *see* SODIUM CELLULOSE PHOSPHATE.

Calcitare (*Armour*) is a proprietary form of the thyroid hormone calcitonin, available only on prescription, used to lower blood levels of calcium (which are significant in maintaining the replication of bone cells) and to treat certain bone diseases. Calcitare is produced in the form of powder for reconstitution in a gelatin diluent as injections.
✚/▲ warning/side-effects: *see* CALCITONIN.

calcitonin is a hormone produced and secreted by the thyroid gland at the base of the neck. Its function is to lower the levels of calcium and phosphate in the blood, and so together with the correspondingly opposite action of a parathyroid hormone to regulate those levels. Therapeutically introduced calcitonin obviously has the same effect, and may thus be used to treat certain bone diseases in which the levels of calcium have become too high. Because these diseases may cause such symptoms as pain or deafness, treatment with calcitonin may give great relief. Administration is ordinarily by injection.
✚ warning: prolonged use of calcitonin derived from animals may eventually lead to the body's producing antibodies against it, and consequent neutralization of its effect. Some patients may be sensitive to animal calcitonin.
▲ side-effects: there may be nausea, with vomiting and flushing; there may also be a tingling sensation in the hands and a peculiar taste in the mouth. Inflammation may arise at the site of injection.
Related article: CALCITARE.

calcitriol is a synthesized form of CALCIFEROL (vitamin D), used to make up body deficiencies, particularly in patients who have had a kidney removed. Calcium levels in the body should be regularly monitored during treatment. Administration is oral in the form of capsules.
✚ warning: overdosage may cause kidney damage. Although an increased amount of vitamin D is necessary

C

during pregnancy, high body levels while lactating may cause corresponding high blood levels of calcium in the breast-fed infant.
Related article: ROCALTROL.

calcium is a metallic element essential in compund form for the normal growth and development of the body, and especially (in the form of calcium phosphate) of the bones and the teeth. It is also a constituent of blood, its level regulated by the opposing actions of the hormones CALCITONIN and parathyroid hormone (parathormone). Its uptake from food ingested is the responsibility of CALCIFEROL (vitamin D). Good food sources are all dairy products. Salts of calcium used therapeutically include the antidiarrhoeal antacid calcium carbonate, the folinic acid supplement calcium folinate, the calcium supplements calcium gluconate and calcium lactate, and the sulphonamide calcium sulphaloxate.
✚ warning: deficiency of vitamin D leads to calcium deficiency, and corresponding bone, blood and nerve disorders. Conversely, excess calcium in the body may cause the formation of stones (calculi, generally composed of calcium oxalate), particularly in the kidney or gall bladder.
see CALCIUM CARBONATE; CALCIUM FOLINATE; CALCIUM GLUCONATE; CALCIUM LACTATE; CALCIUM SULPHALOXATE.

calcium antagonists (calcium channel antagonists; calcium channel blockers) are a relatively new class of drugs used as ANTIHYPERTENSIVES in the treatment of high blood pressure. They act by reducing calcium entry to the heart, which reduces the force of the heart beat and therefore lowers blood pressure. Examples include DILTIAZEM and VERAPAMIL.

calcium carbonate, or chalk, is used therapeutically both as an ANTACID in the treatment of peptic ulcers, and as an ANTIDIARRHOEAL preparation (generally in combination with an astringent). Administration is oral in the form of tablets or as a powder in solution.
✚ warning: prolonged use as an antacid can induce tolerance and eventually cause renewed acid secretion. There may also be abnormally high levels of calcium in the blood. Antacids may impair the absorption of other drugs.
▲ side-effects: treatment with calcium carbonate as an antacid may cause belching (through the liberation of carbon dioxide).
Related articles: NULACIN; RABRO.

calcium carbonate mixture is an ANTACID representing a non-proprietary formulation of calcium carbonate, magnesium carbonate and sodium bicarbonate, together with tincture of cardamom and a dilute syrup.
✚/▲ warning/side-effects: *see* CALCIUM CARBONATE; MAGNESIUM CARBONATE; SODIUM BICARBONATE.

calcium folinate is the usual form in which folinic acid (a derivative of folic acid, a vitamin of the VITAMIN B complex) is administered as a supplement to patients who are susceptible to the toxic effects of certain anticancer drugs – especially METHOTREXATE or PYRIMETHAMINE – and to treat some types of anaemia.
see FOLINIC ACID.

calcium gluconate is one of several common forms in which CALCIUM is administered as a supplement to patients who suffer with calcium deficiency (through dietary insufficiency or disease) or who temporarily need more (as in pregnancy and lactation), with or without the simultaneous administration of CALCIFEROL (vitamin D). It can also be used to treat allergic conditions, such as urticaria, and to relieve the pain of chilblains. Administration is oral in the form of tablets (which may be chewed) or (in solution) by injection or infusion.

✚ warning: calcium gluconate should be administered with caution to patients who suffer from heart disease.

▲ side-effects: following treatment by injection or infusion there may be a slowing of the heart rate together with heartbeat irregularity. There may be irritation at the site of injection.

Related article: SANDOCAL

calcium lactate is one of several common forms in which CALCIUM is administered as a supplement to patients who suffer from calcium deficiency (through dietary insufficiency or disease) or who temporarily need more (as in pregnancy and lactation), with or without the simultaneous administration of CALCIFEROL (vitamin D). Administration is oral in the form of tablets (which may be chewed) or (in solution) by injection or infusion.

✚ warning: calcium lactate should be administered with caution to patients who suffer from heart disease.

▲ side-effects: following treatment by injection or infusion there may be a slowing of the heart rate together with heartbeat irregularity. There may be irritation at the site of injection.

Related article: SANDOCAL.

Calcium Leucovorin (*Lederle*) is a proprietary preparation of folinic acid, available only on prescription, administered as a supplement to patients who are susceptible to the toxic effects of certain anticancer drugs – especially METHOTREXATE or PYRIMETHAMINE – and used to treat various forms of anaemia. It is produced in the form of tablets, and in ampoules or as powder for reconstitution as injections.

✚/▲ warning/side-effects: *see* FOLINIC ACID.

Calcium Resonium (*Winthrop*) is a proprietary non-prescription preparation used to treat high blood POTASSIUM levels, particularly in patients who suffer from fluid retention or who undergo kidney dialysis. It is produced in the form of a powdered resin, as a calcium polystyrene salt.

Calcium-Sandoz (*Sandoz*) is a proprietary CALCIUM supplement, used to treat patients with the neuro-muscular symptoms of calcium deficiency. Produced in the form of (non-prescription) syrup and (available only on prescription) in ampoules for injection, Calcium-Sandoz contains several calcium salts.

calcium sulphaloxate is a SULPHONAMIDE drug that has now largely been replaced by others because it is poorly absorbed. Formerly, however, it was popularly prescribed to treat infections of the intestines and to prevent infection during intestinal surgery. It is still sometimes used to treat chronic diarrhoea. Use may lead to the appearance of rashes.

Calfig (*Sterling Health*) is a proprietary, non-prescription LAXATIVE. Its active constituent is extract of senna leaf.
✚/▲ warning/side-effects: *see* SENNA

Callusolve (*Dermal*) is a proprietary non-prescription preparation, used to treat warts and remove hard, dead skin. Produced in the form of a solute paint, Callusolve is a preparation of the keratolytic benzalkonium chloride as a bromine adduct. Avoid normal skin.
✚ warning: *see* BENZALKONIUM CHLORIDE.

Calmurid (*Pharmacia*) is a proprietary non-prescription preparation, used to treat conditions in which the skin becomes scaly and hardens in layers. Produced in the form of a water- miscible cream for dilution (the cream once dilute retains potency for 14 days), Calmurid is a combination of the diuretic urea and lactic acid.

Calmurid HC (*Pharmacia*) is a proprietary CORTICOSTEROID preparation, available only on prescription, used to treat conditions in which the skin becomes dry and hardens in layers. Produced in the form of a water-miscible cream for dilution (the cream once dilute retains potency for 14 days), Calmurid HC is a combination of the steroid hydrocortisone, the DIURETIC urea and lactic acid.
✚/▲ warning/side-effects: *see* HYDROCORTISONE.

Calogen (*Scientific Hospital Supplies*) is a proprietary non-prescription dietary supplement used in the nutrition of patients with kidney disease. Produced in the form of a gluten-free emulsion, Calogen comprises ARACHIS OIL in water.

Calonutrin (*Geistlich*) is a proprietary non-prescription dietary supplement used in the nutrition of patients who suffer from kidney disease, cirrhosis of the liver or amino acid abnormality (such as phenylketonuria). Produced in the form of powder, Calonutrin comprises many simple sugars (especially glucose).

Caloreen (*Roussel*) is a proprietary non-prescription dietary supplement used in the nutrition of patients who suffer from kidney disease, cirrhosis of the liver or amino-acid abnormality (such as phenylketonuria). Produced in the form of powder, Caloreen comprises many simple sugars (especially glucose).

Calpol (*Calmic*) is a proprietary form of the non- narcotic ANALGESIC paracetamol. It is produced in the form of a suspension in two strengths: the weaker (non-prescription) is produced under the name Calpol Infant; the stronger (not available from the National Health Service) under the name Calpol Six Plus.
✚/▲ warning/side-effects: *see* PARACETAMOL.

Calsynar (*Armour*) is a proprietary synthesized form of calcitonin (salcatonin), one of the two hormones that regulate blood levels of calcium in the body. Available only on prescription, Calsynar is used to treat several types of serious bone disease, including cancer, and is produced

in ampoules (in two strengths) for injection.
✚/▲ warning/side-effects: *see* CALCITONIN; SALCATONIN.

Calthor (*Ayerst*) is a proprietary penicillin-type ANTIBIOTIC, available only on prescription, used to treat bronchitis and infections in the skin and urinary tract. Produced in the form of tablets (in two strengths) and as a syrup for dilution, Calthor is a preparation of ciclacillin. Calthor is not recommended for children aged under 2 months.
✚/▲ warning/side-effects: *see* CICLACILLIN.

CAM (*Rybar*) is a proprietary non-prescription SYMPATHOMIMETIC, a BRONCHODILATOR used to treat patients suffering from asthma and other conditions involving bronchial spasm. Produced in the form of a syrup, CAM's active constituent is EPHEDRINE HYDROCHLORIDE. CAM is not recommended for children aged under 18 months.

Camcolit (*Norgine*) is a proprietary ANTIDEPRESSANT drug, available only on prescription, used to treat acute mania and to prevent manic-depressive bouts. Produced in the form of tablets (in two strengths), Camcolit is a preparation of lithium carbonate. It is not recommended for children.
✚/▲ warning/side-effects: *see* LITHIUM.

Camoquin (*Parke-Davis*) is a proprietary ANTIMALARIAL drug, available only on prescription, used to treat both the benign and the malignant types of malaria. Produced in the form of tablets, Camoquin represents a preparation of amodiaquine hydrochloride.
✚/▲ warning/side-effects: *see* AMODIAQUINE.

Canesten (*Bayer*) is a proprietary non-prescription ANTIFUNGAL and ANTIBACTERIAL preparation, used to treat infections and particularly ones that cause inflammation. Treatment is topical, and for sensitive areas such as the vagina and the penis, but also the outer ear, other areas of the skin, and the nails. Produced in the form of vaginal tablets (pessaries), as a solution, as a spray, as a cream and as a dusting-powder, Canesten is a preparation of clotrimazole. Canesten vaginal cream, vaginal tablets (in two strengths) and a Duopak containing vaginal tablets and cream are available only on prescription.
✚/▲ warning/side-effects: *see* CLOTRIMAZOLE.

Canesten 1 (*Bayer*) is a proprietary ANTIFUNGAL and ANTIBACTERIAL preparation, available only on prescription, used to treat vaginal infections. Produced in the form of vaginal tablets (pessaries), Canesten 1 – which is a stronger version of CANESTEN - is also a preparation of clotrimazole.
✚/▲ warning/side-effects: *see* CLOTRIMAZOLE.

Canesten 10% VC (*Bayer*) is a proprietary ANTIFUNGAL and ANTIBACTERIAL cream, available only on prescription, used to treat vaginal infections. To be inserted through a special applicator, Canesten 10% VC is a preparation of clotrimazole.
✚/▲ warning/side-effects: *see* CLOTRIMAZOLE.

Canesten-HC (*Bayer*) is a proprietary ANTIFUNGAL and ANTIBACTERIAL steroid preparation, available only on prescription, used to treat fungal infections, particularly those that cause inflammation. Produced in

the form of a cream for topical application, Canesten-HC consists of a combination of clotrimazole and hydrocortisone.
✚/▲ warning/side-effects: *see* CLOTRIMAZOLE; HYDROCORTISONE.

cannabis is one name for a drug prepared from the Indian hemp plant Cannabis sativa: other names include bhang, dagga, hashish, marijuana and pot. Its use seems of little therapeutic value, and its social use is illegal although fairly widespread. (It may be prescribed only under licence from the Home Secretary.) A synthetic cannabinoid, NABILONE, is used in cancer chemotherapy to reduce nausea and vomiting.
✚ warning: prolonged use is thought eventually to result in brain damage, and is thought by some to lead a user to experiment with addictive "hard" drugs, although it is difficult to test this theory.
▲ side-effects: smoked or ingested, cannabis is a psychedelic, causing comparatively mild hallucinations with euphoria, heightening awareness and particularly affecting the sense of time. Withdrawal symptoms are rare, but use tends to increase tolerance.

Cantil (*MCP Pharmaceuticals*) is a proprietary ANTICHOLINERGIC drug, available only on prescription, used as a SMOOTH MUSCLE RELAXANT to treat rigidity (spasm) or hyperactivity of the muscles of the colon. Produced in the form of tablets and as an elixir for dilution (the potency of the elixir once dilute is retained for 7 days), Cantil is a preparation of the MUSCLE RELAXANT mepenzolate bromide. It is not recommended for children aged under 6 years.
✚/▲ warning/side-effects: *see* MEPENZOLATE BROMIDE.

Cantil with Phenobarbitone (*MCP Pharmaceuticals*) is a form of the proprietary ANTICHOLINERGIC drug Cantil that additionally contains the BARBITURATE drug phenobarbitone and is on the controlled drugs list. Produced in the form of tablets, it is not recommended for children. Now out of favour due to its barbiturate content.
✚/▲ warning/side-effects: *see* MEPENZOLATE BROMIDE; PHENOBARBITONE.

Capastat (*Dista*) is a proprietary ANTITUBERCULAR drug, available only on prescription, used to treat tuberculosis resistant to other drugs. Produced in the form of powder for reconstitution as intramuscular injections, Capastat represents a preparation of the powerful ANTIBIOTIC capreomycin sulphate. It is not recommended for children.
✚/▲ warning/side-effects: *see* CAPREOMYCIN.

Capitol (*Dermal*) is a proprietary non-prescription ANTIBACTERIAL preparation, used to treat dandruff and other scalp conditions. Produced in the form of a gel applied as a shampoo, Capitol represents a preparation of the antiseptic BENZALKONIUM CHLORIDE.

Caplenal (*Berk*) is a proprietary form of the XANTHINE-OXIDASE INHIBITOR allopurinol, used as a longterm treatment of gout and high levels of uric acid in the bloodstream. It exacerbates symptoms of gout if given during an attack. Available only on prescription, Caplenal is produced in the form of tablets

(in two strengths) and is not recommended for children.
✚/▲ warning/side-effects: *see* ALLOPURINOL.

Capoten (*Squibb*) is a proprietary ANTIHYPERTENSIVE drug, available only on prescription, used accordingly to treat high blood pressure (hypertension) and to slow the heart rate. Although well tolerated, the long-term effects are unknown and so it tends to be used when THIAZIDES or BETA-BLOCKERS have failed or are not tolerated. It works by inhibiting enzymes involved in producing vasoactive hormones in the blood. Produced in the form of tablets (in three strengths), Capoten is a preparation of the powerful drug captopril.
✚/▲ warning/side-effects: *see* CAPTOPRIL.

capreomycin is an ANTIBIOTIC drug used specifically in the treatment of tuberculosis that proves to be resistant to the powerful drugs ordinarily used first, or in cases where those drugs are not tolerated. Administration is by intramuscular injection.
✚ warning: capreomycin should not be administered to patients who are pregnant, and should be administered with caution to those who have impaired function of the liver, kidney or sense of hearing (functions that should be monitored during treatment), or who are already taking other powerful antibiotics, or who are lactating.
▲ side-effects: there may be kidney toxicity and impaired hearing with or without ringing in the ears (tinnitus) or vertigo; sometimes there are sensitivity reactions such as rashes or urticaria.
Related article: CAPASTAT.

Caprin (*Sinclair*) is a proprietary non-prescription preparation of the non-narcotic ANALGESIC aspirin, used particularly to treat headache and rheumatic conditions. Produced in the form of sustained-release tablets, Caprin is not recommended for children aged under 12 years.
✚/▲ warning/side-effects: *see* ASPIRIN.

captopril is a powerful VASODILATOR used in the treatment of high blood pressure (hypertension) particularly when THIAZIDE drugs have failed to be fully effective or are not tolerated. It may also be used to treat heart failure, although a supplementary DIURETIC is then commonly administered. Captopril works by inhibiting enzymes involved in producing vasoactive hormones in the blood thus dilating the smaller arteries. Administration of captopril is oral in the form of tablets.
✚ warning: captopril should not be administered to patients who are pregnant, and administered with caution to those who are lactating. The first dose may cause very rapid reduction in blood pressure, especially if a diuretic is given simultaneously; dosage thereafter may be adjusted for optimum effect. Monitoring of kidney function, white blood cell count and urinary contents during treatment is essential.
▲ side-effects: there may be marked low blood pressure (hypotension); thereafter there may be a loss of the sense of taste and a dry cough; sometimes there is abdominal pain and/or a rash. In patients with impaired kidney function (or who are given a high dosage) there may be changes

C

in the composition of the blood, and protein in the urine.
Related articles: ACEPRIL; CAPOTEN.

carbachol is a PARA-SYMPATHOMIMETIC that is used to treat some heart and circulatory conditions, or to lower pressure in the eyeball while contracting the pupil (in the treatment of glaucoma), but perhaps its most common use is to treat urinary retention, particularly following surgery. Administration is oral in the form of tablets, by injection, or as eye-drops.

✚ warning: carbachol should not be administered to patients who suffer from urinary or intestinal blockage or haemorrhage, or who have recently had a heart attack. It should be administered with caution to those who suffer from heart disease, epilepsy, parkinsonism or thyroid disorders, or who are elderly.

▲ side-effects: there may be sweating and blurred vision, nausea and vomiting, and a slow heart rate.
Related article: ISOPTO.

carbamazepine is an ANTICONVULSANT drug used, sometimes in combination with other drugs, particularly to treat grand mal epilepsy both during seizures and on a maintenance basis. In smaller doses it is effective in reducing attacks of trigeminal neuralgia (a searing pain in paroxysms along the trigeminal nerve in the face) or the neural disorders that may accompany diabetes mellitus, again on a maintenance basis. Surprisingly, it also has DIURETIC properties, and is sometimes alternatively used in that capacity to assist treatment for diabetes insipidus.

✚ warning: carbamazepine should not be administered to patients who suffer from certain heart defects or porphyria, or to those using or having recently used any of the MAO inhibitor drugs; it should be administered with caution to those who suffer from impaired function of the liver or glaucoma, or who are lactating. Dosage should begin at a minimum level and be adjusted upwards for optimum effect. Blood monitoring is essential if high doses are administered.

▲ side-effects: there may be blurring of vision and unsteadiness; high dosage may cause severe dizziness. Sometimes there are gastrointestinal disturbances; occasionally there is a rash.
Related article: TEGRETOL.

carbaryl is an insecticide used in the treatment of scalp or pubic lice. Administration is (in aqueous or alcohol solution) in the form of a lotion, or shampoo which is applied to wet hair, allowed to dry, and then rinsed after a specified time (usually about 12 hours). The procedure may need to be repeated after a week.

✚ warning: keep away from the eyes.
Related articles: CARYLDERM; CLINICIDE; DERBAC-C; SULEO-C.

Carbellon (*Medo*) is a proprietary non-prescription ANTICHOLINERGIC compound that is not available from the National Health Service. It is used to treat muscle spasm (rigidity) of the intestinal walls, and resulting gastrointestinal upsets. Produced in the form of tablets, Carbellon's active constituents are belladonna extract, charcoal and magnesium hydroxide.

✚/▲ warning/side-effects: *see*

BELLADONNA; CHARCOAL; MAGNESIUM HYDROXIDE.

carbenicillin is a penicillin-like ANTIBIOTIC used to treat bacillary infections (particularly) of the urinary tract. Administration is by injection or infusion in the case of systemic infections, or by intramuscular injections for urinary tract infections.

✚ warning: carbenicillin should not be administered to patients known to be sensitive to penicillins, and should be administered with caution to those who suffer from impaired kidney function.

▲ side-effects: there may be sensitivity reactions – serious ones in hypersensitive patients. Body temperature may rise, and there may be pains in the joints and skin rashes or urticaria; potassium and platelet levels in the blood may decline.

Related article: PYOPEN.

carbenoxolone sodium is a compound derivative of a constituent of liquorice used as a treatment for gastric ulcers because it protects the stomach lining from excess acid and enzymes – in a way that is not well understood. Although used primarily to treat gastric or intestinal ulcers, it may also be used locally to soothe mouth ulcers. Administration is oral in the form of tablets (to be chewed or swallowed) as capsules, as a gel, or as a compound liquid.

✚ warning: carbenoxolone sodium should be administered with caution to patients who suffer from impaired function of the liver or kidneys, heart disease, high blood pressure, or who are elderly. The drug is potassium-depleting: potassium supplements should accompany treatment (with or without THIAZIDE diuretics).

▲ side-effects: there may be fluid retention in the tissues (oedema); heartburn is not uncommon. Patients with high blood pressure (hypertension) or muscular weakness may find these conditions aggravated during treatment.

Related articles: BIOGASTRONE; DUOGASTRONE; PYROGASTRONE.

carbidopa is a drug administered in combination with levodopa to treat parkinsonism, but not the parkinsonian symptoms induced by other drugs (*see* ANTIPARKINSONISM).It is levodopa that actually has the major effect. Carbidopa inhibits the breakdown of levodopa (to dopamine) in the body before it reaches the brain, where it carries out its function. The presence of carbidopa allows the dose of levodopa to be at a minimum, thus also minimizing potentially severe side-effects, and speeds the therapeutic response. But it is also responsible for producing involuntary movements. Administration of carbidopa and levodopa is in the form of single compound tablets.

✚/▲ warning/side-effects: *see* LEVODOPA.

Related article: SINEMET.

carbimazole prevents the production or secretion of the hormone thyroxine by the thyroid gland, so treating an excess in the blood of thyroid HORMONES and the symptoms that it causes (thyrotoxicosis). Treatment may be on a maintenance basis over a long period (dosage adjusted to optimum effect), or may be merely preliminary to surgical removal of the thyroid gland. Administration is oral in the form of tablets.

✚ warning: carbimazole should not be administered to patients with obstruction of the upper respiratory tract, and should be administered with extreme caution to patients who are pregnant or lactating.

▲ side-effects: an itching rash is common, but may indicate a need for alternative treatment. There may also be nausea and headache; occasionally there is jaundice or hair loss (alopecia).

Related article: NEO-MERCAZOLE.

carbinoxamine is a short-acting ANTIHISTAMINE that is an anti-allergic constituent in one or two cough linctuses and, because it also has mild ANTINAUSEANT properties, is also found in some proprietary preparations to prevent travel sickness.
Related article: EXTIL COMPOUND.

carbocisteine is a MUCOLYTIC drug, used accordingly to reduce the viscosity of sputum and thus facilitate expectoration (the coughing up of sputum) in patients with disorders of the upper respiratory tract such as asthma and bronchitis. It may also be used to treat accumulations of mucus in the middle ear ("glue ear") in children. Administration is oral in the form of tablets, capsules or syrup.

✚ warning: carbocisteine should not be administered to patients with a peptic ulcer; it should be administered with caution to those who are pregnant.

▲ side-effects: side-effects are uncommon, but there may be gastrointestinal disturbance, with nausea, or a rash.

Related articles: MUCODYNE; MUCOLEX.

Carbo-Cort (*Lagap*) is a proprietary ANTISEPTIC and CORTICOSTEROID preparation, available only on prescription, used to treat serious non-infective skin diseases such as psoriasis and eczema. Produced in the form of a water-miscible cream, Carbo-Cort contains the powerful steroid hydrocortisone together with COAL TAR. In this formulation it is suitable for the face, unlike other formulations of coal tar.

✚/▲ warning/side-effects: *see* HYDROCORTISONE.

Carbo-Dome (*Lagap*) is a proprietary non-prescription ANTISEPTIC used to treat non-infective skin conditions like psoriasis. Produced in the form of a water-miscible cream, Carbo-Dome's active constituent is COAL TAR.

Carbomix (*Penn*) is a proprietary non-prescription adsorbent preparation, used to treat patients suffering from poisoning or a drug overdose. Produced in the form of granulated powder to be mixed with water, Carbomix's active constituent is CHARCOAL.

carboplatin is a CYTOTOXIC drug derived from the ANTICANCER drug cisplatin, and similarly used to treat cancer of the ovary. Side-effects of nausea and vomiting are less than those caused by cisplatin. Administration is by injection.

✚ warning: an anti-emetic may be administered simultaneously to lessen the risk of nausea and vomiting. Monitoring of kidney function and the sense of hearing is advisable.

▲ side-effects: there may be nausea and vomiting, progressive deafness and symptoms of kidney dysfunction. The blood-forming

capacity of the bone-marrow may be suppressed (and treatment should not be repeated within 4 weeks).
Related article: PARAPLATIN

Cardene (*Syntex*) is a proprietary form of the CALCIUM ANTAGONIST ANTIHYPERTENSIVE drug nicardipine hydrochloride, available only on prescription, used to prevent or treat chronic angina and high blood pressure (hypertension). Produced in the form of capsules (in two strengths), Cardene is not recommended for children.
✚/▲ warning/side-effects: *see* NICARDIPINE.

Cardiacap (*Consolidated*) is a proprietary non-prescription vasodilator, used in the prevention or treatment of angina. Produced in the form of sustained-release capsules, Cardiacap is a preparation of pentaerythritol tetranitrate. It is not recommended for children.
✚/▲ warning/side-effects: *see* PENTAERYTHRITOL TETRANITRATE.

cardiac glycosides are a class of drugs that have a pronounced effect on the heart, increasing the force of contraction of cardiac muscle. They therefore have an important use in the treatment of congestive heart failure. Examples include OUABAIN and DIGOXIN.

carfecillin sodium is a penicillin-like ANTIBIOTIC used to treat bacillary infections (particularly) of the urinary tract. Administration is oral in the form of tablets.
✚ warning: carfecillin sodium should not be administered to patients known to be sensitive to penicillins, and should be administered with caution to those with impaired kidney function.
▲ side-effects: there may be sensitivity reactions – serious ones in hypersensitive patients. Body temperature may rise, and there may be pains in the joints and skin rashes or urticaria.
Related article: UTICILLIN.

Carisoma (*Pharmax*) is a proprietary SKELETAL MUSCLE RELAXANT, available only on prescription, used to relieve muscle spasm by direct action on the central nervous system. Produced in the form of tablets (in two strengths), Carisoma is a preparation of carisoprodol. It is not recommended for children.
✚/▲ warning/side-effects: *see* CARISOPRODOL.

carisoprodol is a SKELETAL MUSCLE RELAXANT that works by directly affecting certain areas of the central nervous system, and is used to relieve muscle spasm in muscles used for voluntary movement. Administration is oral in the form of tablets.
✚ warning: carisoprodol should not be administered to patients with porphyria, or who are lactating; it should be administered with caution to those who are epileptic. Withdrawal from treatment must be gradual. Prolonged overdosage may cause muscle atrophy.
▲ side-effects: there is commonly drowsiness and dizziness; there may also be dry mouth, headache, shallow breathing, low blood pressure (hypotension), general debility and gastrointestinal disturbances. Rarely, there are visual disturbances and a rash.
Related article: CARISOMA.

C

carmellose sodium is a substance used as the basis for a paste and a powder that is spread or sprinkled over lesions in or around the mouth in order to protect them while they heal. Both paste and powder also contain soft animal and vegetable proteins.
Related articles: ORABASE; ORAHESIVE.

carmustine is a CYTOTOXIC drug which works by direct interference with DNA, thus preventing normal cell replication. It is used to treat some solid tumours and the lymphatic cancer, Hodgkin's disease. Prolonged treatment may produce considerable toxicity and associated side-effects. Administration is by intravenous injection.
✚ warning: the drug causes permanent sterility in men early in treatment, and prolonged treatment may lead to an early menopause in women; prolonged treatment has also been associated with the incidence of leukaemia following simultaneous irradiation treatment. Blood count monitoring is essential. Dosage should be the minimum still to be effective.
▲ side-effects: there is commonly nausea and vomiting. The blood-producing capacity of the bone-marrow is impaired (although the effect is delayed, and treatment should therefore not be repeated within 4 weeks). There may be hair loss.
Related article: BiCNU.

Carobel, Instant (*Cow & Gate*) is a proprietary non-prescription powder, used to thicken liquid and semi-liquid diets in the treatment of vomiting. Carobel is a preparation of carob seed flour.

carteolol hydrochloride is a BETA-BLOCKER used in the form of eye-drops to treat glaucoma. It is thought to work by slowing the rate of production of the aqueous humour in the eyeball, but it may be absorbed and have systemic effects as well.
✚ warning: because systemic absorption may occur, carteolol hydrochloride should be administered with caution to patients with slow heart rate, heart failure or asthma. (It may interact with verapamil.)
▲ side-effects: there may be periods in which the eyes temporarily become dry; at such times there may be infections such as conjunctivitis or blepharitis.
Related article: TEOPTIC.

Carylderm (*Napp*) is a proprietary non-prescription drug used to treat infestations of the scalp and pubic hair by lice. Produced in the form of a lotion and a shampoo, Carylderm is a preparation of the pediculicide carbaryl.
✚ warning: *see* CARBARYL.

cascara is a slightly old-fashioned but powerful stimulant laxative which acts by increasing the muscular activity of the intestinal walls. It is now used less commonly, not just because of its cumulatively detrimental side-effects but because it may take up to 8 hours to have any relieving effect on constipation. Administration is oral in the form of tablets.
✚ warning: cascara should not be taken by any patient who is breast-feeding, and is not recommended for children.
▲ side-effects: the urine may be coloured red. Prolonged use of such a stimulant can eventually wear out the

muscles on which it works, thus causing severe intestinal problems in terms of motility and absorption.

Casilan (*Farley*) is a proprietary non-prescription protein dietary supplement used to treat patients who are undernourished through lack of food or poor internal absorption. Produced in the form of powder for reconstitution, Casilan contains all essential amino acids and is gluten-free and low in electrolytes.

castor oil is a slightly old-fashioned stimulant LAXATIVE which probably acts by increasing the muscular activity of the intestinal walls. It is now used less commonly because of its cumulatively detrimental side-effects, although its use in hospitals and clinics before surgical examinations and procedures is still well attested. Yet it may take up to 8 hours to relieve constipation. Administration is oral.

✚ warning: castor oil should not be taken by any patient who is menstruating, pregnant or lactating, or who suffers from intestinal obstruction.

▲ side-effects: there may be nausea and vomiting. Prolonged use of such a stimulant can eventually wear out the muscles on which it works, thus causing severe intestinal problems in terms of motility and absorption.

Catapres (*Boehringer Ingelheim*) is a proprietary ANTIHYPERTENSIVE drug, available only on prescription, used to treat high blood pressure (hypertension). Produced in the form of tablets (in two strengths), capsules and ampoules for injection, Catapres is a preparation of clonidine hydrochloride. It is not recommended for children.

✚/▲ warning/side-effects: *see* CLONIDINE HYDROCHLORIDE.

Caved-S (*Tillotts*) is a proprietary non-prescription ANTACID, used to treat the symptoms of peptic ulcers. Produced in the form of tablets, Caved-S contains a compound form of a constituent of liquorice, ALUMINIUM HYDROXIDE gel, MAGNESIUM CARBONATE and SODIUM BICARBONATE. It is not recommended for children under the age of 10 years.

CCNU (*Lundbeck*) is a proprietary CYTOTOXIC drug, available only on prescription, used mainly in cancer chemotherapy. Produced in the form of capsules (in two strengths), CCNU is a preparation of lomustine.

✚/▲ warning/side-effects: *see* LOMUSTINE.

Ceanel Concentrate (*Quinoderm*) is a proprietary non-prescription ANTIBACTERIAL and ANTIFUNGAL preparation, used to treat psoriasis and other non-infective scalp conditions. Produced in the form of a shampoo, Ceanel Concentrate contains the antiseptic CETRIMIDE, the antifungal undecenoic acid, and the astringent ethyl alcohol.

✚/▲ warning/side-effects: *see* CETRIMIDE

Ce-Cobalin (*Paines & Byrne*) is a proprietary non-prescription VITAMIN preparation that is not available from the National Health Service. Produced in the form of a syrup, Ce-Cobalin is a compound of CYANOCOBALAMIN (vitamin B_{12}) and ASCORBIC ACID (vitamin C).

Cedilanid (*Sandoz*) is a proprietary CARDIAC GLYCOSIDE

heart stimulant, available only on prescription, used to treat heart failure and severe heartbeat irregularities. Produced in the form of tablets, Cedilanid is a preparation of LANATOSIDE C (which is converted on ingestion into the better known digoxin).
✚/▲ warning/side-effects: *see* DIGOXIN.

Cedocard (*Tillotts*) represents a series of proprietary forms of the VASODILATOR isosorbide dinitrate, used to prevent and treat angina pectoris. Produced in the form of tablets (in four strengths, under the names Cedocard-5, Cedocard-10, Cedocard-20 and Cedocard-40), as sustained-release tablets (under the name Cedocard Retard) and in flasks (ampoules) for infusion (under the name Cedocard I.V.), not one of these preparations is recommended for children.
✚/▲ warning/side-effects: *see* ISOSORBIDE DINITRATE.

cefaclor is a broad-spectrum ANTIBIOTIC, one of the cephalosporins, used to treat a wide range of bacterial infections, particularly of the skin and soft tissues, the urinary tract, the upper respiratory tract, and the middle ear. Administration is oral in the form of capsules or a dilute suspension.
✚ warning: cefaclor should not be administered to patients who might be sensitive to penicillins in general and cephalosporins in particular. It should be administered with caution to those with impaired kidney function.
▲ side-effects: there may be sensitivity reactions – some of which may be serious. Sometimes there is nausea and vomiting, with diarrhoea.
Related article: DISTACLOR.

cefadroxil is a broad-spectrum ANTIBIOTIC, one of the cephalosporins, used to treat a wide range of bacterial infections, particularly of the skin and soft tissues, the urinary tract, the upper respiratory tract, and the middle ear. Administration is oral in the form of capsules or a dilute suspension.
✚ warning: cefadroxil should not be administered to patients who might be sensitive to penicillins in general and cephalosporins in particular. It should be administered with caution to those who suffer from impaired kidney function.
▲ side-effects: there may be sensitivity reactions – some of which may be serious. Sometimes there is nausea and vomiting, with diarrhoea.
Related article: BAXAN.

Cefizox (*Wellcome*) is a proprietary ANTIBIOTIC, available only on prescription, used to treat gonorrhoea and infections in the upper respiratory tract and urinary tract. Produced in the form of powder for reconstitution as injections, Cefizox is a preparation of ceftizoxime as a salt of sodium. It is not recommended for children aged under 3 months.
✚/▲ warning/side-effects: *see* CEFTIZOXIME.

cefotaxime is a broad-spectrum ANTIBIOTIC, one of the cephalosporins, used to treat a wide range of bacterial infections, particularly of the skin and soft tissues, the urinary tract, the meninges (meningitis) and the blood (septicaemia). It is also used to prevent infection during surgery. Administration is by intravenous or intramuscular injection.
✚ warning: cefotaxime should

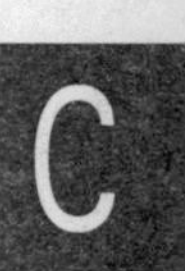

not be administered to patients who might be sensitive to penicillins in general and cephalosporins in particular. It should be administered with caution to those with impaired kidney function, or who are pregnant or lactating.

▲ side-effects: there may be sensitivity reactions – some of which may be serious. Sometimes there is nausea and vomiting, with diarrhoea. *Related article:* CLAFORAN.

cefoxitin is a broad-spectrum ANTIBIOTIC, one of the cephalosporins, used to treat a wide range of bacterial infections, particularly of the skin and soft tissues, the urinary tract, the upper respiratory tract, the peritoneum (peritonitis) and the blood (septicaemia). It is also used to prevent infection during or following gynaecological or obstetric surgery. Administration is by intravenous or intramuscular injection.

✚ warning: cefoxitin should not be administered to patients who might be sensitive to penicillins in general and cephalosporins in particular. It should be administered with caution to those with impaired kidney function.

▲ side-effects: there may be sensitivity reactions – some of which may be serious. Sometimes there is nausea and vomiting, with diarrhoea. *Related article:* MEFOXIN.

cefsulodin is a broad-spectrum ANTIBIOTIC, one of the cephalosporins, used to treat a wide range of bacterial infections, particularly of the skin and soft tissues, the urinary tract, and the upper respiratory tract. Administration is by intravenous or intramuscular injection.

✚ warning: cefsulodin should not be administered to patients who might be sensitive to penicillins in general and cephalosporins in particular. It should be administered with caution to those with impaired kidney function, or who are pregnant. Monitoring of blood counts during treatment is essential.

▲ side-effects: there may be sensitivity reactions – some of which may be serious. Sometimes there is nausea and vomiting, with diarrhoea. *Related article:* MONASPOR.

ceftazidime is a broad-spectrum ANTIBIOTIC, one of the cephalosporins, used to treat a wide range of bacterial infections, particularly of the skin and soft tissues, the urinary tract, the upper respiratory tract, the ear, nose and throat, the bones and the joints, the gastrointestinal tract, the meninges (meningitis) and the blood (septicaemia). It is also used to treat infection in patients whose immune systems are defective. Administration is by intravenous or intramuscular injection.

✚ warning: ceftazidime should not be administered to patients who might be sensitive to penicillins in general and cephalosporins in particular, or to patients who are already taking certain diuretic drugs. It should be administered with caution to those who suffer from impaired kidney function, or who are pregnant.

▲ side-effects: there may be sensitivity reactions – some of which may be serious. Alternatively, sometimes there is nausea and vomiting, with diarrhoea. *Related article:* FORTUM.

C

ceftizoxime is a broad-spectrum ANTIBIOTIC, one of the cephalosporins, used to treat a wide range of bacterial infections, particularly of the skin and soft tissues, the urinary tract, the genital organs, the lower respiratory tract, and the blood (septicaemia). It is also used to treat infection in patients whose immune systems are defective. Administration is by intravenous or intramuscular injection.

✚ warning: ceftizoxime should not be administered to patients who might be sensitive to penicillins in general and cephalosporins in particular. It should be administered with caution to those who suffer from impaired kidney function.

▲ side-effects: there may be sensitivity reactions – some of which may be serious. Alternatively, sometimes there is nausea and vomiting, with diarrhoea.
Related article: CEFIZOX.

cefuroxime is a broad-spectrum ANTIBIOTIC, one of the cephalosporins, used to treat a wide range of bacterial infections, particularly of the skin and soft tissues, the urinary tract, the upper respiratory tract, the genital organs, and the meninges (meningitis). It is also used to prevent infection during surgery. Administration is by intravenous or intramuscular injection.

✚ warning: cefuroxime should not be administered to patients who might be sensitive to penicillins in general and cephalosporins in particular, or to patients who are already taking certain diuretic drugs. It should be administered with caution to those who suffer from impaired kidney function, or who are pregnant.

▲ side-effects: there may be sensitivity reactions – some of which may be serious. Alternatively, sometimes there is nausea and vomiting, with diarrhoea.
Related article: ZINACEF.

Celbenin (*Beecham*) is a proprietary ANTIBIOTIC, available only on prescription, used to treat many forms of infection but particularly those caused by penicillin-resistant bacteria. Produced in the form of powder for reconstitution as injections, Celbenin is a preparation of methicillin sodium.

✚/▲ warning/side-effects: *see* METHICILLIN.

Celevac (*Boehringer Ingelheim*) is a proprietary non-prescription form of the type of LAXATIVE known as a bulking agent, which works by increasing the overall mass of faeces within the rectum, so stimulating bowel movement. It can thus be used to treat either constipation or diarrhoea, to control the consistency of faeces for patients with colostomy, and to reduce appetite in the medical treatment of obesity. Produced in the form of tablets and as granules for solution, Celevac represents a preparation of methylcellulose. (Celevac granules are not available from the National Health Service.)

✚/▲ warning/side-effects: *see* METHYLCELLULOSE.

Cellucon (*Medo*) is a proprietary non-prescription form of the type of LAXATIVE known as a bulking agent, which works by increasing the overall mass of faeces within the rectum, so stimulating bowel movement. It can thus be used to treat either constipation or diarrhoea, and to control the consistency of faeces for patients with colostomy. Produced in the

form of tablets, Cellucon represents a preparation of methylcellulose.
✚/▲warning/side-effects: *see* METHYLCELLULOSE.

Centrax (*Parke-Davis*) is a proprietary ANXIOLYTIC, available on prescription only to private patients. It is used to relieve nervous tension and anxiety in the short term. Produced in the form of tablets, Centrax is a preparation of the BENZODIAZEPINE prazepam. It is not recommended for children.
✚/▲warning/side-effects: *see* PRAZEPAM.

Centyl (*Burgess*) is a proprietary DIURETIC, available only on prescription, used – particularly in combination with ANTIHYPERTENSIVE drugs – to treat an accumulation of fluid in the tissues (oedema) and high blood pressure (hypertension). Produced in the form of tablets (in two strengths), Centyl is a preparation of bendrofluazide.
✚/▲warning/side-effects: *see* BENDROFLUAZIDE.

Centyl-K (*Burgess*) is a proprietary DIURETIC, available only on prescription, used to treat an accumulation of fluid in the tissues (oedema) and high blood pressure (hypertension). Produced in the form of tablets, Centyl-K is a preparation of bendrofluazide with a potassium supplement for sustained release.
✚/▲warning/side-effects: *see* BENDROFLUAZIDE.

cephalexin is a broad-spectrum ANTIBIOTIC, one of the cephalosporins, used to treat a wide range of bacterial infections, particularly of the skin and soft tissues, urinary tract, upper respiratory tract, and middle ear. Administration is oral in the form of capsules, tablets and liquids.
✚ warning: cephalexin should not be administered to patients who might be sensitive to penicillins in general and cephalosporins in particular. It should be administered with caution to those with impaired kidney function.
▲ side-effects: there may be sensitivity reactions – some of which may be serious. Sometimes there is nausea and vomiting, with diarrhoea.
Related articles: CEPOREX; KEFLEX.

cephalosporins are broad-spectrum ANTIBIOTICS used to treat a wide range of bacterial infections. In fact they generally have a wider range than the penicillins, to which they are chemically related. About one patient in ten of those who are sensitive to penicillins are also sensitive to cephalosporins. The drugs tend to interfere with the blood clotting factors of susceptible patients, particularly patients who are elderly or debilitated. Some cephalosporins are not absorbed and may thus be used to treat infections of the urinary tract during their own excretion. Administration is oral or by injection.
✚/▲warning/side-effects: *see* CEFACLOR; CEFADROXIL; CEFOTAXIME; CEFOXITIN; CEFSULODIN; CEFTAZIDIME; CEFTIZOXIME; CEFUROXIME; CEPHALEXIN; CEPHALOTHIN; CEPHAMANDOLE; CEPHAZOLIN; CEPHRADINE; LATAMOXEF DISODIUM.

cephalothin is a broad-spectrum ANTIBIOTIC, one of the cephalosporins, used to treat a wide range of bacterial infections, particularly of the skin and soft tissues, the urinary tract, upper respiratory tract, and middle ear. It is also used to prevent infection during surgery. Administration is by injection.

✚ warning: cephalothin should not be administered to patients who might be sensitive to penicillins in general and cephalosporins in particular, or to those with impaired kidney function.

▲ side-effects: there may be sensitivity reactions – some of which may be serious. Sometimes there is nausea and vomiting, with diarrhoea. *Related article:* KEFLIN.

cephamandole is a broad-spectrum ANTIBIOTIC, one of the cephalosporins, used to treat a wide range of bacterial infections, particularly of the skin and soft tissues, the urinary tract, upper respiratory tract, and middle ear. It is also used to prevent infection during surgery. Administration is by injection.

✚ warning: cephamandole should not be administered to patients who might be sensitive to penicillins in general and cephalosporins in particular. It should be administered with caution to those with impaired kidney function.

▲ side-effects: there may be sensitivity reactions – some of which may be serious. Sometimes there is nausea and vomiting, with diarrhoea. *Related article:* KEFADOL.

cephazolin is a broad-spectrum ANTIBIOTIC, one of the cephalosporins, used to treat a wide range of bacterial infections, particularly of the skin and soft tissues, urinary tract, upper respiratory tract, and middle ear. It is also used to prevent infection during surgery. Administration is by injection.

✚ warning: cephazolin should not be administered to patients who might be sensitive to penicillins in general and cephalosporins in particular. It should be administered with caution to those with impaired kidney function.

▲ side-effects: there may be sensitivity reactions – some of which may be serious. Sometimes there is nausea and vomiting, with diarrhoea. *Related article:* KEFZOL.

cephradine is a broad-spectrum ANTIBIOTIC, one of the cephalosporins, used to treat a wide range of bacterial infections, particularly of the skin and soft tissues, the urinary tract, upper respiratory tract, and middle ear. It is also used to prevent infection during surgery. Administration is oral in the form of capsules or a dilute syrup, or by injection.

✚ warning: cephradine should not be administered to patients who might be sensitive to penicillins in general and cephalosporins in particular. It should be administered with caution to those with impaired kidney function.

▲ side-effects: there may be sensitivity reactions – some of which may be serious. Sometimes there is nausea and vomiting, with diarrhoea. *Related article:* VELOSEF.

Ceporex (*Glaxo*) is a proprietary ANTIBIOTIC, available only on prescription, used to treat infections in the respiratory tract, urogenital area, soft tissues and middle ear. Produced in the form of capsules (in two strengths), as tablets (in two strengths), as drops for children,

as a suspension (in two strengths), and as a syrup (in three strengths) for dilution (the potency of the syrup once diluted is retained for 7 days), Ceporex is a preparation of the CEPHALOSPORIN cephalexin.
✚/▲ warning/side-effects: *see* CEPHALEXIN.

ceratonia is an adsorbent substance which, when mixed with starch and cocoa in a sugar-free mixture, may be taken orally to treat diarrhoea. It works by binding together faecal material into a mass.
Related article: AROBON.

Cerumol (*Laboratories for Applied Biology*) is a proprietary non-prescription preparation used to remove wax from the ear. Produced in the form of ear-drops, Cerumol's active constituent is the ANTIBACTERIAL/ANTIFUNGAL/astringent agent CHLORBUTOL.

Cervagem (*May & Baker*) is a proprietary preparation of the unusual drug gemeprost, available only on prescription. It is used for softening the neck of the womb (cervix) before local surgery, and is produced in the form of vaginal inserts (pessaries).
✚/▲ warning/side-effects: *see* GEMEPROST.

Cesamet (*Lilly*) is a proprietary ANTI-EMETIC, available only on prescription, used to treat nausea in patients undergoing chemical therapy in the treatment of cancer. Produced in the form of capsules, Cesamet's active constituent is the synthetic drug nabilone. It is not recommended for children.
✚/▲ warning/side-effects: *see* NABILONE.

Cetavlex (*Care*) is a proprietary non-prescription ANTISEPTIC, used to treat cuts and abrasions. Produced in the form of a water-based cream, Cetavlex's active constituent is CETRIMIDE.

Cetavlon (*ICI*) is a proprietary non-prescription DISINFECTANT, used to treat skin and scalp conditions, or in cleansing cuts and burns. Produced in the form of a solution, Cetavlon's active constituent is CETRIMIDE.

Cetavlon P.C. (*Care*) is a proprietary non-prescription DISINFECTANT, used to treat dandruff. Produced in the form of a solution to be used as a shampoo, Cetavlon P.C.'s active constituent is CETRIMIDE.

Cetiprin (*KabiVitrum*) is a proprietary ANTICHOLINERGIC, available only on prescription, used to treat bladder disorders and other conditions that cause frequent urination. Produced in the form of tablets, Cetiprin is a preparation of emepronium bromide. It is not recommended for children.
✚/▲ warning/side-effects: *see* EMEPRONIUM BROMIDE.

Cetriclens (*Smith & Nephew Medical*) is a proprietary non-prescription DISINFECTANT, used to clean skin and wounds. Produced in the form of a solution (in two strengths, the stronger under the name Cetriclens Forte), Cetriclens is a compound preparation of two antiseptics, CHLORHEXIDINE GLUCONATE and CETRIMIDE.

cetrimide is a detergent that has ANTISEPTIC properties; therapeutically, it is often combined with the antiseptic CHLORHEXIDINE. It is used in the form of a solution as a disinfectant for the skin and scalp, and in the form of a water-miscible cream as a soap substitute in the care of conditions such as acne and seborrhoea. In use, it should be kept away from the eyes and out of body cavities; some patients find it a mild skin irritant.

cetylpyridinium chloride in mild solution is used as a mouthwash or gargle for oral hygiene. *Related article:* MEROCET.

C-Film (*Arun*) is a proprietary non-prescription SPERMICIDAL contraceptive for use in combination with barrier methods of contraception (such as a condom). Produced in the form of a water-soluble film, C-Film is a preparation of an alcohol ester.

chalk may be used in a non-proprietary formulation ("chalk mixture") to assist in the treatment of diarrhoea. It works by acting as an adsorbent, binding together faecal material. Its bland taste has usually to be disguised with strongly pleasant-tasting or (especially in powdered form – "chalk powder") highly aromatic substances, and an adequate intake of fluids has also to be consciously maintained during treatment.

chalk with opium mixture is a non-proprietary formulation of spiced ("aromatic") chalk powder and MORPHINE in a sugary solution, used when taken orally to treat DIARRHOEA. The chalk is intended to adsorb faecal material, and the morphine to reduce motility within the colon. The mixture may cause sedation. Prolonged use may lead to dependence (addiction).

charcoal is an adsorbent material used medically for its adsorbency in either of two ways. Its primary use is in soaking up poisons in the stomach or small intestine – especially drug overdoses in cases when only a small quantity of the drug may be extremely toxic. Powdered, it is taken in solution, repeated as necessary. But its secondary use is as a constituent in antidiarrhoeal preparations, in which it is effective in binding together faecal material. In this use it is also effective in relieving flatulence.

***chelating agent** is any chemical compound which, when inside the body, binds to itself specific metallic ions before being excreted in the normal way. Chelating agents can thus be used to treat metal poisoning – poisoning by lead, for example. They may be incororated in barrier creams for industrial protection.

Chemocycline (*Consolidated*) is a proprietary ANTIBIOTIC, available only on prescription, used to treat any of many infections. Produced in the form of tablets and as a syrup for dilution (the potency of the syrup once dilute is retained for 14 days), Chemocycline is a preparation of the TETRACYCLINE oxytetracycline.

✚/▲ warning/side-effects: *see* OXYTETRACYCLINE.

Chemotrim Paed (*RP Drugs*) is a proprietary ANTIBACTERIAL, available only on prescription, used to treat infections of the respiratory and gastrointestinal tracts, and to assist in the treatment of skin infections. Produced in the form of a suspension specifically intended for children, Chemotrim Paed. is a compound combination of the SULPHONAMIDE sulphamethoxazole with trimethoprim – a compound itself known as co-trimoxazole.

It is not recommended for children aged under 6 weeks.
✚/▲ warning/side-effects: *see* SULPHAMETHOXAZOLE; TRIMETHOPRIM.

Chendol (*CP Pharmaceuticals*) is a proprietary preparation of chenodeoxycholic acid, available only on prescription, used to dissolve cholesterol gallstones that are radiolucent and not particularly large. Treatment is usually carried out in hospital under suitable monitoring. Produced in the form of capsules and as tablets, Chendol is not recommended for children.
✚/▲ warning/side-effects: *see* CHENODEOXYCHOLIC ACID.

Chenocedon (*Tillotts*) is a proprietary preparation of chenodeoxycholic acid, available only on prescription, used to dissolve cholesterol gallstones that are radiolucent and not particularly large. Treatment is usually carried out in hospital under suitable monitoring. Produced in the form of capsules, Chendocedon is not recommended for children.
✚/▲ warning/side-effects: *see* CHENODEOXYCHOLIC ACID.

chenodeoxycholic acid is an acid that has the capacity to dissolve some cholesterol gallstones in situ; the stones must not be particularly large and must be radiolucent – the drug does not affect radio-opaque calculi. It is used mainly in patients who prefer medical to surgical treatment, or for whom surgery is inadvisable. In one in four patients treated with the acid, however, gallstones recur within 12 months.
Administration is oral in the form of capsules or tablets.
✚ warning: chenodeoxycholic acid should not be administered to patients whose stones are large or radio-opaque or impair gall bladder function; those with chronic liver disease or inflammatory disorders of the intestines; or who are pregnant. Frequent monitoring is essential: treatment should take place in hospital.
▲ side-effects: there is diarrhoea and itching; some patients experience mild dysfunction of the liver.
Related articles: CHENDOL; CHENOCEDON; CHENOFALK.

Chenofalk (*Thames*) is a proprietary preparation of chenodeoxycholic acid, available only on prescription, used to dissolve cholesterol gallstones that are radiolucent and not particularly large. Treatment is usually carried out in hospital under suitable monitoring. Produced in the form of capsules, Chenofalk is not recommended for children.
✚/▲ warning/side-effects: *see* CHENODEOXYCHOLIC ACID.

Chiron (*Downs*) is a proprietary non-prescription barrier cream containing an ANTISEPTIC, used to protect and keep clean a stoma (an outlet on the skin surface following the surgical curtailment of the intestines).

Chironair (*Downs*) is a proprietary non-prescription deodorant solution to be inserted into the appliance or bag that is attached to a stoma (an outlet on the skin surface following the surgical curtailment of the intestines).

Chloractil (*DDSA Pharmaceuticals*) is a proprietary preparation of the powerful PHENOTHIAZINE drug chlorpromazine hydrochloride, used primarily as a major TRANQUILLIZER in patients who are undergoing behavioural disturbances, or who are psychotic (*see* ANTIPSYCHOTIC) particularly schizophrenic. More mundanely, it is used to treat severe anxiety, or as an anti-emetic sedative prior to surgery. Available only on prescription, Chloractil is produced in the form of tablets (in three strengths).

✚/▲ warning/side-effects: *see* CHLORPROMAZINE HYDROCHLORIDE.

chloral hydrate is a water-soluble SEDATIVE and HYPNOTIC that is uncommonly rapid-acting. It is particularly useful in inducing sleep in children or elderly patients, although the drug must be administered in very mild solution in order to minimize gastric irritation. Administration is thus usually oral, although it can alternatively be rectal. Overdosage results in toxic effects; prolonged use may lead to dependence (addiction).

✚ warning: chloral hydrate should not be administered to patients with severe heart disease, inflammation of the stomach, or impaired function of the liver or kidneys. It should be administered with caution to those with lung disease and respiratory depression, who are pregnant or lactating, who are elderly or debilitated, or who have a history of drug abuse. Contact with skin or mucous membranes should be avoided.

▲ side-effects: concentration and speed of thought and movement are affected. There is often drowsiness and dizziness, with dry mouth. Sensitivity reactions are also fairly common, especially in the form of rashes. Susceptible patients may experience excitement or confusion.

Related article: NOCTEC.

chlorambucil is a CYTOTOXIC drug used in the treatment of cancer, particularly leukaemia, the lymphatic cancer Hodgkin's disease, and cancer of the ovaries. It works by interfering with the DNA of new cells, so preventing normal cell replication. However, the drug can also be used as an IMMUNOSUPPRESSANT in connection with rheumatoid arthritis. Administration is oral in the form of tablets.

✚ warning: almost all men are rendered permanently sterile early in treatment although potency is unaffected, and prolonged treatment may cause an early menopause in women. Regular and frequent blood counts are essential.

▲ side-effects: there may be nausea and vomiting; there may also be hair loss and rashes. The capacity of the bone-marrow to produce red blood cells is markedly reduced.

Related article: LEUKERAN.

chloramphenicol is an ANTIBIOTIC that is produced both by derivation from a micro-organism and by synthetic means. It has the capacity to treat many forms of infection effectively, but the serious side-effects that accompany its systemic use demand that it is ordinarily restricted to the treatment of severe infection (such as typhoid fever) after less toxic drugs have failed. In topical application to the eyes, ears or skin, however, the drug is useful in treating such conditions as bacterial conjunctivitis, otitis externa, or many types of skin infection. Topical administration is in the form of eye-drops, ear-drops or a cream. Systemic administration is oral in the form of capsules or a dilute suspension, or by injection or infusion.

✚ warning: chloramphenicol should not be administered to patients who are pregnant or lactating; it should be administered with caution to those with impaired liver or kidney function. In forms for topical application, it should be kept away from open wounds. Prolonged or repeated use should be avoided. Regular blood counts are essential.

▲ side-effects: sensitivity reactions are not uncommon. Systemic treatment may cause serious changes in blood composition with resultant neural damage. There may be nausea and vomiting, with diarrhoea.

Related articles: CHLOROMYCETIN; KEMICETINE; MINIMS; OPULETS; SNO PHENICOL.

Chlorasept 2000 (*Travenol*) is a proprietary disinfectant, available only on prescription, used to cleanse skin and wounds. Produced in sachets of solution (in five strengths), Chlorasept 2000 is a preparation of CHLORHEXIDINE acetate.

Chloraseptic (*Norwich Eaton*) is a proprietary non-prescription disinfectant, used to treat minor mouth and gum disorders, sore throats and mouth ulcers. Produced in the form of a solution for application with a spray or as a gargle, Chloraseptic is a preparation of PHENOL. It is not recommended for children aged under 6 years.

Chlorasol (*Schering-Prebbles*) is a proprietary non-prescription disinfectant and cleanser, used to treat skin infections, and especially in cleansing wounds and ulcers. Produced in the form of a solution in sachets, Chlorasol is a preparation of SODIUM HYPOCHLORITE.

chlorbutol is an ANTIBACTERIAL and ANTIFUNGAL agent that also has astringent and even mildly SEDATIVE properties. It is used in eye-drops and ear-drops, in powder form for topical use, as a constituent in motion sickness preparations, and as a preservative in injection solutions.

Related articles: ASMA-VYDRIN; AURALGICIN; CERUMOL.

chlordiazepoxide is an ANXIOLYTIC drug, one of the BENZODIAZEPINES, used to treat anxiety in the short or long term, and to assist in the treatment of acute alcohol withdrawal symptoms. It may also be used as a SKELETAL MUSCLE RELAXANT. Continued use results in tolerance and may lead to dependence (addiction). Administration is oral in the form of capsules and tablets.

✚ warning: chlordiazepoxide should be administered with caution to patients with respiratory difficulties, glaucoma, or kidney or liver impairment; who are in the last stages of pregnancy; or who are elderly, debilitated, or have a history of drug abuse. Prolonged use or abrupt withdrawal of treatment should be avoided.

▲ side-effects: concentration and speed of thought and movement may be affected; the effects of alcohol consumption may also be enhanced. There may be drowsiness, dizziness, headache, dry mouth and

C

shallow breathing; hypersensitivity reactions may occur.
Related articles: LIBRIUM; TROPIUM.

chlorhexidine is an ANTISEPTIC that is a constituent in many DISINFECTANT preparations, for use especially prior to surgery or in obstetrics, but that is primarily used (in the form of chlorhexidine gluconate, chlorhexidine acetate or chlorhexidine hydrochloride) either as a mouth wash for oral hygiene, or as a dressing for minor skin wounds and infections; it is also used for instillation in the bladder to relieve minor infections.
✚ warning: caution should be exercised in assessing suitable solution concentration for bladder instillation: too high a concentration may lead to the appearance of blood in the urine. Avoid contact with mucous membranes.
▲ side-effects: some patients experience sensitivity reactions.
Related articles: BACTICLENS; BACTIGRAS; CETRICLENS; CHLORASEPT 2000; CORSODIL; CYTEAL; DISPRAY 1 QUICK PREP; ELUDRIL; HIBIDIL; HIBISCRUB; HIBISOL; HIBITANE; INSTILLAGEL; NASEPTIN; NYSTAFORM; pHISO-MED; ROTERSEPT; SAVLOCLENS; SAVLODIL; SAVLON HOSPITAL CONCENTRATE; TISEPT; TRAVASEPT; UNISEPT; URO-TAINER; XYLOCAINE.

chlorinated lime and boric acid solution is a non-proprietary formulation designed for topical application to disinfect and cleanse wounds and ulcers. It is applied as a wet dressing.

chlorinated soda solution is a non-proprietary formulation designed for topical application to disinfect and cleanse wounds and ulcers. Containing boric acid, it is an irritant solution and surrounding tissues should be protected with a layer of petroleum jelly during treatment.

chlormethiazole is a HYPNOTIC drug that also has ANTICONVULSANT properties. It is useful in treating severe insomnia, epilepsy, and for quieting agitated elderly patients, and it is also used under strict medical supervision in the treatment of the withdrawal symptoms of alcohol. Occasionally it is used in the operating theatre as an additional sedative anaesthetic. Administration (in the form of chlormethiazole edisylate) is oral as capsules or dilute syrup, or by injection or infusion.
✚ warning: chlormethiazole should be administered with caution to patients with restricted breathing, or impaired liver or kidney function, who are pregnant or lactating, who are elderly or debilitated, or who have a history of drug abuse. Prolonged use should be avoided; withdrawal of treatment should be gradual.
▲ side-effects: there may be headache, sneezing and gastrointestinal disturbance. High dosage by intravenous infusion may cause depressed breathing and reduced heart rate, and presents a risk of thrombophlebitis.
Related article: HEMINEVRIN.

chlormezanone is an ANXIOLYTIC drug that has HYPNOTIC properties and may also be used as a SKELETAL MUSCLE RELAXANT. It is thus used to treat anxiety and tension in the short term (including premenstrual syndrome), to induce sleep and to relieve muscle spasm. Administration is oral in the form of tablets.

✚ warning: chlormezanone should be administered with caution to patients with respiratory difficulties, closed angle glaucoma, or kidney or liver disease; who are in the last stages of pregnancy; or who are elderly or debilitated. Prolonged use or abrupt withdrawal of treatment should be avoided.

▲ side-effects: concentration and speed of thought and movement may be affected; the effects of alcohol consumption may also be enhanced. There may be drowsiness, dizziness, headache, dry mouth and shallow breathing; hypersensitivity reactions may occur.

Related article: TRANCOPAL.

Chloromycetin (*Parke-Davis*) is a proprietary broad-spectrum ANTIBIOTIC, available only on prescription, used to treat potentially dangerous bacterial infections, such as typhoid fever and meningitis. Produced in the form of capsules, as a suspension for dilution (the potency of the dilute suspension is retained for 14 days), as eye-ointment and eye-drops, as a powder, and in vials for injection, Chloromycetin is a preparation of chloramphenicol.

✚/▲ warning/side-effects: *see* CHLORAMPHENICOL.

Chloromycetin Hydrocortisone (*Parke-Davis*) is a proprietary ANTIBIOTIC and CORTICOSTEROID preparation, available only on prescription, used to treat eye infections. Produced in the form of an eye ointment, Chloromycetin Hydrocortisone contains the antibiotic chloramphenicol and the steroid hydrocortisone.

✚/▲ warning/side-effects: *see* CHLORAMPHENICOL; HYDROCORTISONE.

chloroquine is the major ANTIMALARIAL drug in use, effective against virtually all forms of the malarial organism, Plasmodium, and used both to treat and to prevent contraction of the disease. However, it does not kill those organisms who migrate to the liver, and thus cannot prevent relapses caused by any form of Plasmodium that does so. Moreover, several strains of Plasmodium have recently exhibited resistance to chloroquine in certain areas of the world, and in those areas alternative therapy is now advised. Chloroquine is sometimes also used to treat infection caused by amoebae, or to halt the progress of rheumatic disease. Administration is oral in the form of tablets or a dilute syrup, or by injection or infusion.

✚ warning: chloroquine should not be administered to patients with retinal disease, or who are allergic to quinine; it should be administered with caution to patients with porphyria, psoriasis, or who have impaired kidney or liver function; who are elderly; or who are children. Prolonged treatment should be punctuated by ophthalmic checks.

▲ side-effects: there may be nausea and vomiting, with headache and itching; gastrointestinal disturbance may be severe; some patients break out in a rash. Susceptible patients may undergo psychotic episodes. Prolonged high dosage may cause ringing in the ears

(tinnitus) and damage to the cornea and retina of the eyes.
Related articles: AVLOCLOR; MALARIVON; NIVAQUINE.

chlorothiazide is a DIURETIC, one of the THIAZIDES, used to treat fluid retention in the tissues (oedema), high blood pressure (hypertension) and mild to moderate heart failure. Because all thiazides tend to deplete body reserves of potassium, chlorothiazide may be administered in combination either with potassium supplements or with diuretics that are complementarily potassium-sparing.
Administration is oral in the form of tablets.
✚ warning: chlorothiazide should not be administered to patients with kidney failure or urinary retention, or who are lactating. It should be administered with caution to those who are pregnant. It may aggravate conditions of diabetes or gout.
▲ side-effects: there may be tiredness and a rash. In men, temporary impotence may occur.
Related article: SALURIC.

chloroxylenol is an antiseptic effective in killing some bacteria but not others, and is an established constituent in at least one well-known skin disinfectant. A few patients experience mild skin irritation that may lead to sensitivity reactions, however.
Related article: DETTOL.

chlorpheniramine is an ANTIHISTAMINE, used to treat the symptoms of allergic conditions like hay fever and urticaria; it is also sometimes used in emergencies to treat anaphylactic shock. Administration (as chlorpheniramine maleate) is oral in the form of tablets, sustained-release tablets and a dilute syrup, or by injection.
✚ warning: chlorpheniramine maleate should not be administered to patients who are pregnant, or who have glaucoma, urinary retention, intestinal obstruction, enlargement of the prostate gland, or peptic ulcer; it should be administered with caution to those with epilepsy or liver disease.
▲ side-effects: concentration and speed of thought and movement may be affected. There may be nausea, headaches, and/or weight gain, dry mouth, gastrointestinal disturbances and visual problems. Treatment by injection may cause tissue irritation that leads to a temporary drop in blood pressure.
Related articles: ALUNEX; PIRITON.

chlorpromazine is an ANTIPSYCHOTIC drug used as a major TRANQUILLIZER for patients suffering from schizophrenia and other psychoses, particularly during behavioural disturbances. The drug may also be used in the short term to treat severe anxiety, to soothe patients who are dying, as a premedication prior to surgery, and to remedy an intractable hiccup. It may also be used to relieve nausea and vertigo caused by disorders in the middle or inner ear.
Administration (as chlorpromazine hydrochloride) is oral in the form of tablets or an elixir, as anal suppositories, or by intramuscular injection.
✚ warning: chlorpromazine hydrochloride should not be administered to patients with certain forms of glaucoma, whose blood-cell formation by

the bone-marrow is reduced, or who are taking drugs that depress certain centres of the brain and spinal cord. It should be administered with caution to those with lung disease, cardiovascular disease, epilepsy, parkinsonism, abnormal secretion by the adrenal glands, impaired liver or kidney function, undersecretion of thyroid hormones (hypothyroidism), enlargement of the prostate gland, or any form of acute infection; who are pregnant or lactating; or who are elderly. Prolonged use requires regular checks on eye function and skin pigmentation. Withdrawal of treatment should be gradual.

▲ side-effects: concentration and speed of thought and movement are affected; the effects of alcohol consumption are enhanced. There may be dry mouth and blocked nose, constipation and difficulty in urinating, and blurred vision; menstrual disturbances in women or impotence in men may occur, with weight gain; there may be sensitivity reactions. Some patients feel cold and depressed, and tend to suffer from poor sleep patterns. Blood pressure may be low and the heartbeat irregular. Prolonged high dosage may cause opacity in the cornea and lens of the eyes, and a purple pigmentation of the skin. Treatment by intramuscular injection may be painful.

Related articles: CHLORACTIL; DOZINE; LARGACTIL.

chlorpropamide is a SULPHONYLUREA, used in the treatment of adult-onset diabetes mellitus because it promotes the production of insulin in whatever remains of the pancreas's capacity for it. Its effect lasts longer than that of most similar drugs. Unusually for a sulphonylurea, chlorpropamide can also be used to treat diabetes insipidus, although only mild cases caused by pituitary or thalamic malfunction, because it also reduces frequency of urination. Administration is oral in the form of tablets.

✚ warning: chlorpropamide should not be administered to patients with liver or kidney disease, endocrine disorders, or who are under stress; who are pregnant or lactating; who are already taking corticosteroids or oral contraceptives, oral anticoagulants, or aspirin and other antibiotics.

▲ side-effects: there may be some sensitivity reactions (such as a rash). There may also be mild gastrointestinal disturbance or headache. The consumption of alcohol may cause flushing.

Related articles: DIABINESE; GLYMESE.

chlorprothixene is an ANTIPSYCHOTIC drug used as a major TRANQUILLIZER in patients suffering from schizophrenia and other psychoses, particularly during behavioural disturbances. The drug may also be used in the short term to treat severe anxiety. Administration is oral in the form of tablets. It is not suitable for children.

✚ warning: chlorprothixene should not be administered to patients with certain forms of glaucoma, whose blood-cell formation by the bone-marrow is reduced, or who are taking drugs that depress certain centres of the brain and spinal cord. It should be administered with caution to those with lung disease, cardiovascular disease, epilepsy, parkinsonism, abnormal secretion by the adrenal glands, impaired liver or kidney function, undersecretion of thyroid hormones (hypothyroidism), enlargement of the prostate gland or any form of acute infection; who are pregnant or lactating; or who are elderly. Prolonged use requires regular checks on eye function and skin pigmentation. Withdrawal of treatment should be gradual.

▲ side-effects: concentration and speed of thought and movement are affected; the effects of alcohol consumption are enhanced. There may be dry mouth and blocked nose, constipation and difficulty in urinating, and blurred vision; menstrual disturbances in women or impotence in men may occur, with weight gain; there may be sensitivity reactions. Some patients feel cold and depressed, and tend to suffer from poor sleep patterns. Blood pressure may be low and the heartbeat irregular. Prolonged high dosage may cause opacity in the cornea and lens of the eyes, and a purple pigmentation of the skin. Treatment by intramuscular injection may be painful.

Related article: TARACTAN.

chlortetracycline is a broad-spectrum ANTIBIOTIC used to treat many forms of infection caused by any of several types of micro-organism; conditions it is particularly used to treat include infections of the urinary tract, of the respiratory tract, in and around the eye, of the genital organs, and of the skin, including acne and impetigo. Administration (as chlortetracycline hydrochloride) is oral in the form of capsules or a solution, or topical in the form of a cream, an ointment, and an ophthalmic ointment.

✚ warning: chlortetracycline should not be administered systemically to patients who are aged under 12 years, who are pregnant, or with impaired kidney function; it should be administered with caution to those who are lactating. The cream and the ointment may stain fabric.

▲ side-effects: there may be nausea and vomiting, with diarrhoea. Occasionally, there is sensitivity to light or some other sensitivity reaction. These side-effects may still occur even if the causative organism of the disorder proves to be resistant to the drug.

Related article: AUREOMYCIN.

chlorthalidone is a DIURETIC related to the THIAZIDES, used to treat fluid retention in the tissues (oedema), high blood pressure (hypertension) and diabetes insipidus. Because all thiazides tend to deplete body reserves of potassium, chlorthalidone may be administered in combination either with potassium supplements or with diuretics that are complementarily potassium-sparing. Administration is oral in the form of tablets.

✚ warning: chlorthalidone should not be administered to patients with kidney failure or urinary retention, or who are lactating. It should be administered with caution to those who are pregnant. It may aggravate conditions of diabetes or gout.

▲ side-effects: there may be tiredness and a rash. In men,

temporary impotence may occur.
Related article: HYGROTON.

Chocovite (*Medo*) is a proprietary non-prescription CALCIUM supplement that is not available from the National Health Service. Produced in the form of tablets, Chocovite contains CALCIUM GLUCONATE and a form of CALCIFEROL (vitamin D).

cholecalciferol is one of the natural forms of calciferol (vitamin D), formed in humans by the action of sunlight on the skin.
see CALCIFEROL.

Choledyl (*Parke-Davis*) is a proprietary non-prescription BRONCHODILATOR, used to treat bronchitis and asthma. Produced in the form of tablets (in two strengths) and as a syrup for dilution (the potency of the syrup once diluted is retained for 14 days), Choledyl is a preparation of choline theophyllinate. It is not recommended for children aged under 3 years.
✚/▲ warning/side-effects: *see* CHOLINE THEOPHYLLINATE.

cholera vaccine is a suspension containing non-infective versions of the bacteria that cause the dangerous intestinal epidemic disease cholera. Administration is initially by subcutaneous or intramuscular injection, followed 2 to 4 weeks later by a booster shot. The vaccine cannot guarantee total protection, and travellers should be warned still to take great care over the hygiene of the food and drink they consume. In any case, what protection is afforded lasts only for about 6 months.

cholestyramine is a resin which, when taken orally, binds to itself bile salts in the intestines that can then be excreted in the normal way. This is a useful property in the treatment of high blood fat, especially cholesterol, levels (hyperlipidaemia), and of the itching associated with obstruction in the bile ducts. The property can also be utilized in the treatment of diarrhoea following intestinal disease or surgery. Administration is oral in the form of a powder taken with liquids.
✚ warning: cholestyramine should not be administered to patients who suffer from complete blockage of the bile ducts, who are already taking any other drug, or who are pregnant. High dosage may require simultaneous administration of fat-soluble vitamins.
▲ side-effects: there may be nausea, heartburn, flatulence with abdominal discomfort, constipation or diarrhoea, and a rash.
Related article: QUESTRAN.

choline is a natural compound used in the body in the synthesis of various forms of protein and of the neurotransmitter acetylcholine. It is also essential to the transportation of fats within the body. Because it is synthesized in the body, however, it cannot really be classed as a vitamin (of the B group) as some authorities would specify.

choline magnesium trisalicylate is an non-narcotic ANALGESIC with ANTI-INFLAMMATORY properties very similar to aspirin, used to treat the pain and inflammation of rheumatic disease and other musculo-skeletal disorders. Administration is oral in the form of tablets.
✚ warning: choline magnesium trisalicylate should not be

administered to patients who are aged under 12 years, or who have peptic ulcers; it should be administered with caution to those with impaired liver or kidney function, dehydration or any form of allergy, who are pregnant or lactating, who are elderly, or who are already taking oral anticoagulant drugs.

▲ side-effects: there may be gastrointestinal problems involving ulceration or bleeding, nausea, and disturbances in hearing and in vision; some patients experience serious sensitivity reactions.
Related article: TRILISATE.

choline salicylate is a mild ANALGESIC and local ANAESTHETIC that is used primarily in topical application in the mouth or in the ears. In the mouth it may be used to relieve the pain of teething, of aphthous ulcers or of minor scratches. Administration is in the form of an oral gel or ear-drops.

✚ warning: prolonged treatment may result in salicylate poisoning.
Related articles: AUDAX; BONJELA; TEEJEL.

choline theophyllinate is a modified form of the BRONCHODILATOR theophylline used to treat conditions such as asthma and bronchitis. It is thought to be slightly better tolerated than theophylline. Administration is oral in the form of tablets, sustained-release tablets, or a dilute syrup.

✚ warning: treatment should initially be gradually progressive in the quantity administered. Choline theophyllinate should be administered with caution to epileptics, and patients with heart or liver disease, or a peptic ulcer; or who are pregnant or lactating.

▲ side-effects: there may be nausea and gastrointestinal disturbances, and increase or irregularity in the heartbeat, and/or insomnia.
Related articles: CHOLEDYL; SABIDAL SR 270.

Choloxin (*Travenol*) is a proprietary form of the drug dextrothyroxine sodium, available only on prescription, used to treat high blood levels of fats (hyperlipidaemia). It is no longer the drug of choice because of the possibility of its causing heart problems.

✚/▲ warning/side-effects: *see* DEXTROTHYROXINE SODIUM.

cho/vac is an abbreviation for cholera vaccine.
see CHOLERA VACCINE.

Chymar (*Armour*) is a proprietary preparation of the digestive enzyme alpha-chymotrypsin, available only on prescription, used therapeutically to help treat inflammation and fluid retention (oedema). It is thought to work by facilitating the removal of coagulated blood and cellular debris from sites of inflammation, and is produced in the form of powder for reconstitution as a medium for intramuscular injections.

✚/▲ warning/side-effects: *see* CHYMOTRYPSIN.

Chymar-Zon (*Armour*) is a proprietary form of an enzymatic preparation used to dissolve the little ligament that suspends the lens of the eye within the eyeball (the zonule of Zinn) in order to facilitate the surgical removal of a lens that has become opaque through cataract. Available only on prescription, Chymar-Zon is produced as a powder for reconstitution as a medium for injection; the fluid – in which the active constituent is alpha-chymotrypsin – is injected behind the iris a minute or so before the lens is removed, and affects no other part of the eye.

✚/▲ warning/side-effects: *see* CHYMOTRYPSIN.

Chymocyclar (*Armour*) is a proprietary tetracycline ANTIBIOTIC, available only on prescription, used to treat many forms of infection. Produced in the form of capsules, Chymocyclar contains tetracycline hydrochloride and the pancreatic enzymes trypsin and chymotrypsin. It is not recommended for children.

✚/▲ warning/side-effects: *see* CHYMOTRYPSIN; TETRACYCLINE; TRYPSIN.

Chymoral (*Armour*) is a proprietary non-prescription enzymatic preparation, used to treat acute inflammatory fluid retention (oedema). It is thought to work by facilitating the removal of coagulated blood and cellular debris from sites of inflammation. Produced in the form of tablets (in two strengths, the stronger under the name Chymoral Forte), Chymoral contains the enzymes trypsin and alpha-chymotrypsin.

✚/▲ warning/side-effects: *see* CHYMOTRYPSIN; TRYPSIN.

chymotrypsin is a protein-digesting enzyme secreted in one form by the pancreas and converted into another within the duodenum by the presence of the other enzyme trypsin. It has more than one therapeutic use. Its primary use is in treating inflammation, especially in conditions of fluid retention (oedema), in which it is thought to work by facilitating the removal of coagulated blood and cellular debris from sites of inflammation. But it is also used very specifically as the medium to dissolve the tiny ligament that suspends the lens within the eyeball in surgery to remove the lens because of cataract. Administration is oral in the form of tablets, or by injection.

✚ warning: chymotrypsin should be administered with caution to patients who are already taking oral anticoagulants. Injection should not take place before testing a patient for sensitivity.

▲ side-effects: there may be nausea and vomiting, with diarrhoea. Some patients experience sensitivity reactions – which may be serious.

Related articles: CHYMAR; CHYMAR-ZON; CHYMORAL; DEANASE D.C.

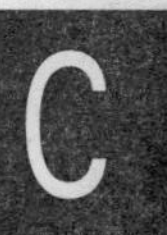

Cicatrin (*Calmic*) is a proprietary ANTIBIOTIC drug, available only on prescription, used in topical application to treat skin infections. Produced in the form of a cream, as a dusting-powder and as an aerosol powder-spray, Cicatrin's major active constituents include the antiseptics neomycin sulphate and bacitracin zinc.

✚/▲ warning/side-effects: *see* NEOMYCIN.

ciclacillin is an ANTIBIOTIC, a PENICILLIN used to treat infections of the upper respiratory tract, of the urinary tract, and of the soft tissues. Administration is oral in the form of tablets or a dilute suspension.

✚ warning: ciclacillin should not be administered to patients known to be allergic to penicillins; it should be administered with caution to

those with impaired kidney function.
▲ side-effects: the drug may cause diarrhoea if given in tablet form; there may be sensitivity reactions ranging from a minor rash to urticaria and joint pains, and (occasionally) to high temperature and anaphylactic shock. High dosage may in any case cause convulsions.
Related article: CALTHOR.

Cidomycin (*Roussel*) is a proprietary ANTIBIOTIC, available only on prescription, used to treat many forms of infection. Produced in ampoules for injection (in two strengths), in vials for the treatment of children, in ampoules for intrathecal injections, as a powder for reconstitution as a medium for injection, as ear- and eye-drops, as an eye ointment, and as a cream and an ointment for topical application, Cidomycin is a preparation of the aminoglycoside gentamicin sulphate.
✚/▲ warning/side-effects: *see* GENTAMICIN.

Cidomycin Topical (*Roussel*) is a proprietary ANTIBIOTIC preparation, available only on prescription, used in topical application to treat skin infections. Produced in the form of a water-miscible cream and a paraffin-based ointment, Cidomycin Topical is a preparation of gentamicin sulphate.
✚/▲ warning/side-effects: *see* GENTAMICIN.

cimetidine is an ulcer healing drug that reduces the secretion of gastric acids, and is thus used primarily to assist in the healing of peptic ulcers in the stomach and duodenum. It works by blocking histamine H_2 receptors. It is well tolerated, and side-effects are comparatively rare. Administration is oral in the form of tablets or a dilute syrup, or by injection or infusion.
✚ warning: cimetidine should be administered with caution to patients with impaired liver or kidney function. Treatment of undiagnosed dyspepsia may potentially mask the onset of stomach or duodenal cancer and is therefore undesirable.
▲ side-effects: the drug may enhance the effects of benzodiazepines or beta-blockers taken simultaneously. In men, because the drug also affects androgen receptors, there may be some minor and temporary feminization. In elderly patients there may be mild (and reversible) confusion.
Related article: TAGAMET.

cinchocaine is a local ANAESTHETIC used to relieve pain particularly in dental surgery, but also in topical application to the skin or mucous membranes. It can also be injected into the spinal membranes to effect epidural anaesthesia. Administration is thus in the form of an ointment or by injection.
▲ side-effects: there may be nausea, vomiting and diarrhoea; some patients experience yawning or excitement. Rarely, there are sensitivity reactions.
Related article: NUPERCAINAL.

cinnarizine is an ANTIHISTAMINE used primarily as an ANTI-EMETIC in the treatment or prevention of motion sickness and vomiting caused either by chemotherapy for cancer or by infection of the middle or inner ear. But it is also a VASODILATOR that affects the blood vessels of the hands and feet and may also be used to improve circulation in those areas. Administration is oral in the form of tablets. Not recommended for children under 6 years.

✚ warning: cinnarizine should be administered with caution to patients with epilepsy, liver disease, glaucoma or enlargement of the prostate gland. Drowsiness may be increased by alcohol consumption.

▲ side-effects: concentration and speed of thought and movement may be affected. There is commonly drowsiness and dry mouth; there may also be headache, blurred vision and gastrointestinal disturbances.
Related article: STUGERON.

Cinobac (*Lilly*) is a proprietary ANTIBACTERIAL drug, available only on prescription, used primarily to treat infections in the urinary tract. Produced in the form of capsules, Cinobac is a preparation of cinoxacin. It is not recommended for children.

✚/▲ warning/side-effects: *see* CINOXACIN.

cinoxacin is an ANTIBACTERIAL drug used primarily to treat infections in the urinary tract. Administration is oral in the form of capsules.

✚ warning: cinoxacin should be administered with caution to patients with even only slightly impaired kidney function.

▲ side-effects: there may be nausea and vomiting, with gastrointestinal distrubances and weight loss, diarrhoea and cramps. Some patients experience sensitivity reactions, including a rash, dizziness, a headache and tinnitus.
Related article: CINOBAC.

cisplatin is an unusual CYTOTOXIC drug that contains an organic complex of platinum. It works by damaging the DNA of newly-forming cells, and is used to treat cancers that are metastatic and have failed to respond to other forms of therapy, particularly cancers of the testes or ovaries. Side-effects may be severe. Administration is by injection.

✚ warning: cisplatin should be administered with caution to patients with impaired kidney function. Regular, frequent monitoring of blood levels is essential, and specialist consultancy is advised at all times during treatment.

▲ side-effects: there is severe nausea and vomiting. There may also be disturbances in hearing, loss of sensation at the fingertips, and reduced blood levels in many normal factors. Toxic effects may require withdrawal of treatment.
Related articles: NEOPLATIN; PLATINEX; PLATOSIN.

Citanest (*Astra*) is a proprietary local ANAESTHETIC, available only on prescription. Produced in vials (in two strengths) for injection, Citanest is a preparation of prilocaine hydrochloride.

✚/▲ warning/side-effects: *see* PRILOCAINE.

Citanest with Octapressin (*Astra*) is a proprietary local ANAESTHETIC, available only on prescription, used as a dental anaesthetic and as premedication before surgery. Produced in cartridges and self-aspirating cartridges for injection (in two strengths), Citanest with Octapressin contains prilocaine hydrochloride and the minor VASOCONSTRICTOR felypressin.

✚/▲ warning/side-effects: *see* PRILOCAINE.

Claforan (*Roussel*) is a proprietary ANTIBIOTIC preparation, available only on prescription, used to treat many forms of infection, including meningitis. Produced in vials as a powder for reconstitution as a medium for injection, Claforan is a preparation of the CEPHALOSPORIN cefotaxime.
✚/▲ warning/side-effects: *see* CEFOTAXIME.

Clairvan (*Sinclair*) is a proprietary respiratory stimulant, available only on prescription, used to treat patients about to lapse into unconsciousness or coma and who are unable, for one reason or another, to tolerate the more usual forms of ventilatory support. Produced in the form of a solution to be taken orally, and in ampoules for injection, Clairvan's active constituent is ethamivan.
✚/▲ warning/side-effects: *see* ETHAMIVAN.

Claradin (*Nicholas*) is a proprietary non-prescription non-narcotic ANALGESIC that is not available from the National Health Service; it can be used to treat rheumatic pain and high body temperature. Produced in the form of effervescent tablets, Claradin is a preparation of ASPIRIN. It is not recommended for children under 12 years.

clavulanic acid is an enzymatic substance which has the effect of inhibiting bacterial resistance in bacteria that have become resistant to some penicillin-type antibiotics, notably amoxycillin and ticarcillin. It is therefore used in combination with amoxycillin or ticarcillin to treat infective conditions in which the penicillin alone might be unsuccessful, and has the additional effect of extending the activity of the antibiotic.
Related articles: AUGMENTIN; TIMENTIN.

clemastine is an ANTIHISTAMINE used in the relief of allergic disorders such as hay fever, urticaria and some rashes. Administration is oral in the form of tablets or a dilute elixir.
✚ warning: clemastine should not be administered to patients who are pregnant, or with glaucoma, urinary retention, intestinal obstruction, enlargement of the prostate gland, or peptic ulcer; it should be administered with caution to those with epilepsy or liver disease.
▲ side-effects: concentration and speed of thought and movement may be affected; there may be nausea, headaches, and/or weight gain, dry mouth, gastrointestinal disturbances and visual problems.
Related articles: ALLER-EZE; TAVEGIL.

clindamycin is an ANTIBIOTIC used to treat infections of bones and joints, and to assist in the treatment of peritonitis (inflammation of the peritoneal lining of the abdominal cavity). Administration is oral in the form of capsules or a dilute suspension, or by injection.
✚ warning: clindamycin should not be administered to patients suffering from diarrhoea; and if diarrhoea or other symptoms of colitis appear during treatment, administration must be halted at once. This is because clindamycin's comparatively high toxicity is especially disposed towards promoting colitis (particularly in mature

or elderly women), causing potentially severe symptoms. It should be administered with caution to those with impaired liver or kidney function.

▲ side-effects: if diarrhoea or other symptoms of colitis appear during treatment, administration must be halted at once (see above). There may also be nausea and vomiting. *Related article:* DALACIN C.

Clinicide (*De Witt*) is a proprietary non-prescription preparation used to treat scalp and pubic infestations of lice (pediculosis). Produced in the form of a lotion, Clinicide's active constituent is CARBARYL.

Clinifeed (*Roussel*) is a proprietary non-prescription nutritionally complete feed, used as a dietary supplement for patients whose metabolic processes are unable to break down protein. Produced in four formulations, Clinifeed contains protein, carbohydrate, fat and vitamins and minerals, but it is free of gluten. It is unsuitable for children aged under 12 months.

Clinitar (*Smith & Nephew Pharmaceuticals*) is a proprietary non-prescription medicated shampoo used to treat dandruff and psoriasis: its active constituent is COAL TAR.

Clinitar Cream (*Smith & Nephew Pharmaceuticals*) is a proprietary non-prescription tar preparation, used in topical application to treat severe non-infective skin conditions such as eczema and psoriasis. Produced in the form of cream and a gel, Clinitar Cream's active constituent is COAL TAR.

Clinium (*Janssen*) is a proprietary coronary VASODILATOR, available only on prescription, used to treat angina pectoris (heart pain). Produced in the form of tablets, Clinium is a preparation of lidoflazine. It is not recommended for children.

✚/▲ warning/side-effects: *see* LIDOFLAZINE.

Clinoril (*Merck, Sharp & Dohme*) is a proprietary anti-inflammatory non-narcotic ANALGESIC, available only on prescription, used to treat rheumatic conditions and acute gout. Produced in the form of tablets (in two strengths), Clinoril is a preparation of sulindac.

✚/▲ warning/side-effects: *see* SULINDAC.

clioquinol is an ANTISEPTIC compound that contains iodine and is effective in treating infections by amoebae and some other micro-organisms. Consequently, its primary use is to treat infections of the skin, the intestines, and the outer ear, and administration is oral or topical (in the form of drops, creams, ointments and anal suppositories).

✚ warning: prolonged or excessive use encourages the onset of fungal infection. The drug stains skin and fabric.

▲ side-effects: some patients experience sensitivity reactions. *Related article:* LOCORTEN-VIOFORM.

clobazam is an ANXIOLYTIC drug, one of the BENZODIAZEPINES, used to treat anxiety in the short term, and sometimes to assist in the treatment of some forms of epilepsy. Administration is oral in the form of capsules.

✚ warning: clobazam should be administered with caution to patients with depressed respiration, closed angle glaucoma, or impaired kidney or liver function; who are in the last stages of pregnancy; or who are elderly or debilitated. Prolonged use and abrupt withdrawal of treatment should be avoided.

▲ side-effects: concentration and speed of thought and movement may be affected; the effects of alcohol consumption may be enhanced. There is often drowsiness and dry mouth; there may also be dizziness, headache, and shallow breathing, and sensitivity reactions may occur.
Related article: FRISIUM.

clobetasol propionate is an extremely powerful CORTICOSTEROID, used in topical application on severe non-infective skin inflammations such as eczema, especially in cases where less powerful steroid treatments have failed. Administration is in the form of an aqueous cream, a paraffin-based ointment or an alcohol-based scalp lotion.

✚ warning: as with all corticosteroids, clobetasol propionate treats the symptoms of inflammation but has no effect on any underlying infection. Undetected infection may thus become worse even as its effects are masked by the steroid. The steroid should not in any case be administered to patients with untreated skin lesions; use on the face is best avoided.

▲ side-effects: topical application may result in local thinning of the skin, with possible whitening, and an increased local growth of hair. Some young patients experience the outbreak of a kind of inflammatory dermatitis on the face or at the site of application.
Related articles: DERMOVATE; DERMOVATE-NN.

clobetasone butyrate is a powerful CORTICOSTEROID, used in topical application on severe non-infective skin inflammations such as eczema, especially in cases where less powerful steroid treatments have failed. Administration is in the form of a water-miscible cream, and a paraffin-based ointment.

✚ warning: as with all corticosteroids, clobetasone butyrate treats the symptoms of inflammation but has no effect on any underlying infection. Undetected infection may thus become worse even as its effects are masked by the steroid. The steroid should not in any case be administered to patients with untreated skin lesions; use on the face is best avoided.

▲ side-effects: topical application may result in local thinning of the skin, with possible whitening, and an increased local growth of hair. Some young patients experience the outbreak of a kind of inflammatory dermatitis on the face or at the site of application.
Related articles: EUMOVATE; TRIMOVATE.

clofazimine is a drug used as part of the treatment of the major form of leprosy, in combination with dapsone and rifampicin. That the treatment requires no fewer than three drugs is due to the increasing resistance shown by the leprotic bacterium. Administration is oral in the form of capsules.

✚ warning: clofamizine should be administered with caution to patients with impaired kidney or liver function. Regular tests on both functions are essential.

▲ side-effects: there may be nausea and giddiness, diarrhoea and headache. High dosage may cause the skin and the urine to take on a reddish tinge and a blue-black discoloration of skin lesions.
Related article: LAMPRENE.

clofibrate is a hypolipidaemic drug used to reduce the level of fats (lipids) such as cholesterol in the bloodstream in patients with hyperlipidaemia. It works by altering the metabolism of fats. Generally, it is administered only to patients in whom a strict and regular dietary regime is not having the desired effect, although during treatment such a regime should additionally be adhered to. Administration is oral in the form of capsules.

✚ warning: clofibrate should not be administered to patients with severely impaired kidney or liver function, disease of the gall bladder, or associated blood disorders, or who are pregnant.

▲ side-effects: there may be nausea and abdominal pain; rarely, there may be itching or urticaria. In men, impotence occasionally occurs.
Related article: ATROMID-S.

Clomid (*Merrell Dow Pharmaceuticals*) is a proprietary HORMONE preparation, available only on prescription, used to treat infertility due to ovulatory failure. Produced in the form of tablets, Clomid is a preparation of the anti-oestrogen clomiphene citrate, and should be administered only under specialist supervision.

✚/▲ warning/side-effects: *see* CLOMIPHENE CITRATE.

clomiphene citrate is a substance that is an anti-oestrogen: although it is not actually an androgen (a male sex hormone), it neutralizes the effect of any oestrogen (female sex hormone) present. This property can be useful in treating infertility in women whose condition is linked to the persistent presence of oestrogens and a consequent failure to ovulate. Administration is oral in the form of tablets.

✚ warning: clomiphene citrate should not be administered to patients with ovarian cysts, cancer of the womb lining, liver disease, or with abnormal uterine bleeding, or who are pregnant.

▲ side-effects: multiple births are not uncommon following successful treatment. Hot flushes, nausea, vomiting, visual disturbances, dizziness and insomnia, breast tenderness, weight gain, rashes and hair loss may occur.
Related articles: CLOMID; SEROPHENE.

clomipramine hydrochloride is an ANTIDEPRESSANT drug that has mild sedative properties. It is used primarily to treat depressive illness, but can be used to assist in treating phobic or obsessional states, and to try to reduce the incidence of cataplexy in narcoleptic patients. Administration is oral in the form of capsules, sustained-release tablets, and a dilute syrup, or by injection.

✚ warning: clomipramine hydrochloride should not be administered to patients with heart disease; it should be administered with caution to those with diabetes, epilepsy, liver or thyroid disease, glaucoma, or urinary retention; or who are pregnant or lactating. Withdrawal of treatment must be gradual.

▲ side-effects: concentration and speed of thought and movement are affected; there is also dry mouth. There may also be blurred vision, difficulty in urinating, sweating, and irregular heartbeat, behavioural disturbances, a rash, a state of confusion, and/or a loss of libido. Rarely, there are also blood deficiencies.
Related article: ANAFRANIL.

clomocycline sodium is a broad-spectrum ANTIBIOTIC, one of the tetracyclines used to treat many forms of infection caused by any of several types of micro-organism. It is used particularly to treat infections of the urinary tract, the respiratory tract, and genital organs, and acne. Administration is oral in the form of capsules.

✚ warning: clomocycline sodium should not be administered to patients who are aged under 12 years, who are pregnant, or with impaired kidney function; it should be administered with caution to those who are lactating.

▲ side-effects: there may be nausea and vomiting, with diarrhoea. Occasionally there is sensitivity to light or other sensitivity reaction. These side-effects may still occur even if the causative organism of the disorder being treated proves to be resistant to the drug.
Related article: MEGACLOR.

clonazepam is a drug related to DIAZEPAM and the BENZODIAZEPINES but is in effect an ANTICONVULSANT drug used to treat all forms of epilepsy. Administration is oral in the form of tablets.

✚ warning: clonazepam should be administered with caution to patients who are lactating. The drug is more sedative than most drugs used to treat epilepsy.

▲ side-effects: concentration and speed of thought and movement are affected; in susceptible patients the degree of sedation may be marked. It also enhances the effects of alcohol consumption. There may also be dizziness, fatigue and muscular weakness. Again in susceptible patients, there may be mood changes.
Related article: RIVOTRIL.

clonidine hydrochloride is an ANTIHYPERTENSIVE drug used to treat moderate to severe high blood pressure (hypertension). Although controversial, use of the drug has also been extended to assisting in the prevention of migraine attacks. It is thought to work by reducing release of the neurotransmitter NORADRENALINE both in the brain and in blood vessels. Administration is oral in the form of tablets and sustained-release capsules, or by injection.

✚ warning: clonidine hydrochloride should not be administered to patients who have a history of depression. Treatment must be withdrawn gradually (in order to avoid a hypertensive crisis).

▲ side-effects: there is sedation and dry mouth; there may also be fluid retention (oedema), a reduced heart rate, and depression.
Related article: CATAPRES.

clopamide is a DIURETIC, one of the THIAZIDES, used to treat fluid retention in the tissues (oedema) and high blood pressure (hypertension). Because all thiazides tend to deplete body reserves of potassium, clopamide

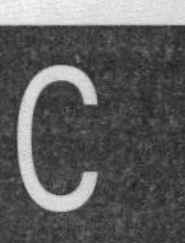

may be administered in combination either with potassium supplements or with diuretics that are complementarily potassium-sparing. Administration is oral in the form of tablets.

✚ warning: clopamide should not be administered to patients with kidney failure or urinary retention, or who are lactating. It should be administered with caution to those who are pregnant. The drug may aggravate conditions of diabetes or gout.

▲ side-effects: there may be tiredness and a rash. In men, impotence may occur that is reversible on cessation of treatment.

Related articles: BRINALDIX K; VISKALDIX.

Clopenthixol is an alternative proprietary name for the powerful ANTIPSYCHOTIC drug zuclopenthixol.
see ZUCLOPENTHIXOL.

Clopixol (*Lundbeck*) is a proprietary ANTIPSYCHOTIC drug, available only on prescription, used to treat and restrain psychotic patients, particularly the more aggressive or agitated schizophrenic ones. Produced in the form of tablets (in three strengths), Clopixol is a preparation of zuclopenthixol dihydrochloride; produced in ampoules and vials for injection (in two strengths, the stronger under the name Clopixol Conc.), Clopixol is a preparation of zuclopenthixol decanoate. It is not recommended for children.

✚/▲ warning/side-effects: *see* ZUCLOPENTHIXOL.

clorazepate dipotassium is an ANXIOLYTIC drug, one of the BENZODIAZEPINES, used to treat anxiety in the short term. Administration is oral in the form of capsules.

✚ warning: clorazepate dipotassium should not be administered to patients with depressed respiration; it should be administered with caution to those with glaucoma, or impaired kidney or liver function; who are in the last stages of pregnancy; or who are elderly or debilitated. Prolonged use and abrupt withdrawal of treatment should be avoided.

▲ side-effects: concentration and speed of thought and movement may be affected; the effects of alcohol consumption may be enhanced. There is often drowsiness and dry mouth; there may also be dizziness, headache, and shallow breathing, and sensitivity reactions may occur.

Related article: TRANXENE.

clotrimazole is an ANTIFUNGAL drug used in topical application to treat fungal infection on the skin and mucous membranes (especially the vagina and the outer ear). Administration is in the form of a water-miscible cream, a dusting-powder, a spray, vaginal inserts (pessaries), and a lotion (solution).

▲ side-effects: rarely, there is a burning sensation or irritation; a very few patients experience sensitivity reactions.

Related article: CANESTEN.

cloxacillin is an ANTIBIOTIC, a semisynthetic PENICILLIN used primarily to treat forms of infection which other penicillins are incapable of countering. This is because cloxacillin is not inactivated by the enzymes produced, for example, by certain Staphylococci. Administration is

C

oral in the form of capsules and a dilute syrup, and by injection.

✚ warning: cloxacillin should not be administered to patients who are known to be allergic to penicillins; it should be administered with caution to those with impaired kidney function.

▲ side-effects: there may be sensitivity reactions ranging from a minor rash to urticaria and joint pains, and (occasionally) to high body temperature or anaphylactic shock. High dosage may in any case cause convulsions.
Related articles: AMPICLOX; ORBENIN.

coal tar is a black, viscous liquid obtained by the distillation of coal: it has both anti-itching and keratolytic properties, and works by speeding up the rate at which the surface scale of skin is lost naturally. Therapeutically employed primarily to treat psoriasis and eczema, coal tar is used in solution in which the concentration is decided by each individual patient's condition and response. It is a constituent in many non-proprietary and proprietary formulations, especially pastes, some of which are not suitable for the treatment of facial conditions.

✚ warning: avoid contact with broken or inflamed skin. Coal tar stains skin, hair and fabric.

▲ side-effects: some patients experience skin irritation and an acne-like rash. Rarely, there is sensitivity to light.
Related articles: ALPHOSYL; CARBO-CORT; CARBO-DOME; CLINITAR; COLTAPASTE; GELCOTAR; GENISOL; IONIL T; MEDITAR; POLYTAR; PRAGMATAR; PSORIDERM; PSORIGEL; TARBAND; TARCORTIN; T/GEL.

Cobadex (*Cox Pharmaceuticals*) is a proprietary CORTICOSTEROID preparation, available only on prescription, used to treat mild inflammatory skin conditions, and itching in the anal and vulval regions. Produced in the form of a water-miscible cream (in two strengths), Cobadex contains the steroid hydrocortisone and the antifoaming agent DIMETHICONE.

✚/▲ warning/side-effects: *see* HYDROCORTISONE.

Cobalin-H (*Paines & Byrne*) is a proprietary VITAMIN preparation, available on prescription only to private patients. Produced in ampoules for injection, Cobalin-H is a preparation of hydroxocobalamin (vitamin B_{12}).

✚/▲ warning/side-effects: *see* HYDROXOCOBALAMIN.

Co-betaloc (*Astra*) is a proprietary compound ANTIHYPERTENSIVE drug, available only on prescription, used to treat high blood pressure. Produced in the form of tablets, Co-betaloc contains the BETA-BLOCKER metoprolol tartrate and the THIAZIDE DIURETIC hydrochlorothiazide. It is not recommended for children.

✚/▲ warning/side-effects: *see* HYDROCHLOROTHIAZIDE; METOPROLOL.

Co-betaloc SA (*Astra*) is a proprietary compound ANTIHYPERTENSIVE drug, available only on prescription, used to treat high blood pressure. Produced in the form of tablets, Co-betaloc SA contains the BETA-BLOCKER metoprolol tartrate (in a form that guarantees sustained release) and the THIAZIDE DIURETIC hydrochlorothiazide.

✚/▲ warning/side-effects: *see* HYDROCHLOROTHIAZIDE; METOPROLOL.

Cobutolin (*Cox Pharmaceuticals*) is a proprietary BETA-RECEPTOR STIMULANT BRONCHODILATOR, available only on prescription, used to treat bronchial asthma and chronic bronchitis. It is produced in the form of tablets (in two strengths) and in an aerosol that emits metered doses; in this form dosage should be strictly adhered to. Cobutolin is a preparation of the selective beta$_2$-adrenoceptor stimulant salbutamol. It is not recommended for children aged under 2 years.
✚/▲ warning/side-effects: *see* SALBUTAMOL.

cocaine is a central nervous system STIMULANT that rapidly causes dependence (addiction). Therapeutically it is used mainly as a local ANAESTHETIC for topical application, particularly (as cocaine hydrochloride, with or without the atropine derivative homatropine) in eye-drops. Its use as an analgesic, and especially as a constituent in elixirs prescribed to treat pain in terminal care (including the BROMPTON COCKTAILS), is now virtually discontinued.

co-codamol is a compound ANALGESIC combining the OPIATE codeine phosphate with paracetamol in a ratio of 2:125. As a compound it forms a constituent in a number of proprietary analgesic preparations, but although it has the advantages of both drugs, it also has the disadvantages.
✚/▲ warning/side-effects: *see* CODEINE PHOSPHATE; PARACETAMOL.

co-codaprin is a compound ANALGESIC combining the OPIATE codeine phosphate with aspirin in a ratio of 1:50. As a compound it forms a constituent in a number of proprietary analgesic preparations, but although it has the advantages of both drugs, it also has the disadvantages.
✚/▲ warning/side-effects: *see* ASPIRIN; CODEINE PHOSPHATE.

Codanin (*Whitehall Laboratories*) is a proprietary, non-prescription ANALGESIC produced in the form of tablets and as a powder. It is a preparation of codeine phosphate and paracetamol.
✚/▲ warning/side-effects: *see* CODEINE PHOSPHATE; PARACETAMOL.

co-danthrusate is a compound LAXATIVE combining the stimulant laxative danthron together with the surfactant laxative DIOCTYL SODIUM SULPHOSUCCINATE (also called docusate sodium). As a compound it is produced in the form of capsules, but although it has the advantage of both drugs, it also has the disadvantages.
✚/▲ warning/side-effects: *see* DANTHRON.

codeine phosphate is an OPIATE, a narcotic ANALGESIC that also has the properties of a cough suppressant. As an analgesic, codeine is a common, but often minor, constituent in non-proprietary and proprietary preparations to relieve pain (a majority of which are not available from the National Health Service), although some authorities dislike any combined form that contains codeine. Even more authorities disapprove of the drug's use as a cough suppressant. The drug also has the capacity to reduce intestinal motility (and so treat diarrhoea). Administration is oral or by injection.
✚ warning: codeine phosphate should not be administered to patients who suffer from

depressed breathing, or who are aged under 12 months.
▲ side-effects: tolerance occurs readily, although dependence (addiction) is relatively unusual. Constipation is common. There may be sedation and dizziness, especially following injection. The effects of alcohol consumption may be enhanced.
Related articles: ANTOIN; BENYLIN EXPECTORANT; CODIS; DIARREST; DIMOTANE WITH CODEINE; GALCODINE; HYPON; KAODENE; MEDOCODENE; MIGRALEVE; MYOLGIN; NEURODYNE; PANADEINE; PARACODOL; PARADEINE; PARAHYPON; PARAKE; PARAMOL; PARDALE; PHARMIDONE; PHENSEDYL; PROPAIN; SAFAPRYN-CO; SOLPADEINE; SYNDOL; TERCODA; TERCOLIX; TERPOIN; UNIFLU; VEGANIN.

Codelsol (*Merck, Sharp & Dohme*) is a proprietary CORTICOSTEROID, available only on prescription, used to treat inflammation in joints and soft tissues, and to relieve the symptoms of allergic disorders. Produced in vials for injection, Codelsol is a preparation of the steroid prednisolone.
✚/▲ warning/side-effects: *see* PREDNISOLONE.

co-dergocrine mesylate is a VASODILATOR that affects the blood vessels of the brain. It is sometimes claimed to improve brain function, but clinical results of psychological tests during and following treatment have neither proved nor disproved that claim, and patients with senile dementia seem to derive little, if any, benefit. It is for the treatment of senile dementia that the drug is most frequently prescribed.
✚ warning: co-dergocrine mesylate should be administered with caution to patients who have a particularly slow heart rate.
▲ side-effects: there may be nausea and vomiting, flushing, a blocked nose, and a rash. Low blood pressure may cause dizziness on standing up from a lying or sitting position.
Related article: HYDERGINE.

Codis (*Reckitt & Colman*) is a proprietary compound ANALGESIC that is not available from the National Health Service. Used to relieve pain and high body temperature, and produced in the form of soluble (dispersible) tablets, Codis contains a combination of ASPIRIN with CODEINE PHOSPHATE (a combination itself known as co-codaprin). It is not recommended for children.
✚/▲ warning/side-effects: *see* CO-CODAPRIN.

co-dydramol is a compound ANALGESIC combining the OPIATE dihydrocodeine tartrate together with paracetamol in a ratio of 1:50. As a compound it forms a constituent in a number of proprietary analgesic preparations, but although it has the advantages of both drugs, it also has the disadvantages.
✚/▲ warning/side-effects: *see* DIHYDROCODEINE TARTRATE; PARACETAMOL.

Cogentin (*Merck, Sharp & Dohme*) is a proprietary preparation of the ANTICHOLINERGIC drug benztropine mesylate, available only on prescription, used in the treatment of parkinsonism (*see* ANTIPARKINSONISM) AND TO CONTROL TREMORS WITHIN DRUG-INDUCED STATES INVOLVING INVOLUNTARY MOVEMENT

(dyskinesia). Produced in the form of tablets and in ampoules for injection, Cogentin is not recommended for children aged under 3 years.
✚/▲ warning/side-effects: *see* BENZTROPINE MESYLATE.

colchicine is a drug derived from the meadow saffron plant, used to treat gout, particularly as an introductory measure to prevent acute gout attacks during initial treatment with other drugs that reduce blood levels of uric acid. Administration is oral in the form of tablets.
✚ warning: colchicine should be administered with caution to patients with heart or gastrointestinal disease, or who have impaired kidney function, who are pregnant or lactating, or who are elderly or debilitated.
▲ side-effects: there is often nausea, vomiting and abdominal pain. High or excessive dosage may lead to gastrointestinal bleeding and diarrhoea, and even kidney damage. Prolonged treatment may eventually result in blood deficiencies and hair loss in some patients.

Coldrex (*Sterling Health*) is a proprietary, non-prescription cold relief preparation produced in the form of tablets and as a powder. It contains paracetamol, phenylephrine and ascorbic acid. The tablet formulation also contains caffeine.
✚/▲ warning/side-effects: *see* ASCORBIC ACID; CAFFEINE; PARACETAMOL; PHENYLEPHRINE.

Colestid (*Upjohn*) is a proprietary form of the resin colestipol hydrochloride, available only on prescription, used to treat high levels of fats (hyperlipidaemia) in the blood. Produced in the form of granules (to be taken orally with liquid), Colestid is not recommended for children.
✚/▲ warning/side-effects: *see* COLESTIPOL HYDROCHLORIDE.

colestipol hydrochloride is a resin which, when taken orally, binds to itself bile salts in the intestines that can then be excreted in the normal way. This is a useful property in the treatment of high blood fat (especially cholesterol) levels and of the itching associated with obstruction in the bile ducts. The property can also be utilized in the treatment of diarrhoea following intestinal disease or surgery. Administration is oral in the form of granules to be taken with liquid.
✚ warning: colestipol hydrochloride should not be administered to patients with complete blockage of the bile ducts, who are already taking any other drug, or who are pregnant. High dosage may require simultaneous administration of fat-soluble vitamins.
▲ side-effects: there may be nausea, heartburn, flatulence with abdominal discomfort, constipation or diarrhoea, and a rash.
Related article: COLESTID.

Colifoam (*Stafford-Miller*) is a proprietary CORTICOSTEROID, available only on prescription, used to treat inflammation in the rectum and piles (haemorrhoids). Produced in the form of foam and applied with an aerosol, Colifoam is a preparation of the steroid hydrocortisone acetate. It is not recommended for children.
✚/▲ warning/side-effects: *see* HYDROCORTISONE.

colistin is a comparatively toxic

ANTIBIOTIC that is used in topical application (in the form of colistin sulphate) to treat infections of the skin, and particularly the ears. However, in certain conditions and under strict supervision, the drug may be administered orally (primarily to treat intestinal infection) or by injection (primarily to treat urinary infection).

✚ warning: colistin should not be administered to patients who suffer from the neuromuscular disease myasthenia gravis; it should be administered with caution to those who suffer from impaired kidney function. Dosage by injection is in millions of units.

▲ side-effects: there may be breathlessness, vertigo, numbness round the mouth, and muscular weakness. Treatment by injection may cause symptoms of nerve or kidney disease.

Related article: COLOMYCIN.

Colofac (*Duphar*) is a proprietary ANTICHOLINERGIC drug available only on prescription, used to treat gastrointestinal disturbance caused by spasm of the muscles of the intestinal walls (irritable bowel syndrome). Produced in the form of tablets and as a sugar-free suspension, Colofac is a preparation of the ANTISPASMODIC drug mebeverine hydrochloride. It is not recommended for children aged under 10 years.

✚/▲ warning/side-effects: *see* MEBEVERINE HYDROCHLORIDE.

Cologel (*Lilly*) is a proprietary non-prescription LAXATIVE that is not available from the National Health Service. Used to treat constipation that results from inadequate fibre intake, it acts as a bulking agent to form a mass of faecal material that stimulates bowel movement. Produced in the form of sugar-free syrup for dilution (the potency of the syrup once diluted is retained for 14 days), Cologel is a preparation of METHYLCELLULOSE.

Colomycin (*Pharmax*) is a proprietary form of the ANTIBIOTIC colistin sulphate, available only on prescription. In powder form, it used mainly in topical application to treat skin infections, burns and wounds. It is also produced in the form of tablets, and as a syrup for dilution (the potency of the syrup once dilute is retained for 14 days), and (in the form of colistin sulphomethate sodium) as a powder for reconstitution as a medium for injection.

✚/▲ warning/side-effects: *see* COLISTIN.

Colostomy Plus (*Shannon*) is a proprietary non-prescription deodorant, used to freshen and sanitize the appliance or bag attached to a stoma (an outlet on the skin surface following the surgical curtailment of the intestines).

Colpermin (*Tillotts*) is a proprietary non-prescription SMOOTH MUSCLE RELAXANT, used to treat gastrointestinal disturbance caused by spasm of the muscles of the intestinal walls. Produced in the form of capsules, Colpermin is a preparation of peppermint oil. It is not recommended for children.

✚/▲ warning/side-effects: *see* PEPPERMINT OIL.

Coltapaste (*Smith & Nephew*) is a proprietary non-prescription form of impregnated bandaging, used to dress and treat serious non-infective skin diseases (such as eczema and psoriasis). The bandaging is impregnated with COAL TAR and ZINC paste.

Colven (*Reckitt & Colman*) is a proprietary ANTICHOLINERGIC SMOOTH MUSCLE RELAXANT, available only on prescription, used to treat gastrointestinal disturbance caused by spasm of the muscles of the intestinal walls. Produced in the form of effervescent granules in sachets, Colven is a preparation of the ANTISPASMODIC drug mebeverine hydrochloride with the ANTIDIARRHOEAL bulking agent ispaghula husk. It is not recommended for children.
✚/▲ warning/side-effects: *see* ISPAGHULA HUSK; MEBEVERINE HYDROCHLORIDE.

Combantrin (*Pfizer*) is a proprietary ANTHELMINTIC preparation, available only on prescription, used to treat infestations by roundworm, threadworm, hookworm and whipworm. Produced in the form of tablets, Combantrin is a preparation of pyrantel embonate. It is not recommended for children aged under 6 months.
✚/▲ warning/side-effects: *see* PYRANTEL.

Comfeel (*Coloplast*) is a proprietary non-prescription barrier cream, used for the protection, freshening and sanitization of a stoma (an outlet in the skin surface following the surgical curtailment of the intestines).

Comox (*Norton*) is a proprietary broad-spectrum ANTIBACTERIAL drug, available only on prescription, used to treat infections of the urinary tract, the sinuses or the middle ear, and diseases such as typhoid fever or chronic bronchitis. Produced in the form of tablets, (in two strengths, the stronger under the name Comox Forte), as soluble (dispersible) tablets, and as a suspension for children, Comox is a compound of the SULPHONAMIDE sulphamethoxazole and the ANTIBACTERIAL agent trimethoprim – a compound itself known as CO-TRIMOXAZOLE.
✚/▲ warning/side-effects: *see* SULPHAMETHOXAZOLE; TRIMETHOPRIM.

Complоment Continus (*Napp*) is a proprietary non-prescription VITAMIN preparation that is not available from the National Health Service. Produced in the form of sustained-release tablets, Complоment Continus contains PYRIDOXINE hydrochloride (vitamin B_6). It is not recommended for children.

Concavit (*Wallace*) is a proprietary non-prescription multivitamin compound that is not available from the National Health Service. Produced in the form of capsules, as drops and as a syrup, Concavit contains RETINOL (vitamin A), several forms of vitamin B (THIAMINE, RIBOFLAVINE, PYRIDOXINE, CYANOCOBALAMIN, NICOTINAMIDE and PANTOTHENIC ACID), ASCORBIC ACID (vitamin C), CALCIFEROL (vitamin D), and TOCOPHEROL (vitamin E).

Concordin (*Merck, Sharp & Dohme*) is a proprietary ANTIDEPRESSANT available only on prescription, used to treat depressive illness and especially in apathetic or withdrawn patients. Produced in the form of tablets (in two strengths), Concordin is a preparation of protriptyline hydrochloride. It is not recommended for children.
✚/▲ warning/side-effects: *see* PROTRIPTYLINE.

Conjuvac Mite (*Dome/Hollister-Stier*) is a proprietary preparation

C

of allergens associated with the house dust mite, for use in desensitizing patients who are allergic to it. Available only on prescription and administered by injection, Conjuvac Mite is produced in sets of treatment or for maintenance.

✚ warning: Close medical supervision is required for a minimum of 2 hours after the injection; administration should take place in locations where emergency facilities for full cardio-respiratory resuscitation are immediately available. Patients should not have had a large meal before treatment.

Conjuvac Two Grass (*Dome/Hollister-Stier*) is a proprietary set of two grass pollen preparations (Timothy and Cocksfoot) for use in desensitizing patients who are allergic to such pollen (and so suffer from hay fever). Available only on prescription and administered by injection, Conjuvac pollen preparations are of carefully annotated different allergenic effect, so that the process of desensitization, as regulated by a doctor, can be progressive.

✚ warning: close medical supervision is required for a minimum of 2 hours after the injection; administration should take place in locations where emergency facilities for full cardio-respiratory resuscitation are immediately available. Patients should not have had a large meal before treatment.

Conotrane (*Boehringer Ingelheim*) is a proprietary non-prescription ANTISEPTIC preparation, used to treat rash and sores and for skin protection. Produced in the form of cream, Conotrane represents a preparation of BENZALKONIUM CHLORIDE and DIMETHICONE '350' and a fragrance.

Conova 30 (*Gold Cross*) is a proprietary low-oestrogen combined ORAL CONTRACEPTIVE, available only on prescription. Produced in the form of tablets, Conova 30 is a preparation of the PROGESTOGEN ethynodiol diacetate and the OESTROGEN ethinyloestradiol (30mg).

✚/▲ warning/side-effects: *see* ETHINYLOESTRADIOL.

Contac 400 (*Menley & James*) is a proprietary, non-prescription cold relief preparation. It contains the ANTIHISTAMINE chlorpheniramine and the DECONGESTANT propanolamine.

✚/▲ warning/side-effects: *see* CHLOROPHENIRAMINE.

***contraceptives** are the means of preventing conception. Methods that involve drugs include oral contraceptives (the "Pill") which contain either a hormonal combination of a PROGESTOGEN and an OESTROGEN or just a progestogen; and SPERMICIDAL preparations which contain drugs that kill sperm and/or prevent motility within the vagina or cervix. Spermicides are for use in combination with barrier methods of contraceptives (such as a condom or diaphragm), and a new spermicide-impregnated sponge to be inserted into the vagina is now available over the counter. A progestogen-only injection is prescribed by some doctors, and is renewable at intervals of three months. Post-coital contraception is also possible in an emergency, and consists of high-dose oestrogen preparations. All contraceptives that involve the use of drugs produce side-effects, and a form

that is ideally suited to a patient is not always possible.
see ORAL CONTRACEPTIVES.

Controvlar (*Schering*) is a proprietary combined sex HORMONE preparation, available only on prescription, used to treat menstrual disorders. Produced in the form of tablets, Controvlar is a preparation of the PROGESTOGEN norethisterone acetate and the OESTROGEN ethinyloestradiol.
✚/▲ warning/side-effects: *see* ETHINYLOESTRADIOL; NORETHISTERONE.

Coparvax (*Calmic*) is a proprietary preparation of a VACCINE available only on prescription, used to prompt the immune system to form antibodies and so assist in the treatment of malignant effusions in the abdominal or chest cavity. Produced in the form of powder for reconstitution as a medium for injection, Coparvax's active constituent is inactivated Corynebacterium parvum bacteria.
✚/▲ warning/side-effects: *see* CORYNEBACTERIUM PARVUM VACCINE.

Copholco (*Radiol Chemicals*) is a proprietary non- prescription EXPECTORANT and cough mixture that is not available from the National Health Service. Produced in the form of a linctus, Copholco is a preparation that includes the OPIATE pholcodine and MENTHOL. It is not recommended for children aged under 5 years.
✚/▲ warning/side-effects: *see* PHOLCODINE.

Coppertone Supershade 15 (*Scholl*) is a proprietary non-prescription sunscreening preparation, used to help protect the skin from ultraviolet radiation, as in radiotherapy. Produced in the form of a lotion, Coppertone Supershade 15 contains para- AMINOBENZOIC ACID ester and OXYBENZONE.

co-proxamol is a compound ANALGESIC combining the NARCOTIC dextropropoxyphene with paracetamol in a ratio of 1:10. As a compound it forms a constituent in a number of proprietary analgesic preparations, but although it has the advantages of both drugs, it also has the disadvantages.
✚/▲ warning/side-effects: *see* DEXTROPROPOXYPHENE; PARACETAMOL.

Cordarone X (*Labaz*) is a proprietary ANTIARRHYTHMIC drug, available only on prescription, used to treat heartbeat irregularities. Produced in the form of tablets (in two strengths) and in ampoules for injections, Cordarone X is a preparation of amiodarone hydrochloride.
✚/▲ warning/side-effects: *see* AMIODARONE.

Cordilox (*Abbott*) is a proprietary ANTIARRHYTHMIC, ANTIHYPERTENSIVE drug, available only on prescription, used to treat heartbeat irregularities, angina pectoris (heart pain) and high blood pressure (hypertension). Produced in the form of tablets (in four strengths, the strongest under the name Cordilox 160) and in ampoules for injection, Cordilox is a preparation of the calcium antagonist verapamil hydrochloride. It is not recommended for the treatment of angina in children.
✚/▲ warning/side-effects: *see* VERAPAMIL HYDROCHLORIDE.

Corgard (*Squibb*) is a proprietary BETA-BLOCKER ANTIHYPERTENSIVE

drug, available only on prescription, used to treat heartbeat irregularities, angina pectoris (heart pain), and high blood pressure (hypertension), to prevent migraine, and to assist in the treatment of excess levels of thyroid hormones in the blood (thyrotoxicosis). Produced in the form of tablets (in two strengths), Corgard is a preparation of nadolol. It is not recommended for children.
✚/▲ warning/side-effects: *see* NADOLOL.

Corgaretic (*Squibb*) is a proprietary compound ANTIHYPERTENSIVE drug, available only on prescription, used to treat high blood pressure (hypertension). Produced in the form of tablets (in two strengths, under the names Corgaretic 40 and Corgaretic 80), it is a combination of the BETA-BLOCKER nadolol and the THIAZIDE DIURETIC bendrofluazide. It is not recommended for children.
✚/▲ warning/side-effects: *see* BENDROFLUAZIDE; NADOLOL.

Corlan (*Glaxo*) is a proprietary CORTICOSTEROID, available only on prescription, used in topical application to treat ulcers and sores in the mouth. Produced in the form of lozenges, Corlan's active constituent is the steroid hydrocortisone.
✚/▲ warning/side-effects: *see* HYDROCORTISONE.

Coro-nitro Spray (*MCP Pharmaceuticals*) is a proprietary non-prescription VASODILATOR used to treat and prevent angina pectoris (heart pain). Produced in the form of an aerosol spray in metered doses, for application on or under the tongue, Coro-nitro Spray is a preparation of glyceryl trinitrate. It is not recommended for children.
✚/▲ warning/side-effects: *see* GLYCERYL TRINITRATE.

Corsodyl (*ICI*) is a proprietary non-prescription ANTIBACTERIAL drug, used in topical application to treat inflammations and infections of the mouth. Produced in the form of a gel and as a mouth-wash, Corsodyl is a preparation of CHLORHEXIDINE gluconate.

Cortacream (*Smith & Nephew*) is a proprietary brand of dressings, available only on prescription, used to treat mild inflammatory skin conditions. Produced in the form of an impregnated bandage, it requires additional bandaging to keep it in place. It should be applied only to the affected area. Cortacream's active constituent is the CORTICOSTEROID hydrocortisone acetate.
✚/▲ warning/side-effects: *see* HYDROCORTISONE.

Cortelan (*Glaxo*) is a proprietary preparation of the CORTICOSTEROID hormone cortisone acetate, available only on prescription, used less commonly now in replacement therapy to make up hormonal deficiency following surgical removal of one or both of the adrenal glands. It is produced in the form of tablets.
✚/▲ warning/side-effects: *see* CORTISONE ACETATE.

Cortenema (*Bengué*) is a proprietary CORTICOSTEROID preparation, available only on prescription, used to treat inflammation in the tissues around the kidney or the colon. Produced in the form of a retention enema, Cortenema is a preparation of partly solubilized hydrocortisone. It is not recommended for children.
✚/▲ warning/side-effects: *see* HYDROCORTISONE.

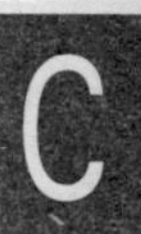

***corticosteroids** are STEROID HORMONES produced and secreted by the cortex (the outer portion) of the adrenal glands, or substances produced synthetically that resemble them. There are two main types: glucocorticoids and mineralocorticoids. The glucocorticoids assist in the metabolism of fats, carbohydrate and protein in the body, and contribute to the neuromuscular and tissue processes that convey the body's reaction to stress. The mineralocorticoids assist in maintaining the balance of salt and water in the body. Therapeutically, the glucocorticoids are far more important, used particularly for their anti-inflammatory properties – it is they that are the basis of almost all therapy with corticosteroids. Best known are HYDROCORTISONE (cortisol), CORTISONE, TRIAMCINOLONE, BETAMETHASONE, PREDNISONE, PREDNISOLONE and DEXAMETHASONE. Mineralocorticoids include FLUDROCORTISONE acetate.

corticotrophin, or adrenocorticotrophic hormone (ACTH), is a hormone produced and secreted by the pituitary gland in order to control the production and secretion of other hormones – CORTICOSTEROIDS – in the adrenal glands, generally as a response to stress. Therapeutically, corticotrophin may be administered to make up for hormonal deficiency in the pituitary gland, to cause the production of extra corticosteroids in the treatment of inflammatory conditions such as rheumatism and asthma, or to test the function of the adrenal glands.

cortisol is another name for the CORTICOSTEROID hormone hydrocortisone.
✚/▲ warning/side-effects: *see* HYDROCORTISONE.

cortisone acetate is a CORTICOSTEROID hormone that has the properties both of glucocorticoids and of mineralocorticoids. It can thus theoretically be used both to treat inflammatory conditions caused, for instance, by allergy or rheumatism, and to make up for hormonal deficiency (especially relating to the salt and water balance in the body) following surgical removal of the adrenal glands. In practice, however, it is not generally used for the suppression of inflammation because it has a tendency to cause fluid retention. Administration is oral in the form of tablets.
✚ warning: cortisone acetate should not be administered to patients with psoriasis. It should be administered with caution to the elderly (in whom overdosage can cause osteoporosis, "brittle bones"), those with kidney disease peptic ulcer, hypertension, glaucoma, epilepsy or diabetes, or who are pregnant. In children, administration of cortisone acetate may lead to stunting of growth. The effects of potentially serious infections may be masked by the drug during treatment. Withdrawal of treatment must be gradual.
▲ side-effects: treatment of susceptible patients may engender euphoria, or a state of confusion or depression. Rarely, there is peptic ulcer.
Related articles: CORTELAN; CORTISTAB; CORTISYL.

Cortistab (*Boots*) is a proprietary preparation of the

CORTICOSTEROID hormone cortisone acetate, available only on prescription, used less commonly now in replacement therapy to make up hormonal deficiency following surgical removal of one or both of the adrenal glands; it is even less commonly used to treat allergic and rheumatic inflammation. It is produced in the form of tablets (in two strengths).
✚/▲ warning/side-effects: *see* CORTISONE ACETATE.

Cortisyl (*Roussel*) is a proprietary preparation of the corticosteroid hormone cortisone acetate, available only on prescription, used less commonly now in replacement therapy to make up hormonal deficiency following surgical removal of one or both of the adrenal glands. Produced in the form of tablets, it is not recommended for children.
✚/▲ warning/side-effects: *see* CORTISONE ACETATE.

Cortucid (*Nicholas*) is a proprietary CORTICOSTEROID ointment, available only on prescription, used in topical application to treat inflammations in and around the eye. It is a combination of the steroid hydrocortisone acetate together with the ANTIBIOTIC SULPHACETAMIDE sodium.
✚/▲ warning/side-effects: *see* HYDROCORTISONE.

Corynebacterium parvum vaccine is a suspension of inactivated Corynebacterium parvum bacteria prepared as a VACCINE that may be injected into a body cavity in order to promote the formation of antibodies that then assist in the treatment of malignant effusions. It is known as an immunostimulant.
✚ warning: injection of the vaccine should not take place within 10 days of surgery on the chest wall.
▲ side-effects: there is high body temperature; there may also be nausea and vomiting, with abdominal pain.
Related article: COPARVAX.

Cosmegen Lyovac (*Merck, Sharp & Dohme*) is a proprietary CYTOTOXIC drug that also has ANTIBIOTIC properties. Available only on prescription, it is used mainly to treat cancers in children, and is produced in the form of a powder for reconstitution as a medium for injection. It may also be used as an immunosuppressant during or following transplant surgery in order to limit tissue rejection. Cosmegen Lyovac is a preparation of actinomycin D.
✚/▲ warning/side-effects: *see* ACTINOMYCIN D.

Cosuric (*DDSA Pharmaceuticals*) is a proprietary form of the XANTHINE-OXIDASE INHIBITOR allopurinol, used to treat high levels of uric acid in the bloodstream (which may cause gout). Available only on prescription, Cosuric is produced in the form of tablets (in two strengths).
✚/▲ warning/side-effects: *see* ALLOPURINOL.

Cosylan (*Parke-Davis*) is a proprietary non-prescription cough mixture that is not available from the National Health Service. Used to treat persistent dry cough, and produced in the form of a syrup for dilution (the potency of the syrup once diluted is retained for 14 days), Cosylan is a preparation of the OPIATE dextromethorphan hydrobromide. It is not recommended for children aged under 12 months.
✚/▲ warning/side-effects: *see* DEXTROMETHORPHAN.

Cotazym (*Organon*) is a proprietary non-prescription preparation of digestive enzymes, used to make up a deficiency of digestive juices normally supplied by the pancreas. This may be required following surgery on the alimentary canal or be necessitated by disease. It is produced in the form of capsules to be sprinkled on food.

co-trimoxazole is the name for a combination of the SULPHONAMIDE sulphamethoxazole and the similar but not related trimethoprim (a folic acid inhibitor). Together they have more than twice the individual effect of either alone. The compound is used to treat and to prevent the spread of infections of the urinary tract, the nasal passages and upper respiratory tract, and the bones and joints, and such diseases as typhoid fever or gonorrhoea (particularly in patients allergic to penicillin): it is a constituent of many proprietary antibiotic preparations. Administration is oral in the form of tablets or suspension, or by injection or infusion.

✚ warning: co-trimoxazole should not be administered to patients who are pregnant or with blood disorders, jaundice, or impaired liver or kidney function. It should be administered with caution to infants under 6 weeks and those who are elderly or lactating. Adequate fluid intake must be maintained. Prolonged treatment requires regular blood counts.

▲ side-effects: there may be nausea and vomiting; rashes are not uncommon. Blood disorders may occur.
Related articles: BACTRIM; CHEMOTRIM; COMOX; FECTRIM; LARATRIM; SEPTRIN.

***counter-irritants** are preparations that are applied topically to produce an irritation of the sensory nerve endings, which offsets underlying muscle or joint pain.

Covermark (*Stiefel*) is the name of a proprietary non-prescription brand of camouflaging preparations designed for topical application to mask scars and other skin disfigurements. Produced in the form of a cream rouge (in three shades), a spotstick (in seven shades), a grey toner (as a cream), a masking or covering cream (in ten shades), a shading cream and a finishing powder, they may be obtained on prescription if the skin disfigurement is the result of surgery or is giving rise to emotional disturbance.

Cradocap (*Napp*) is a proprietary non-prescription ANTISEPTIC, used to treat the infants' skin conditions cradle cap or scurf cap. Produced in the form of a shampoo, Cradocap represents a 10% solution of CETRIMIDE.

Cremalgin (*Berk*) is a proprietary non-prescription COUNTER-IRRITANT which, in the form of a cream applied to the skin, produces an irritation of sensory nerve endings that offsets the pain of underlying muscle or joint ailments. It contains various vegetable extracts and alcohol esters.

✚ warning: cremalgin should not be used on inflamed or broken skin, or on mucous membranes.

Creon (*Duphar*) is a proprietary non-prescription preparation of digestive enzymes, used to make up a deficiency of digestive juices normally supplied by the pancreas. This may be required

C

following surgery on the alimentary canal or be necessitated by disease. It is produced in the form of capsules.

crotamiton is a drug used both to relieve itching and to kill parasitic mites on the skin (as in scabies). It is applied to the skin in the form of a lotion or a cream, usually following a bath; the application should be left in position for as long as possible – ideally 24 hours for treatment of parasitic mites – before being washed off.
✚ warning: crotamiton should not be used on broken skin or near the eyes.

crystal violet is another name for gentian violet.
see GENTIAN VIOLET.

Crystapen (*Glaxo*) is a proprietary ANTIBIOTIC, available only on prescription, used to treat infections of the skin, of the middle ear, and of the respiratory tract (such as tonsillitis), and certain severe systemic infections (such as meningitis). Produced as a powder for reconstitution in any of three forms suited to specific sites of injection, Crystapen is a preparation of benzylpenicillin sodium.
✚/▲ warning/side-effects: *see* BENZYLPENICILLIN.

Crystapen V (*Glaxo*) is a proprietary ANTIBIOTIC, available only on prescription, used to treat many forms of infection and to prevent rheumatic fever. Produced in the form of a syrup (in two strengths) for dilution (the potency of the syrup once dilute is retained for 7 days), Crystapen V is a preparation of phenoxymethylpenicillin.
✚/▲ warning/side-effects: *see* PHENOXYMETHYLPENICILLIN.

Cuplex (*Smith & Nephew*) is a proprietary non-prescription preparation used to remove warts and hard skin (a keratolytic). Produced in the form of a gel, Cuplex's active constituents are salicylic acid and lactic acid.

cyanocobalamin is a form of VITAMIN B_{12} found in most normal diets – in eggs, diary products and meats – and is essential for the functioning of nerve cells and the growth of red blood cells. Really strict vegetarians who eat no animal products whatever may eventually suffer from deficiency of this vitamin in a condition that is a form of anaemia; the condition is also found in patients who for one reason or another cannot absorb food properly. Therapeutically, however, cyanocobalamin has recently been replaced by HYDROXOCOBALAMIN as the version of the vitamin for medical use. Supplements of vitamin B_{12} are administered mainly by injection (because vitamin B_{12} deficiency arises most often through malabsorption – possibly following gastrectomy – which renders oral administration futile). But whereas hydroxocobalamin can be retained in the body for more than 3 months following injection, cyanocobalamin must be re-injected at least once a month.
Related articles: BC 500; CALCIMAX; CE-COBALIN; CONCAVIT; CYTACON; CYTAMEN; HEPACON; KETOVITE; OCTOVIT; SOLIVITO; VERDIVITON.

cyclandelate is a VASODILATOR that specifically affects the blood vessels of the brain. It is sometimes claimed to improve brain function, but clinical results of psychological tests during and following treatment have neither proved nor disproved that claim, and patients suffering from senile dementia seem to derive little benefit if any. It is to assist in the treatment of senile dementia that the drug is most prescribed, although it can also be used to improve circulatory disorders of the limbs.

✚ warning: cyclandelate should not be administered to patients who are suffering from brain injury.

▲ side-effects: there may be nausea and flushing; high doses may cause dizziness.
Related articles: CYCLOBRAL; CYCLOSPASMOL.

Cyclimorph (*Calmic*) is a proprietary form of the narcotic ANALGESIC morphine tartrate together with the anti-emetic ANTIHISTAMINE cyclizine tartrate, and is on the controlled drugs list. Used to treat moderate to severe pain, especially in serious conditions of fluid within the lungs, it is produced in ampoules (in two strengths, under the names Cyclimorph-10 and Cyclimorph-15) for injection. It is not recommended for children or for those in terminal care because of the anti-emetic content.

✚/▲ warning/side-effects: *see* CYCLIZINE; MORPHINE.

cyclizine is an ANTIHISTAMINE used primarily as an ANTI-EMETIC in the treatment or prevention of motion sickness and vomiting caused either by chemotherapy for cancer or by infection of the middle or inner ear. Administration (as cyclizine hydrochloride, cyclizine lactate or cyclizine tartrate) is oral in the form of tablets, or by injection.

✚ warning: cyclizine should be administered with caution to patients with epilepsy, liver disease, glaucoma or enlargement of the prostate gland. Drowsiness may be increased by alcohol consumption.

▲ side-effects: concentration and speed of thought and movement may be affected. There is commonly drowsiness and dry mouth; there may also be headache, blurred vision and gastrointestinal disturbances.
Related articles: CYCLIMORPH; DICONAL; MIGRIL; VALOID.

cyclobarbitone calcium is a HYPNOTIC BARBITURATE used only when absolutely necessary, to treat severe and intractable insomnia. Administration is oral in the form of tablets. The proprietary form is on the controlled drugs list.

✚ warning: cyclobarbitone calcium should not be administered to patients whose insomnia is caused by pain, who have porphyria, who are pregnant or lactating, who are elderly or debilitated, or who have a history of drug (including alcohol) abuse. It should be administered with caution to those with kidney, liver, or lung disease. Use of the drug should be avoided as far as possible. Repeated doses are cumulative in effect, and may lead to real sedation; abrupt withdrawal of treatment, on the other hand, may cause serious withdrawal symptoms. Tolerance and dependence (addiction) occur readily.

▲ side-effects: concentration and the speed of thought and movement are affected. There may be drowsiness, dizziness and shallow breathing, with headache. Some patients

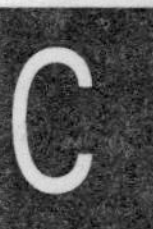

experience hypersensitivity reactions. (The drug enhances the effects of alcohol consumption.)
Related article: PHANODORM.

Cyclobral (*Norgine*) is a proprietary non-prescription VASODILATOR, used to improve blood circulation to the brain (particularly to assist in the treatment of senile dementia) and to the extremities. Produced in the form of capsules, Cyclobral is a preparation of cyclandelate.
✚/▲ warning/side-effects: *see* CYCLANDELATE.

cyclofenil is an ANTI-OESTROGEN. Although it is not actually an androgen (a male sex hormone), it neutralizes the effect of any oestrogen (female sex hormone) present. This property can be useful in treating infertility or sparse or infrequent menstrual periods in women whose condition is linked to the persistent presence of oestrogens and a consequent failure to ovulate. Administration is oral in the form of tablets.
✚ warning: cyclofenil should not be administered to patients with ovarian cysts, cancer of the womb lining, or liver disease, or who are pregnant.
▲ side-effects: there may be nausea and hot flushes, with abdominal discomfort; rarely, there is jaundice.
Related article: REHIBIN.

Cyclogest (*Hoechst*) (Cox Pharmaceuticals) is a proprietary preparation of the female sex HORMONE progesterone, available only on prescription, used to treat premenstrual problems and depression after childbirth. It is produced in the form of (vaginal or anal) suppositories (in two strengths).
✚/▲ warning/side-effects: *see* PROGESTERONE.

cyclopenthiazide is a DIURETIC, one of the THIAZIDES, used to treat fluid retention in the tissues (oedema) and high blood pressure (hypertension). Because all thiazides tend to deplete body reserves of potassium, cyclopenthiazide may be administered in combination either with potassium supplements or with diuretics that are complementarily potassium-sparing. Administration is oral in the form of tablets.
✚ warning: cyclopenthiazide should not be administered to patients with kidney failure or urinary retention, or who are lactating. It should be administered with caution to those who are pregnant. It may aggravate conditions of diabetes or gout.
▲ side-effects: there may be tiredness and a rash. In men, temporary impotence may occur; this is reversible on stopping treatment.
Related article: NAVIDREX.

cyclopentolate hydrochloride is an ANTICHOLINERGIC drug that is used in eye-drops to dilate the pupil and paralyse the ciliary muscle (which alters the curvature of the lens). Used to prepare a patient for ophthalmic examination and, less commonly, to assist in the treatment of eye inflammations, cyclopentolate's action may last for up to 24 hours.
✚ warning: cyclopentolate hydrochloride should be administered with caution to patients with pressure within the eyeball. Contact dermatitis may appear where the drug touches the skin.
▲ side-effects: vision may be affected to some degree for the duration of the drug's action. Susceptible patients may

experience raised intra-ocular pressure.
Related articles: MINIMS; MYDRILATE; OPULETS.

cyclophosphamide is a CYTOTOXIC drug that is widely used in the treatment of some forms of leukaemia and lymphoma, and some solid tumours. It works by interfering with the DNA of new cells, so preventing normal cell replication, but it remains inactive until metabolised by the liver. The drug may also be used as an IMMUNOSUPPRESSANT to limit tissue rejection during and following transplant surgery, or to assist in the treatment of complicated rheumatoid arthritis. Administration is oral in the form of tablets, or by injection, and should be accompanied by increased fluid intake.
✚ warning: cyclophosphamide should be administered with caution to patients with impaired kidney function. It may in susceptible patients cause an unpleasant form of cystitis (inflammation of the bladder): greatly increased fluid intake or the simultaneous administration of the synthetic drug mesna may help to avoid the problem. Prolonged treatment may cause an early menopause in women, and men may be rendered permanently sterile early in treatment.
▲ side-effects: there is commonly nausea and vomiting; there is often also hair loss.
Related article: ENDOXANA.

Cyclo-progynova (*Schering*) is a proprietary preparation of female sex hormones, available only on prescription, used to treat menopausal problems. Produced in the form of tablets (in two strengths, under the names Cyclo-progynova 1mg and Cyclo-progynova 2mg), Cyclo-progynova is a combination of the OESTROGEN oestradiol valerate and the PROGESTOGEN norgestrel (or its stronger analogue, levonorgestrel).
✚/▲ warning/side-effects: *see* LEVONORGESTREL; NORGESTREL; OESTRADIOL.

cyclopropane is a gas used as an inhalant general ANAESTHETIC for both induction and maintenance of general anaesthesia. It has some MUSCLE RELAXANT properties too, although in practice a muscle relaxant drug is usually administered simultaneously. However, it has the great disadvantage of being potentially explosive in air, and must be used via closed-circuit systems.
✚ warning: cyclopropane causes respiratory depression, and some form of assisted pulmonary ventilation may be necessary during anaesthesia.
▲ side-effects: although recovery afterwards is rapid, there may be vomiting and agitation.

cycloserine is an ANTIBIOTIC drug used specifically in the treatment of tuberculosis that proves to be resistant to the powerful drugs ordinarily used first, or in cases where those drugs are not tolerated. Administration is oral in the form of capsules.
✚ warning: cycloserine should not be administered to patients with epilepsy, alcoholism, depressive illness, anxiety or psychosis; it should be administered with caution to those with impaired kidney function.
▲ side-effects: there may be headache, dizziness and drowsiness; possible sensitivity reactions include a rash or, rarely, convulsions.

C

Cyclospasmol (*Brocades*) is a proprietary non-prescription VASODILATOR, used to improve blood circulation to the brain (particularly to assist in the treatment of senile dementia) and to the extremities. Produced in the form of capsules, as tablets and as a suspension for dilution (the potency of the suspension once dilute is retained for 14 days), Cyclospasmol is a preparation of cyclandelate.
✚/▲ warning/side-effects: *see* CYCLANDELATE.

cyclosporin is a powerful IMMUNOSUPPRESSANT that is particularly used to limit tissue rejection during and following transplant surgery. Unusually, it has very little effect on the blood-cell producing capacity of the bone-marrow. Administration is oral in the form of an oily solution, or by dilute intravenous infusion.
✚ warning: treatment with cyclosporin inevitably leaves the body much more open to infection, in that part of the immune system – its defence mechanism against microbial invasion – is rendered non-functional. It should be administered with caution to patients who are breast-feeding.
▲ side-effects: treatment may result in impaired liver and kidney function, with gastrointestinal disturbances; some patients experience tremor or excessive hair growth.
Related article: SANDIMMUN.

Cyklokapron (*KabiVitrum*) is a proprietary HAEMOSTATIC, available only on prescription, used to staunch blood flow (for instance in menstruation, or following the extraction of a tooth, in haemophiliac patients). Produced in the form of tablets, as a syrup (the potency of the syrup once dilute is retained for 14 days) and in ampoules for injection, Cyklokapron is a preparation of the styptic tranexamic acid.
✚/▲ warning/side-effects: *see* TRANEXAMIC ACID.

cyproheptadine hydrochloride is a powerful ANTIHISTAMINE that has the unusual distinction of inhibiting not only allergic responses resulting from the release of histamine in the body, but also those allergic responses resulting from the similar release of serotonin. Cyproheptadine is thus capable of treating a much wider range of allergic symptoms than almost any other antihistamine. Moreover, it is sometimes also used to treat migraine and – under medical supervision – to stimulate the appetite (especially in children). Administration is oral in the form of tablets or a dilute syrup.
✚ warning: cyproheptadine hydrochloride should be administered with caution to patients with epilepsy, glaucoma, liver disease or enlargement of the prostate gland.
▲ side-effects: there may be a sedative effect (or, in susceptible patients – especially children – excitement), a headache, and/or weight gain; some patients experience dry mouth, blurred vision, gastrointestinal disturbances and/or urinary retention.
Related article: PERIACTIN.

Cyprostat (*Schering*) is a proprietary preparation of the drug cyproterone acetate, available only on prescription, used to treat cancer of the prostate gland. In combination with the administration of OESTROGENS, Cyprostat works by neutralizing the effects of the male sex hormones (androgens) that contribute to the cancer. It is produced in the form of tablets.

✚/▲ warning/side-effects: *see* CYPROTERONE ACETATE.

cyproterone acetate is an anti-androgen, a drug that neutralizes or otherwise modifies the effects of male sex hormones (androgens) in the body. It is used in the treatment of cancer of the prostate gland, a cancer that advances because of the presence of androgens; in the treatment of masculinization in women, whose symptoms may for example be excessive hair growth or acne; and in the treatment of hypersexuality or sexual deviation in men, in whom the drug causes a condition of reversible sterility through a reduction in the formation of sperm and the creation of non-viable forms of sperm. Administration is oral in the form of tablets.

✚ warning: cyproterone acetate should not be administered to patients with non-sex-linked cancers, liver disease, or severe depression; who have a history of thrombosis; who are pregnant; or who are adolescent boys (in whom bone growth and testicular development may be arrested). It should be administered with caution to those with diabetes or insufficient secretion of adrenal hormones, or who are lactating. Regular checks on liver function, adrenal gland function, and blood levels of glucose are essential. The drug has no effect on patients who are chronic alcoholics due to its interaction with alcohol.

▲ side-effects: concentration and speed of thought and movement are affected, with fatigue and lethargy. Hormonal effects include changes in hair growth patterns and in men the growth of the breasts. Rarely, there is osteoporosis ("brittle bones").

Related articles: ANDROCUR; CYPROSTAT; DIANE.

Cytacon (*Duncan, Flockhart*) is a proprietary non-prescription VITAMIN preparation that is not available from the National Health Service. It is used to treat vitamin deficiency disorders (including anaemia), especially those caused by the malabsorption of food. Produced in the form of tablets and as an elixir, Cytacon is a preparation of CYANOCOBALAMIN (vitamin B_{12}).

Cytamen (*Duncan Flockhart*) is a proprietary VITAMIN preparation, available on prescription only to private patients, used to treat different forms of anaemia. Produced in ampoules for injection, Cytamen is a preparation of CYANOCOBALAMIN (vitamin B_{12}).

cytarabine is an ANTICANCER drug used primarily in the treatment of leukaemia. It works by combining with new-forming cells in a way that prevents normal cell replication (it is cytostatic rather than cytotoxic). Administration is by injection.

✚ warning: cytarabine has a severely depressive effect upon the blood-cell forming capacity of the bone-marrow: constant blood counts are essential. Treatment may cause sterility in men and an early menopause in women if prolonged. Leakage of the drug into the tissues at the site of injection or infusion may cause tissue damage.

▲ side-effects: there is commonly nausea and vomiting; there is often also hair loss.
Related articles: ALEXAN; CYTOSAR.

Cyteal (*Concept*) is a proprietary non-prescription ANTISEPTIC skin cleanser. Produced in the form of a liquid that can (but need not) be diluted, Cyteal contains three disinfectants, including CHLORHEXIDINE gluconate.

Cytosar (*Upjohn*) is a proprietary ANTICANCER drug, available only on prescription, used to treat acute forms of leukaemia. Produced in the form of a powder for reconstitution as a medium for injection (in vials in two strengths, with or without diluent), Cytosar is a preparation of the cytostatic drug cytarabine.
✚/▲ warning/side-effects: *see* CYTARABINE.

***cytotoxic** drugs are used mainly in the treatment of cancer (and thus form a major group of the ANTICANCER drugs). They have the essential property of preventing normal cell replication, and so inhibiting the growth of tumours or of excess cells in body fluids. There are several mechanisms by which they do this. However, in every case they inevitably also affect the growth of normal healthy cells and cause toxic side-effects, generally in the form of nausea and vomiting, with hair loss. Most used cytotoxic drugs are the alkylating agents, which work by interfering with the action of DNA in cell replication; they include CYCLOPHOSPHAMIDE, CHLORAMBUCIL, BUSULPHAN, LOMUSTINE, MELPHALAN, THIOTEPA and CISPLATIN. The VINCA ALKALOIDS damage part of the metabolic features of new-forming cells; they too are effective cytotoxic drugs but tend to have severely limiting neural side-effects. Some cytotoxic drugs have additional antibiotic properties: such drugs include DOXORUBICIN, ACTINOMYCIN D, EPIRUBICIN and BLEOMYCIN. Not all cytotoxic drugs are used in cancer treatment; some, for example AZATHIOPRINE, are used as immunosuppressants to limit tissue rejection during and following transplant surgery.

dacarbazine is a CYTOTOXIC drug that is used comparatively rarely because of its high toxicity. But in combination with other ANTICANCER drugs it may be used to treat the skin (mole) cancer melanoma, some soft-tissue sarcomas, and the lymphatic cancer Hodgkin's disease. Administration is by injection.
✚ warning: an antiemetic should be administered simultaneously to lessen the risk of nausea and vomiting. Monitoring of kidney function and the sense of hearing is essential. Care must be taken in handling the drug: it is a skin irritant.
▲ side-effects: there may be severe nausea and vomiting, progressive deafness, and symptoms of kidney dysfunction. The blood-forming capacity of the bone-marrow is generally suppressed (and treatment should not be repeated within 4 weeks). Skin disorders are not uncommon.
Related article: DTIC-DOME.

Dactil (*MCP Pharmaceuticals*) is a proprietary ANTISPASMODIC drug, available only on prescription, used to assist in the treatment of gastrointestinal disorders arising from muscular spasm of the intestinal walls. Produced in the form of tablets, Dactil is a preparation of the ANTICHOLINERGIC drug piperidolate hydrochloride.
✚/▲ warning/side-effects: *see* PIPERIDOLATE HYDROCHLORIDE.

Dactinomycin is an alternative form of the name of actinomycin D, a drug that is both ANTIBIOTIC and CYTOTOXIC.
see ACTINOMYCIN D.

Daktacort (*Janssen*) is a proprietary cream for topical application, available only on prescription, that contains the CORTICOSTEROID hydrocortisone and the ANTIFUNGAL agent miconazole nitrate in a water-miscible base. It is used to treat skin inflammation in which fungal infection is also present.
✚/▲ warning/side-effects: *see* HYDROCORTISONE; MICONAZOLE.

Daktarin (*Janssen*) is a proprietary ANTIFUNGAL drug, available only on prescription, used to treat both systemic and skin-surface fungal infections. Produced in the form of tablets and as a solution for infusion (after dilution), Daktarin is a preparation of the IMIDAZOLE miconazole. Three other versions are available without prescription, in the form of a sugar-free gel for oral treatment, and a water-miscible cream and a spray powder in an aerosol for topical application.
✚/▲ warning/side-effects: *see* MICONAZOLE.

Dalacin C (*Upjohn*) is a proprietary ANTIBIOTIC, available only on prescription, used to treat staphylococcal infections of bones and joints, and peritonitis (inflammation of the peritoneal lining of the abdominal cavity). Produced in the form of capsules (in two strengths), as a paediatric suspension for dilution (the potency of the suspension once dilute is retained for 14 days), and in ampoules for injection, Dalacin C is a preparation of the rather toxic drug clindamycin. Side-effects are potentially severe.
✚/▲ warning/side-effects: *see* CLINDAMYCIN.

Dalivit (*Paines & Byrne*) is a proprietary non-prescription MULTIVITAMIN compound that is

D

not available from the National Health Service. Produced in the form of tablets, as oral drops, and as a syrup, Dalivit contains RETINOL (vitamin A), many forms of vitamin B (THIAMINE, RIBOFLAVINE, PYRIDOXINE, NICOTINAMIDE and PANTOTHENIC ACID), ASCORBIC ACID (vitamin C), and CALCIFEROL (vitamin D).

Dalmane (*Roche*) is a proprietary HYPNOTIC, available on prescription only to private patients, used to treat insomnia in cases where some degree of daytime sedation is acceptable. Produced in the form of capsules (in two strengths), Dalmane is a preparation of the long-acting BENZODIAZEPINE flurazepam.
✚/▲ warning/side-effects: *see* FLURAZEPAM.

danazol is a derivative of the PROGESTOGEN ethisterone that inhibits the release of gonadotrophins from the pituitary gland, thus in turn preventing the release of sex HORMONES. It is used to treat conditions such as precocious puberty, endometriosis (the presence of areas of womb-lining – endometrium – outside the womb, within the abdominal cavity), gynaecomastia (the development of feminine breasts on a male), and menorrhagia (excessive menstrual flow). Administration is oral in the form of capsules.
✚ warning: danazol should not be administered to patients who are pregnant; it should be administered with caution to those with impaired heart, liver or kidney function, diabetes, epilepsy or migraine, or who are lactating. Non-hormonal contraceptive methods should be used where applicable.
▲ side-effects: there may be nausea, backache and muscle spasm, dizziness and flushing, a rash, and hair loss; in women patients there may be a mild form of masculinization (possibly including a deepening of the voice, and acne).
Related article: DANOL.

Daneral SA (*Hoechst*) is a proprietary non-prescription ANTIHISTAMINE used to treat the symptoms of allergy, such as hay fever or urticaria. Produced in the form of sustained-release tablets, Daneral SA is a preparation of pheniramine maleate.
✚/▲ warning/side-effects: *see* PHENIRAMINE MALEATE.

Danol (*Winthrop*) is a proprietary preparation of the HORMONAL drug danazol, a derivative of the PROGESTOGEN ethisterone that inhibits the release of gonadotrophins from the pituitary gland, thus in turn preventing the release of sex hormones. Available only on prescription, it is used to treat conditions such as precocious puberty, endometriosis (the presence of areas of womb-lining – endometrium – outside the womb, within the abdominal cavity), gynaecomastia (the development of feminine breasts on a male), and menorrhagia (excessive menstrual flow). It is produced in the form of capsules (in two strengths, the weaker under the name Danol-½).
✚/▲ warning/side-effects: *see* DANAZOL.

danthron is a powerful stimulant LAXATIVE which works by increasing the muscular activity of the intestinal walls. Used not only to relieve constipation but also to prepare patients for intestinal examination or surgery, danthron is administered (generally in combination with dioctyl sodium sulphosuccinate) orally in the form of capsules.

✚ warning: danthron should not be taken by any patient who is breast-feeding (because it may be excreted in breast milk). Prolonged contact with the skin may cause irritation and excoriation.

▲ side-effects: the urine may be coloured red. Prolonged use of such a stimulant can eventually wear out the muscles on which it works, thus causing severe intestinal problems in terms of motility and absorption.
Related articles: CO-DANTHRUSATE; NORMAX.

Dantrium (*Norwich Eaton*) is a proprietary SKELETAL MUSCLE RELAXANT, available only on prescription, used to treat long-term rigidity of muscles in disorders such as multiple sclerosis, cerebral palsy and similar conditions resulting from stroke or spinal injury. It is also used in emergencies (in combination with MANNITOL) to treat anaesthetized patients who enter the potentially lethal state of hyperthermia. Produced in the form of capsules (in two strengths), and as a powder for reconstitution as a medium for intravenous injection (under the name Dantrium Intravenous), Dantrium represents a preparation of dantrolene sodium.

✚/▲ warning/side-effects: *see* DANTROLENE SODIUM.

dantrolene sodium is a SKELETAL MUSCLE RELAXANT used to treat long-term rigidity of muscles in disorders such as multiple sclerosis, cerebral palsy and similar conditions resulting from stroke or spinal injury. It is also used in emergencies (in combination with the diuretic MANNITOL) to treat anaesthetized patients who enter the potentially lethal state of hyperthermia. Administration is oral in the form of capsules, or by injection.

✚ warning: dantrolene sodium should not be administered to children; it should be administered with caution to patients who suffer from impaired heart, liver or lung function. Full therapeutic effect of the drug administered orally may take up to 6 weeks to develop - if no effect is manifest then, treatment should be discontinued. Leakage into the tissues from the site of injection may cause severe symptoms.

▲ side-effects: concentration and speed of reaction are initially affected. There may be drowsiness, dizziness, weakness and general malaise; some patients experience diarrhoea. Rarely there is a rash, urinary difficulty, or muscle pain.
Related article: DANTRIUM.

Daonil is a proprietary preparation of the SULPHONYLUREA glibenclamide, available only on prescription, used to treat adult-onset diabetes mellitus. It works by augmenting what remains of insulin production in the pancreas, and is produced in the form of tablets (at twice the strength of SEMI-DAONIL tablets).

✚/▲ warning/side-effects: *see* GLIBENCLAMIDE.

dapsone is an ANTIBIOTIC compound of SULPHONES used specifically to treat leprosy (in both lepromatous and tuberculoid forms); it is also sometimes used to treat severe forms of

D

dermatitis, or, in combination with the enzyme-inhibitor pyrimethamine (under the trade name Maloprim), to prevent tropical travellers from contracting malaria. Administration is oral in the form of tablets, or by injection.

✚ warning: dapsone should be administered with caution to patients with heart or lung disease, or who are pregnant or lactating.

▲ side-effects: side-effects are rare at low doses (as for leprosy), but with higher dosage there may be nausea, vomiting and headache, insomnia and increased heart rate, severe weight loss, anaemia and/or hepatitis.

Related article: MALOPRIM.

Daranide (*Merck, Sharp & Dohme*) is a proprietary preparation of the drug dichlorphenamide, available only on prescription, used to treat glaucoma. It is a weak DIURETIC and works by reducing the fluid within the aqueous humour in the eyeball, but there are some potentially troublesome side-effects. Daranide is produced in the form of tablets.

✚/▲ warning/side-effects: *see* DICHLORPHENAMIDE.

Daraprim (*Wellcome*) is a proprietary non-prescription ANTIMALARIAL drug used to prevent tropical travellers from contracting malaria. It works by interfering with the cellular composition of the parasitic organism that causes malaria, but treatment must be continued for 4 weeks after leaving the area of exposure. Representing a preparation of pyrimethamine, Daraprim is not recommended for children aged under 5 years.

✚/▲ warning/side-effects: *see* PYRIMETHAMINE.

Davenol (*Wyeth*) is a proprietary non-prescription cough linctus that is not available from the National Health Service. Orange-flavoured, it contains the BRONCHODILATOR ephedrine hydrochloride, the OPIATE cough suppressant pholcodine, and the antihistamine carbinoxamine maleate, and is produced as a syrup for dilution (the potency of the dilute linctus is retained for 15 days).

✚/▲ warning/side-effects: *see* EPHEDRINE HYDROCHLORIDE; PHOLCODINE.

Day Nurse (*Beecham Health Care*) is a proprietary, non-prescription cold relief preparation produced in the form of tablets and as a syrup. It contains paracetamol, the DECONGESTANT phenylpropanolamine and the ANTITUSSIVE dextromethorphan.

✚/▲ warning/side-effects: *see* PARACETAMOL; PHENYLPROPANOLAMINE; DEXTROMETHORPHAN.

DDAVP (*Ferring*) is a proprietary preparation of the antidiuretic hormone vasopressin in the form of its analogue DESMOPRESSIN. Available only on prescription, it is administered primarily to diagnose or to treat pituitary-originated diabetes insipidus, although it can be used for some other diagnostic tests and even (in specialist centres) to boost blood concentration of blood-clotting factors in haemophiliac patients. It is produced in ampoules for injection, and in the form of nose-drops.

✚/▲ warning/side-effects: *see* VASOPRESSIN.

Deanase D.C. (*Consolidated*) is a proprietary non-prescription preparation of the enzyme deoxyribonuclease, used to treat

inflammation (particularly of veins, or in and around the eye), bruising or swelling. Thought to work by promoting the removal of coagulated blood, dead tissue and exudate, Deanase is also used to treat bronchitis. It is produced in the form of tablets, and also as Deanase (consolidated) powder for reconstitution as a medium for injection, solution, instillation or inhalation. Deanase is not recommended for children.
▲ side-effects: *see* DEOXYRIBONUCLEASE.

Debrisan (*Pharmacia*) is a proprietary DEXTRAN-derivative, available only on prescription, used in the form of powder or paste (applied topically in a dressing) as an absorbent for open wounds and surface ulcers that are seeping or suppurating.

debrisoquine is an ANTIHYPERTENSIVE drug that works by inhibiting the release in the body of the neurotransmitter NORADRENALINE. In combination with a DIURETIC (such as a thiazide) or a BETA-BLOCKER, debrisoquine is used to treat moderate to severe high blood pressure (hypertension), especially when other forms of treatment have failed. Administration is oral in the form of tablets.
✚ warning: debrisoquine should not be administered to patients with disease of the adrenal glands or with kidney failure; it should be administered with caution to those who are pregnant. Resultant low blood pressure, especially on rising from sitting or lying down, may cause falls in the elderly.
▲ side-effects: there may be low blood pressure (hypotension), nasal congestion and fluid retention leading to weight gain, and failure of ejaculation in men.
Related article: DECLINAX.

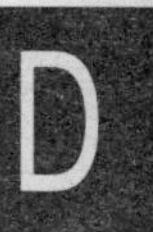

Decadron (*Merck, Sharp & Dohme*) is a proprietary CORTICOSTEROID preparation, available only on prescription, used to treat inflammation especially in rheumatic or allergic conditions. Produced in the form of tablets, it comprises the glucocorticoid steroid dexamethasone.
✚/▲ warning/side-effects: *see* DEXAMETHASONE.

Decadron Injection (*Merck, Sharp & Dohme*) is a proprietary CORTICOSTEROID preparation (produced in vials), available only on prescription, used primarily in emergencies to replace steroid loss; but the injection – comprising dexamethasone sodium phosphate – can also be used to treat inflammation in the joints or in soft tissues.
✚/▲ warning/side-effects: *see* DEXAMETHASONE.

Decadron Shock-pak (*Merck, Sharp & Dohme*) is a proprietary CORTICOSTEROID preparation of dexamethasone sodium phosphate (produced in greater concentration and larger vials than Decadron Injection), available only on prescription, used in emergencies to replace steroid loss and thus to assist in the treatment of shock. Administered by intravenous injection, it is not recommended for children.
✚/▲ warning/side-effects: *see* DEXAMETHASONE.

Deca-Durabolin (*Organon*) is a proprietary form of the anabolic steroid nandrolone, available only on prescription, used to assist the metabolic synthesis of

protein in – that is, build up – the body following major surgery or long-term debilitating disease, or to treat osteoporosis ("brittle bones"). Sometimes administered also to treat sex-hormone-linked cancers, it is additionally used in the treatment of certain forms of anaemia, although how it works in this respect – and even whether it works – remains the subject of some debate: variations in patient response are wide. It is produced in ampoules or syringes for intramuscular injection.
✚/▲ warning/side-effects: *see* NANDROLONE.

Deca-Durabolin 100 (*Organon*) is a form of Deca-Durabolin containing NANDROLONE decanoate, used to treat certain forms of anaemia.
see DECA-DURABOLIN.

Decaserpyl (*Roussel*) is a proprietary ANTIHYPERTENSIVE drug, available only on prescription, used to treat high blood pressure (hypertension). Produced in the form of tablets (in two strengths), Decaserpyl is a preparation of methoserpidine, a derivative of Rauwolfia serpentina that is one of the Rauwolfia alkaloids. It is not recommended for children.
✚/▲ warning/side-effects: *see* RAUWOLFIA ALKALOIDS.

Decaserpyl Plus (*Roussel*) is a proprietary ANTIHYPERTENSIVE drug, available only on prescription, used to treat high blood pressure (hypertension). Produced in the form of tablets (in two strengths), Decaserpyl Plus is a compound preparation of methoserpidine (a derivative of Rauwolfia serpentina that is one of the Rauwolfia alkaloids) together with the THIAZIDE diuretic benzthiazide. It is not recommended for children.
✚/▲ warning/side-effects: *see* RAUWOLFIA ALKALOIDS.

Declinax (*Roche*) is a proprietary ANTIHYPERTENSIVE drug, available only on prescription, used to treat moderate to severe high blood pressure (hypertension), especially when other forms of treatment have failed. Administered in combination with a DIURETIC or a BETA-BLOCKER, Declinax works by inhibiting the release in the body of the neurotransmitter NORADRENALINE. It represents a preparation of debrisoquine, is produced in the form of tablets, and is not recommended for children.
✚/▲ warning/side-effects: *see* DEBRISOQUINE.

***decongestants** are drugs administered to relieve or reduce nasal congestion. Generally applied in the form of nose-drops or as a nasal spray – although some are administered orally – most decongestants are SYMPATHOMIMETIC drugs, which work by constricting the blood vessels within the mucous membranes of the nasal cavity, so reducing the membranes' thickness and creating more room for drainage and ventilation. Nasal congestion caused by allergy, as in hay fever, however, is usually dealt with by using ANTIHISTAMINES, which inhibit the allergic response, or CORTICOSTEROIDS, which inhibit the allergic response and reduce any inflammation.

Decortisyl (*Roussel*) is a proprietary CORTICOSTEROID preparation, available only on prescription, used to treat inflammation especially in

rheumatic or allergic conditions. Produced in the form of tablets, it contains the glucocorticoid steroid prednisone. It is not recommended for children aged under 12 months.
✚/▲ warning/side-effects: *see* PREDNISONE.

dehydrocholic acid is a drug that is administered after surgery on or near the bile ducts. It stimulates the production of thin, watery bile that then flushes the common bile duct, washing away any small calculi (stones) that may remain. It may also be used to clear the gall bladder in preparation for X-ray or endoscope examination. Administration is oral in the form of tablets.
✚ warning: dehydrocholic acid should not be administered to patients with completely blocked bile ducts, chronic liver disease or hepatitis.

Delfen (*Ortho-Cilag*) is a proprietary non-prescription SPERMICIDAL preparation, for use only in combination with barrier methods of contraception (such as a condom or diaphragm). Produced in the form of a cream, and as a foam in an aerosol, Delfen is a preparation of the alcohol ester nonoxinol.

Delial Factor 10 (*Bayer*) is a proprietary non-prescription preparation containing constituents that are able to help protect the skin from ultraviolet radiation. Patients whose skin condition is such as to require this sort of protection, or who are undergoing therapies that might require it, may be prescribed Delial Factor 10 at the discretion of their doctors. It is produced in the form of a cream and a lotion (milk) for topical application.

Delimon (*Consolidated*) is a proprietary compound non-narcotic ANALGESIC, available on prescription only to private patients. Used for the relief of pain anywhere in the body, Delimon's major active constituent is paracetamol.
✚/▲ warning/side-effects: *see* PARACETAMOL.

Deltacortril (*Pfizer*) is a proprietary CORTICOSTEROID preparation, available only on prescription, used to treat allergic conditions, inflammation or collagen disorders requiring systemic treatment with corticosteroids. Produced in the form of tablets in two strengths, (also under the name Deltacortril Enteric), it contains the glucocorticoid steroid prednisolone.
✚/▲ warning/side-effects:*see* PREDNISOLONE.

Deltalone (*DDSA Pharmaceuticals*) is a proprietary CORTICOSTEROID preparation, available only on prescription, used to treat inflammation especially in rheumatic and allergic conditions. Produced in the form of tablets (in two strengths), it contains the glucocorticoid steroid prednisolone.
✚/▲ warning/side-effects: *see* PREDNISOLONE.

Delta-Phoricol (*Wallace*) is a proprietary CORTICOSTEROID preparation, available only on prescription, used to treat inflammation especially in rheumatic and allergic conditions. Produced in the form of tablets, it contains the glucocorticoid steroid prednisolone.
✚/▲ warning/side-effects: *see* PREDNISOLONE.

D

Deltastab (*Boots*) is a proprietary CORTICOSTEROID preparation, available only on prescription, used to treat inflammation especially in allergic and rheumatic conditions, particularly those affecting the joints, and collagen disorders. It may also be used for systemic corticosteroid therapy. Produced in the form of tablets (in two strengths), and in vials for injection (as an aqueous solution), it contains the glucocorticoid steroid prednisolone.

✚/▲ warning/side-effects: *see* PREDNISOLONE.

demecarium bromide is a drug used to treat glaucoma. Applied (in solution) in the form of eye-drops, it works by reducing the formation of aqueous humour within the eyeball.

✚ warning: demecarium bromide should not be administered to patients with peptic ulcers, asthma, or a slow heart rate.

▲ side-effects: some patients experience a burning sensation in eyes treated for a short time following administration (which may in turn be treated with analgesics). Possible sensitivity reactions include nausea and sweating.

Related article: TOSMILEN.

demeclocycline hydrochloride is a broad-spectrum ANTIBIOTIC, one of the TETRACYCLINES, used to treat infections of many kinds. Administration is oral in the form of tablets and capsules.

✚ warning: demeclocycline hydrochloride should not be administered to patients with kidney failure, who are pregnant, or who are aged under 12 years. It should be administered with caution to those who are lactating, or with impaired liver function.

▲ side-effects: there may be nausea and vomiting, with diarrhoea. Some patients experience a sensitivity to light. Rarely, there are allergic reactions.

Related articles: DETECLO; LEDERMYCIN.

Demser (*Merck, Sharp & Dohme*) is a proprietary ANTIHYPERTENSIVE drug, available only on prescription, used to treat symptoms of a disorder of the adrenal glands (phaeochromocytoma) and certain acute forms of high blood pressure (hypertension). Produced in the form of capsules, and usually administered only in hospitals and clinics, Demser is a preparation of the unusual drug metirosine.

✚/▲ warning/side-effects: *see* METIROSINE.

De-Nol (*Brocades*) is a proprietary non-prescription preparation of tripotassium dicitratobismuthate (an inert bismuth compound) which promotes the healing of peptic ulcers in the stomach and duodenum. It is thought to work by forming a protective coating over the ulcer under which the ulcer is then able to heal. It is produced in the form of an elixir with what has been described as a pungent ammoniacal odour.

✚ warning: because the elixir may need time to achieve a coating over an ulcer, it is advised that food and drink should be avoided for two hours before and for half an hour after administration.

De-Noltab (*Brocades*) is a proprietary non-prescription preparation of tripotassium dicitratobismuthate (an inert bismuth compound) which promotes the healing of peptic ulcers in the stomach and duodenum. It is thought to work by forming a protective coating over the ulcer under which the ulcer is then able to heal. It is produced in the form of tablets (which are said to be more palatable than the liquid form, DE-NOL).

✚ warning: because the tablets may need time to achieve a coating over an ulcer, it is advised that food and drink should be avoided for two hours before and for half an hour after administration.

deoxycortone pivalate is a CORTICOSTEROID administered therapeutically to make up for a deficiency of mineralocorticoids (the kind of corticosteroids that regulate salt and water, sodium and potassium levels in the body) resulting from a disorder of the adrenal glands.

✚ warning: deoxycortone pivalate administered to children may restrict growth; administered to pregnant women it may prevent adrenal development in the fetus. As with all corticosteroids, administration may also mask the effects of infection, which may then spread undiagnosed and unchecked. Prolonged usage may cause severe physical symptoms.

▲ side-effects: there may be sodium and water retention leading to weight gain, high blood pressure (hypertension) and muscle weakness. Some patients experience psychological symptoms, such as euphoria or mild confusion.

deoxyribonuclease is an enzyme used therapeutically as an ANTI-INFLAMMATORY (particularly in the veins, or in and around the eye), bruising and swelling. It is thought to work by promoting the removal of coagulated blood, dead tissue and exudate, and is administered orally in the form of tablets, topically in the form of an instillation or by inhalation from an aerosol, or by injection.

▲ side-effects: local injection may cause skin irritation; inhalation may give rise to irritation in the throat. Prolonged use may evoke sensitivity reactions.
Related article: DEANASE.

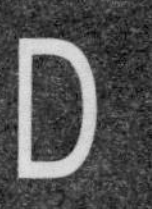

Depixol (*Lundbeck*) is a proprietary ANTIPSYCHOTIC drug, available only on prescription, used to tranquillize patients suffering from psychosis (including schizophrenia), especially patients with forms of psychosis that render them apathetic and withdrawn. It may also be used in the short term to treat severe anxiety. Produced in the form of tablets, or in ampoules for injection (in two strengths, the stronger under the name Depixol Conc.), Depixol is a preparation of flupenthixol.

✚/▲ warning/side-effects: *see* FLUPENTHIXOL.

Depocillin (*Brocades*) is a proprietary ANTIBIOTIC, available only on prescription, used to treat serious infections such as gonorrhoea, syphilis and gas gangrene following amputation, where long-term treatment is envisaged. Produced in the form of powder for reconstitution as a medium for depot injection, Depocillin is a preparation of the penicillin-type antibiotic procaine penicillin.

✚/▲ warning/side-effects: *see* PROCAINE PENICILLIN.

Depo-Medrone (*Upjohn*) is a proprietary CORTICOSTEROID preparation, available only on prescription, used to treat inflammation and relieve allergic disorders (such as rheumatoid

arthritis, osteoarthrosis, hay fever and asthma), and sometimes used additionally to treat shock. Produced in vials and pre-prepared syringes for intramuscular depot injection, Depo-Medrone is a preparation of the steroid methylprednisolone acetate (in aqueous solution).
✚/▲ warning/side-effects: *see* METHYLPREDNISOLONE.

Depo-Medrone with Lidocaine (*Upjohn*) is a proprietary CORTICOSTEROID preparation, available only on prescription, used to treat inflammation in the joints (as in rheumatic disease). Produced in vials for intra-articular injection, Depo-Medrone with Lidocaine is a preparation of the steroid methylprednisolone acetate (in aqueous solution) containing the local ANAESTHETIC lignocaine hydrochloride.
✚/▲ warning/side-effects: *see* LIGNOCAINE; METHYLPREDNISOLONE.

Deponit (*Schwarz*) is a proprietary, non-prescription, self-adhesive skin-coloured dressing (patch) containing the VASODILATOR glyceryl trinitrate which, when placed on the chest wall, is absorbed through the skin and helps to give lasting relief from attacks of angina pectoris (heart pain). Patches are replaced daily, and each should be sited in a surface location different from the preceding patch. Deponit is not recommended for children.
✚/▲ warning/side-effects: *see* GLYCERYL TRINITRATE.

Depo-provera (*Upjohn*) is a proprietary HORMONE preparation of the synthetic PROGESTOGEN medroxyprogesterone acetate in aqueous suspension, available only on prescription. It has three major uses: as a long-lasting contraceptive preparation, administered as an intramuscular injection every 3 months; as a relatively non-masculinizing hormonal supplement in women whose progestogen level requires boosting, such as at the menopause, or to treat recurrent miscarriage; and (in higher doses) to treat sex-hormone-linked cancer (such as cancer of the breast or of the womb-lining). It is produced in vials (in two strengths).
✚/▲ warning/side-effects: *see* MEDROXYPROGESTERONE.

Depostat (*Schering*) is a proprietary preparation of the synthetic HORMONE PROGESTOGEN gestronol hexanoate, available only on prescription, used in women to treat sex-hormone-linked cancers (such as cancer of the breast or of the womb-lining), or in men to treat benign enlargement of the prostate gland or malignant enlargement of the kidneys. It is produced in ampoules for intramuscular injection.
✚/▲ warning/side-effects: *see* GESTRONOL HEXANOATE.

Dequacaine (*Farley*) is the name of a proprietary non-prescription lozenge containing the local ANAESTHETIC benzocaine together with the ANTIFUNGAL agent DEQUALINIUM CHLORIDE, to be sucked slowly until it dissolves, so affording relief from the pain of mouth ulcers or other oral lesions.
✚ warning: *see* BENZOCAINE.

Dequadin (*Farley*) is the name of a proprietary non-prescription lozenge containing the ANTIFUNGAL agent DEQUALINIUM CHLORIDE, to be sucked slowly until it dissolves, so treating oral infections.

dequalinium chloride is an antiseptic ANTIFUNGAL agent that also has some antibacterial properties. It is used primarily to treat fungal infections of the mouth and throat (such as thrush). Administration is oral in the form of lozenges, or topical in the form of a paint.

Derbac-C (*International Labs*) is a proprietary non-prescription antiparasitic drug used to treat infestations of the scalp and pubic hair by lice (pediculosis). Produced in the form of a shampoo, Derbac-C (also called Derbac Shampoo) is a preparation of the pediculicide carbaryl.
✚ warning: *see* CARBARYL.

Derbac-M (*International Labs*) is a proprietary non-prescription antiparasitic drug used to treat infestations of the scalp and pubic hair by lice (pediculosis), or of the skin by the itch-mite (scabies). Produced in the form of a lotion, Derbac-M is a preparation of the insecticide malathion.
✚ warning: *see* MALATHION.

Derbac Shampoo is another name for Derbac-C.
see DERBAC-C.

Dermacolor (*Fox*) is the name of a proprietary non-prescription camouflage cream, in any of 30 shades, designed for use in masking scars and other skin disfigurements; there is an additional fixing powder (in 5 shades). It may be obtained on prescription if the skin disfigurement is the result of surgery or is giving rise to emotional disturbance.

Dermalex (*Labaz*) is a proprietary non-prescription skin lotion and emollient (soother and softener), used to treat nappy rash and to prevent bedsores. Its major active constituent is the antiseptic hexachlorophane. It is not recommended for children aged under 2 years.
✚/▲ warning/side-effects: *see* HEXACHLOROPHANE.

Dermonistat (*Ortho-Cilag*) is a proprietary non-prescription antifungal cream used to treat infections of the skin and the nails. Topical treatment must be continued for 10 days after the infective lesions have disappeared. Dermonistat is a preparation of the IMIDAZOLE miconazole nitrate.
✚/▲ warning/side-effects: *see* MICONAZOLE.

Dermovate (*Glaxo*) is an extremely powerful CORTICOSTEROID preparation for topical application, available only on prescription, used (in the short term only) to treat severe exacerbations in serious inflammatory skin disorders such as discoid lupus erythematosus. Produced in the form of a water-miscible cream for dilution (the potency of the cream once dilute is retained for 14 days), as an ointment in an anhydrous base for dilution with liquid paraffin (the potency of the ointment once dilute is retained for 14 days), and as a scalp application in an alcohol base, Dermovate is in all forms a preparation of the steroid clobetasol propionate.
✚/▲ warning/side-effects: *see* CLOBETASOL PROPIONATE.

Dermovate-NN (*Glaxo*) is an extremely powerful CORTICOSTEROID preparation for topical application, available only on prescription, used (in the short term only) to treat severe exacerbations in serious inflammatory skin disorders such as discoid lupus erythematosus.

Produced in the form of a cream, and as an ointment in an anhydrous base for dilution with white soft paraffin (the potency of the ointment once dilute is retained for 14 days), Dermovate-NN is in both forms a preparation of the steroid clobetasol propionate with the broad-spectrum antibiotic neomycin sulphate and the antifungal agent nystatin.

✚/▲ warning/side-effects: *see* CLOBETASOL PROPIONATE; NEOMYCIN; NYSTATIN.

***desensitizing vaccines** are preparations of particular allergens (substances to which a patient has an allergic reaction). They are administered to reduce the degree of allergic reaction the patient suffers when exposed to the allergen. For example, preparations of grass pollens are administered for the treatment of hay fever. The mechanism by which they work is unclear.

✚ warning: administration should be under close medical supervision.

Deseril (*Sandoz*) is a proprietary preparation of the potentially dangerous drug methysergide, available only on prescription (and generally only in hospitals under strict medical supervision). It is used primarily to prevent severe recurrent migraine and similar headaches in patients for whom other forms of treatment have failed. But the drug may also be used to treat patients who suffer from tumours of the intestinal glands that have metastasized to the liver: the liver then produces excess serotonin in the bloodstream – and it is the symptoms of that excess that methysergide treats. Deseril is produced in the form of tablets.

✚/▲ warning/side-effects: *see* METHYSERGIDE.

Desferal (*Ciba*) is a proprietary form of the CHELATING AGENT desferrioxamine mesylate, available only on prescription, used to treat iron poisoning (by ingestion or through anaemia) and the symptoms associated with it (vomiting of blood, diarrhoea, bleeding from the anus and low blood pressure, then if untreated, liver, pancreas and endocrine gland damage, a bronze coloration of the skin, and a form of diabetes). It is produced as a powder for reconstitution as a medium for injection.

✚/▲ warning/side-effects: *see* DESFERRIOXAMINE MESYLATE.

desferrioxamine mesylate is a CHELATING AGENT used to treat iron poisoning (by ingestion or through anaemia) and the symptoms associated with it (vomiting of blood, diarrhoea, bleeding from the anus and low blood pressure, then if untreated, liver, pancreas and endocrine gland damage, a bronze coloration of the skin, and a form of diabetes). Administration is oral (in water) following initial emptying of the stomach either by induction of vomiting or by stomach pump; absorbed iron can also be chelated by an intramuscular injection of desferrioxamine mesylate.

✚ warning: over-rapid injection of the drug can lead to sensitivity reactions and low blood pressure (hypotension).

▲ side-effects: there may be pain at the site of injection.

Related article: DESFERAL.

desipramine hydrochloride is an ANTIDEPRESSANT drug of a type that has fewer sedative properties than many others. Used to treat depressive illness, it is thus suited more to the treatment of withdrawn and apathetic patients than to those who are agitated and restless. Administration is oral in the form of tablets.

✚ warning: desipramine hydrochloride should not be administered to patients with heart disease or liver failure; it should be administered with extreme caution to those with epilepsy, psychoses or glaucoma, or who are pregnant. Treatment may take up to four weeks to achieve full effect; premature withdrawal of treatment thereafter may cause the return of symptoms.

▲ side-effects: dry mouth, drowsiness, blurred vision, constipation and urinary retention are all fairly common; there may also be heartbeat irregularities accompanying low blood pressure (hypotension). Concentration and speed of reaction are affected. Elderly patients may enter a state of confusion; younger patients may experience behavioural disturbances. Not recommended for children. There may be alteration in blood sugar levels, and weight gain.

Related article: PERTOFRAN.

desmopressin is one of two major forms of the ANTIDIURETIC hormone vasopressin, which reduces urine production. It is used primarily to diagnose or to treat pituitary-originated diabetes insipidus, although it can be used for some other diagnostic tests and even (in specialist centres) to boost blood concentration of blood-clotting factors in haemophiliac patients. Administration is topical in the form of nose-drops, or by injection. Dosage is adjusted to individual patient response (with special care being taken in patients with hypertension or who are pregnant).

✚/▲ warning/side-effects: *see* VASOPRESSIN.

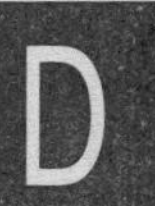

desonide is a powerful CORTICOSTEROID, used in topical application on severe skin inflammations (such as eczema), especially in cases where less powerful steroid treatments have failed. Administration is in the form of a dilute aqueous cream or a dilute paraffin-based ointment.

✚ warning: as with all corticosteroids, desonide treats the symptoms of inflammation but has no effect on any underlying infection; undetected infection may thus become worse even as its effects are masked by the steroid. Desonide should not in any case be administered to patients who suffer from untreated skin lesions; use on the face should also be avoided; caution is advised in treatment for children.

▲ side-effects: topical application may result in the thinning of skin, with possible whitening, and an increased local growth of hair. Some young patients experience the outbreak of a kind of inflammatory dermatitis on the face or at the site of application.

Related article: TRIDESILON.

desoxymethasone is a CORTICOSTEROID drug used to treat acute inflammatory conditions resulting from skin disorders and allergic reactions. Administration is topical in the form of an oily cream.

✚ warning: as with all corticosteroids, desoxymethasone treats the symptoms of inflammation but has no effect on any underlying infection; undetected infection may thus become worse even as its effects are masked by the steroid. Desoxymethasone should not in any case be administered to patients with untreated skin lesions; use on the face should also be avoided; caution is advised in treatment for children.

▲ side-effects: topical application may result in the thinning of skin, with possible whitening, and an increased local growth of hair. Some young patients experience the outbreak of a kind of inflammatory dermatitis on the face or at the site of application when they use desoxymethasone.

Related article: STIEDEX.

Destolit (*Merrell*) is a proprietary preparation of the acidic drug ursodeoxycholic acid, used to dissolve relatively small, light, cholesterol gallstones. X-ray monitoring of treatment is required to supervise progress. The course may last for up to two years, and treatment must be continued for at least three months after stones have been dissolved. Destolit is produced in the form of tablets.

✚/▲ warning/side-effects: *see* URSODEOXYCHOLIC ACID.

Deteclo (*Lederle*) is a proprietary compound ANTIBIOTIC preparation, available only on prescription, used to treat many kinds of infection, but especially those of the respiratory tract, the ear, nose, and throat, the gastrointestinal tract and the urinary tract, and the soft tissues. Deteclo consists of a combination of TETRACYCLINES – chlortetracycline hydrochloride, tetracycline hydrochloride and demeclocycline hydrochloride – is produced in the form of tablets, and is not recommended for children.

✚/▲ warning/side-effects: *see* CHLORTETRACYCLINE; DEMECLOCYCLINE HYDROCHLORIDE; TETRACYCLINE.

Dettol (*Reckitt & Colman*) is a well-known proprietary non-prescription ANTISEPTIC lotion, used for ordinary disinfectant purposes or in treating abrasions and minor wounds. But it is also particularly used in obstetrics for the antisepsis of hands, gloves and forceps, and as a vaginal lubricant during labour. It is a preparation of CHLOROXYLENOL (in mild solution).

dexamethasone is a synthesized CORTICOSTEROID used, as are most corticosteroids, in the treatment of non-infective inflammation. Accordingly, it is used to treat many conditions, ranging from the suppression of allergic disorders and shock (in the form of dexamethasone or dexamethasone sodium phosphate), and the relief of pain in inflamed joints and tissues (as dexamethasone sodium phosphate), to the soothing of eye inflammations (as dexamethasone) or nasal congestion (as dexamethasone isonicotinate). Administration is in the form of tablets, eye-drops and ointment, and by injection or infusion.

✚ warning: dexamethasone should not be administered to patients with psoriasis; it should be administered with caution to the elderly (in whom overdosage can cause osteoporosis, "brittle bones"). In children, administration of dexamethasone may lead to stunting of growth. As with all corticosteroids, dexamethasone treats only inflammatory symptoms; an undetected and potentially serious infection

may have its effects masked by the drug until it is well established.
▲ side-effects: systemic treatment of susceptible patients may engender a euphoria – or a state of confusion or depression. Rarely, there is peptic ulceration. Treatment of eye inflammations may in susceptible patients lead to a form of glaucoma (and should therefore be carried out under careful supervision).
Related articles: DECADRON; DECADRON SHOCK-PAK; DEXA-RHINASPRAY; MAXIDEX; MAXITROL; ORADEXON; SOFRADEX.

dexamphetamine sulphate is an AMPHETAMINE, a powerful STIMULANT drug, used primarily to treat narcolepsy (a condition marked by irresistible attacks of sleep during the daytime), although it is sometimes also used under specialist supervision to treat children who are medically hyperactive. Tolerance and dependence (addiction) are major hazards. Administration is oral in the form of tablets and sustained-release capsules.
✚ warning: dexamphetamine sulphate should not be administered to patients who suffer from cardiovascular disease, glaucoma, or an excess of thyroid hormones in the bloodstream (thyrotoxicosis); it should be administered with caution to those with impaired kidney function, anorexia, insomnia, an unstable personality or during pregnancy.
▲ side-effects: tolerance and dependence (addiction) occur readily. There may also be agitation, insomnia, headache and dizziness. Some patients experience heartbeat irregularities, dry mouth, diarrhoea or constipation. There may also be tremor and a personality change. In children, drastic weight loss may be accompanied by inhibition of growth. Overdoses may result in psychoses, convulsions, or even death.
Related articles: DEXEDRINE; DUROPHET.

Dexa-Rhinaspray (*Boehringer Ingelheim*) is a proprietary nasal inhalation, available only on prescription, used to treat hay fever (allergic rhinitis). Produced in a metered-dose aerosol, it represents a preparation of the CORTICOSTEROID dexamethasone isonicotinate together with the ANTIBIOTIC neomycin sulphate and the SYMPATHOMIMETIC tramazoline hydrochloride. It is not recommended for children aged under 5 years.
✚/▲ warning/side-effects: *see* DEXAMETHASONE; NEOMYCIN.

Dexedrine (*Smith, Kline & French*) is a proprietary preparation of the powerful stimulant drug dexamphetamine sulphate, which is on the controlled drugs list. It is used primarily to treat narcolepsy (a condition marked by irresistible attacks of sleep during the daytime), although it is sometimes also used under specialist supervision to treat children who are medically hyperactive. Tolerance and dependence (addiction) are major hazards. Produced in the form of tablets, it is not generally recommended for children.
✚/▲ warning/side-effects: *see* DEXAMPHETAMINE SULPHATE.

dextran is a carbohydrate chemically consisting of glucose units, used in solution as a plasma substitute – that is, as a substitute for the straw-coloured fluid in which blood cells are normally suspended. It is most used in infusion to increase a patient's overall volume of blood following drastic haemorrhage or other forms of shock (such as burns or septicaemia). Generally, administration is on an emergency basis only, until properly tissue-matched blood can be infused. Even so, dextran in a patient's circulation may interfere with the cross-matching process and such tissue-typing should ideally take place first. There are two major preparations of dextran: dextran 40 and dextran 70. Dextran 40 represents a 10% concentration in glucose or saline solution, and is used mostly to improve blood flow in the limbs and extremities (so treating ischaemic conditions and preventing thrombosis or embolism). Dextran 70 represents a 6% concentration in glucose or saline solution, and is used mostly as outlined initially above to expand a patient's overall blood volume. There is also a proprietary form of dextran 110 which is to all intents and purposes very much the same as dextran 70.

✚ warning: dextran should not be administered to patients with severe congestive heart failure or kidney failure, or who may experience blood clotting difficulties.

▲ side-effects: rarely, there are hypersensitivity reactions.
Related articles: DEXTRAVEN 110; GENTRAN; LOMODEX; MACRODEX; RHEOMACRODEX.

Dextraven 110 (*CP Pharmaceuticals*) is a proprietary preparation of dextran 110, available only on prescription, used in infusion to boost the overall volume of a patient's blood circulation in emergency circumstances. It is produced in flasks (bottles).

✚/▲ warning/side-effects: *see* DEXTRAN.

Dextrolyte (*Cow & Gate*) is a proprietary non-prescription sodium supplement, used to treat mild or moderate degrees of sodium depletion in the body (as may happen in cases of dehydration or in illnesses – particularly kidney disease – in which salt is lost in some quantity). Dextrolyte is produced in the form of a solution (for swallowing) containing SODIUM CHLORIDE (salt), POTASSIUM CHLORIDE, GLUCOSE and SODIUM LACTATE.

dextromethorphan is an ANTITUSSIVE, an opiate that is used singly or in combination with other drugs in linctuses, syrups and lozenges to relieve dry or painful coughs.

✚ warning: dextromethorphan should not be administered to patients who suffer from liver disease. Used as a linctus, it may cause sputum retention which may be injurious to patients with asthma, chronic bronchitis or bronchiectasis (two conditions for which linctuses are commonly prescribed).

▲ side-effects: constipation is a comparatively common side-effect.
Related articles: ACTIFED COMPOUND LINCTUS; COSYLAN; TANCOLIN.

dextromoramide is a synthesized derivative of morphine, and like morphine used as a narcotic ANALGESIC to counter severe and intractable pain, particularly in the final stages of terminal illness. Proprietary forms are on the controlled drugs list because, also like morphine, dextromoramide is potentially addictive.

✚ warning: dextromoramide should not be administered to patients who suffer from head injury or intracranial pressure; it should be administered with caution to those with impaired kidney or liver function, asthma, depressed respiration, insufficient secretion of thyroid hormones (hypothyroidism) or low blood pressure (hypotension), or who are pregnant or lactating. Dosage should be decreased for the elderly or debilitated.

▲ side-effects: shallow breathing, urinary retention, constipation, and nausea are all common; tolerance and dependence (addiction) occur fairly readily. There may also be drowsiness, and pain at the site of injection (where there may also be tissue damage).
Related article: PALFIUM.

dextropropoxyphene is a weak ANALGESIC that is nevertheless similar to a narcotic, used to treat pain anywhere in the body. It is usually combined with other analgesics (especially paracetamol or aspirin) for compound effect. Administration of the drug alone is oral in the form of capsules.

✚ warning: dextropropoxyphene should not be administered to patients who suffer from head injury or intracranial pressure; it should be administered with caution to those with impaired kidney or liver function, asthma, depressed respiration, insufficient secretion of thyroid hormones (hypothyroidism) or low blood pressure (hypotension), or who are pregnant or lactating. Dosage should be decreased for the elderly or debilitated.

▲ side-effects: shallow breathing, urinary retention, constipation, and nausea are all common; in high overdosage tolerance and dependence (addiction) occur fairly readily, leading possibly to psychoses and convulsions.
Related article: DOLOXENE.

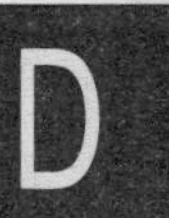

dextrose, or dextrose monohydrate, is another term for glucose.
see GLUCOSE.

dextrothyroxine sodium is a drug that was formerly used to reduce high levels of fats (lipids) in the blood, in patients for whom simple dietary measures were not sufficient. Although the drug does reduce cholesterol levels, it also has the effect of increasing the heart rate which, for patients with heart disease (as many patients with high blood fat levels are), could lead to angina pectoris (heart pain). Administration is/was oral in the form of tablets.

✚ warning: dextrothyroxine sodium should not be administered to patients with heart disease involving deficient blood supply to the heart, or from severe liver or kidney disease.

▲ side-effects: the heart rate is increased.
Related article: CHOLOXIN.

DF118 (*Duncan, Flockhart*) is a proprietary narcotic ANALGESIC available on prescription only to private patients, used to treat moderate to severe pain anywhere in the body. Produced in the form of tablets and as an elixir for dilution (the potency of the elixir once dilute is retained for 14 days) and in ampoules (as a controlled drug) for injection,

D

DF118 is a preparation of the narcotic dihydrocodeine tartrate.
✚/▲ warning/side-effects: *see* DIHYDROCODEINE TARTRATE.

Diabinese (*Pfizer*) is a proprietary SULPHONYLUREA, available only on prescription, which has the effect of reducing blood levels of glucose by promoting the secretion of INSULIN within the pancreas. It is thus useful in treating the hyperglycaemia that is associated with adult-onset diabetes mellitus (in which the pancreas still has some capacity for insulin production). Produced in the form of tablets (in two strengths), Diabinese represents a preparation of chlorpropamide.
✚/▲ warning/side-effects: *see* CHLORPROPAMIDE.

Dialamine (*Scientific Hospital Supplies*) is a proprietary non-prescription nutritional supplement for patients who need extra amino acids (perhaps following kidney failure). Produced in the form of a powder for reconstitution as an orange-flavoured liquid, Dialamine contains essential amino acids, carbohydrate, ascorbic acid (vitamin C), minerals and trace elements.

Diamicron (*Servier*) is a proprietary SULPHONYLUREA, available only on prescription, which has the effect of reducing blood levels of glucose by promoting the secretion of INSULIN within the pancreas. It is useful in treating the hyperglycaemia that is associated with adult-onset diabetes mellitus (in which the pancreas still has some capacity for insulin production). Produced in the form of tablets, Diamicron is a preparation of gliclazide.
✚/▲ warning/side-effects: *see* GLICLAZIDE.

diamorphine is the chemical name of heroin, a white crystalline powder that is a derivative of morphine. Like morphine, it is a powerful NARCOTIC ANALGESIC useful in the treatment of moderate to severe pain, although it has a shorter duration of effect; and like morphine it is also sometimes used – generally in the form of diamorphine hydrochloride – as a cough suppressant in compound linctuses (especially in the treatment of terminal lung cancer). Again like morphine, its use quickly tends to tolerance and then dependence (addiction). Administration is oral in the form of tablets or an elixir, or by injection.
✚ warning: diamorphine should not be administered to patients with renal or liver disease; it should be administered with caution to those with asthma (because it tends to cause sputum retention).
▲ side-effects: there may be euphoria, depending on dosage. There may also be constipation and low blood pressure. In some patients there is respiratory depression with high dosage.

Diamox (*Lederle*) is a proprietary DIURETIC, available only on prescription, used to treat an accumulation of fluid in the tissues (oedema), especially in association with congestive heart failure, to assist in the prevention of epileptic seizures, and to treat the symptoms of premenstrual syndrome. Like many diuretics, it may additionally be used in the treatment of glaucoma, having the effect of reducing the moisture of the aqueous humour in the eyeball. Produced in the form of tablets, as capsules

(under the trade name Diamox Sustets), and as a powder for reconstitution as a medium for injection or infusion, Diamox is a preparation of acetazolamide. It is not recommended for children.
✚/▲ warning/side-effects: *see* ACETAZOLAMIDE.

Diane (*Schering*) is a proprietary compound that combines the oestrogen (female sex hormone) ethinyloestradiol with the anti-ANDROGEN cyproterone acetate. It is used to treat women who suffer from skin conditions that are androgen-linked, particularly acne (and especially in cases where antibacterial treatment is not tolerated or has failed) or hirsutism. It is produced in the form of tablets presented, like many oral contraceptives, in packs of 21 corresponding to one complete menstrual cycle.
✚/▲ warning/side-effects: *see* CYPROTERONE ACETATE; ETHINYLOESTRADIOL.

Diarrest (*Galen*) is a proprietary drug, available only on prescription, that is a preparation of the OPIATE codeine phosphate together with sodium and potassium salts as supplements to replace minerals lost through vomiting or diarrhoea. (The opiate has the capacity to reduce intestinal motility.) Diarrest is produced in the form of a liquid (for swallowing); prolonged use must be avoided.
✚/▲ warning/side-effects: *see* CODEINE PHOSPHATE.

Diatensec (*Gold Cross*) is a proprietary DIURETIC, available only on prescription, used to treat the symptoms of cirrhosis of the liver or of kidney disease, and to assist in the treatment of high blood pressure (hypertension), especially in association with congestive heart failure or diabetes mellitus. Produced in the form of tablets, it is a preparation of the mild but potassium-sparing diuretic spironolactone.
✚/▲ warning/side-effects: *see* SPIRONOLACTONE.

Dia-tuss (*Lipha*) is a proprietary non-prescription ANTITUSSIVE (cough suppressant) used to stop a dry or painful cough. It works by directly affecting the cough centre of the brain. Produced in the form of a sugar-free orange syrup for dilution with sorbitol (the potency of the syrup once dilute is retained for 14 days), Dia-tuss is a preparation of the opiate pholcodine.
✚/▲ warning/side-effects: *see* PHOLCODINE.

Diazemuls (*KabiVitrum*) is a proprietary ANXIOLYTIC drug, available only on prescription, used to treat anxiety in the short or long term, to relieve insomnia, and to assist in the treatment of alcohol withdrawal symptoms and migraine. It may be used additionally to provide sedation for very minor surgery or as a premedication prior to surgical procedures and, because it also has some SKELETAL MUSCLE RELAXANT properties, to treat the spasm of tetanus or poisoning, or to relieve the bronchospasm of severe conditions of asthma. Continued use results in tolerance and may lead to dependence (addiction). Produced as an emulsion in ampoules for injection, Diazemuls is a preparation of the BENZODIAZEPINE diazepam.
✚/▲ warning/side-effects: *see* DIAZEPAM.

diazepam is an ANXIOLYTIC drug, one of the BENZODIAZEPINES, used to treat anxiety in the short or long term, to relieve insomnia, and to assist in the treatment of alcohol withdrawal symptoms and migraine. It may be used additionally to provide sedation for very minor surgery or as a premedication prior to surgical procedures and, because it also has some SKELETAL MUSCLE RELAXANT properties, to treat the spasm of tetanus or poisoning, or to relieve the bronchospasm of severe conditions of asthma. Continued use results in tolerance and may lead to dependence (addiction), especially in patients with a history of drug (including alcohol) abuse. Administration is oral in the form of tablets or capsules or a dilute elixir, topical as anal suppositories, or by injection.

✚ warning: concentration and speed of thought and movement are often affected; the effects of alcohol consumption may also be enhanced. Diazepam should be administered with caution to patients with respiratory difficulties, glaucoma, or kidney or liver damage; who are in the last stages of pregnancy; or who are elderly or debilitated. Prolonged use of the drug or abrupt withdrawal from treatment should be avoided.

▲ side-effects: there may be drowsiness, dizziness, headache, dry mouth, urinary retention, and shallow breathing; hypersensitivity reactions may occur.
Related articles: ALUPRAM; ATENSINE; DIAZEMULS; EVACALM; SOLIS; STESOLID; TENSIUM; VALIUM.

diazoxide is a hypoglycaemic drug used to treat chronic conditions involving a deficit of glucose in the bloodstream (as occurs, for example, if a pancreatic tumour causes excessive secretion of insulin). It is also useful in treating an acute hypertensive crisis (apoplexy). Administration is by injection.

✚ warning: diazoxide should be administered with caution to patients with reduced blood supply to the heart or impaired kidney function, or who are pregnant or in labour. During prolonged treatment, regular monitoring of blood constituents and pressure is essential.

▲ side-effects: there may be nausea and vomiting, an increased heart rate with low blood pressure (hypotension), loss of appetite accumulation of fluid in the tissues (oedema), arrhythmias, and hyperglycaemia.
Related article: EUDEMINE.

Dibenyline (*Smith, Kline & French*) is a proprietary VASODILATOR used (in combination with a BETA-BLOCKER) in the treatment of the high blood pressure (*see* ANTIHYPERTENSIVE) caused by tumours in the adrenal glands and the resulting secretion of the hormones adrenaline and noradrenaline. Under specialist supervision it may be used to treat urinary retention due to nerve damage in the bladder. Produced in the form of capsules and in ampoules for injection, Dibenyline is a preparation of phenoxybenzamine hydrochloride.

✚/▲ warning/side-effects: *see* PHENOXYBENZAMINE HYDROCHLORIDE.

dichloralphenazone is a HYPNOTIC drug used to treat insomnia, particularly in children or elderly patients. Prolonged use leads to tolerance and dependence (addiction). Administration is oral in the

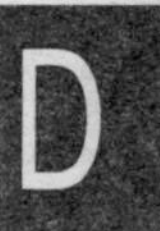

form of tablets or a dilute elixir.
✚ warning: concentration and speed of movement and thought are affected. Dichloralphenazone should be administered with caution to patients with lung disease, who are pregnant or lactating, or who have a history of drug abuse. Dosage should be reduced for elderly or debilitated patients, or for those with impaired liver or kidney function, cardiac disease or gastritis. Keep the drug off the skin and the mucous membranes.
▲ side-effects: there is commonly drowsiness, dizziness headache and dry mouth. More rarely there may be gastrointestinal disturbance or a rash.
Related article: WELLDORM.

dichlorphenamide is a drug that has the effect of a DIURETIC; in particular, it reduces the fluid (aqueous humour) in the eyeball, and is therefore used to treat glaucoma. Administration is oral in the form of tablets.
✚ warning: side-effects are marked in elderly patients.
▲ side-effects: there may be tingling in the nerve endings, drowsiness, headache, constipation, loss of appetite and a low potassium blood level. Some patients experience depression.
Related article: DARANIDE.

diclofenac sodium is a non-steroidal ANTI-INFLAMMATORY non-narcotic ANALGESIC drug used to treat pain and inflammation in rheumatic disease and other musculo-skeletal disorders (such as arthritis and gout). Administration is oral in the form of tablets, topical in the form of anal suppositories, or by injection.
✚ warning: diclofenac sodium should be administered with caution to patients with gastric ulcers, impaired kidney or liver function, or allergic disorders particularly induced by aspirin or anti-inflammatory drugs, or to those who are pregnant.
▲ side-effects: there may be nausea and gastrointestinal disturbance (to avoid which a patient may be advised to take the drug with food or milk), headache and ringing in the ears (tinnitus). Some patients experience sensitivity reactions (such as a rash or the symptoms of asthma). Fluid retention and/or blood disorders may occur.
Related article: VOLTAROL.

dicobalt edetate is used solely as an antidote to poisoning with cyanides – it is actually toxic in the absence of cyanides. Administration is by intravenous injection.
▲ side-effects: the heart rate is increased and the blood pressure reduced; there may be vomiting.
Related article: KELOCYANOR.

Diconal (*Calmic*) is a proprietary narcotic ANALGESIC that is on the controlled drugs list. Used to treat moderate to severe pain, and produced in the form of tablets, Diconal represents a compound of the narcotic and OPIATE dipipanone hydrochloride together with the ANTIHISTAMINE and ANTINAUSEANT cyclizine hydrochloride. It is not recommended for children.
✚/▲ warning/side-effects: *see* CYCLIZINE; DIPIPANONE.

dicyclomine hydrochloride is a synthetic ANTICHOLINERGIC ANTISPASMODIC used primarily to assist in the treatment of gastrointestinal disorders caused by spasm (rigidity) in the muscular walls of the stomach or intestines. Administration is oral in the form of tablets, gel, or dilute syrup.

✚ warning: dicyclomine hydrochloride should not be administered to patients with glaucoma; it should be administered with caution to those with heart problems and rapid heart rate, ulcerative colitis, urinary retention or enlargement of the prostate gland; who are elderly; or who are lactating.

▲ side-effects: there is commonly dry mouth and thirst; there may also be visual disturbances, flushing, irregular heartbeat and constipation. Rarely, there may be high temperature accompanied by delirium.
Related articles: KOLANTICON; KOLANTYL; MERBENTYL.

Dicynene (*Delandale*) is a proprietary HAEMOSTATIC drug, available only on prescription, used to treat haemorrhage from small blood vessels or to relieve excessive menstrual flow. Produced in the form of tablets (in two strengths) and in ampoules for injection (in two strengths), Dicynene represents a preparation of ethamsylate.

✚/▲ warning/side-effects: *see* ETHAMSYLATE.

Didronel (*Norwich Eaton*) is a CHELATING AGENT, available only on prescription, used to treat the condition known as Paget's disease of bone (osteitis deformans: a severely and continuously painful condition in which the larger bones of the body thicken while their structure becomes disorganized). It works by inhibiting the demineralization process inherent in the disease. Treatment may last for 6 months, and require a simultaneous dietary regimen. Produced in the form of tablets, Didronel represents a preparation of disodium etidronate. Not recommended for children.

✚/▲ warning/side-effects: *see* DISODIUM ETIDRONATE.

dienoestrol is a synthetic OESTROGEN, a female sex hormone used in the form of a cream to make up hormonal deficiency in and around the vagina (especially following the menopause). Dosage should be adjusted to be the minimum that still retains effect, and should be discontinued as soon as possible, in order to minimize the absorption of the oestrogen

✚ warning: absorption of oestrogen following prolonged use may eventually lead to increased risk of thrombosis or even of endometrial cancer.

▲ side-effects: absorption may result in weight gain through sodium and fluid retention; there may also be nausea and headache, and a rash.
Related articles: HORMOFEMIN; ORTHO DIENOESTROL.

diethyl ether is the now old-fashioned 'ether' used as a general ANAESTHETIC. Powerful as it is, it is now unpopular both because it is flammable and explosive in the presence of oxygen, and because it tends to cause nausea and vomiting in a patient. All the same, it is an effective anaesthetic under the influence of which body processes – in particular the heart rhythm – are generally well maintained.

diethylcarbamazine citrate is an antifilarial agent used to treat infestation by worm-parasites (such as those that cause elephantiasis, lymphangitis,

loiasis and onchocerciasis). Side-effects are inevitable but are generally treated in turn with other drugs; close monitoring is essential throughout treatment, particularly at first. Several courses of treatment may be necessary, but the drug is almost always successful.
Administration is oral in the form of tablets.

✚ warning: the destruction of the worm-parasites causes the release of antigens and the corresponding allergic response which manifest themselves in skin irritation and inflammation, and visual disturbances because the eyes are also affected. Antihistamines and corticosteroids may be prescribed to deal with these.

▲ side-effects: there may be nausea and vomiting, with headache. Skin and eye inflammations may be aggravated.
Related article: BANOCIDE.

diethylpropion hydrochloride is a drug used under medical supervision to aid slimming regimes because it acts to suppress the appetite. But it is also a stimulant and potentially represents the basis for drug abuse, although the stimulant action may in fact be useful in the treatment of lethargic and/or depressed patients. Proprietary preparations are therefore on the controlled drugs list.
Administration is oral in the form of sustained-release tablets.

✚ warning: diethylpropion hydrochloride should not be administered to patients who suffer from glaucoma or any medical condition (such as thyrotoxicosis) that disposes towards excitability; it should be administered with caution to those with heart disease, diabetes, epilepsy, peptic ulcer, depression or unstable personality, and to those with a history of alcohol or drug abuse.

▲ side-effects: there is commonly rapid heart rate, nervous agitation and insomnia, tremor, gastrointestinal disturbance, dry mouth, dizziness and headache. Tolerance and dependence may occur. Susceptible patients may undergo psychotic episodes.
Related articles: APISATE; TENUATE DOSPAN.

Difflam (*Riker*) is a proprietary non-prescription preparation of the ANALGESIC benzydamine hydrochloride. It is produced both as a cream which, when applied to the skin, produces an irritation of sensory nerve endings that offsets the pain of underlying muscle or joint ailments, and as a mouthwash or spray to relieve the pain of mouth ulcers and other sores or inflammations in the mouth or throat. Prolonged use in any form should be avoided.

✚/▲ warning/side-effects: *see* BENZYDAMINE HYDROCHLORIDE.

diflucortolone valerate is a powerful and popular CORTICOSTEROID, used in topical application on severe non-infective skin inflammations (such as eczema), especially in cases where less powerful steroid treatments have failed.
Administration is in the form of a dilute water-miscible cream, a dilute hydrous ointment (or oily cream), or an anhydrous paraffin-based ointment.

✚ warning: as with all corticosteroids, diflucortolone valerate treats the symptoms of inflammation but has no effect on any underlying infection; undetected infection may thus become worse even as its effects are masked by the steroid. The drug should not in any case be administered to patients with untreated skin lesions; use on the face should be avoided. Not for use in children under 4.

▲ side-effects: topical application may result in the local thinning of skin, with possible whitening, and an increased local growth of hair. Some young patients experience the outbreak of a kind of inflammatory dermatitis on the face or at the site of application.
Related articles: NERISONE; TEMETEX.

diflunisal is a non-steroidal ANTI-INFLAMMATORY non-narcotic ANALGESIC drug derived from aspirin, used to treat pain and inflammation especially in rheumatic disease and other musculo- skeletal disorders. Administration is oral in the form of tablets.

✚ warning: diflunisal should be administered with caution to patients with gastric ulcers, impaired kidney or liver function, or allergic disorders particularly those induced by aspirin or anti- inflammatory agents, or those who are pregnant or lactating.

▲ side-effects: there may be nausea and gastrointestinal disturbance (to avoid which a patient may be advised to take the drug with food or milk), headache and ringing in the ears (tinnitus). Some patients experience sensitivity reactions (such as the symptoms of asthma). Fluid retention and/or blood disorders may occur.
Related article: DOLOBID.

Digibind (*Wellcome*) is an antidote to overdosage of the heart stimulant digoxin, representing digoxin-specific antibody fragments for emergency injection.
see DIGOXIN.

Digitalin Nativelle (*Lewis*) is a proprietary form of the powerful heart stimulant digitoxin (a CARDIAC GLYCOSIDE), available only on prescription, used to treat heart failure and severe heartbeat irregularity. It is produced in the form of tablets and as an elixir (the use of which requires some counselling).

✚/▲ warning/side-effects: *see* DIGITOXIN.

digitoxin is the most powerful heart stimulant derived from the leaf of the digitalis plant, and is a CARDIAC GLYCOSIDE. The effect is to regularize and strengthen a heartbeat that is either too fast or too slow. Useful as it is, however, the drug has common toxic side-effects, the severity of which depends on each individual patient's specific condition. Monitoring of kidney function is particularly advisable. Digitoxin is administered orally in the form of tablets or an elixir.

✚ warning: digitoxin should be administered with caution to patients who suffer from under-secretion of thyroid hormones (hypothyroidism) or who have recently undergone a heart attack. Dosage should be reduced for the elderly and for those with impaired kidney function. Regular monitoring of the blood potassium level is also recommended.

▲ side-effects: there is commonly a loss of appetite, nausea and vomiting, with a consequent weight loss (resulting in some cases in anorexia). There may also be visual disturbances.

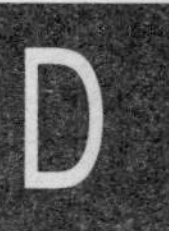

Overdosage may lead to heart block.
Related article: DIGITALIN NATIVELLE.

digoxin is a heart stimulant derived from the leaf of the digitalis plant, and is a CARDIAC GLYCOSIDE. The effect is to regularize and strengthen a heartbeat that is either too fast or too slow. Useful as it is, however, the drug has common toxic side-effects, the severity of which depends on each individual patient's specific condition. Monitoring of kidney function is particularly advisable. (Overdosage can be corrected by the administration of an antidote called Digibind.) Digoxin is administered orally in the form of tablets or an elixir, or by injection.

✚ warning: digoxin should be administered with caution to patients who suffer from under-secretion of thyroid hormones (hypothyroidism) or who have recently undergone a heart attack. Dosage should be reduced for the elderly and for those with impaired kidney function. Regular monitoring of the blood potassium level is also recommended.

▲ side-effects: there is commonly a loss of appetite, nausea and vomiting, with a consequent weight loss (resulting in some cases in anorexia). There may also be visual disturbances. Overdosage may lead to heart block.
Related article: LANOXIN.

Dihydergot (*Sandoz*) is a proprietary preparation, available only on prescription, that is used specifically either to treat or to prevent migraine attacks (prevention demands a regular regimen for administration, whether or not attacks occur). It also has ANTINAUSEANT properties. Produced in the form of tablets, as an oral solution, and in ampoules for injection, Dihydergot is a preparation of the ergotamine derivative dihydroergotamine mesylate

✚/▲ warning/side-effects: *see* DIHYDROERGOTAMINE MESYLATE.

dihydrocodeine tartrate is a NARCOTIC ANALGESIC that is similar to CODEINE. It is used to relieve pain, especially in cases where continued mobility is required, although it may cause some degree of dizziness and constipation. It is commonly used before and after surgery. Administration is oral in the form of tablets or a dilute elixir, or by injection.

✚ warning: dihydrocodeine tartrate should not be administered to patients with respiratory depression, obstructive airways disease, or to children aged under 12 months. Tolerance and dependence (addiction) readily occur.

▲ side-effects: there is dizziness, headache, and sedation; often there is also nausea and constipation. The effects of alcohol consumption may be increased.
Related article: DF 118.

dihydroergotomine mesylate is an anti-migraine drug, a derivative of ergotamine that also has ANTINAUSEANT properties. It is used specifically either to treat or to prevent migraine attacks (prevention demands a regular regimen for administration whether or not attacks occur), and is administered orally in the form of tablets or a solution, or by injection.

D

✚ warning: dihydroergotamine mesylate should not be administered to patients with any infection or circulatory disorders of the limbs, or who are pregnant or lactating; it should be administered with caution to those with heart, liver or kidney disease, or an excess of thyroid hormones in the bloodstream (thyrotoxicosis).

▲ side-effects: there may be nausea and vomiting, with headache, and paraesthesia, and possibly vascular spasm.
Related article: DIHYDERGOT.

dihydrotachysterol is a synthetic form of CALCIFEROL (vitamin D), used to make up body deficiencies. Calcium levels in the body should be regularly monitored during treatment. Administration is oral in the form of tablets and a solution.

✚ warning: overdosage may cause kidney damage. Although an increased amount of vitamin D is necessary during pregnancy, high body levels while lactating may also cause high levels of calcium in the breast-fed infant.
Related articles: A.T. 10; TACHYROL.

Dijex (*Crookes*) is a proprietary non-prescription ANTACID that is not available from the National Health Service. A compound used to reduce stomach acidity and aid digestion, it contains ALUMINIUM HYDROXIDE and MAGNESIUM CARBONATE, and is produced in the form of tablets and as an oral liquid.

diloxanide furoate is an AMOEBICIDAL drug used to treat chronic infection of the intestine by amoebae, causing amoebic dysentery. Administration is oral in the form of tablets; the drug is given in combination with the antibiotic metronidazole in acute cases.

✚ warning: treatment with diloxanide furoate alone usually lasts 10 days; with metronidazole 15 days.

▲ side-effects: there is usually flatulence; there may also be vomiting, itching (pruritus) and/or urticaria.
Related article: FURAMIDE.

diltiazem hydrochloride is a VASODILATOR that is a CALCIUM-ANTAGONIST drug used in the prevention and treatment of angina pectoris (heart pain), especially in cases where beta-blockers are not tolerated or have been ineffective. Administration is oral in the form of sustained-release tablets.

✚ warning: diltiazem hydrochloride should not be administered to patients with slow heart rate or progressive heart disease, or who are pregnant; it should be administered with caution to those with impaired liver or kidney function.

▲ side-effects: there may be slowed heart rate and low blood pressure, with an accumulation of fluid (oedema) at the ankles. Occasionally, there may be nausea and headache, and a rash.
Related article: TILDIEM.

Dimelor (*Lilly*) is a proprietary SULPHONYLUREA, available only on prescription, which has the effect of reducing blood levels of glucose by promoting the secretion of INSULIN within the pancreas. It is thus useful in treating the hyperglycaemia that is associated with adult-onset diabetes mellitus (in which the pancreas still has some capacity for insulin production). Produced in the form

of tablets, Dimelor is a preparation of acetohexamide.
✚/▲ warning/side-effects: *see* ACETOHEXAMIDE.

dimenhydrinate is an ANTIHISTAMINE that is effective in quelling nausea, and useful in preventing vomiting caused by travelling in a moving vehicle, by pregnancy, or by chemotherapy or radiation sickness. It is also used to assist in the treatment of the vertigo and loss of balance that accompanies infections of the middle or inner ear. Administration is oral in the form of tablets.
✚ warning: dimenhydrinate should be administered with caution to patients who suffer from liver disease, epilepsy, enlargement of the prostate gland or glaucoma, and during pregnancy. Concentration and speed of thought and movement are affected – and these symptoms may be made worse by alcohol consumption.
▲ side-effects: there may be dry mouth, drowsiness and headache, with blurred vision. Some patients experience gastroinetstinal disturbances.
Related article: DRAMAMINE.

dimercaprol is a CHELATING AGENT used as an antidote to poisoning with antimony, arsenic, bismuth, gold, mercury or thallium. Administration is by injection.
▲ side-effects: there is an increase in heart rate and blood pressure, sweating, weeping and agitation, nausea and vomiting, constriction of the throat and chest, and a burning sensation – all temporary unless too high a dosage is administered.

dimethicone is a water-repellent silicone used as an antifoaming agent and, when taken orally, thought to reduce flatulence while protecting mucous membranes. It is also a constituent in many barrier creams intended to protect against irritation or chapping (as in nappy rash). Not for use on acutely inflamed or weeping skin.
Related articles: ACTONORM; ALTACAPS; ALTACITE PLUS; ANDURSIL; ANTASIL; ASILONE; KOLANTICON; LOASID; MAALOX; PHAZYME; PIPTALIN; POLYCROL; SILOXYL; SIOPEL; VASOGEN.

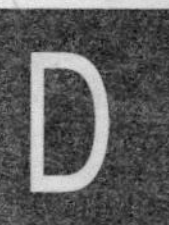

dimethindene maleate is an ANTIHISTAMINE, used to treat the symptoms of allergic conditions such as hay fever and urticaria; it is also used, in combination with other drugs, in expectorants to loosen a dry cough. Administration is oral in the form of sustained-release tablets.
✚ warning: dimethindene maleate should not be administered to patients who are pregnant, or with glaucoma, urinary retention, intestinal obstruction, enlargement of the prostate gland, or peptic ulcer; it should be administered with caution to those with epilepsy or liver disease.
▲ side-effects: sedation may affect patients' capacity for speed of thought and movement; there may be nausea, headaches and/or weight gain, dry mouth, gastrointestinal disturbances and visual problems.
Related articles: FENOSTIL RETARD; VIBROSIL.

Dimotane (*Robins*) is a proprietary non-prescription ANTIHISTAMINE, used to treat the symptoms of allergic conditions such as hay fever and urticaria. Produced as tablets, as sustained-release tablets (under the name

D

Dimotane LA), and as an elixir for dilution (the potency of the elixir once dilute is retained for 14 days), Dimotane is a preparation of brompheniramine maleate.
✚/▲ warning/side-effects: *see* BROMPHENIRAMINE MALEATE.

Dimotane Expectorant (*Robins*) is a proprietary non-prescription EXPECTORANT that is not available from the National Health Service. Intended to promote the expulsion of excess bronchial secretions, it contains the ANTIHISTAMINE brompheniramine maleate and the VASOCONSTRICTOR phenylephrine hydrochloride, and is produced as a sugar-free elixir for dilution (the potency of the elixir once diluted is retained for 14 days).
✚/▲ warning/side-effects: *see* BROMPHENIRAMINE MALEATE; PHENYLEPHRINE.

Dimotane Plus (*Robins*) is a proprietary non-prescription oral preparation intended to clear a stuffed nose. It represents a combination of the ANTIHISTAMINE brompheniramine maleate and the SYMPATHOMIMETIC pseudoephedrine hydrochloride, and is produced as a sugar-free liquid (in two strengths, the weaker labelled for children) for dilution with glycerol (the potency of the liquid once diluted is retained for 14 days).
✚/▲ warning/side-effects: *see* BROMPHENIRAMINE MALEATE; EPHEDRINE HYDROCHLORIDE.

Dimotane with Codeine (*Robins*) is a proprietary non-prescription cough linctus that is not available from the National Health Service. Intended both to promote the expulsion of excess bronchial secretions and to suppress a cough, it contains the OPIATE codeine phosphate, the ANTIHISTAMINE brompheniramine maleate and the SYMPATHOMIMETIC pseudoephedrine hydrochloride, and is produced as a sugar-free elixir (in two strengths, the weaker labelled for children) for dilution with glycerol (the potency of the elixir once diluted is retained for 14 days).
✚/▲ warning/side-effects: *see* BROMPHENIRAMINE MALEATE; CODEINE PHOSPHATE; EPHEDRINE HYDROCHLORIDE.

Dimotapp (*Robins*) is a proprietary non-prescription oral preparation intended to clear a stuffed nose; it is not available from the National Health Service. It contains the ANTIHISTAMINE brompheniramine maleate, the SYMPATHOMIMETIC VASOCONSTRICTOR phenylephrine hydrochloride, and the SYMPATHOMIMETIC phenylpropanolamine, and is produced as a sugar-free elixir (in two strengths, the weaker labelled for children) for dilution (the potency of the elixir once diluted is retained for 14 days), and in the form of sustained-release tablets (under the trade name Dimotapp LA).
✚/▲ warning/side-effects: *see* BROMPHENIRAMINE MALEATE; PHENYLEPHRINE; PHENYLPROPANOLAMINE.

Dimyril (*Fisons*) is a proprietary cough linctus that is available on prescription only to private patients. It represents a preparation of the cough suppressant isoaminile citrate, and is produced in the form of a syrup for dilution (the potency of the syrup once dilute is retained for 14 days).
✚/▲ warning/side-effects: *see* ISOAMINILE CITRATE.

Dindevan (*Duncan, Flockhart*) is

a proprietary ANTICOAGULANT, available only on prescription, used primarily to treat deep-vein thrombosis. Produced in the form of tablets (in three strengths), Dindevan is a preparation of phenindione, and produces sensitivity reactions in a number of patients.

✚/▲ warning/side-effects: *see* PHENINDIONE.

Dinneford's (*Beecham Health Care*) is a proprietary, non-prescription magnesia gripe mixture. It contains citric acid, sucrose, ALCOHOL and the ANTACIDS sodium bicarbonate and magnesium carbonate.

✚/▲ warning/side-effects: *see* SODIUM BICARBONATE; MAGNESIUM CARBONATE.

dinoprost is a drug, a HORMONE-like prostaglandin, that has the effect of causing contractions in the muscular walls of the womb. It is used virtually solely to induce termination of pregnancy (abortion). Administration is by injection, generally into the amniotic sac that surrounds the fetus.

✚ warning: dinoprost should not be administered to patients with uterine muscular disorders or infections, or in whom there is some obstruction between the womb and the outside world or signs of fetal distress. It should be administered with caution to those with asthma or glaucoma, or in whom there is more than one fetus. Overdosage may cause rupture of the womb.

▲ side-effects: there may be nausea, vomiting, flushing and shivering, headache and dizziness, a raised temperature and diarrhoea. These effects are all related to the dosage, and are especially liable to occur if treatment is (unusually) by intravenous infusion.

Related article: PROSTIN F2 ALPHA.

dinoprostone is a drug, a HORMONE-like prostaglandin, that has the effect of causing contractions in the muscular walls of the womb. It is used virtually solely to induce or to assist in termination of pregnancy (abortion). Administration is oral in the form of tablets, topical in the form of a gel or vaginal inserts, or by injection, generally into the amniotic sac that surrounds the fetus.

✚ warning: dinoprostone should not be administered to patients with uterine muscular disorders or uterine or vaginal infections, or in whom there is some obstruction between the womb and the outside world or signs of fetal distress. It should be administered with caution to those with asthma or glaucoma, or in whom there is more than one fetus. Overdosage may cause rupture of the womb.

▲ side-effects: there may be nausea, vomiting, flushing and shivering, headache and dizziness, a raised temperature and diarrhoea. These effects are all related to the dosage, and are especially liable to occur if treatment is (unusually) by intravenous infusion.

Related article: PROSTIN E2.

Diocalm (*Beecham Health Care*) is a proprietary, non-prescription ANTIDIARRHOEAL preparation, containing the OPIATE morphine and attapulgite (magnesium aluminium silicate).

✚/▲ warning/side-effects: *see* MORPHINE.

D

Dioctyl (*Medo*) is a proprietary non-prescription LAXATIVE used to relieve constipation and also to evacuate the rectum prior to abdominal X-ray procedures. Produced in the form of tablets, and as a syrup (in two strengths, the weaker for children) for dilution (the potency of the syrup once diluted is retained for 14 days), Dioctyl is a preparation of DIOCTYL SODIUM SULPHOSUCCINATE (also called docusate sodium).

Dioctyl Ear Drops (*Medo*) is a proprietary non-prescription preparation of DIOCTYL in the form of ear-drops, used for the dissolution and removal of ear wax. Not for patients with perforated ear drum. Dioctyl Ear Drops is a preparation of dioctyl sodium sulphosuccinate (also called docusate sodium).

dioctyl sodium sulphosuccinate, or docusate sodium, is primarily a LAXATIVE that is used not only to relieve constipation but also to evacuate the rectum prior to abdominal X-rays. It is a constituent of many proprietary compound laxatives because it appears to have few, if any, side-effects. It works as a surfactant, applying a very thin film of low surface tension (like a detergent) over the intestinal wall surface. Dioctyl sodium sulphosuccinate is also used in the form of ear-drops to dissolve and remove ear wax; again it is a constituent in many proprietary ear-drop preparations.
Related articles: DIOCTYL; DIOCTYL EAR DROPS; DULCODOS; FLETCHER'S ENEMETTE; KLYX; MOLCER; NORMAX; SOLIWAX; WAXSOL.

Dioderm (*Dermal*) is a proprietary, water-miscible, CORTICOSTEROID cream for topical application, used to treat mild inflammation of the skin. Available only on prescription, its major active constituent is the steroid hydrocortisone.
✚/▲ warning/side-effects: *see* HYDROCORTISONE.

Dioralyte (*Armour*) is a proprietary non-prescription sodium supplement, used to treat mild or moderate degrees of sodium depletion (as may happen in cases of dehydration or in illnesses - particularly in kidney disease – in which salt is lost in some quantity). Dioralyte is produced in the form of sachets containing a powder for solution, consisting of a compound of SODIUM CHLORIDE, POTASSIUM CHLORIDE, SODIUM BICARBONATE and GLUCOSE; flavours are plain, cherry or pineapple.

Diovol (*Pharmax*) is a proprietary non-prescription ANTACID used to relieve acid stomach and flatulence, and to assist digestion in patients with peptic ulcers or hiatus hernia. Produced in the form of tablets for chewing or sucking, and as a mint- or fruit-flavoured suspension, Diovol is a compound preparation of ALUMINIUM HYDROXIDE together with the antifoaming agent DIMETHICONE. It is not recommended for children aged under 6 years.

diphenhydramine hydrochloride is an ANTIHISTAMINE, one of the first to be discovered, used to treat allergic conditions such as hay fever and urticaria, some forms of dermatitis, and some sensitivity reactions to drugs. Its additional sedative properties are useful in the treatment of some allergic conditions, but the fact that it is also an ANTINAUSEANT makes it useful in the treatment or prevention of travel sickness, vertigo, and infections of the inner and middle ears too. Administration is oral in the form of capsules.

✚ warning: diphenhydramine hydrochloride should not be administered to patients with glaucoma, urinary retention, intestinal obstruction, enlargement of the prostate gland, or peptic ulcer, or who are pregnant; it should be administered with caution to those who suffer from epilepsy or liver disease.

▲ side-effects: sedation may affect patients' capacity for speed of thought and movement; there may be headache and/or weight gain, dry mouth, gastrointestinal disturbances and visual problems.
Related articles: BENADRYL; BENILYN DECONGESTANT; BENILYN EXPECTORANT; HISTALIX.

diphenoxylate hydrochloride is a powerful ANTIDIARRHOEAL drug, an OPIATE used to treat chronic diarrhoea. It works by reducing the speed at which material travels along the intestines. Overdosage is uncommon but does occur, particularly in young children – however, the symptoms of overdosage (chiefly sedation) do not appear until some 48 hours after treatment, so monitoring of patients for at least that time is necessary. Because long-term treatment with diphenoxylate hydrochloride is liable to induce dependence (addiction), the drug is usually administered in combination with the belladonna alkaloid ATROPINE, which reduces its potential for abuse. Administration is oral in the form of tablets or as a sugar-free dilute liquid.

✚ warning: fluid intake must be maintained during treatment. In elderly patients, monitoring is essential to detect possible faecal impaction. The drug should not be used in patients with gastrointestinal obstruction or jaundice. Care should be taken in patients with ulcerative colitis, or hepatic disorders

▲ side-effects: overdosage causes sedation. Prolonged usage may lead to impaired gastrointestinal function and eventual dependence. The presence of atropine may cause dry mouth, thirst and some visual disturbance in susceptible patients.
Related article: LOMOTIL.

diphenylpyraline hydrochloride is an ANTIHISTAMINE used to treat allergic conditions such as hay fever and urticaria, some forms of dermatitis, and some sensitivity reactions to drugs. Its additional sedative properties are useful in the treatment of some allergic conditions. Administration of the drug is oral in the form of sustained-release capsules (spansules) or tablets.

✚ warning: diphenylpyraline hydrochloride should not be administered to patients with glaucoma, urinary retention, intestinal obstruction, enlargement of the prostate gland, or peptic ulcer, or who are pregnant; it should be administered with caution to those who suffer from epilepsy or liver disease.

▲ side-effects: sedation may affect patients' capacity for speed of thought and movement; there may be nausea, headache and/or weight gain, dry mouth, gastrointestinal disturbances and visual problems.
Related articles: ESKORNADE; HISTRYL; LERGOBAN.

D

diphtheria vaccine is a VACCINE preparation of an antitoxin – that is, an antibody produced in response to the presence of the toxin of the diphtheria bacterium, rather than to the presence of the bacterium itself – prepared in horses, and adsorbed on to a mineral carrier (almost always aluminium hydroxide). Available only on prescription, the vaccine is produced in ampoules for injection. However, far more commonly, it is administered as one constituent in a triple vaccine (additionally against whooping cough – known as pertussis – and tetanus, often called the DPT vaccine) or, when patients do not want vaccination against whooping cough, in a double vaccine (with TETANUS VACCINE). Administered singly or in combination, diphtheria vaccine often causes allergic reactions.

diphtheria-pertussis-tetanus (DPT) vaccine is a combination of VACCINES against diphtheria, whooping cough and tetanus used for the routine immunization of infants at the ages of 3 months, 4-1B-+-1C- months and 6 months. Repeat vaccination with this triple vaccine is not usual, although booster vaccinations of the diphtheria and tetanus vaccines are relatively common.
see DIPHTHERIA VACCINE; PERTUSSIS VACCINE; TETANUS VACCINE.

diphtheria-tetanus vaccine is a combination of VACCINES against diphtheria and tetanus used for the routine immunization of infants at the ages of 3 months, 4½ months and 6 months in children whose parents do not wish them to have the triple vaccine that additionally contains pertussis (whooping cough) vaccine. This double vaccine is also used as a booster shot for children at the age of school entry
✚/▲ warning/side-effects: *see* DIPHTHERIA VACCINE; TETANUS VACCINE.

dipipanone is a rapidly-acting and powerful OPIATE narcotic ANALGESIC drug, that is used in combination with an ANTINAUSEANT drug (the antihistamine cyclizine) for the relief of acute moderate to severe pain. Its proprietary form is on the controlled drugs list and is not recommended for children. Administration (in the form of dipipanone hydrochloride) is oral as tablets.
✚ warning: dipipanone should not be administered to patients who have any blockage of the respiratory passages or any form of depressed breathing; it should be administered with caution to those with severely impaired kidney or liver function, or who are pregnant. The consumption of alcohol must be avoided during treatment.
▲ side-effects: the mouth may become dry, vision may blur, and the patient may become drowsy. Tolerance may rapidly be followed by dependence (addiction).
Related article: DICONAL.

dipivefrine is a derivative of the HORMONE (catecholamine) adrenaline which is in fact converted internally into adrenaline; it is used – like adrenaline – in ophthalmic treatment to reduce the formation of aqueous humour in the eyeball and to promote its drainage away, so lessening intra-ocular pressure and relieving the main symptoms of glaucoma. However, the drug should not be used in cases of

closed-angle glaucoma or soft lens. Treatment may cause transient stinging and mild sensitivity reactions. Administration (in the form of a mild solution of dipivefrine hydrochloride) is topical in the form of eye-drops.
✚/▲ warning/side-effects: *see* ADRENALINE.
Related article: PROPINE.

dipotassium clorazepate is a drug better known simply as clorazepate.
see CLORAZEPATE.

Diprivan (*ICI*) is a proprietary form of the general ANAESTHETIC propofol, used primarily for the induction of anaesthesia at the start of a surgical operation, but sometimes also for its maintenance thereafter. Available only on prescription, it is produced as an emulsion in ampoules for injection.
✚/▲ warning/side-effects: *see* PROPOFOL.

Diprobase (*Kirby-Warrick*) is a proprietary non-prescription form of OINTMENT used as a base for medications; it is a combination of paraffins (and is intended for particular use with DIPROSONE).

Diprosalic (*Kirby-Warrick*) is a proprietary CORTICOSTEROID preparation, available only on prescription, used to treat severe non-infective skin inflammations such as eczema, particularly in patients who are not responding to less powerful steroids. Produced in the form of an ointment and an alcohol-based lotion for topical application, Diprosalic is a compound preparation of the steroid betamethasone dipropionate together with the antibacterial/antifungal drug salicylic acid.
✚/▲ warning/side-effects: *see* BETAMETHASONE DIPROPIONATE; SALICYLIC ACID.

Diprosone (*Kirby-Warrick*) is a proprietary CORTICOSTEROID preparation, available only on prescription, used to treat severe non-infective skin inflammation such as eczema. particularly in patients who are not responding to less powerful steroids. Produced in the form of a water-miscible cream, as an ointment and as an alcohol-based lotion for topical application, Diprosone is a preparation of the steroid betamethasone dipropionate.
✚/▲ warning/side-effects: *see* BETAMETHASONE DIPROPIONATE.

dipyridamole is a drug used to prevent thrombosis, but does not have the usual action of an ANTICOAGULANT. Instead it works by inhibiting the adhesiveness of blood platelets so that they stick neither to themselves nor to the walls of valves or tubes surgically inserted. Administration is oral in the form of tablets, or by injection.
✚ warning: treatment may make low blood pressure (hypotension) or migraine worse. Care is required in patients suffering from angina pectoris or other heart conditions associated with poor cardiovascular blood flow.
▲ side-effects: there may be nausea and diarrhoea, with a throbbing headache. Blood pressure may fall.
Related article: PERSANTIN.

Dirythmin IV (*Astra*) is a proprietary form of DIRYTHMIN SA prepared in a form suitable for intravenous injection. The method of administration is, however, long and complicated.
see DISOPYRAMIDE.

D

Dirythmin SA (*Astra*) is a proprietary ANTIARRHYTHMIC drug, available only on prescription, used to regularize the heartbeat especially following a heart attack. Produced in the form of sustained-release tablets ("Durules"), it is a preparation of disopyramide phosphate. It is not recommended for children.
✚/▲ warning/side-effects: *see* DISOPYRAMIDE.

Disadine DP (*Stuart*) is a proprietary non-prescription form of the compound DISINFECTANT POVIDONE-IODINE, prepared as a powder within an aerosol. For topical application, it is used to treat or prevent infection of the skin following injury or surgery, or to cleanse bedsores.

Disalcid (*Riker*) is a proprietary NON-NARCOTIC ANALGESIC, available only on prescription, used to relieve pain – particularly the pain of rheumatic disease in and around the joints. Produced in the form of tablets, it represents a preparation of the aspirin-like drug salsalate, and is not recommended for children.
✚/▲ warning/side-effects: *see* SALSALATE.

***disinfectants** are agents that destroy micro-organisms, or inhibit their activity to a level such that they are less or no longer harmful to health. The term is applied to agents used on inanimate objects as well as to those used to treat the skin and living tissue, and in the latter case is often used synonymously with ANTISEPTIC.

Disipal (*Brocades*) is a proprietary ANTICHOLINERGIC drug, available only on prescription, used in ANTIPARKINSONISM treatment to relieve some of the symptoms of parkinsonism, specifically the tremor of the hands, the overall rigidity of the posture, and the tendency to produce an excess of saliva. (The drug also has the capacity to treat these conditions in some cases where they are produced by drugs.) It is thought to work by compensating for the lack of dopamine in the brain that is the major cause of such parkinsonian symptoms. Produced in the form of tablets and in ampoules for injection, Disipal is a preparation of orphenadrine hydrochloride. Counselling of patients is advised.
✚/▲ warning/side-effects: *see* ORPHENADRINE HYDROCHLORIDE.

Di-sipidin (*Paines & Byrne*) is a proprietary preparation of a pituitary extract in powder form, used as snuff by patients who suffer from diabetes insipidus and urinary incontinence. It is available only on prescription, and presented in the form of insufflation capsules.
✚ warning: di-Sipidin should not be administered to patients who suffer from high blood pressure (hypertension) or chronic nephritis. Dosage of Di-sipidin should initially be adjusted according to individual response: optimum response level should then become the maintenance level.
▲ side-effects: there may be nausea, internal muscular cramps, constriction of the coronary arteries and an urge to defecate. Some patients experience the symptoms of hay fever or asthma.

disodium etidronate is a drug used virtually solely to treat the condition known as Paget's disease of bone (osteitis deformans: a severely and continuously painful condition in which the larger bones of the body thicken while their structure becomes disorganized). It works by inhibiting the demineralization process inherent in the disease. Treatment may last for 6 months. Administration is oral in the form of tablets. Dietary counselling of patients is advised.

✚ warning: disodium etidronate should be administered with caution to patients with impaired kidney function or intestinal inflammation. Treatment should be withdrawn if the patient suffers a fracture.

▲ side-effects: there may be nausea and diarrhoea. High dosage increases both bone pain and the risk of fractures. *Related article:* DIDRONEL.

disopyramide is an ANTIARRHYTHMIC drug used to regularize the heartbeat especially following a heart attack. Dosage must be adjusted to suit the response of each individual patient. Administration (as disopyramide or as disopyramide phosphate) is oral in the form of capsules, sustained-release capsules or sustained-release tablets, or by slow intravenous injection that has to be monitored using an electrocardiograph (and followed by further dosage by mouth or by infusion).

✚ warning: disopyramide should be administered with caution to patients with depressed heart function (i.e. heart failure and impaired cardiac output) reduced kidney function, or glaucoma.

▲ side-effects: there may be slow heart rate and low blood pressure (hypotension). Many patients experience dry mouth, blurred vision and urinary retention. Rarely, there is heart block. *Related articles:* DIRYTHMIN IV; DIRYTHMIN SA; RYTHMODAN.

Dispray 1 Quick Prep (*Stuart*) is a proprietary non-prescription DISINFECTANT used primarily to cleanse the skin prior to surgery or injection. Produced in an aerosol for immediate topical application, it represents a solution of CHLORHEXIDINE GLUCONATE.

Disprin (*Reckitt & Colman*) is a proprietary non-prescription non-narcotic ANALGESIC containing paracetomol.

✚/▲ warning/side-effects: *see* PARACETAMOL.

Disprol (*Reckitt & Colman*) is a proprietary non-prescription non-narcotic ANALGESIC for children that also helps to reduce high body temperature. Produced in the form of a sugar-free suspension, it is a preparation of paracetamol. Even as a paediatric preparation, however, it is not recommended for children aged under 3 months.

✚/▲ warning/side-effects: *see* PARACETAMOL.

Distaclor (*Dista*) is a proprietary broad-spectrum ANTIBIOTIC, available only on prescription, used to treat a wide range of bacterial infections, particularly of the skin and soft tissues, urinary tract, upper respiratory tract, and middle ear. Produced in the form of capsules and as a suspension (in two strengths) for dilution (the potency of the suspension once dilute is retained for 14 days), Distaclor is a preparation of the cephalosporin cefaclor.

✚/▲ warning/side-effects: *see* CEFACLOR.

D

Distalgesic (*Dista*) is a proprietary ANALGESIC available on prescription only to private patients. Used to relieve pain anywhere in the body, and produced in the form of tablets, Distalgesic is a preparation of the narcotic-like analgesic dextropropoxyphene together with paracetamol (a compound known as co-proxamol). It is not recommended for children.
✚/▲ warning/side-effects: *see* DEXTROPROPOXYPHENE; PARACETAMOL.

Distamine (*Dista*) is a proprietary preparation, available only on prescription, used specifically to relieve the pain of rheumatoid arthritis, and potentially to halt the progress of the disease. Patients should be warned that treatment may take up to 12 weeks for any improvement to be manifest, and up to a year before full effect is achieved. The drug may also be used as a long-term CHELATING AGENT to treat poisoning by the metals copper or lead. Produced in the form of tablets (in three strengths), Distamine is a preparation of the penicillin derivative penicillamine.
✚/▲ warning/side-effects: *see* PENICILLAMINE.

Distaquaine V-K (*Dista*) is a proprietary preparation of the penicillin-type ANTIBIOTIC phenoxymethylpenicillin, used mainly to treat infections of the head and throat, and some skin conditions; it may also be used to reduce high body temperature. Available only on prescription, it is produced in the form of tablets (in two strengths) or as an elixir (in three strengths) for dilution (the potency of the elixir once dilute is retained for 7 days).
✚/▲ warning/side-effects: *see* PHENOXYMETHYLPENICILLIN.

distigmine bromide is an anticholinesterase drug that enhances the transmission of neural impulses from the brain to the muscles. It is primarily used, perhaps surprisingly, as a PARASYMPATHOMIMETIC to treat urinary retention caused by lesions in the brain or following surgery; but it may also be used to treat constipation due to paralytic ileus, and also to treat the systemic neuromuscular transmission disorder myasthenia gravis. Administration is oral in the form of tablets, or by injection.
✚ warning: distigmine bromide should not be administered to patients who suffer from urinary or intestinal blockage, or who have recently had a heart attack; it should be administered with caution to those with parkinsonism, epilepsy, cardiovascular disease, overactivity of the thyroid glands or asthma, or who are elderly or pregnant.
▲ side-effects: there may be nausea and vomiting, sweating and blurred vision, slow heart rate and colic.
Related article: UBRETID.

Distran (*Whitehall Laboratories*) is a proprietary, non-prescription DECONGESTANT, produced in the form of tablets and as a nasal spray. The nasal spray contains oxymetazoline, and the tablets contain caffeine, aspirin, phenylephrine and the ANTIHISTAMINE chlorpheniramine.
✚/▲ warning/side-effects: *see* ASPIRIN; CAFFEINE; CHLORPHENIRAMINE; OXYMETAZOLINE; PHENYLEPHRINE.

disulfiram is a drug that, in combination with the consumption of even small quantities of alcohol, gives rise to rather unpleasant, even dangerous, reactions – such as flushing, headache, palpitations, nausea and vomiting. This is because disulfiram and alcohol together cause an accumulation in the body of acetaldehyde. The drug is quite well known under its proprietary name. Administration is oral in the form of tablets.

✚ warning: disulfiram should not be administered to patients with heart disorders, or during pregnancy, or to patients with drug dependence or mental illness. Simultaneous use of medications containing forms of alcohol should also be avoided.

▲ side-effects: taken with a large amount of alcohol, the drug may cause low blood pressure, serious heartbeat irregularities, and eventual collapse.

Related article: ANTABUSE.

dithranol is the most powerful drug presently used to treat chronic or milder forms of psoriasis in topical application. For about an hour at a time, lesions are covered with a dressing on which there is a preparation of the drug in mild solution. Concentration is adjusted not only to suit individual response but also in relation to each patient's tolerance of the associated skin irritation. Healthy skin (and the eyes) must be avoided. The drug may be used in combination with others that have a moisturizing effect.

✚ warning: dithranol is not suitable for the treatment of acute forms of psoriasis. The drug stains skin, hair and fabrics.

▲ side-effects: irritation and a local sensation of burning are common.

Related articles: ANTHRANOL; ANTRADERM; DITHOCREAM; DITHROLAN; PSORADRATE; PSORIN.

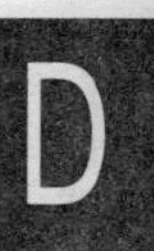

dithranol triacetate, as a salt of dithranol, is used for the same purpose – the treatment of psoriasis – but is less effective and may be compared in this respect with COAL TAR.

✚/▲ warning/side-effects: *see* DITHRANOL.

Related article: EXOLAN.

Dithrocream (*Dermal*) is a proprietary non-prescription preparation of the powerful drug dithranol, in dilute solution, used in topical application on dressings to treat chronic and mild forms of psoriasis. It is produced in the form of a water-miscible cream (in four strengths).

✚/▲ warning/side-effects: *see* DITHRANOL.

Dithrolan (*Dermal*) is a proprietary non-prescription preparation of the powerful drug dithranol, in dilute solution, together with the ANTIBACTERIAL/ANTIFUNGAL drug salicylic acid, and is used in topical application on dressings to treat chronic and mild forms of psoriasis. It is produced in the form of a paraffin-based ointment for dilution (the potency of the ointment once dilute is retained for 14 days).

✚/▲ warning/side-effects: *see* DITHRANOL; SALICYLIC ACID.

Diumide-K Continus (*Degussa*) is a proprietary DIURETIC, available only on prescription, used to treat the accumulation of fluid in the tissues (oedema) associated with heart, liver or kidney disorders, especially in cases where a potassium supplement is deemed necessary. Produced in the form

of tablets, Diumide-K Continus is a compound preparation of the diuretic frusemide together with POTASSIUM CHLORIDE.
✚/▲ warning/side-effects: *see* FRUSEMIDE.

D

Diuresal (*Lagap*) is a proprietary DIURETIC, available only on prescription, used to treat the accumulation of fluid in the tissues (oedema) associated with heart, liver or kidney disorders. Produced in the form of tablets and in ampoules for injection, Diuresal is a preparation of frusemide.
✚/▲ warning/side-effects: *see* FRUSEMIDE.

***diuretics** are drugs that rid the body of fluids, generally by promoting their excretion in the form of urine. Accumulation of fluid in the tissues (oedema) is a common symptom of many disorders, particularly chronic disorders of the heart, liver, kidneys or lungs. Treatment with diuretics can thus assist in remedying such disorders. Salt and water retention also occurs in high blood pressure (hypertension), and diuretics are particularly used to treat that condition (as ANTIHYPERTENSIVE therapy), often in combination with a potassium supplement. Some diuretics are also useful in reducing the aqueous content of the eyeballs, so relieving internal pressure (as in glaucoma). Diuretics are commonly also used for premedication prior to surgery. Best known and most used diuretics are the thiazides; other non-thiazide diuretics include ACETAZOLAMIDE, FRUSEMIDE, SPIRONOLACTONE and TRIAMTERENE.
see THIAZIDES.

Diurexan (*Merck*) is a proprietary DIURETIC, available only on prescription, used mainly to relieve the accumulation of fluids in the tissues (oedema) due to heart failure, and in lower dosages or in combination, to relieve high blood pressure (*see* ANTIHYPERTENSIVE). Produced in the form of tablets, Diurexan is a preparation of the THIAZIDE xipamide. It is not recommended for children.
✚/▲ warning/side-effects: *see* XIPAMIDE.

Dixarit (*WB Pharmaceuticals*) is a proprietary preparation of the ANTIHYPERTENSIVE drug clonidine hydrochloride, used in low dosage sometimes to try to prevent recurrent migraine and similar headaches, and to relieve flushing during the menopause in women. It is produced in the form of tablets, and is not recommended for children.
✚/▲ warning/side-effects: *see* CLONIDINE HYDROCHLORIDE.

dobutamine hydrochloride is a SYMPATHOMIMETIC drug used to treat cardiogenic shock and other serious heart disorders. It works by increasing the heart's force of contraction without affecting the heart rate. Administration is by injection or infusion.
✚ warning: dobutamine hydrochloride should be administered with caution to patients with severe low blood pressure (hypotension).
▲ side-effects: the heart rate following treatment may increase too rapidly and result in high blood pressure (hypertension).
Related article: DOBUTREX.

Dobutrex (*Lilly*) is a proprietary preparation of the SYMPATHOMIMETIC drug dobutamine hydrochloride, used to treat cardiogenic shock and other serious heart disorders.

Available only on prescription, Dobutrex is produced in the form of powder for reconstitution as a medium for intravenous infusion.
✚/▲ warning/side-effects: *see* DOBUTAMINE HYDROCHLORIDE.

docusate sodium is an alternative term for dioctyl sodium sulphosuccinate, a constituent in many LAXATIVES. *see* DIOCTYL SODIUM SULPHOSUCCINATE.

Dolmatil (*Squibb*) is a proprietary ANTIPSYCHOTIC drug used to treat the symptoms of schizophrenia. In low doses it increases an apathetic, withdrawn patient's awareness and tends to generate a true consciousness of events. In high doses it is used also to treat other conditions that may cause tremor, tics, involuntary movements or involuntary utterances (such as the relatively uncommon Giles de la Tourette syndrome). Produced in the form of tablets, Dolmatil is a preparation of sulpiride. It is not recommended for children aged under 14 years.
✚/▲ warning/side-effects: *see* SULPIRIDE.

Dolobid (*Morson*) is a proprietary ANTI-INFLAMMATORY non-narcotic ANALGESIC, available only on prescription, used to treat the pain of rheumatic disease and other musculo-skeletal disorders. Produced in the form of tablets (in two strengths), Dolobid is a preparation of the aspirin-like anti-inflammatory drug diflunisal. It is not recommended for children.
✚/▲ warning/side-effects: *see* DIFLUNISAL.

Doloxene (*Lilly*) is a proprietary narcotic ANALGESIC, available on prescription only to private patients, used to treat mild to moderate pain anywhere in the body. Produced in the form of capsules, Doloxene is a preparation of the OPIATE-like dextropropoxyphene napsylate. It is not recommended for children.
✚/▲ warning/side-effects: *see* DEXTROPROPOXYPHENE.

Doloxene Compound (*Lilly*) is a proprietary compound ANALGESIC, available on prescription only to private patients, used to treat mild to moderate pain anywhere in the body. Produced in the form of capsules, Doloxene represents a preparation of the OPIATE-like dextropropoxyphene napsylate, together with aspirin and caffeine. It is not recommended for children.
✚/▲ warning/side-effects: *see* ASPIRIN; CAFFEINE; DEXTROPROPOXYPHENE.

Dome-Acne (*Lagap*) is a proprietary non-prescription KERATOLYTIC preparation used to treat acne. Produced in the form of a cream and as a lotion for topical application, Dome-Acne contains the powerful astringent resorcinol together with SULPHUR. Another version is produced (under the name Dome-Acne Cleanser) and instead of resorcinol contains salicylic acid, which has both keratolytic and ANTIFUNGAL properties.
✚/▲ warning/side-effects: *see* RESORCINOL.

Dome-Cort (*Lagap*) is a proprietary, water-miscible, CORTICOSTEROID cream for topical application, used to treat mild inflammations of the skin. Available only on prescription, its major active constituent is the steroid hydrocortisone.
✚/▲ warning/side-effects: *see* HYDROCORTISONE.

Domical (*Berk*) is a proprietary

ANTIDEPRESSANT drug, available only on prescription, administered to treat depressive illness (and especially in cases where some degree of sedation is deemed necessary). Like many such drugs, it is also used to treat bedwetting by children at night. Produced in the form of tablets (in three strengths), Domical is a preparation of amitriptyline.
✚/▲ warning/side-effects: *see* AMITRIPTYLINE.

domperidone is an ANTINAUSEANT drug that works by inhibiting the action of the substance dopamine on the vomiting centre of the brain; this can be useful in patients undergoing treatment with CYTOTOXIC drugs. It also has the effect of stimulating the emptying of the stomach and promoting the passage of nutritional debris through the small intestine; this can be useful in facilitating rapid barium-meal examination via radiotherapy. Administration is oral in the form of tablets or in suspension, or as anal suppositories.
✚ warning: domperidone should not be administered to patients in accordance with any form of routine schedule, or immediately after any abdominal surgery; it should be administered with caution to those who suffer from impaired kidney function.
▲ side-effects: there may be muscle spasms in the face and other voluntary muscles (which can in turn be treated by the administration of anti-parkinsonian drugs). Occasionally, spontaneous lactation in women or the development of feminine breasts in men may occur.
Related article: MOTILIUM.

Dopamet (*Berk*) is a proprietary ANTIHYPERTENSIVE drug, available ONLY ON PRESCRIPTION, USED (GENERALLY IN COMBINATION WITH A DIURETIC) to treat moderate to severe high blood pressure (hypertension). Produced in the form of tablets, Dopamet is a preparation of methyldopa.
✚/▲ warning/side-effects: *see* METHYLDOPA.

dopamine is a neurotransmitter substance (a catecholamine) that is an intermediate in the synthesis of noradrenaline, acts as a neurotransmitter (relaying nerve "messages"), and is particularly concentrated in the brain and in the adrenal glands. It is possible that some psychoses may in part be caused by abnormalities in the metabolism of dopamine because drugs that antagonize its activity as a neurotransmitter (such as chlorpromazine) tend to relieve schizophrenic symptoms. It may be administered therapeutically (in the form of dopamine hydrochloride) in the treatment of the cardiogenic shock associated with a heart attack or in those who have undergone heart surgery. Administration is by injection or infusion.
✚ warning: dopamine hydrochloride should not be administered to patients who suffer from disruptive disorder of the adrenal glands (phaeochromocytoma) or from heartbeat irregularities involving very rapid heart rate. Dosage to treat shock after a heart attack need only be low.
▲ side-effects: there may be nausea and vomiting, with changes in heart rate and blood pressure – the fingertips and toes may become cold.
Related articles: INTROPIN; SELECT-A-JET DOPAMINE.

Dopram (*Robins*) is a proprietary

preparation of the respiratory stimulant drug doxapram hydrochloride, available only on prescription, used in some instances to relieve severe respiratory difficulties in patients with chronic disease of the respiratory tract or who undergo respiratory depression following major surgery, particularly in cases where ventilatory support is for one reason or another not applicable. It is produced in flasks (bottles) for infusion (in dextrose solution) or in ampoules for injection.

✚/▲ warning/side-effects: *see* DOXAPRAM HYDROCHLORIDE.

Dor (*Simpla*) is a proprietary non-prescription deodorant solution used (in drops) to freshen and sanitize the appliance (bag) placed over a stoma (an outlet, in the skin surface, of the surgical curtailment of the intestines or of the ureters).

Dormonoct (*Roussel*) is a proprietary HYPNOTIC drug, available only on prescription, used in the short term to treat insomnia. Produced in the form of tablets, it is a preparation of the BENZODIAZEPINE loprazolam mesylate. It is not recommended for children.

✚/▲ warning/side-effects: *see* LOPRAZOLAM.

dothiepin hydrochloride is an ANTIDEPRESSANT drug used to treat depressive illness, especially in cases where some degree of sedation is deemed to be necessary. Administration is oral in the form of capsules or tablets.

✚ warning: dothiepin hydrochloride should not be administered to patients with heart disease or psychosis; it should be administered with caution to those who are pregnant or lactating, and to those with epilepsy, diabetes, liver or thyroid disease, glaucoma, or urinary retention. Withdrawal of treatment must be gradual.

▲ side-effects: concentration and speed of reaction are commonly affected; there may also be dry mouth and blurred vision, difficulty in urinating, a rash, sweating and irregular heartbeat. Some patients experience behavioural disturbance, a state of confusion and/or a loss of libido. Rarely, there are also blood deficiencies.

Related article: PROTHIADEN.

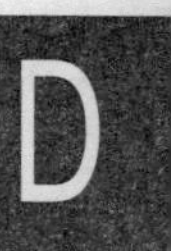

Double Check (*Family Planning Sales*) is a proprietary non-prescription SPERMICIDAL preparation, for use only in combination with barrier methods of contraception (such as a condom). Produced in the form of vaginal inserts (pessaries), Double Check is a preparation of an alcohol ester.

doxapram hydrochloride is a respiratory stimulant drug, used with care in some instances, to relieve severe respiratory difficulties in patients who suffer from chronic disease of the respiratory tract or who undergo respiratory depression following major surgery, particularly in cases where ventilatory support is not applicable. Administration is by injection or by infusion (in dextrose solution).

✚ warning: doxapram hydrochloride should not be administered to patients who suffer from very high blood pressure (hypertension), from cardiovascular disease, from an excess of thyroid hormones in the blood (thyrotoxicosis), or from severe asthma; it should be administered with caution to those who suffer from

D

epilepsy or who are taking antidepressant drugs that affect mood.

▲ side-effects: the blood pressure and heart rate may increase; some patients experience dizziness.

Related article: DOPRAM.

Doxatet (*Cox Pharmaceuticals*) is a proprietary broad-spectrum ANTIBIOTIC, available only on prescription, used to treat infections of many kinds. Produced in the form of tablets, Doxatet represents a preparation of the tetracycline doxycycline hydrochloride. It is not recommended for children.

✚/▲ warning/side-effects: *see* DOXYCYCLINE.

doxepin is an ANTIDEPRESSANT drug used to treat depressive illness, especially in cases where some degree of sedation is deemed to be necessary. Administration is oral in the form of capsules (comprising doxepin hydrochloride).

✚ warning: doxepin hydrochloride should not be administered to patients with heart disease or psychosis; it should be administered with caution to those who are pregnant or lactating, and to those with epilepsy, diabetes, liver or thyroid disease, glaucoma, or urinary retention. Withdrawal of treatment must be gradual.

▲ side-effects: concentration and speed of reaction are commonly affected; there may also be dry mouth and blurred vision, difficulty in urinating, a rash, sweating and irregular heartbeat. Some patients experience behavioural disturbance, a state of confusion and/or a loss of libido. Rarely, there are also blood deficiencies.

Related article: SINEQUAN.

doxorubicin hydrochloride is a powerful and widely used CYTOTOXIC drug that also has ANTIBIOTIC properties, used to treat leukaemia, lymphomas and some solid tumours, especially those situated in the bladder. Administration is by fast-running infusion (usually at intervals of 21 days, although a low dose weekly may result in fewer toxic side-effects).

✚ warning: doxorubicin hydrochloride should be administered with caution to patients with heart disease, who are elderly, or who are receiving radiotherapy in the cardiac region. Heart monitoring is essential throughout treatment: high doses tend to cause eventual heart dysfunction. Leakage of the drug from the site of infusion into the tissues may cause tissue damage.

▲ side-effects: nausea and vomiting, hair loss and reduction in the blood-forming capacity of the bone-marrow are all fairly common side-effects. Rarely, there is also an increased heart rate. In the treatment of bladder tumours, side-effects may include urgency or difficulty in urinating, and possible reduction in bladder capacity.

Related article: ADRIAMYCIN.

doxycycline is a broad-spectrum ANTIBIOTIC, one of the tetracyclines, used to treat severe infections of many kinds. Administration is oral in the form of tablets and capsules, soluble (dispersible) tablets for solution, and as a dilute syrup.

✚ warning: doxycycline should be administered with care to patients with kidney failure, who are pregnant, or who are aged under 12 years. It should be administered with caution

to those who are lactating, or with impaired liver function.
▲ side-effects: there may be nausea and vomiting, with diarrhoea. Some patients experience a sensitivity to light. Rarely, there are allergic reactions.
Related articles: DOXATET; DOXYLAR; NORDOX; VIBRAMYCIN.

Doxylar (*Lagap*) is a proprietary broad-spectrum ANTIBIOTIC, available only on prescription, used to treat infections of many kinds. Produced in the form of capsules, Doxylar represents a preparation of the tetracycline doxycycline hydrochloride.
✚/▲ warning/side-effects: *see* DOXYCYCLINE.

Dozic (*RP Drugs*) is a proprietary ANTIPSYCHOTIC drug, available only on prescription, used to treat psychosis (especially schizophrenia or the hyperactive, euphoric condition, mania) and to tranquillize patients undergoing behavioural disturbance. It may also be used in the short term to treat severe anxiety. Produced in the form of a sugar-free liquid (for swallowing, in two strengths), Dozic is a preparation of the powerful drug haloperidol.
✚/▲ warning/side-effects: *see* HALOPERIDOL.

Dozine (*RP Drugs*) is a proprietary ANTIPSYCHOTIC drug, available only on prescription, used to treat psychosis (especially schizophrenia) and to tranquillize patients undergoing behavioural disturbance. It may also be used in the short term to treat severe anxiety (especially in the case of terminal disease) or to treat an intractable hiccup. Produced in the form of an elixir for dilution (the potency of the elixir once dilute is retained for 14 days), Dozine is a preparation of the powerful drug chlorpromazine hydrochloride.
✚/▲ warning/side-effects: *see* CHLORPROMAZINE HYDROCHLORIDE.

Dramamine (*Searle*) is a proprietary non-prescription ANTI-EMETIC, used to treat nausea and vomiting, to prevent forms of motion sickness, and to relieve the loss of balance and vertigo experienced by patients with infections of the middle or inner ear or who have radiation sickness. Produced in the form of tablets, Dramamine is a preparation of dimenhydrinate. It is not recommended for children aged under 12 months.
✚/▲ warning/side-effects: *see* DIMENHYDRINATE.

Drapolene (*Wellcome*) is a proprietary non-prescription ANTISEPTIC cream used primarily to treat nappy rash, although it can also be used to dress abrasions and minor wounds. It contains the antiseptics BENZALKONIUM CHLORIDE and CETRIMIDE in very dilute solution.

Driclor (*Stiefel*) is a proprietary medicated ANTIPERSPIRANT, available only on prescription, used to treat abnormally heavy sweating (hyperhidrosis) of the armpits, hands and feet. Produced in a roll-on bottle, Driclor represents a 20% solution of aluminium chloride.
✚/▲ warning/side-effects: *see* ALUMINIUM CHLORIDE.

Droleptan (*Janssen*) is a proprietary preparation of the powerful tranquillizer droperidol, available only on prescription, used primarily in emergencies to subdue or soothe psychotic (particularly manic) patients during behavioural disturbances,

D

although it is also used on patients about to undergo certain diagnostic procedures that may be difficult or painful, because it promotes a sensation of dispassionate detachment. It is produced in the form of tablets, as a sugar-free liquid for dilution (the potency of the liquid once dilute is retained for 14 days), and in ampoules for injection.

✚/▲ warning/side-effects: *see* DROPERIDOL.

Dromoran (*Roche*) is a proprietary NARCOTIC ANALGESIC which, because it is a preparation of the powerful OPIATE and NARCOTIC levorphanol tartrate, is on the controlled drugs list. It is used to relieve severe pain anywhere in the body, and to enhance general anaesthesia, and is produced in the form of tablets and in ampoules for injection. It is not recommended for children.

✚/▲ warning/side-effects: *see* LEVORPHANOL.

droperidol is a powerful TRANQUILLIZER and ANTIPSYCHOTIC, used primarily in emergencies to subdue or soothe psychotic (particularly manic) patients during behavioural disturbances, although it is also used on patients about to undergo certain diagnostic procedures that may be difficult or painful, because it promotes a sensation of dispassionate detachment. Administration is oral in the form of tablets or as a sugar-free dilute liquid, or by injection.

✚ warning: droperidol should not be administered to patients with a reduction in the bone-marrow's capacity to produce blood cells, or with certain types of glaucoma. It should be administered only with caution to those with heart or vascular disease, kidney or liver disease, parkinsonism, or depression; or who are pregnant or lactating.

▲ side-effects: concentration and speed of reaction is usually affected. There may also be restlessness, insomnia and nightmares, rashes and jaundice, dry mouth, gastrointestinal disturbances, difficulties in urinating, and blurred vision. Muscles in the neck and back, and sometimes in the arms, may undergo spasms. Rarely, there is weight loss and impaired kidney function.

Related articles: DROLEPTAN; THALAMONAL.

drostanolone propionate is a synthesized steroid that has many of the properties of an ANDROGEN (a male sex hormone) and of an anabolic steroid, used therapeutically to treat the sex-hormone-related cancer of the breast in women. Administration is by injection.

✚ warning: drostanolone propionate should not be administered to patients with impaired liver function or who are pregnant; it should be administered with caution to those with impaired heart or kidney function, epilepsy, diabetes, high blood pressure (hypertension) or migraine. In patients young enough still to be growing, bone development should be monitored.

▲ side-effects: there is usually a degree of masculinization, involving at least menstrual irregularity. High levels of calcium in the blood are also usual. There may be acne and fluid retention leading to weight gain.

Related article: MASTERIL.

Droxalin (*Sterling Health*) is a proprietary non-prescription ANTACID that is not available

from the National Health Service. Used to treat acid stomach and indigestion, peptic ulcer and hiatus hernia, it is produced in the form of tablets for chewing that contain magnesium trisilicate and ALEXITOL SODIUM. It is not recommended for children.
✚ warning: see MAGNESIUM TRISILICATE.

Dryptal (*Berk*) is a proprietary DIURETIC, available only on prescription, used to treat fluid retention in the tissues (oedema) and mild to moderate high blood pressure (*see* ANTIHYPERTENSIVE). In high dosage it may also be used to assist a failing kidney. Produced in the form of tablets (in two strengths, the stronger for hospital use only), Dryptal is a preparation of the powerful but short-acting diuretic frusemide.
✚/▲ warning/side-effects: *see* FRUSEMIDE.

DTIC-Dome (*Bayer*) is a proprietary CYTOTOXIC drug, available only on prescription, used (infrequently) to treat the skin (mole) cancer melanoma, some soft-tissue sarcomas, and the lymphatic cancer Hodgkin's disease. Produced in vials for injection, DTIC-Dome is a preparation of dacarbazine.
✚/▲ warning/side-effects: *see* DACARBAZINE.

Dubam (*Norma*) is a proprietary non-prescription COUNTER-IRRITANT compound which, in the form of a spray (in an aerosol) applied to the skin, produces an irritation of sensory nerve endings that offsets the pain of underlying muscle or joint ailments. It contains several salts of SALICYLIC ACID in solution.

Dulcodos (*Boehringer Ingelheim*) is a proprietary non-prescription compound LAXATIVE that is not available from the National Health Service. Produced in the form of tablets, it is a combination of the stimulant laxative bisacodyl together with the faecal softener DIOCTYL SODIUM SULPHOSUCCINATE (also called docusate sodium). It is not recommended for children.
✚/▲ warning/side-effects: *see* BISACODYL.

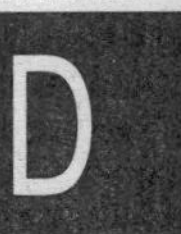

Dulcolax (*Boehringer Ingelheim*) is a proprietary non-prescription LAXATIVE that is not available from the National Health Service. Produced in the form of tablets and as anal suppositories (in two strengths), it is a preparation of the stimulant laxative bisacodyl. It is not recommended for children.
✚/▲ warning/side-effects: *see* BISACODYL.

Duo-autohaler (*Riker*) is a proprietary SYMPATHOMIMETIC compound bronchodilator, available only on prescription, used to treat bronchospasm in asthma and chronic bronchitis. Produced in a metered-dose aerosol, it is a combination of isoprenaline hydrochloride together with the VASOCONSTRICTOR phenylephrine bitartrate.
✚/▲ warning/side-effects: *see* ISOPRENALINE; PHENYLEPHRINE.

Duofilm (*Stiefel*) is a proprietary non-prescription liquid preparation intended to remove warts, particularly verrucas (on the soles of the feet). For daily topical application, avoiding normal skin surfaces, it is a compound in which the major active constituent is SALICYLIC ACID.

Duogastrone (*Winthrop*) is a proprietary ANTACID that has ANTI-INFLAMMATORY and ANALGESIC

D

properties. Available only on prescription, it is used to treat duodenal ulcer. It is produced in the form of capsules especially formulated for release in the duodenum, and contains carbenoxolone sodium, which is thought to create a protective coating over the mucous lining of the duodenum. It is not recommended for children.
✚/▲ warning/side-effects: *see* CARBENOXOLONE SODIUM.

Duovent (*Boehringer Ingelheim*) is a proprietary compound BRONCHODILATOR, available only on prescription, used to treat bronchospasm in asthma and chronic bronchitis. Produced in a metered-dose aerosol with mouthpiece, it is a combination of the SYMPATHOMIMETIC fenoterol hydrobromide together with the ANTICHOLINERGIC drug ipratropium bromide. It is not recommended for children aged under 6 years.
✚/▲ warning/side-effects: *see* FENOTEROL; IPRATROPIUM.

Duphalac (*Duphar*) is a proprietary non-prescription LAXATIVE that is not available from the National Health Service. It works by maintaining a volume of fluid within the intestines through osmosis, so lubricating the faeces and reducing levels of ammonia-producing organisms. Produced in the form of a syrup, Duphalac is a preparation of the semi-synthetic disaccharide lactulose.
✚/▲ warning/side-effects: *see* LACTULOSE.

Duphaston (*Duphar*) is a proprietary preparation of the PROGESTOGEN dydrogesterone, an analogue of the sex hormone PROGESTERONE. Available only on prescription, it is used to treat many conditions of hormonal deficiency in women, including menstrual difficulty, premenstrual syndrome, displacement of womb-lining tissue (endometriosis), recurrent miscarriage and infertility. It is produced in the form of tablets.
✚/▲ warning/side-effects: *see* DYDROGESTERONE.

Durabolin (*Organon*)is a proprietary form of the anabolic STEROID nandrolone, available only on prescription, used to assist the metabolic synthesis of protein, e.g., in building up the body following major surgery or long-term debilitating disease, or to treat osteoporosis ("brittle bones"). Sometimes administered also to treat sex-hormone-linked cancers, it is additionally used in the treatment of certain forms of anaemia, although how it works in this respect – and even whether it works – remains the subject of some debate: variations in patient response are wide. It is produced in ampoules or syringes for intramuscular injection.
✚/▲ warning/side-effects: *see* NANDROLONE.

Duracreme (*Family Planning Sales*) is a proprietary non-prescription SPERMICIDAL preparation, for use only in combination with barrier methods of contraception (such as a condom). Produced in the form of a cream, its active constituent is an alcohol ester.

Duragel (*LRC Products*) is a proprietary non-prescription SPERMICIDAL preparation, for use only in combination with barrier methods of contraception (such as a condom). Produced in the form of a gel, its active constituent is an alcohol ester.

Duromine (*Riker*) is a proprietary preparation of phentermine

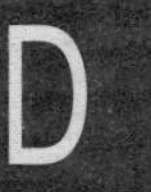

which, as a strong stimulant drug, is on the controlled drugs list. Used as an APPETITE SUPPRESSANT in the medical treatment of obesity, it is produced in the form of sustained-release tablets (in two strengths), and is not recommended for children.
✚/▲ warning/side-effects: *see* PHENTERMINE.

Duromorph (*L A B*) is a proprietary narcotic ANALGESIC which, because it represents a preparation of the OPIATE and NARCOTIC morphine (in aqueous solution), is on the controlled drugs list. It is used primarily to relieve pain following surgery, or the pain experienced during the final stages of terminal malignant disease, and is produced in ampoules for injection. It is not recommended for children.
✚/▲ warning/side-effects: *see* MORPHINE.

Durophet (*Riker*) is a proprietary preparation of amphetamine and dexamphetamine, and is on the controlled drugs list. It is an immensely powerful stimulant, and is used primarily to treat narcolepsy (a condition marked by irresistible attacks of sleep during the daytime), although it is sometimes also used to treat children who are medically hyperactive. Tolerance and dependence are major hazards. Produced in the form of sustained-release capsules (in three strengths), Durophet is not generally recommended for children.
✚/▲ warning/side-effects: *see* AMPHETAMINE; DEXAMPHETAMINE.

Duvadilan (*Duphar*) is a proprietary VASODILATOR that affects principally the blood vessels of the feet and hands, but also affects the blood supply to the brain. It is therefore used to relieve the symptoms of both cerebral and peripheral vascular disease. The drug also has the effect of inhibiting contractions of the womb, and is thus additionally used to prevent or stall premature labour. A preparation of isoxsuprine hydrochloride, it is produced in the form of tablets and (under the name Duvadilan Retard) sustained-release tablets, and in ampoules for injection.
✚/▲ warning/side-effects: *see* ISOXSUPRINE HYDROCHLORIDE.

Dyazide (*Smith, Kline & French*) is a proprietary compound DIURETIC, available only on prescription, used to treat severe fluid retention in the tissues (oedema) and mild to moderate high blood pressure (hypertension). Produced in the form of tablets, Dyazide is a preparation of two powerful diuretics, triamterene and (the THIAZIDE) hydrochlorothiazide.
✚/▲ warning/side-effects: *see* HYDROCHLOROTHIAZIDE; TRIAMTERENE.

dydrogesterone is a PROGESTOGEN, an analogue of the sex hormone PROGESTERONE, and is used to treat many conditions of hormonal deficiency in women, including menstrual difficulty, premenstrual syndrome, displacement of womb-lining tissue (endometriosis), recurrent miscarriage and infertility. Administration is oral in the form of tablets.
✚ warning: dydrogesterone should not be administered to patients who suffer from cancer of the breast, thrombosis, or undiagnosed bleeding from the vagina; it should be administered with

D

caution to those with diabetes, heart, liver or kidney disease, or high blood pressure (hypertension), or who are lactating.

▲ side-effects: there may be breast tenderness and irregular menstruation, fluid retention and consequent weight gain, a change in libido, and gastrointestinal disturbances. Some patients also experience acne or urticaria.

Related article: DUPHASTON.

Dynese (*Galen*) is a proprietary non-prescription ANTACID that is not available from the National Health Service. Produced in the form of a (mint- or orange-flavoured) suspension, it is a preparation of the complex MAGALDRATE, and is not recommended for children aged under 6 years.

Dytac (*Smith, Kline & French*) is a proprietary DIURETIC, available only on prescription, used to treat fluid retention in the tissues (oedema) especially when caused by kidney or liver disease, or by congestive heart failure. Produced in the form of capsules, Dytac is a preparation of the powerful potassium- sparing diuretic triamterene. It is not recommended for children.

✚/▲ warning/side-effects: *see* TRIAMTERENE.

Dytide (*Smith, Kline & French*) is a proprietary compound DIURETIC, available only on prescription, used to treat fluid retention in the tissues (oedema). Produced in the form of capsules, Dytide represents a preparation of the powerful potassium-sparing diuretic triamterene together with the THIAZIDE diuretic benzthiazide. It is not recommended for children.

✚/▲ warning/side-effects: *see* BENZTHIAZIDE; TRIAMTERENE.

E45 Cream (*Crookes*) is a proprietary non-prescription skin emollient (softener and soother) containing a mixture of paraffins and fats, including wool fat.
✚ warning: wool fat causes sensitivity reactions in some patients.

Ebufac (*DDSA Pharmaceuticals*) is a proprietary non-narcotic ANALGESIC that has additional ANTI-INFLAMMATORY properties. Available only on prescription, Ebufac is used to relieve pain – particularly the pain of rheumatic disease and other musculo-skeletal disorders – and is produced in the form of tablets consisting of a preparation of ibuprofen.
✚/▲ warning/side-effects: *see* IBUPROFEN.

Econacort (*Squibb*) is a proprietary preparation that combines the CORTICOSTEROID hydrocortisone with the ANTI-BACTERIAL and ANTIMICROBIAL econazole nitrate. Available only on prescription and produced in the form of a cream for topical application, Econacort is used to treat inflammation in which infection is also diagnosed. The cream, applied sparingly, should be massaged into the skin; prolonged use should be avoided, as should use during pregnancy.
✚/▲ warning/side-effects: *see* ECONAZOLE NITRATE; HYDROCORTISONE.

econazole nitrate is an ANTI-BACTERIAL and ANTIFUNGAL agent; one of the IMIDAZOLES used particularly in topical applications to treat fungal infections of the skin or mucous membranes. Administration is in the form of creams or ointments, as vaginal inserts (pessaries or tampons), or as lotions, sprays or dusting-powders.
▲ side-effects: there may be local skin irritation, even to the extent of a burning sensation and redness.
Related articles: ECOSTATIN; GYNO-PEVARYL; PEVARYL.

Econocil VK (*DDSA Pharmaceuticals*) is a proprietary preparation of the penicillin-type ANTIBIOTIC phenoxymethyl-penicillin, used mainly to treat infections of the head and throat, and some skin conditions; it may also be used to reduce high body temperature. Available only on prescription, it is produced in the form of capsules and tablets (in two strengths).
✚/▲ warning/side-effects: *see* PHENOXYMETHYLPENICILLIN.

Economycin (*DDSA Pharmaceuticals*) is a proprietary ANTIBIOTIC, available only on prescription, used to treat many kinds of infection, but especially those of the respiratory tract, ear, nose and throat, gastrointestinal tract, urinary tract, and soft tissues. Produced in the form of capsules and tablets, Economycin is a preparation of the TETRACYCLINE tetracycline hydrochloride.
✚/▲ warning/side-effects: *see* TETRACYCLINE.

Econosone (*DDSA Pharmaceuticals*) is a proprietary CORTICOSTEROID preparation, available only on prescription, used to treat inflammation especially in cases where it is caused by allergy. Produced in the form of tablets (in two strengths), it is a form of the steroid prednisone.
✚/▲ warning/side-effects: *see* PREDNISONE.

Ecostatin (*Squibb*) is a proprietary non-prescription ANTIFUNGAL preparation of

E

econazole nitrate, used primarily to treat yeast infections of the skin and mucous membranes, especially in the urogenital areas. It is produced (in solution) in the form of a water-miscible cream, as a lotion, as a spray for topical application, as a dusting-powder, as a talc-based powder in a spray container, and as vaginal inserts (pessaries). Treatment should continue for at least a fortnight after lesions have disappeared.
▲ side-effects: *see* ECONAZOLE NITRATE.

ecothiopate iodide is a miotic drug (that is, it causes the pupil of the eye to contract) used to reduce pressure in the eyeball and so relieve the symptoms of glaucoma. It is an anticholinesterase and is more powerful than some other drugs used for the purpose, and its duration of effect longer, but associated side-effects prevent its common use. Administration is in the form of eye-drops.
✚ warning: ecothiopate iodide should not be administered to patients who suffer from retinal damage, inflammation in the eye, or asthma, or who are already taking muscle relaxant drugs.
▲ side-effects: there may be irritation on initial administration. Some patients then experience an ache across the eyebrow and blurred vision (because the accommodation of the eye is affected). But there is also a risk of cataract and/or blockage of the tear-ducts.
Related article: PHOSPHOLINE IODIDE.

Eczederm (*Quinoderm*) is a proprietary non-prescription skin emollient (softener and soother) in the form of a cream that contains CALAMINE (zinc carbonate) and starch, of use in the treatment of eczematous dermatotes.

Eczederm with Hydrocortisone (*Quinoderm*) is a proprietary form of the emollient skin cream ECZEDERM that also contains the CORTICOSTEROID hydrocortisone. Available only on prescription, it is used to soften and soothe dry or cracked skin and to treat local inflammation. Prolonged use should be avoided.
✚/▲ warning/side-effects: *see* HYDROCORTISONE.

Edecrin (*Merck, Sharp & Dohme*) is a proprietary DIURETIC, available only on prescription, used to treat fluid retention within the tissues (oedema), especially when related to congestive heart failure or liver or kidney disorders. Produced in the form of tablets, and in vials for injection, Edecrin is a preparation of ethacrynic acid. The tablets are not recommended for children aged under 2 years; the injection is not suitable for children.
✚/▲ warning/side-effects: *see* ETHACRYNIC ACID.

edrophonium chloride is a drug that has the effect of enhancing the transmission of neural impulses between the nerves and the muscles they serve because it is an anticholinesterase that prolongs the duration of the neurotransmitter. But its effect is of only very brief duration, and so it is used mainly for the diagnosis of neural disorders such as myasthenia gravis, and to check on the efficacy of cholinergic drugs prescribed to treat them. Administration is by injection.
✚ warning: edrophonium chloride should not be

administered to patients who suffer from intestinal or urinary blockage. It should be administered only with caution to those with asthma, epilepsy, parkinsonism, slow heart rate or low blood pressure (hypotension); who have respiratory depression; who have recently had a heart attack; or who are pregnant. Some doctors administer atropine (or a similar drug) simultaneously to forestall some side-effects.

▲ side-effects: there may be nausea and vomiting with an excess of saliva in the mouth, diarrhoea and abdominal cramps. High dosage may cause gastrointestinal disturbance and sweating; and overdosage may result in urinary and faecal incontinence, loss of coordination in vision, nervous agitation and weakness amounting to paralysis.

Related article: TENSILON.

Efcortelan (*Glaxo*) is a proprietary preparation of the CORTICOSTEROID hydrocortisone, available only on prescription, used to treat inflammation especially where it is caused by allergy, to relieve itching in the urogenital areas, or to promote the healing of dermatitis. It is produced in the form of a cream, as an ointment, and as a lotion for topical application (undiluted).

✚/▲ warning/side-effects: *see* HYDROCORTISONE.

Efcortelan Soluble (*Glaxo*) is a proprietary preparation of the CORTICOSTEROID hydrocortisone, available only on prescription, used to treat inflammation especially where it is caused by allergy, to treat shock, or to make up a deficiency of steroid hormones in a patient. It is produced in the form of a powder for reconstitution (in water) as a medium for injection.

✚/▲ warning/side-effects: *see* HYDROCORTISONE.

Efcortesol (*Glaxo*) is a proprietary preparation of the CORTICOSTEROID hydrocortisone, available only on prescription, used to treat inflammation especially where it is caused by allergy, to treat shock, or to make up a deficiency of steroid hormones in a patient. It is produced in ampoules for injection.

✚/▲ warning/side-effects: *see* HYDROCORTISONE.

Effercitrate (*Typharm*) is a proprietary non-prescription alkalizing agent used to render a patient's urine alkaline in cases of cystitis (inflammation and/or infection of the bladder). Produced in the form of tablets for effervescent solution, it represents a compound of citric acid and potassium bicarbonate. It is not recommended for children aged under 12 months.

✚ warning: Effercitrate should not be administered to patients who suffer from ulceration or obstruction of the small intestine; it should be administered with caution to those with impaired kidney function.

▲ side-effects: there may be mild diuresis, reduction in blood potassium levels and gastric irritation.

Effico (*Pharmax*) is a proprietary non-prescription tonic that is not available from the National Health Service. Used primarily to stimulate the appetite, Effico contains the stimulant CAFFEINE, vitamin B in the form of THIAMINE hydrochloride and NICOTINAMIDE, and an infusion of gentian. It is produced in the form of a syrup for dilution (the potency of the syrup once dilute is retained for 14 days).

E

Efudix (*Roche*) is a proprietary CYTOTOXIC drug, available only on prescription, used in the form of a cream for topical application to treat malignant skin lesions. Consisting of a preparation of the drug fluorouracil, it works by being incorporated into new-forming cells and so preventing normal cell reproduction.
✚/▲ warning/side-effects: *see* FLUOROURACIL.

Elantan (*Schwarz*) is a proprietary preparation of the VASODILATOR isosorbide mononitrate, available only on prescription, used to prevent or treat angina pectoris (heart pain). Produced in the form of tablets (in two strengths, under the names Elantan 20 and Elantan 40), it is not recommended for children.
✚/▲ warning/side-effects: *see* ISOSORBIDE MONONITRATE.

Elavil (*DDSA Pharmaceuticals*) is a proprietary ANTIDEPRESSANT drug, available only on prescription, administered to treat depressive illness (and especially in cases where some degree of sedation is deemed necessary). Like many such drugs, it has also been used to treat bedwetting by children at night although this use is now becoming less common. Produced in the form of tablets (in two strengths), Elavil is a preparation of amitriptyline hydrochloride.
✚/▲ warning/side-effects: *see* AMITRIPTYLINE.

Eldepryl (*Britannia*) is a proprietary preparation of the drug selegiline, available only on prescription, used to assist in the treatment of the symptoms of parkinsonism (see ANTIPARKINSONISM). It has the effect of reducing the breakdown of dopamine in the brain, and is used in combination with the amino acid LEVODOPA (which is converted to dopamine in the brain) to supplement and extend levodopa's action through its action as a monoamine oxidase inhibitor (MAO INHIBITOR). In many patients it has the additional effect of lessening some side-effects. It is produced in the form of tablets.
✚/▲ warning/side-effects: *see* SELEGILINE.

Eldisine (*Lilly*) is a proprietary CYTOTOXIC drug, available only on prescription, used to treat leukaemia, lymphomas and some solid tumours (such as cancer of the breast or lung). Produced in the form of a powder for reconstitution as a medium for injection, Eldisine is a preparation of the VINCA ALKALOID vindesine sulphate.
✚/▲ warning/side-effects: *see* VINDESINE SULPHATE.

Electrosol (*Macarthys*) is a proprietary non-prescription sodium supplement, used to treat mild or moderate degrees of sodium depletion (as may happen in cases of dehydration or in illnesses – particularly kidney disease – in which salt is lost in some quantity). Electrosol is produced in the form of tablets for effervescent solution, containing SODIUM CHLORIDE, POTASSIUM CHLORIDE and SODIUM BICARBONATE.

Elemental 028 (*Scientific Hospital Supplies*) is a proprietary nutritional supplement for patients who are severely undernourished or who are suffering from some problem with the absorption of food (such as following gastrectomy); it may also be used to feed patients who require a liquid diet through injury or disease. Produced in the form of orange-flavoured or plain powder in sachets for solution in water, Elemental 028 contains amino acids, carbohydrate, fats, VITAMINS and minerals. It is not suitable for children aged under 12 months.

Eltroxin (*Glaxo*) is a proprietary preparation of the thyroid hormone thyroxine, used to make up a hormonal deficiency, and to treat associated symptoms (myxoedema). It is produced in the form of tablets (in two strengths) containing thyroxine sodium, and has a delayed effect and cumulative action.

✚/▲ warning/side-effects: *see* THYROXINE SODIUM.

Eludril (*Concept*) is a proprietary non-prescription mouth-wash that has ANTIBACTERIAL and ANTIFUNGAL properties and inhibits the formation of plaque on the teeth. It is also used in the treatment of gum disease and mouth ulcers. Containing the antiseptic chlorhexidine gluconate and the chlorbutol, Eludril is not recommended for children aged under 6 years. An aerosol spray version is also available.

✚/▲ warning/side-effects: *see* CHLORHEXIDINE.

emepronium bromide is a powerful ANTICHOLINERGIC drug used to treat patients who suffer from excessive frequency of urination or from incontinence. It works by acting on the muscles at the base of the bladder both to inhibit the involuntary release of urine and to expand the bladder's overall capacity. However, emepronium is poorly absorbed by the stomach and intestines, and even before reaching that stage may cause ulceration of the gums, mouth, throat or oesophagus unless sufficient fluid is taken simultaneously.

✚ warning: emepronium bromide should not be administered to patients with disorders of or injury to the oesophagus, or from glaucoma; it should be administered with caution to those with abnormal retention of food in the stomach, or enlargement of the prostate gland. It is essential that adequate fluid intake is maintained, or ulceration may occur.

▲ side-effects: there may be dry mouth and difficulty in swallowing; the pupils may be dilated, causing blurred vision and sensitivity to light; pressure may increase inside the eyeballs. Flushing may be followed by heart rate disturbance and heartbeat irregularities. There may also be constipation. Rarely, there is fever.

Related article: CETIPRIN.

Emeside (*L A B*) is a proprietary preparation of the ANTI-EPILEPTIC drug ethosuximide, available only on prescription, used to treat and suppress petit mal ("absence") seizures – the mild form of epilepsy. Produced in the form of capsules and as a blackcurrant- or orange-flavoured syrup for dilution (the potency of the syrup once diluted is retained for 14 days), Emeside's effects should be monitored following the initiation of treatment so that an optimum treatment level can be established.

✚/▲ warning/side-effects: *see* ETHOSUXIMIDE.

***emetic** is any agent that causes

vomiting. Emetics are used mostly to treat poisoning by non-acidic non-corrosive substances, especially drugs in overdose. Some affect the vomiting centre in the brain; others irritate the stomach nerves. Among the best known and most used is IPECACUANHA, but several drugs similarly used as constituents in expectorant preparations can in higher concentrations also cause effective emesis.

Emetrol (*Radiol*) is a proprietary non-prescription ANTI-EMETIC drug, used to treat nausea and vomiting (especially morning sickness during pregnancy), or to prevent regurgitation in babies, and travel sickness. Produced in the form of a solution, its major active constituents are the sugars FRUCTOSE and GLUCOSE, together with some phosphoric acid.

Emko (*Syntex*) is a proprietary non-prescription SPERMICIDAL preparation, for use only in combination with barrier methods of contraception (such as a condom). Produced in the form of a foam in an aerosol with an applicator, Emko's active constituent is an alcohol ester.

Emla (*Astra*) is a proprietary local ANAESTHETIC in the form of a cream for topical application. Available only on prescription, it is used primarily to relieve localized pain (caused, for example, by skin disease or sensitivity reaction), but may also be used to prepare patients for a painful injection. It is a combined preparation of the anaesthetics lignocaine and prilocaine, and is presented in a pack that includes dressings.
✚/▲ warning/side-effects: *see* LIGNOCAINE; PRILOCAINE.

Emtexate (*Nordic*) is a proprietary CYTOTOXIC drug, available only on prescription, used in the treatment of leukaemia, lymphomas and some solid tumours (such as cancer of the breast, or a hydatidiform mole). It works by being incorporated into new- forming cells and so preventing normal cell reproduction. Produced in the form of tablets, in vials for injection (in four strengths) and as a powder for reconstitution as a medium for injection, Emtexate is a preparation of methotrexate.
✚/▲ warning/side-effects: *see* METHOTREXATE.

Emulsiderm (*Dermal*) is a proprietary non-prescription skin emollient (softener and soother) in the form of a liquid emulsion that contains benzalkonium chloride and liquid paraffin. It can be rubbed into the skin or added to a bath.
✚ warning: *see* BENZALKONIUM CHLORIDE.

emulsifying ointment is a non-proprietary formulation comprising a combination of wax together with white soft paraffin and liquid paraffin. It is used as a base for medications that require topical application.

enalapril is an ANTIHYPERTENSIVE drug used to treat all forms of high blood pressure (hypertension), especially when more standard forms of therapy have failed or are not tolerated, and to assist in the treatment of congestive heart failure. It works by inhibiting the action of a certain peptide in the blood (angiotensin) that normally constricts the blood vessels. Administration (in the form of enalapril maleate) is oral, as tablets; some patients may require simultaneous administration of a DIURETIC (such as a THIAZIDE).

✚ warning: enalapril should be administered with caution to patients with impaired kidney function, or who are pregnant. The initial dose may cause a rapid fall in blood pressure to low blood pressure (hypotension), especially in patients who are also taking diuretics or who are dehydrated.

▲ side-effects: there may be a dry cough, headache, fatigue, dizziness, nausea, an alteration in the sense of taste, muscle cramps, diarrhoea, low blood pressure and renal failure. Some patients develop a rash.
Related article: INNOVACE.

En-De-Kay (*Stafford-Miller*) is a proprietary non-prescription form of fluoride supplement for administration in areas where the water supply is not fluoridated, especially to growing children. Produced in the form of tablets (in three strengths, labelled for children of different ages), as a sugar-free liquid to be used in drops, and as a mouthwash for dilution, En-De-Kay's active constituent is SODIUM FLUORIDE.

Endoxana (*Boehringer Ingelheim*) is a proprietary CYTOTOXIC drug, available only on prescription, used in the treatment of leukaemia, lymphomas and some solid tumours. It works by disrupting the DNA in new-forming cells and so preventing normal cell reproduction. Produced in the form of tablets (in two strengths) and as a powder for reconstitution as a medium for injection, Endoxana is a preparation of cyclophosphamide; it is sometimes prescribed in combination with the drug MESNA. It is not recommended for children.

✚/▲ warning/side-effects: *see* CYCLOPHOSPHAMIDE.

Enduron (*Abbott*) is a proprietary DIURETIC, available only on prescription, used to treat an accumulation of fluid within the tissues (oedema) and high blood pressure (hypertension). Produced in the form of tablets, Enduron is a preparation of the THIAZIDE methyclothiazide.

✚/▲ warning/side-effects: *see* METHYCLOTHIAZIDE.

Ener-G (*General Designs*) is a proprietary non-prescription gluten-free brown rice bread, for patients whose metabolisms are unable to tolerate the compound cereal protein gluten (as with coeliac disease). The bread is made without milk, eggs, wheat, soya or refined sugar.

enflurane is a volatile general ANAESTHETIC usually given to supplement nitrous oxide-oxygen mixtures (in a concentration of between 1 and 5%) for the induction and maintenance of anaesthesia during major surgery. Only a small proportion of the drug is metabolized by a patient, making it particularly safe for repeated use. Administration is by inhalation through a calibrated vaporizer.

✚ warning: enflurane slows both the heart and the breathing rate. Shallow breathing may tend to build up carbon dioxide levels in the body. The drug should not be administered to patients who have respiratory disorders.

▲ side-effects: reduced heart function results in low blood pressure.
Related article: ETHRANE.

Enrich (*Abbott*) is a proprietary

nutritional supplement for patients who are severely undernourished (such as with anorexia nervosa) or who are suffering from some problem with the absorption of food (such as following gastrectomy); it may also be used to feed patients who require a liquid diet through injury or disease. Produced in the form of a lactose- and gluten-free liquid in cans, Enrich contains protein, carbohydrate (including dietary fibre), fats, vitamins and minerals. It is not suitable for children aged under 12 months, or as a sole source of nutrition for children under 5 years.

Ensure (*Abbott*) is a proprietary nutritional supplement for patients who are severely undernourished (such as with anorexia nervosa) or who are suffering from some problem with the absorption of food (such as following gastrectomy); it may also be used to feed patients who require a liquid diet through injury or disease. Produced in the form of a lactose- and gluten-free liquid in cans and bottles (or as a powder for reconstitution in identical form), Ensure contains protein, carbohydrate, fats, vitamins and minerals, and comes in vanilla, coffee and eggnog flavours. It is not suitable for children aged under 12 months. A version with a higher proportion of protein, carbohydrate and fats is also available (under the name Ensure Plus).

Enteromide (*Consolidated*) is a proprietary ANTIBACTERIAL drug, available only on prescription, formerly used to treat inflammation and infection of the intestines, to relieve food poisoning, or to reduce bacterial levels in the intestines before surgery or examination, but now used less commonly and generally only to relieve chronic diarrhoea. Produced in the form of tablets, Enteromide is a preparation of the SULPHONAMIDE drug CALCIUM SULPHALOXATE.

Enterosan (*Windsor Pharmaceuticals*) is a proprietary, non-prescription ANTIDIARRHOEAL preparation containing morphine, kaolin and belladonna.
✚/▲ warning/side-effects: *see* BELLADONNA; MORPHINE.

Entrotabs (*Wallis*) is a proprietary, non-prescription ANTIDIARRHOEAL preparation containing the ANTACIDS aluminium hydroxide and magnesium aluminium silicate (attapulgite), and the fruit substance pectin.
✚/▲ warning/side-effects: *see* ALUMINIUM HYDROXIDE.

Epanutin (*Parke-Davis*) is a proprietary ANTICONVULSANT drug, available only on prescription, used to treat and prevent grand mal (tonic-clonic) and partial (focal) epileptic seizures. It is sometimes alternatively used to treat or prevent attacks of migraine or trigeminal (facial) neuralgia. Produced in the form of capsules (in three strengths), as chewable tablets (under the name Epanutin Infatabs), and as a suspension for dilution (the potency of the suspension once dilute is retained for 14 days), Epanutin is a preparation of the effective but non-hypnotic drug phenytoin.
✚/▲ warning/side-effects: *see* PHENYTOIN.

Epanutin Ready Mixed Parenteral (*Parke-Davis*) is a form of the proprietary ANTICONVULSANT drug EPANUTIN that is administered to treat the

emergency epileptic condition status epilepticus. It may, however, also be used to prevent convulsive seizures during neurosurgical operations and, perhaps more mundanely, to treat and regularize heartbeat irregularities. Produced in ampoules for injection, it is a solution of phenytoin sodium with propylene glycol. Not recommended for children.
✚/▲ warning/side-effects: *see* PHENYTOIN.

ephedrine hydrochloride is a SYMPATHOMIMETIC drug used as a VASOCONSTRICTOR and BRONCHODILATOR, used mainly in the treatment of asthma, chronic bronchitis and similar conditions (especially allergy-based ones). (This is also the major use of the closely related drug pseudoephedrine.) Its effect as a vasoconstrictor is sometimes utilized to counteract the fall in blood pressure in the blood vessels of the hands and feet that may occur in general anaesthesia. Other uses are in treating whooping cough, in inhibiting urinary incontinence in adults and bedwetting by children, to treat nasal congestion, and to dilate the pupil of the eye for ophthalmic examination or surgery. Administration is oral in the form of tablets or as an elixir, or topical in the form of nose-drops.
✚ warning: ephedrine hydrochloride should not be administered to patients who are already taking drugs that affect the action of the heart; it should be administered with caution to those with diabetes, reduced blood supply to the heart, high blood pressure (hypertension), disorder of the thyroid gland, and during pregnancy and lactation. Prolonged use as a bronchodilator or as a nasal decongestant may eventually result in tolerance.
▲ side-effects: there may be changes in heart rate and blood pressure, anxiety, restlessness, tremor, insomnia, dry mouth, and cold fingertips and toes. Used as a nasal decongestant, there may be local irritation.
Related articles: ARGOTONE; AURALGICIN; CAM; DAVENOL; EXPULIN; EXPURHIN; FRANOL; FRANOL EXPECT; FRANOL PLUS; HAYMINE; LOTUSSIN; NORADRAN; PHENSEDYL; RUBELIX; TAUMASTHMAN; TEDRAL.

Ephynal (*Roche*) is a proprietary non-prescription form of vitamin E (TOCOPHEROL) supplement, used to make up for vitamin deficiency. It is produced in the form of tablets (in four strengths) consisting of a preparation of alpha tocopheryl acetate.

Epifoam (*Stafford-Miller*) is a proprietary CORTICOSTEROID preparation with mild local ANAESTHETIC properties, available only on prescription, in the form of a foam for topical application in the perineal region of the body (the vulva in women, between the anus and the scrotum in men), especially on women patients who have undergone an episiotomy during childbirth. It is a combination of the steroid hydrocortisone and the mild local anaesthetic pramoxine hydrochloride, and is applied on a pad.
✚/▲ warning/side-effects: *see* HYDROCORTISONE.

Epifrin (*Allergan*) is a proprietary preparation of the natural hormone adrenaline hydrochloride, available only on prescription. It is used (in very

E

dilute solution) in the form of eye-drops as a SYMPATHOMIMETIC to treat glaucoma. Prolonged use should be avoided.
✚/▲ warning/side-effects: *see* ADRENALINE.

Epilim (*Labaz*) is a proprietary ANTICONVULSANT drug, available only on prescription, used to treat all forms of epilepsy. Considerable monitoring of body functions is necessary during treatment for the first 6 months. Produced in the form of crushable tablets, as enteric-coated tablets (in two strengths), as a sugar-free liquid, and as a syrup for dilution (the potency of the syrup once dilute is retained for 14 days), Epilim is a preparation of the carboxylic acid derivative sodium valproate.
✚/▲ warning/side-effects: *see* SODIUM VALPROATE.

epirubicin hydrochloride is an ANTIBIOTIC and CYTOTOXIC drug, and is used both to treat cancer and as an IMMUNOSUPPRESSANT following tissue grafting or transplantation in order to prevent tissue rejection. Dosage is critical to each individual patient. Administration is by injection.
✚ warning: suppression of the bone-marrow's function of producing red blood cells is inevitable, and regular blood counts are essential. The drug is also a skin irritant.
▲ side-effects: hair loss is common, even to total baldness; there may be inflammation of the mucous lining of the mouth (stomatitis), nausea and vomiting. There is also increased sensitivity to radiotherapy (which in most cases should be avoided).
Related article: PHARMORUBICIN.

Epodyl (*ICI*) is a proprietary CYTOTOXIC drug, available only on prescription, used primarily in the treatment of recurrent but only mildly malignant tumours of the bladder. Produced in the form of a liquid solution for instillation into the bladder (for retention there for at least one hour), Epodyl is a preparation of ethoglucid.
✚/▲ warning/side-effects: *see* ETHOGLUCID.

epoprostenol, or prostacyclin, is a prostaglandin present in the walls of blood vessels. Administered therapeutically, by intravenous infusion, it constitutes an ANTICOAGULANT that inhibits blood coagulation by preventing the aggregation of platelets, in addition having the effect of a VASODILATOR. Its major uses are to preserve platelet function in heart by-pass operations, and to act as a substitute for HEPARIN if required during kidney dialysis.
✚ warning: epoprostenol's half-life is only about 3 minutes, so the drug must be administered in continous intravenous infusion. Blood count monitoring is essential, especially when there is simultaneous administration of heparin.
▲ side-effects: there is commonly flushing and low blood pressure (hypotension); there may also be headache. High dosage may cause pallor and sweating.
Related article: FLOLAN.

Eppy (*Smith & Nephew*) is a proprietary preparation of the hormone adrenaline, available only on prescription. It is used (in very dilute solution) in the form of eye-drops as a SYMPATHOMIMETIC to treat

glaucoma. Prolonged use should be avoided.
✚/▲ warning/side-effects: *see* ADRENALINE.

Equagesic (*Wyeth*) is a proprietary compound ANALGESIC that is on the controlled drugs list and is not available from the National Health Service. Used primarily in the short-term treatment of rheumatic pain or the symptoms of other musculo-skeletal disorders, and produced in the form of tablets, Equagesic contains the (potentially addictive) TRANQUILLIZER meprobamate, the SKELETAL MUSCLE RELAXANT ethoheptazine citrate, and aspirin. It is not recommended for children. There are interactions with a wide variety of drugs including alcohol and nervous system depressants.
✚/▲ warning/side-effects: *see* ASPIRIN; MEPROBAMATE.

Equanil (*Wyeth*) is a proprietary ANXIOLYTIC drug that is on the controlled drugs list. Used in the short-term treatment of nervous anxiety and associated muscular tension, and produced in the form of tablets (in two strengths), Equanil is a preparation of the, potentially addictive, TRANQUILLIZER meprobamate. It is not recommended for children, and is contraindicated in acute porphyria and alcoholism.
✚/▲ warning/side-effects: *see* MEPROBAMATE.

Eradacin (*Sterling Research*) is a proprietary preparation of the unusual ANTIBIOTIC drug acrosoxacin, available only on prescription, used to treat the sexually transmitted disease gonorrhoea in patients who are allergic to penicillin, or whose strain of gonorrhoea is resistant to penicillin-type antibiotics. Produced in the form of capsules, Eradacin is not recommended for children.
✚/▲ warning/side-effects: *see* ACROSOXACIN.

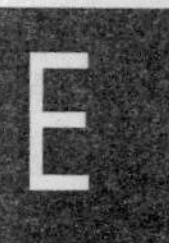

Eraldin (*ICI*) is a proprietary ANTI-ARRHYTHMIC drug, available only on prescription, used to treat fast heart rate, especially following a heart attack. It works by inhibiting the contractile capacity of the heart muscle. Produced in ampoules for slow intravenous injection, Eraldin is a preparation of practolol.
✚/▲ warning/side-effects: *see* PRACTOLOL.

ergocalciferol is one of the two natural forms of calciferol (vitamin D), formed in plants by the action of sunlight.
see CALCIFEROL.

ergometrine maleate is an alkaloid VASOCONSTRICTOR and uterine stimulant drug administered to women in childbirth during the third stage of labour: the delivery of the placenta. A measure to prevent excessive postnatal bleeding. The drug is generally administered by injection when the baby is half-way delivered, although it is produced also in the form of tablets.
✚ warning: ergometrine maleate must not in any circumstances be administered to patients who are still in the first and early second stages of labour; it should not be administered to those with vascular disease, or impaired kidney, liver or lung function. Caution must be exercised in administration to those with heart disease and high blood pressure (hypertension) or with any infection, who have toxaemia of pregnancy, or who have just undergone a multiple birth.
▲ side-effects: there may be

nausea and vomiting, with temporary high blood pressure.
Related article: SYNTOMETRINE.

E

ergotamine tartrate is a drug administered to patients who suffer from migraine that is not relieved by the ordinary forms of pain-killing drug. A vegetable alkaloid, it is most effectively administered during the aura – the initial symptoms – of an attack, and probably works by constricting the cranial arteries. However, although the pain may be relieved, other symptoms, such as the visual disturbances and nausea, may not (although other drugs may be administered to treat those separately). Repeated treatment may in some patients eventually lead to habituation (addiction); in others it may cause ergot poisoning, resulting in gangrene of the fingers and toes, and confusion. Administration is oral in the form of tablets either for swallowing or to be held under the tongue to dissolve, or as an aerosol inhalant; one proprietary compound preparation is in the form of anal suppositories.

✚ warning: ergotamine tartrate should not be administered to patients who suffer from vascular disease or any infection, or who are pregnant or lactating. It should be administered with caution to those with kidney, liver or heart disease, or with thyroid gland overactivity. Dosage should be carefully monitored; treatment should not be repeated within 4 days. It should never be administered on a prophylactic (preventative) basis. Treatment should be withdrawn at once if the patient experiences tingling or numbness at the extremities.

▲ side-effects: there may be abdominal pain and muscle cramps that may lead to nausea and vomiting. Overdosage or rapid withdrawal of the drug may in turn cause headache.
Related articles: CAFERGOT; LINGRAINE; MEDIHALER-ERGOTAMINE; MIGRIL.

Ermysin (*Britannia*) is a proprietary ANTIBIOTIC, available only on prescription, used to treat many forms of infection (particularly pneumonia and legionnaires' disease) and to prevent others (particularly sinusitis, diphtheria and whooping cough), and as an alternative to penicillin-type antibiotics in patients who are allergic or whose infections are resistant. Produced in the form of tablets (in two strengths), Ermysin is a preparation of the macrolide erythromycin. It is not recommended for children.

✚/▲ warning/side-effects: *see* ERYTHROMYCIN.

Ervevax (*Smith, Kline & French*) is a proprietary VACCINE against German measles (rubella) in the form of a solution containing live but attenuated viruses of the Wistar RA27/3 strain. Available only on prescription, it is administered in the form of an injection.

Erycen (*Berk*) is a proprietary ANTIBIOTIC, available only on prescription, used to treat many forms of infection (particularly pneumonia and legionnaires' disease) and to prevent others (particularly sinusitis, diphtheria and whooping cough), and as an alternative to penicillin-type antibiotics in patients who are allergic or whose infections are resistant. Produced in the form of tablets (in two strengths), Erycen

is a preparation of the macrolide erythromycin. It is not recommended for children.
✚/▲ warning/side-effects: *see* ERYTHROMYCIN.

Erymax (*Parke-Davis*) is a proprietary ANTIBIOTIC, available only on prescription, used to treat many forms of infection (particularly pneumonia and legionnaires' disease) and to prevent others (particularly sinusitis, diphtheria and whooping cough), and as an alternative to penicillin-type antibiotics in patients who are allergic or whose infections are resistant. Produced in the form of capsules, Erymax is a preparation of the macrolide erythromycin.
✚/▲ warning/side-effects: *see* ERYTHROMYCIN.

Erythrocin (*Abbott*) is a proprietary ANTIBIOTIC, available only on prescription, used to treat many forms of infection (particularly pneumonia and legionnaires' disease) and to prevent others (particularly sinusitis, diphtheria and whooping cough), and as an alternative to penicillin-type antibiotics in patients who are allergic or whose infections are resistant. Produced in the form of tablets (in two strengths), and as a powder for reconstitution as a medium for injection, Erythrocin is a preparation of salts of the macrolide erythromycin. The tablets are not recommended for children.
✚/▲ warning/side-effects: *see* ERYTHROMYCIN.

Erythrolar (*Lagap*) is a proprietary ANTIBIOTIC, available only on prescription, used to treat many forms of infection (particularly pneumonia and legionnaires' disease) and to prevent others (particularly sinusitis, diphtheria and whooping cough), and as an alternative to penicillin-type antibiotics in patients who are allergic or whose infections are resistant. Produced in the form of tablets (in two strengths), and as a suspension for dilution (the potency of the suspension once dilute is retained for 5 days), Erythrolar is a preparation of salts of the macrolide erythromycin.
✚/▲ warning/side-effects: *see* ERYTHROMYCIN.

Erythromid (*Abbott*) is a proprietary ANTIBIOTIC, available only on prescription, used to treat many forms of infection (particularly pneumonia and legionnaires' disease) and to prevent others (particularly sinusitis, diphtheria and whooping cough), and as an alternative to penicillin-type antibiotics in patients who are allergic or whose infections are resistant. Produced in the form of tablets (in two strengths, the stronger under the name Erythromid DS), Erythromid is a preparation of the macrolide erythromycin. It is not recommended for children.
✚/▲ warning/side-effects: *see* ERYTHROMYCIN.

erythromycin is a broad-spectrum ANTIBIOTIC, one of the macrolides, used to treat many forms of infection (particularly pneumonia and legionnaires' disease) and to prevent others (particularly sinusitis, diphtheria and whooping cough), and as an alternative to penicillin-type antibiotics in patients who are allergic or whose infections are resistant. Administration is oral in the form of tablets, as capsules, or as a dilute suspension (mixture), or by injection. Tablets have to be enteric- or film-coated because the drug is inactivated by gastric secretions.

▲ side-effects: one salt of erythromycin (the estolate), a constituent in a proprietary suspension, should not be administered to patients with liver disease; all forms of the drug should be administered with caution to those with impaired liver function.

✚ warning: large doses may cause nausea and vomiting, and possibly diarrhoea.

Related articles: ARPIMYCIN; ERMYSIN; ERYCEN; ERYMAX; ERYTHROCIN; ERYTHROLAR; ERYTHROMID; ERYTHROPED; ILOSONE; ILOTYCIN; RETCIN.

Erythroped (*Abbott*) is a proprietary ANTIBIOTIC, available only on prescription, used to treat many forms of infection (particularly pneumonia and legionnaires' disease) and to prevent others (particularly sinusitis, diphtheria and whooping cough), and as an alternative to penicillin-type antibiotics in patients who are allergic or whose infections are resistant. Produced in the form of a suspension (in three strengths) for dilution (the potency of the suspension once dilute is retained for 5 days), as sugar-free granules in sachets for solution, and as tablets (under the name Erythroped A), Erythroped is a preparation of salts of the macrolide erythromycin.

✚/▲ warning/side-effects: *see* ERYTHROMYCIN.

Esbatal (*Calmic*) is a proprietary ANTIHYPERTENSIVE drug, available only on prescription, used to treat very high blood pressure (hypertension). Produced in the form of tablets (in two strengths), it is a preparation of bethanidine sulphate.

✚/▲ warning/side-effects: *see* BETHANIDINE SULPHATE.

Esidrex (*Ciba*) is a proprietary DIURETIC, available only on prescription, used to treat an accumulation of fluid in the tissues (oedema) and high blood pressure (hypertension). Produced in the form of tablets (in two strengths), Esidrex is a preparation of the THIAZIDE hydrochlorothiazide.

✚/▲ warning/side-effects: *see* HYDROCHLOROTHIAZIDE.

Esidrex K (*Ciba*) is a proprietary DIURETIC, available only on prescription, used to treat an accumulation of fluid in the tissues (oedema) and high blood pressure (hypertension). Produced in the form of double-layered tablets, Esidrex K is a preparation of the THIAZIDE hydrochlorothiazide (which is potassium-depleting) with the potassium supplement POTASSIUM CHLORIDE.

✚/▲ warning/side-effects: *see* HYDROCHLOROTHIAZIDE.

Eskamel (*Smith, Kline & French*) is a proprietary non-prescription cream used to treat acne. It contains the KERATOLYTIC agent resorcinol together with SULPHUR.

✚ warning: *see* RESORCINOL.

Eskornade (*Smith, Kline & French*) is a proprietary non-prescription nasal DECONGESTANT that is not available from the National Health Service. It is used particularly to treat the symptoms of the common cold, sinusitis and flu. Produced in the form of spansules (sustained-release capsules) and as a sugar-free syrup for dilution (the potency of the syrup once dilute is retained for 14 days), Eskornade is a combination of the SYMPATHOMIMETIC

phenylpropanolamine hydrochloride with the ANTIHISTAMINE diphenylpyraline hydrochloride. In the form of spansules, (sustained-release capsules), the preparation is not recommended for children.
✚/▲ warning/side-effects: *see* DIPHENYLPYRAMINE HYDROCHLORIDE; PHENYLPROPANOLAMINE HYDROCHLORIDE.

Esoderm (*Napp*) is a proprietary non-prescription preparation of the drug lindane, used to treat parasitic infestation by lice (pediculosis) or by itch-mites (scabies) on the skin surface, particularly under the hair. However, strains of head-lice resistant to lindane have recently emerged, and the drug is not now recommended for use on the scalp. It is produced in the form of a (flammable) alcohol-based lotion, and as a cream shampoo.
✚/▲ warning/side-effects: *see* LINDANE.

Estracyt (*Lundbeck*) is a proprietary CYTOTOXIC drug, available only on prescription, an OESTROGEN used to treat cancer of the prostate gland. Because this type of cancer is sex-hormone-linked (with respect to androgens, male sex hormones), administration of a female sex hormone – although it produces some feminization – is an effective counter-measure. Produced in the form of capsules (not to be taken with milk or with any other dairy product), Estracyt is a preparation of estramustine phosphate.
✚/▲ warning/side-effects: *see* ESTRAMUSTINE PHOSPHATE.

Estradurin (*Lundbeck*) is a proprietary CYTOTOXIC drug, available only on prescription, a compound OESTROGEN used to treat cancer of the prostate gland. Because this type of cancer is sex-hormone-linked (with respect to androgens, male sex hormones), administration of female sex hormones – although it produces some feminization – is an effective counter-measure. Produced in vials for injection, Estradurin is a combination of the oestrogen preparation polyestradiol phosphate with the local ANAESTHETIC mepivacaine and the B vitamin NICOTINAMIDE.
✚/▲ warning/side-effects: *see* POLYESTRADIOL PHOSPHATE.

estramustine phosphate is a CYTOTOXIC drug, an OESTROGEN used to treat cancer of the prostate gland. Because this type of cancer is sex-hormone-linked (with respect to androgens, male sex hormones), administration of a female sex hormone – although it produces some feminization – is an effective counter-measure. Administration is oral in the form of capsules.
✚ warning: treatment causes sterility; prolonged treatment may increase a disposition towards leukaemia especially if there is simultaneous irradiation treatment. Estramustine phosphate should be administered with caution to patients who suffer from diabetes, epilepsy, severe migraine, kidney or heart disease, or high blood pressure (hypertension). Blood count monitoring is essential.
▲ side-effects: there is commonly nausea and vomiting, and sodium retention with a consequent weight gain. The breasts may develop. The blood-producing capacity of the bone-marrow is impaired. And there is hair loss.
Related article: ESTRACYT.

Estrovis (*Parke-Davis*) is a

proprietary preparation of the synthetic OESTROGEN quinestrol, available only on prescription, formerly used to inhibit or suppress lactation in women following childbirth. (Such use was almost entirely discontinued when an association was made between the use of oestrogens and some forms of thrombosis.) Estrovis is produced in the form of tablets.

✚/▲ warning/side-effects: *see* QUINESTROL.

ethacrynic acid is a DIURETIC used to treat fluid retention in the tissues (oedema) or to assist a failing kidney by promoting the excretion of urine. Administration is oral in the form of tablets (effective in 1 hour, full diuresis in 6 hours) or by injection (peak effect in half an hour). Patients with kidney failure may require large doses – but large doses imply worse side-effects, especially if the doses are applied intravenously.

✚ warning: ethacrynic acid should not be administered to patients who suffer from cirrhosis of the liver; it should be administered with caution to those who are pregnant. Treatment may aggravate existing conditions of diabetes, gout or those involving the prostrate gland.

▲ side-effects: there may be a rash. High doses administered to patients who suffer from kidney failure may cause deafness, ringing in the ears (tinnitus) and gastrointestinal disturbances.
Related article: EDECRIN.

ethambutol hydrochloride is an ANTIBIOTIC that is one of the major forms of treatment for tuberculosis. Even so, it is used generally in combination (to cover resistance and for maximum effect) with other antitubercular drugs such as ISONIAZID or rifampicin. Treatment lasts for between 6 and 18 months depending on severity and on the specific drug combination, but the use of ethambutol tends to imply the shorter duration. The drug is also used to prevent the contraction of tuberculosis by relatives. Administration is oral in the form of tablets or as a powder.

✚ warning: ethambutol hydrochloride should not be administered to children aged under 6 years, to patients who are elderly, or to those who suffer from nervous disorders of the eyes.

▲ side-effects: side-effects are rare, and are mostly in the form of visual disturbances (such as loss of acuity or colour-blindness) which should prove temporary if treatment is withdrawn. A regular ophthalmic check is advised during treatment.
Related articles: MYAMBUTOL; MYNAH.

ethamivan is a respiratory stimulant drug, used to relieve severe respiratory difficulties in patients who have been gassed (particularly with carbon dioxide), who suffer from chronic disease of the respiratory tract, or who undergo respiratory depression following major surgery – especially in cases where for one reason or another ventilatory support is not applicable. Administration is oral in the form of a solution (intended for paediatric use), or by injection.

✚ warning: ethamivan should not be administered to patients who have respiratory failure due to drug overdose or neurological disease, or with coronary artery disease, severe asthma, or an excess of thyroid hormones in the blood (thyrotoxicosis). It should be administered with caution to those with severe high blood pressure (hypertension) or a reduced supply of blood to the heart.

▲ side-effects: there may be nausea, restlessness and tremor, leading possibly to convulsions and heartbeat irregularities.
Related article: CLAIRVAN.

ethamsylate is a drug that reduces bleeding, although how it does so is not perfectly understood – it may correct abnormal adhesion by the blood platelets on the fibrin matrix (so coagulating the blood). As a HAEMOSTATIC, it is used particularly to treat haemorrhage from small blood vessels or to relieve excessive menstrual flow. Administration is oral in the form of tablets, or by injection.

✚ warning: ethamsylate should not be administered to patients who are known to have platelet deficiency in the blood.

▲ side-effects: there may be nausea with headache; some patients come out in a rash.
Related article: DICYNENE.

ethanol, or ethyl alcohol, is the form of alcohol found in alcoholic drinks, produced by the fermentation of sugar by yeast. *see* ALCOHOL.

ethanolamine oleate is a drug used in sclerotherapy – a technique to treat varicose veins by the injection of an irritant solution. The resultant inflammation of the vein promotes the obliteration of the vein by thrombosis. Leakage of the drug into the tissues at the site of injection may cause severe tissue damage.

✚ warning: ethanolamine oleate should not be injected into patients whose varicose veins are already inflamed or so painful as to prevent walking, who are obese, or who are taking oral contraceptives.

▲ side-effects: some patients experience sensitivity reactions.

ethinyloestradiol is a major female sex HORMONE, a synthetic OESTROGEN, used to make up hormonal deficiencies – sometimes in combination with a PROGESTOGEN – to treat menstrual, menopausal or other gynaecological problems (such as oestrogen-related infertility). It is also a constituent of many ORAL CONTRACEPTIVES. Administration is oral in the form of tablets.

✚ warning: ethinyloestradiol should not be administered to patients who have cancers proved to be sex-hormone-linked, who have a history of thrombosis or inflammation of the womb, or who have porphyria or impaired liver function. Prolonged treatment increases the risk of cancer of the endometrium (the lining of the womb). Caution should be exercised in administering ethinyloestradiol to patients who are diabetic or epileptic, who have heart or kidney disease, who are pregnant or lactating, or who have high blood pressure (hypertension) or recurrent severe migraine.

▲ side-effects: there may be nausea and vomiting. A common effect is weight gain, generally through fluid or sodium retention in the tissues. The breasts may become tender and enlarge slightly. There may also be headache and/or depression;

sometimes a rash breaks out.
Related articles: ANOVLAR; BINOVUM; BREVINOR; CONOVA 30; CONTROVLAR; DIANE; EUGYNON; GYNOVLAR; LOESTRIN; LOGYNON; MARVELON; MICROGYNON; MINILYN; MINOVLAR; MIXOGEN; NEOCON-1/35; NORIMIN; OVRAN; OVRANETTE; OVYSMEN; PC4; SYNPHASE; TRINORDIOL; TRINOVUM.

ethoglucid is a CYTOTOXIC drug used primarily in the treatment of recurrent but only mildly malignant tumours of the bladder. It works by damaging the DNA of newly-forming cells, thus preventing normal cell replication. Administration is by instillation into the bladder of a solution that remains in the bladder for as long as possible (at least an hour); treatment is commonly once a week for 3 months, then once a month for 12.

✚ warning: blood count monitoring is essential; a reduction in the blood level of white blood cells is to be expected.

▲ side-effects: treatment may cause frequency of, or difficulty in, urinating. Almost all males are rendered sterile.
Related article: EPODYL.

ethosuximide is an ANTICONVULSANT drug used to treat and suppress petit mal ("absence" and myoclonic) seizures – the mild form of epilepsy. It may be used singly or in combination with other drugs, and is particularly useful in successfully treating some patients on whom other anticonvulsants have no effect. Dosage must be adjusted to the optimum level for each individual patient. Administration is oral in the form of capsules or as a dilute elixir.

✚ warning: ethosuximide should not be administered to patients with porphyria. Withdrawal of treatment, if undertaken, must be gradual. Special monitoring of blood levels of the drug are required for a patient who is pregnant or lactating.

▲ side-effects: there may be gastrointestinal disturbances, drowsiness, headache and/or dizziness; some patients experience depression or euphoria. Rarely, there are haematological disorders or psychotic states.
Related articles: EMESIDE, ZARONTIN.

ethyl alcohol, or ETHANOL, is the form of alcohol found in alcoholic drinks, produced by the fermentation of sugar by yeast. *see* ALCOHOL.

Ethrane (*Abbott*) is a proprietary preparation of the general ANAESTHETIC enflurane, usually administered to supplement nitrous oxide-oxygen mixtures for the induction and maintenance of anaesthesia during major surgery. It is produced in gas bottles for administration through a calibrated vaporizer.

✚/▲ warning/side-effects: *see* ENFLURANE.

etodolac is a non-steroidal ANTI-INFLAMMATORY non-narcotic ANALGESIC used primarily to treat rheumatoid arthritis. Administration is oral in the form of tablets and capsules.

✚ warning: etodolac should not be administered to patients known to be allergic to aspirin, who suffer from peptic ulcer or from gastrointestinal bleeding, or who are pregnant or lactating. It should be administered with caution to those who suffer from impaired kidney or liver function.

▲ side-effects: there may be gastrointestinal disturbance (which may be decreased by taking the drug with food). Some patients experience sensitivity reactions, such as a rash, and CNS side-effects, including headaches, vertigo or hearing disturbances. There may be fluid retention and consequent weight gain. Blood disorders have occurred. *Related articles:* LODINE; RAMODAR.

etomidate is a general ANAESTHETIC used specifically for the initial induction of anaesthesia. Recovery after treatment is rapid and without any hangover effect, and it causes less of a fall in blood pressure than many other anaesthetics. But there is pain on injection, when there may also be simultaneous extraneous muscle movements.

✚ warning: pain on injection may be overcome by prior administration of suitable premedication (such as a narcotic analgesic). Intravenous injection must be carried out with caution in order to avoid thrombophlebitis.

▲ side-effects: repeated doses may suppress the secretion of corticosteroid hormones by the adrenal glands. *Related article:* HYPNOMIDATE.

etoposide is an ANTICANCER drug used primarily to treat small cell lung cancer, or cancer of the testes that proves resistant to other forms of therapy; it may also be used to treat some lymphomas. A unique drug, it works in much the same way as the VINCA ALKALOIDS in disrupting a specific phase in cell replication, thus preventing further growth. Administration is oral in the form of capsules, or by injection.

✚ warning: the use of etoposide must be closely monitored in relation to each individual patient's tolerance of the toxicity of the drug.

▲ side-effects: there is commonly nausea and vomiting, and hair loss. The capacity of the bone-marrow for producing red blood cells is reduced: regular blood count monitoring is essential. High dosage may cause loss of sensation at the extremities and other neural symptoms. *Related article:* VEPESID.

etretinate is a powerful drug, a derivative of RETINOL (vitamin A), used in the treatment of severe psoriasis and complex skin conditions involving keratinization. Treatment may take up to 4 weeks to achieve full effect, but should be continued on a strict regime for between 6 and 9 months; more prolonged treatment is not recommended, although a second course of treatment may be begun after an interval of 3 or 4 months if necessary. It should be prescribed only by a consultant dermatologist, and treatment take place under clinical supervision. Administration is oral in the form of capsules.

✚ warning: etretinate should not be administered to patients who are pregnant (it may cause congenital abnormality in the fetus) or likely to become pregnant; contraception must be practised by women patients for a year after completion of a course of treatment.

▲ side-effects: there is commonly dryness of the mouth with cracking of the lips. Sometimes there is also hair

loss, generalized itching, and nose-bleeds. Fat levels in the blood may rise.
Related article: TIGASON.

E

Eudemine (*Allen & Hanburys*) is a proprietary preparation of the hyperglycaemic drug diazoxide, available only on prescription, used to treat chronic conditions involving a deficiency of glucose in the bloodstream. Such a condition might occur, for example, if a pancreatic tumour caused excessive secretion of insulin. Also useful in treating an acute hypertensive crisis (apoplexy), Eudemine is produced in the form of tablets and in ampoules for rapid intravenous injection.
✚/▲ warning/side-effects: *see* DIAZOXIDE.

Euglucon (*Roussel*) is a proprietary form of the SULPHONYLUREA drug glibenclamide, used to treat adult-onset diabetes; it works by promoting insulin secretion in whatever remains of the capacity of the pancreas for it, and increasing the number of insulin receptors. Available only on prescription, Euglucon is produced in the form of tablets (in two strengths).
✚/▲ warning/side-effects: *see* GLIBENCLAMIDE.

Eugynon 30 (*Schering*) is a combination ORAL CONTRACEPTIVE, available only on prescription, that combines the OESTROGEN ethinyloestradiol with the PROGESTOGEN levonorgestrel in a ratio of 30:250. It is produced in packs of 21 tablets corresponding to one complete menstrual cycle.
✚/▲ warning/side-effects: *see* ETHINYLOESTRADIOL; LEVONORGESTREL.

Eugynon 50 (*Schering*) is a combination ORAL CONTRACEPTIVE, available only on prescription, that combines the OESTROGEN ethinyloestradiol with the PROGESTOGEN norgestrel in a ratio of 50:500. It is produced in packs of 21 tablets corresponding to one complete menstrual cycle.
✚/▲ warning/side-effects: *see* ETHINYLOESTRADIOL; NORGESTREL.

Eumovate (*Glaxo*) is a proprietary CORTICOSTEROID preparation, available only on prescription, used in topical application to treat non-infective inflammation, especially in cases where less powerful steroid treatments have failed. Produced in the form of a water-miscible cream and an anhydrous ointment to treat inflammatory skin disorders, such as eczema and some types of dermatitis, and in the form of eye-drops (in two preparations, one additionally containing the ANTIBIOTIC NEOMYCIN SULPHATE under the name Eumovate-N) to treat ophthalmic inflammations, Eumovate is a preparation of the steroid clobetasone butyrate.
✚/▲ warning/side-effects: *see* CLOBETASONE BUTYRATE.

Eumydrin (*Winthrop*) is a proprietary preparation of the ANTICHOLINERGIC ANTISPASMODIC drug atropine methonitrate, used primarily to relieve muscle spasm in the valve-like sphincter between the stomach and the duodenum (the pylorus) in infants. It is produced in the form of a solution in a dropper bottle (and should be stored in a cool place).
✚/▲ warning/side-effects: *see* ATROPINE METHONITRATE.

Eurax (*Geigy*) is a proprietary non-prescription form of the drug crotamiton, used to treat itching, especially in relation to the

effects of infestation by the itch-mite (scabies). It is produced in the form of a lotion and a cream. Another version is available (only on prescription) additionally containing the CORTICOSTEROID hydrocortisone, and used also to treat itching that results from skin inflammation.
✚/▲ warning/side-effects: *see* CROTAMITON; HYDROCORTISONE.

Evacalm (*Unimed*) is a proprietary ANXIOLYTIC drug, available on prescription only to private patients, used to treat anxiety and insomnia, or to assist in the treatment of acute alcohol withdrawal symptoms. Produced in the form of tablets (in two strengths), Evacalm is a preparation of the long-acting BENZODIAZEPINE diazepam.
✚/▲ warning/side-effects: *see* DIAZEPAM.

Evadyne (*Ayerst*) is a proprietary ANTIDEPRESSANT drug, available only on prescription, used to treat depression with the added complication of anxiety. Produced in the form of tablets (in two strengths), Evadyne is a preparation of butriptyline. It is not recommended for children.
✚/▲ warning/side-effects: *see* BUTRIPTYLINE.

Exelderm (*ICI*) is a proprietary ANTIFUNGAL cream, available only on prescription, used for topical application to skin infections, such as athlete's foot or thrush. The cream should be massaged into the skin; treatment should continue for at least a fortnight after lesions have disappeared. Exelderm is a preparation of the IMIDAZOLE sulconazole nitrate.
✚/▲ warning/side-effects: *see* SULCONAZOLE NITRATE.

Exirel (*Pfizer*) is a proprietary BRONCHODILATOR, available only on prescription, used to treat conditions such as asthma and chronic bronchitis. Produced in the form of capsules (in two strengths), as an aerosol inhalant, and as a syrup, Exirel is a preparation of the SYMPATHOMIMETIC pirbuterol. It is not recommended for children aged under 6 years.
✚/▲ warning/side-effects: *see* PIRBUTEROL.

Ex-Lax (*Intercare*) is a proprietary, non-prescription LAXATIVE produced in the form of chocolate and as tablets. It contains phenolphthalein.
✚/▲ warning/side-effects: *see* PHENOLPHTHALEIN.

Exolan (*Dermal*) is a proprietary non-prescription preparation of the drug dithranol triacetate in mild solution, used to treat psoriasis. It is produced in the form of a water-miscible cream for topical application.
✚/▲ warning/side-effects: *see* DITHRANOL.

***expectorant** is a medicated liquid intended to increase the viscosity of sputum and so make it easier to cough up phlegm; expectorants are used particularly in the case of bronchial congestion. (They are not the same as linctuses, which merely comprise liquids thick and soothing enough to relieve sore throats or to loosen a cough. Nor is an expectorant necessarily an elixir, which disguises a potentially horrible taste with a sweetening substance like glycerol or alcohol.) Many expectorants work by irritating the lining of the stomach, so stimulating the reflex secretion of sputum by the glands in the mucous membranes of the upper respiratory tract. In high dosage, most expectorants can be used as EMETICS (to provoke vomiting).

Expulin (*Galen*) is a proprietary non-prescription cough linctus that is not available from the National Health Service. It is produced as a linctus in two strengths (the weaker labelled as a paediatric version) for dilution (the potency of the linctus once dilute is retained for 14 days), and is a combination of the OPIATE pholcodine, the SYMPATHOMIMETIC ephedrine hydrochloride, the ANTIHISTAMINE chlorpheniramine maleate, and GLYCEROL and menthol. Even the paediatric linctus is not recommended for children aged under 3 months.
✚/▲ warning/side-effects: *see* CHLORPHENIRAMINE; EPHEDRINE HYDROCHLORIDE; PHOLCODINE.

Expurhin (*Galen*) is a proprietary non-prescription nasal DECONGESTANT for children that is not available from the National Health Service. It is used to relieve all forms of congestion in the upper respiratory tract. Produced in the form of a sugar-free linctus, Expurhin is a comination of the SYMPATHOMIMETIC ephedrine hydrochloride together with the ANTIHISTAMINE chlorpheniramine maleate and MENTHOL. Even as a paediatric linctus, it is not recommended for children aged under 3 months.
✚/▲ warning/side-effects: *see* CHLORPHENIRAMINE; EPHEDRINE HYDROCHLORIDE.

Exterol (*Dermal*) is a proprietary non-prescription preparation of a urea-hydrogen peroxide complex designed to dissolve and wash out wax in the ears. To be held in the ear with cotton wool for as long as possible, Exterol is produced in the form of ear-drops also containing GLYCEROL.

Extil Compound (*Evans*) is a proprietary cough linctus that is available on prescription only to private patients. Not to be diluted or shaken, it is a combination of the OPIATE noscapine, the SYMPATHOMIMETIC PSEUDOEPHEDRINE and the ANTIHISTAMINE CARBINOXAMINE maleate.
✚/▲ warning/side-effects: *see* NOSCAPINE.

Fabahistin (*Bayer*) is a proprietary ANTIHISTAMINE, available only on prescription, used to treat allergic symptoms in such cases as hay fever and urticaria. Produced in the form of tablets and as a suspension (in either of two diluents), Fabahistin's active constituent is mebhydrolin.
✚/▲ warning/side-effects: *see* MEBHYDROLIN.

Fabrol (*Zyma*) is a proprietary MUCOLYTIC, available on prescription only to private patients. Used to reduce the viscosity of sputum and thus facilitate expectoration in patients with asthma or bronchitis, Fabrol is produced in the form of sachets of granules (for solution in water) consisting of a preparation of acetylcysteine.
✚/▲ warning/side-effects: *see* ACETYLCYSTEINE.

Fansidar (*Roche*) is a proprietary ANTIMALARIAL drug, available only on prescription, used to treat patients who are seriously ill with malaria, particularly with strains resistant to the standard drug chloroquine. (A very few strains are resistant also to Fansidar.) It is sometimes alternatively used prophylactically to try to prevent tropical travellers from contracting the disease. Produced in the form of tablets, Fansidar is a compound of (the antimalarial) pyrimethamine together with (the ANTIBACTERIAL sulphonamide drug) SULFADOXINE. Dosage is critical, and must be carefully monitored.
✚/▲ warning/side-effects: *see* PYRIMETHAMINE.

Farlutal (*Farmitalia Carlo Erba*) is a proprietary preparation of the synthetic PROGESTOGEN (female sex hormone) medoxyprogesterone acetate, available only on prescription, used in women primarily to support drug treatments against breast cancer or cancer of the womb, or occasionally cancer of the kidney. In men it may be used to treat cancer of the prostate. Produced in the form of tablets (in any of three strengths) and in vials for injection, Farlutal should not be administered in high doses.
✚/▲ warning/side-effects: *see* MEDOXYPROGESTERONE.

Fasigyn (*Pfizer*) is a proprietary ANTIMICROBIAL drug, available only on prescription, used to treat infections by anaerobic bacteria and protozoa, particularly in the vagina or on the gums, and to ensure asepsis during surgery. Produced in the form of tablets and as fluid in (two sizes of) flasks for intravenous infusion, Fasigyn is a preparation of the nitroimidazole drug tinidazole.
✚/▲ warning/side-effects: *see* TINIDAZOLE.

Fe-Cap (*MCP Pharmaceuticals*) is a proprietary non-prescription preparation of the drug ferrous glycine sulphate, used as an IRON supplement in the treatment of iron deficiency anaemia, and produced in the form of capsules. It should not be taken simultaneously with tetracycline antibiotics.
✚/▲ warning/side-effects: *see* FERROUS GLYCINE SULPHATE.

Fe-Cap C (*MCP Pharmaceuticals*) is a proprietary non-prescription mineral-and-VITAMIN compound, consisting of capsules containing iron in the form of FERROUS GLYCINE SULPHATE together with ASCORBIC ACID (vitamin C).

Fe-Cap Folic (*MCP Pharmaceuticals*) is a proprietary

F

non- prescription mineral-and-VITAMIN compound used primarily as an iron supplement in the treatment of iron deficiency anaemia, and prophylactically during pregnancy. Produced in the form of capsules, Fe-Cap Folic is a preparation of ferrous glycine sulphate with FOLIC ACID (a vitamin of the B complex). It is not recommended for children, and should not be taken simultaneously with tetracycline antibiotics.
✚/▲ warning/side-effects: *see* FERROUS GLYCINE SULPHATE.

Fectrim (*DDSA Pharmaceuticals*) is a proprietary ANTIBACTERIAL drug available only on prescription, used especially in infections of the urinary tract, infections of the such as sinusitis and bronchitis, and infections of bones and joints. Produced in the form of soluble (dispersible) tablets (in any of three strengths), Fectrim represents a preparation of the compound drug co-trimoxazole, made up of the SULPHONAMIDE SULPHAMETHOXAZOLE together with the antibacterial agent TRIMETHOPRIM.
✚/▲ warning/side-effects: *see* CO-TRIMOXAZOLE.

Fefol (*Smith, Kline & French*) is a proprietary non-prescription mineral-and-VITAMIN compound used primarily as an IRON supplement during pregnancy. Produced in the form of spansules (sustained- release capsules), Fefol is a preparation of ferrous sulphate together with FOLIC ACID (a vitamin of the B complex). It is not recommended for children, and should not be taken simultaneously with tetracycline antibiotics.
✚/▲ warning/side-effects: *see* FERROUS SULPHATE.

Fefol-Vit (*Smith, Kline & French*) is a proprietary non-prescription mineral-and-VITAMIN compound used primarily as a supplement during pregnancy. Produced in the form of spansules (sustained-release capsules), Fefol-Vit represents a preparation of ferrous sulphate together with THIAMINE (vitamin B_1), RIBOFLAVINE (vitamin B_2), PYRIDOXINE (vitamin B_6), NICOTINAMIDE (of the B complex), FOLIC ACID (of the B complex) and ASCORBIC ACID (vitamin C). It is not recommended for children, and should not be taken simultaneously with tetracycline antibiotics.
✚/▲ warning/side-effects: *see* FERROUS SULPHATE.

Fefol Z (*Smith, Kline & French*) is a proprietary non-prescription mineral-and-VITAMIN compound used primarily as an IRON and ZINC supplement during pregnancy. Produced in the form of spansules (sustained-release capsules), Fefol is a preparation of ferrous sulphate together with FOLIC ACID (a vitamin of the B complex) and zinc sulphate. It is not recommended for children, and should not be taken simultaneously with tetracycline antibiotics.
✚/▲ warning/side-effects: *see* FERROUS SULPHATE.

Feldene (*Pfizer*) is a proprietary, NON-STEROIDAL ANTI-INFLAMMATORY DRUG available only on prescription, used to treat gout, arthritic and rheumatic pain, and other musculo-skeletal disorders. Produced in the form of capsules (in two strengths), soluble (dispersible) tablets (in two strengths), and as anal suppositories, Feldene's active constituent is piroxicam. It is not recommended for children.
✚/▲ warning/side-effects: *see* PIROXICAM.

Femerital (*MCP Pharmaceuticals*) is a proprietary non-prescription compound ANALGESIC that is not available from the National Health Service. Used to treat menstrual pain (dysmenorrhoea), and produced in the form of tablets, it is a preparation of ambucetamide and paracetamol.
✚/▲ warning/side-effects: *see* PARACETAMOL.

Feminax (*Nicholas Kiwi*) is a proprietary non-prescription ANALGESIC preparation, produced specifically for the relief of menstrual pain. Produced in the form of tablets, it contains paracetamol, codeine, caffeine, and the atropine-like drug hyoscine.
✚/▲ warning/side-effects: *see* CAFFEINE, CODEINE, HYOSCINE, PARACETAMOL.

Femulen (*Gold Cross*) is a proprietary ORAL CONTRACEPTIVE, available only on prescription, that consists of a preparation of the PROGESTOGEN ethynodiol acetate. It is produced in the form of tablets, and comes in a calendar pack of 28 corresponding to one complete menstrual cycle.
✚/▲ warning/side-effects: *see* ETHYNODIOL.

Fenbid (*Smith, Kline & French*) is a proprietary ANTI-INFLAMMATORY non-narcotic ANALGESIC, available only on prescription, used to treat pain of all kinds, especially pain from arthritis and rheumatism, and other musculo-skeletal disorders. Produced in the form of spansules (sustained-release capsules), Fenbid's active constituent is ibuprofen. It is not recommended for children or patients suffering from peptic ulcer.
✚/▲ warning/side-effects: *see* IBUPROFEN.

fenbufen is an, ANTI-INFLAMMATORY non-narcotic ANALGESIC drug with effects similar to those of aspirin. It is used particularly in the treatment of pain from rheumatoid arthritis and osteoarthritis.
✚ warning: fenbufen should not be administered to patients who are pregnant or lactating; who are allergic to aspirin or other anti- inflammatory drugs; or who are already taking aspirin or an anticoagulant.
▲ side-effects: there may be a skin rash; rarely, there is an allergic response, headache, disturbance of the sense of balance, gastrointestinal bleeding (though less than with some others of this class) or kidney dysfunction.
Related article: LEDERFEN.

fenfluramine hydrochloride is a drug used to aid slimming regimes because it acts as an appetite suppressant. Not a stimulant – unlike most other appetite suppressants – fenfluramine hydrochloride instead has sedative properties that may affect a patient's intricacy of thought and movement, and is potentially addictive (although dependence is rare).
✚ warning: fenfluramine hydrochloride may affect mental concentration; it enhances the effect of alcohol.
▲ side-effects: there may be depression; sedation, with headache, vertigo and gastric upsets, is not uncommon. Sometimes there is insomnia, dry mouth, fluid retention, increased frequency of urination and speeding of the heart rate. Treatment is only in the short term, tolerance and/or dependence may occur;

dosage should be tapered off gradually to avoid withdrawal depression.
Related article: PONDERAX.

fenoprofen is an ANTI-INFLAMMATORY non-narcotic ANALGESIC drug with effects similar to those of aspirin. It is used particularly in the treatment of pain from rheumatoid arthritis and osteoarthritis, and to reduce fever.

✚ warning: fenoprofen should not be administered to patients who are suffering from gastric or intestinal bleeding (as with a peptic ulcer); who are pregnant or lactating; who are allergic to aspirin or other anti-inflammatory drugs; who have reduced kidney function; who are asthmatic; or who are already taking aspirin, an anticoagulant or a drug to control the blood level of glucose.

▲ side-effects: there may be a skin rash; rarely, there is an allergic response or gastrointestinal bleeding.
Related articles: FENOPRON; PROGESIC.

Fenopron (*Dista*) is a proprietary, ANTI-INFLAMMATORY non-narcotic ANALGESIC drug available only on prescription, used to relieve pain – particularly arthritic and rheumatic pain – and to treat other musculo-skeletal disorders. Its active constituent is fenoprofen, and it is produced in the form of tablets (in either of two strengths). Not recommended for children, Fenopron should not be administered to patients with a peptic ulcer, gastrointestinal haemorrhage or asthma, or who are pregnant or lactating.

✚/▲ warning/side-effects: *see* FENOPROFEN.

Fenostil Retard (*Zyma*) is a proprietary non-prescription ANTIHISTAMINE used to treat allergic symptoms in such cases as hay fever. Produced in the form of tablets, Fenostil Retard's active constituent is dimethindene maleate.

✚/▲ warning/side-effects: *see* DIMETHINDENE MALEATE.

fenoterol is a SYMPATHOMIMETIC drug used as a BRONCHODILATOR to treat asthmatic attacks and other respiratory problems caused by airway obstruction. Administration is by aerosol spray, nebulizer or ventilator; less commonly, injection or infusion is used.

✚ warning: fenoterol should not be administered to patients who have heart disease or high blood pressure (hypertension); or who are pregnant. Elderly patients should be given a reduced dosage. Diabetics may be treated by intravenous infusion, with careful monitoring of blood sugar levels.

▲ side-effects: there may be tremor of the hands, nervous tension and headache; the heart rate may increase; the potassium level in the bloodstream may drop (hypokalaemia), following an injected dose.
Related article: BEROTEC.

fentanyl is a narcotic ANALGESIC, used primarily for analgesia during surgery and to supplement other anaesthetics; it may be used also to slow the breathing of an anaesthetized patient. As a narcotic, its proprietary forms are on the controlled drugs list.

✚ warning: fentanyl should not be administered to patients whose respiration is already impaired by disease or those

with myasthenia gravis, hypothyroidism or chronic liver disease. Use on a mother during childbirth may cause respiratory depression in the newborn. Elderly patients should be given a reduced dosage.
▲ side-effects: post-operatively there may be respiratory depression, low blood pressure, slowing of the heart, and nausea (with or without vomiting).
Related articles: SUBLIMAZE; THALAMONAL.

Fentazin (*Allen & Hanburys*) is a powerful proprietary ANTIPSYCHOTIC drug, available only on prescription, used to treat and tranquillize patients who are undergoing behavioural disturbances, or who are psychotic, particularly schizophrenic. It is also used to treat severe anxiety, or as an ANTI-EMETIC sedative prior to surgery. Produced in the form of tablets (in three strengths) and in ampoules for injection, Fentazin is a preparation of perphenazine. It is not recommended for children.
✚/▲ warning/side-effects: *see* PERPHENAZINE.

Feospan (*Smith, Kline & French*) is a proprietary non-prescription preparation of the drug ferrous sulphate, used as an IRON supplement in the treatment of iron deficiency anaemia, and produced in the form of spansules (sustained-release capsules). It is not recommended for children aged under 12 months, and should not be taken simultaneously with tetracycline antibiotics.
✚/▲ warning/side-effects: *see* FERROUS SULPHATE.

Feospan Z (*Smith, Kline & French*) is a proprietary non-prescription mineral-and-VITAMIN compound used primarily as an IRON and ZINC supplement during pregnancy. Produced in the form of spansules (sustained-release capsules), Feospan Z is a preparation of ferrous sulphate together with zinc sulphate. It is not recommended for children aged under 12 months, and should not be taken simultaneously with tetracycline antibiotics.
✚/▲ warning/side-effects: *see* FERROUS SULPHATE.

Ferfolic SV (*Sinclair*) is a proprietary mineral-and-VITAMIN compound, available only on prescription, used primarily as an IRON supplement in the treatment of iron deficiency anaemia, and prophylactically during pregnancy. Produced in the form of tablets, Ferfolic SV represents a preparation of ferrous gluconate together with FOLIC ACID (a vitamin of the B complex). It is not recommended for children, and should not be taken simultaneously with tetracycline antibiotics. A vitamin-enriched version, additionally containing other forms of vitamin B together with vitamin C, is available – on prescription only to private patients – under the name Ferfolic.
✚/▲ warning/side-effects: *see* FERROUS GLUCONATE.

Fergluvite (*Sinclair*) is a proprietary non-prescription mineral-and-VITAMIN compound that is not available from the National Health Service. It is used primarily as a supplement to treat the effects of anaemia. Produced in the form of tablets, Fergluvite is a preparation of ferrous gluconate with THIAMINE (vitamin B_1), RIBOFLAVINE (vitamin B_2), NICOTINAMIDE (of the

F

B complex) and ASCORBIC ACID (vitamin C). It is not recommended for children, and should not be taken simultaneously with tetracycline antibiotics.
✚/▲ warning/side-effects: *see* FERROUS GLUCONATE.

Fergon (*Winthrop*) is a proprietary non-prescription preparation of the drug ferrous gluconate, used as an IRON supplement in the treatment of iron deficiency anaemia, and produced in the form of tablets. It is not recommended for children aged under 6 years, and should not be taken simultaneously with tetracycline antibiotics.
✚/▲ warning/side-effects: *see* FERROUS GLUCONATE.

Ferrocap (*Consolidated Chemicals*) is a proprietary non-prescription preparation of the drug ferrous fumarate and THIAMINE HYDROCHLORIDE, used as an IRON supplement in the treatment of iron deficiency anaemia, and produced in the form of capsules. It is not recommended for children aged under 6 years, and should not be taken simultaneously with tetracycline antibiotics.
✚/▲ warning/side-effects: *see* FERROUS FUMARATE.

Ferrocap-F 350 (*Consolidated Chemicals*) is a proprietary non-prescription mineral-and-VITAMIN compound used primarily as an IRON supplement prophylactically during pregnancy. Produced in the form of capsules, Ferrocap-F 350 is a preparation of ferrous fumarate with FOLIC ACID (a vitamin of the B complex). It is not recommended for children, and should not be taken simultaneously with tetracycline antibiotics.
✚/▲ warning/side-effects: *see* FERROUS FUMARATE.

Ferrocontin Continus (*Degussa*) is a proprietary non-prescription preparation of the drug ferrous glycine sulphate, used as an IRON supplement in the treatment of iron deficiency anaemia, and produced in the form of tablets. It is not recommended for children, and should not be taken simultaneously with tetracycline antibiotics.
✚/▲ warning/side-effects: *see* FERROUS GLYCINE SULPHATE.

Ferrocontin Folic Continus (*Degussa*) is a proprietary non-prescription mineral-and-VITAMIN compound used primarily as an IRON supplement in the treatment of iron deficiency anaemia, and prophylactically during pregnancy. Produced in the form of tablets, Ferrocontin Folic Continus is a preparation of ferrous glycine sulphate with FOLIC ACID (a vitamin of the B complex). It is not recommended for children, and should not be taken simultaneously with tetracycline antibiotics.
✚/▲ warning/side-effects: *see* FERROUS GLYCINE SULPHATE.

Ferrograd (*Abbott*) is a proprietary non-prescription preparation of the drug ferrous sulphate, used as an IRON supplement in the treatment of iron deficiency anaemia, and produced in the form of sustained-release capsules. It is not recommended for children, and should not be taken simultaneously with tetracycline antibiotics, or by patients with diverticular disease or intestinal obstruction.
✚/▲ warning/side-effects: *see* FERROUS SULPHATE.

Ferrograd C (*Abbott*) is a proprietary non-prescription mineral-and-VITAMIN compound

used primarily as an IRON supplement in the treatment of iron deficiency anaemia. Produced in the form of sustained-release capsules, Ferrograd C is a preparation of ferrous sulphate with ASCORBIC ACID (vitamin C). It is not recommended for children, and should not be taken by patients with diverticular disease or from intestinal obstruction.
✚/▲ warning/side-effects: *see* FERROUS SULPHATE.

Ferrograd Folic (*Abbott*) is a proprietary non-prescription mineral-and-VITAMIN compound used primarily as an IRON supplement in the treatment of iron deficiency anaemia. Produced in the form of sustained-release capsules, Ferrograd Folic is a preparation of ferrous sulphate with FOLIC ACID (a vitamin of the B complex). It is not recommended for children, and should not be taken by patients with diverticular disease, intestinal obstruction, or a dietary deficiency of CYANOCOBALAMIN (vitamin B_{12}).
✚/▲ warning/side-effects: *see* FERROUS SULPHATE.

Ferromyn (*Calmic*) is a proprietary non-prescription preparation of the drug ferrous succinate, used as an IRON supplement in the treatment of iron deficiency anaemia, and produced in the form of tablets and as an elixir. It should not be taken simultaneously with tetracycline antibiotics or antacids.
✚/▲ warning/side-effects: *see* FERROUS SUCCINATE.

Ferromyn S (*Calmic*) is a form of Ferromyn with additional succinic acid.
see FERROMYN.

ferrous fumarate is an IRON-rich drug used to restore iron to the blood in cases of iron deficiency anaemia. Once a patient's blood haemoglobin level has reached normal, treatment should continue for at least 3 months to replenish fully the stores of iron in the body. Some preparations combine ferrous fumarate with various vitamins, for use particularly as supplements during pregnancy.
✚ warning: ferrous fumarate should not be administered to patients already taking tetracycline antibiotics or antacids; or to patients with a peptic ulcer.
▲ side-effects: large doses may cause gastrointestinal upset and diarrhoea; there may be vomiting. Prolonged treatment may result in constipation.
Related articles: B.C. 500 WITH IRON; FERROCAP; FERROCAP-F 350; FERSADAY; FERSAMAL; FOLEX-350; GALFER; GALFER F.A.; GALFERVIT; GIVITOL; METERFER; METERFOLIC; PREGADAY.

ferrous gluconate is an IRON-rich drug used to restore iron to the blood in cases of iron deficiency anaemia. Once a patient's blood haemoglobin level has reached normal, treatment should continue for at least 3 months to replenish fully the stores of iron in the body. Some preparations combine ferrous gluconate with various VITAMINS, for use particularly as supplements during pregnancy.
✚ warning: ferrous gluconate should not be administered to patients already taking tetracycline antibiotics.
▲ side-effects: large doses may cause gastrointestinal upset and diarrhoea; there may be vomiting. Prolonged treatment may result in constipation.

Related articles: FERFOLIC SV; FERGLUVITE; FERGON.

ferrous glycine sulphate is a drug used to restore IRON to the blood in cases of iron deficiency anaemia. Once a patient's blood haemoglobin level has reached normal, treatment should continue for at least 3 months to replenish fully the stores of iron in the body. Some preparations combine ferrous glycine sulphate with various VITAMINS, for use particularly as supplements during pregnancy.
✚ warning: ferrous glycine sulphate should not be administered to patients already taking tetracycline antibiotics.
▲ side-effects: large doses may cause gastrointestinal upset and diarrhoea; there may be vomiting. Prolonged treatment may result in constipation.
Related articles: FE-CAP; FE-CAP FOLIC; FERROCONTIN CONTINUS; FERROCONTIN FOLIC CONTINUS; KELFERON; KELFOLATE; PLESMET.

ferrous succinate is an IRON-rich drug used to restore iron to the blood in cases of iron deficiency anaemia. Once a patient's blood haemoglobin level has reached normal, treatment should continue for at least 3 months to replenish fully the stores of iron in the body.
✚ warning: ferrous succinate should not be administered to patients already taking tetracycline antibiotics or antacids.
▲ side-effects: large doses may cause gastrointestinal upset and diarrhoea; there may be vomiting. Prolonged treatment may result in constipation.
Related articles: FERROMYN FERROMYN S

ferrous sulphate is a drug used to restore IRON to the blood in cases of iron deficiency anaemia. Once a patient's blood haemoglobin level has reached normal, treatment should nevertheless continue for at least 3 months to replenish fully the stores of iron in the body. Some preparations combine dried ferrous sulphate with various vitamins, or with zinc, for use particularly as tonic supplements.
✚ warning: ferrous sulphate should not be administered to patients already taking tetracycline antibiotics.
▲ side-effects: large doses may cause gastrointestinal upset and diarrhoea; there may be vomiting. Prolonged treatment may result in constipation.
Related articles: FEFOL; FEFOL-VIT; FEFOL Z; FEOSPAN; FEOSPAN Z; FERROGRAD; FERROGRAD C; FERROGRAD FOLIC; FESOVIT; FESOVIT Z; FOLICIN; IROFOL C; IRONORM; PREGNAVITE FORTE F; SLOW-FE; SLOW-FE FOLIC.

Fersaday (*Duncan, Flockhart*) is a proprietary non-prescription preparation of the drug ferrous fumarate. Used as an IRON supplement in the treatment of iron deficiency anaemia, it is produced in the form of tablets. It is not recommended for children, and should not be taken simultaneously with tetracycline antibiotics or antacids.
✚/▲ warning/side-effects: *see* FERROUS FUMARATE.

Fersamal (*Duncan, Flockhart*) is a weaker version of Fersaday, permitting its administration to children. In addition to tablets, it is produced in the form of a syrup. Like Fersaday, Fersamal should not be taken simultaneously with

tetracycline antibiotics or antacids.
see FERSADAY.

Fertiral (*Hoechst*) is a proprietary preparation of GONADOTROPHIN-RELEASING HORMONE, available only from clinics and hospitals, used to treat women for infertility or lack of menstruation (amenorrhoea) due to hormonal insufficiency. In such cases, it is sometimes additionally used to try to determine whether it is the pituitary gland or the hypothalamus that is at fault, but with little success. Administration is by pulsed infusion.

✚ warning: Fertiral should not be administered to patients with cysts on the lining of the womb or on an ovary. Maximum duration of treatment is 6 months.

▲ side-effects: rarely, there is abdominal pain, with headache and nausea; there may be irritation at the site of infusion.

Fesovit (*Smith, Kline & French*) is a proprietary non-prescription compound of the drug ferrous sulphate together with ASCORBIC ACID (vitamin C) and several forms of VITAMIN B. It is not available from the National Health Service. Used as a mineral-and-vitamin supplement in the treatment of iron deficiency anaemia, it is produced in the form of spansules (sustained-release capsules). It is not recommended for children aged under 12 months, and should not be taken simultaneously with tetracycline antibiotics.

✚/▲ warning/side-effects: *see* FERROUS SULPHATE.

Fesovit Z (*Smith, Kline & French*) is a proprietary non-prescription compound of the drug ferrous sulphate with ZINC SULPHATE, ASCORBIC ACID (vitamin C) and several forms of VITAMIN B. It is not available from the National Health Service. Used as a mineral-and-vitamin supplement in the treatment of iron deficiency anaemia, it is produced in the form of spansules (sustained-release capsules). It is not recommended for children aged under 12 months, and should not be taken simultaneously with tetracycline antibiotics.

✚/▲ warning/side-effects: *see* FERROUS SULPHATE.

***fibrinolytic** drugs act to break up or dissolve blot clots, and are used to treat conditions such as thrombosis and embolism. Examples include STREPTOKINASE and UROKINASE.

figs elixir is a non-proprietary compound LAXATIVE used to relieve mild constipation. It is not available from the National Health Service. Made up as a syrup, it contains the powerful stimulant laxatives CASCARA and SENNA. Prolonged use should be avoided; treatment of children is not advised.

Finalgon (*Boehringer Ingelheim*) is a proprietary non-prescription ointment which, smoothed on to the skin using an applicator, produces an irritation of sensory nerve endings that offsets the pain of underlying muscle or joint ailments.

✚ warning: Finalgon should not be used on inflamed or broken skin, or on mucous membranes.

Fisherman's Friend (*Lofthouse of Fleetwood*) is a proprietary non-prescription lozenge for the relief of cold symptoms. It contains liquorice, MENTHOL and aniseed oil.

Flagyl (*May & Baker*) is a proprietary form of the AMOEBICIDAL drug metronidazole, available only on prescription, used to treat amoebic dysentery, infection by the organism Entamoeba histolytica, and abscesses on the liver. It is produced in the form of capsules (in two strengths). Simultaneous treatment with anticoagulants or barbiturates should be avoided; during treatment patients should not consume alcohol.
✚/▲ warning/side-effects: *see* METRONIDAZOLE.

Flagyl Compak (*May & Baker*) is a proprietary form of the drug metronidazole, available only on prescription, used to treat protozoan or bacterial infections of the vagina. It is produced in the form of tablets together with vaginal inserts (pessaries) also containing the ANTIFUNGAL drug NYSTATIN.
✚/▲ warning/side-effects: *see* METRONIDAZOLE.

Flagyl S (*May & Baker*) is a proprietary form of the AMOEBICIDAL drug metronidazole, available only on prescription, used to treat amoebic dysentery, infection by the organism Entamoeba histolytica, and abscesses on the liver; it is also used to treat acute inflammation of the gums (for which purpose it is not recommended for children aged under 12 months). Flagyl S is produced in the form of a suspension for dilution. Simultaneous treatment with anticoagulants or barbiturates should be avoided; during treatment patients should not consume alcohol.
✚/▲ warning/side-effects: *see* METRONIDAZOLE.

Flagyl 400 (*May & Baker*) is a proprietary form of the drug metronidazole, available only on prescription, used to treat protozoan or bacterial infections (such as trichomoniasis and non-specific vaginitis). It is produced in the form of tablets.
✚/▲ warning/side-effects: *see* METRONIDAZOLE.

Flamazine (*Smith & Nephew*) is a proprietary ANTIBACTERIAL cream, available only on prescription, used to treat wounds, burns and ulcers, bedsores and skin-graft donor sites. It is a preparation of silver sulphadiazine in a water-soluble base.
✚/▲ warning/side-effects: *see* SILVER SULPHADIAZINE.

Flar (*Consolidated Chemicals*) is a proprietary ANTIDIARRHOEAL preparation comprised largely of vitamins of the B complex together with lactic acid bacilli (thought to assist by acidifying the intestinal walls). It is produced in the form of capsules.

flavoxate hydrochloride is a form of drug used to treat problems of frequent urination, incontinence, and associated pain. Administration is oral, in the form of tablets.
✚ warning: flavoxate hydrochloride should not be administered to patients who suffer from infection or muscular disorder in the oesophagus, or from ulceration of the intestinal walls.
▲ side-effects: there may be ulceration of the oesophagus; reduced secretion of digestive juices in the stomach, and diarrhoea. Vision may blur; there may be a pressure build-up in the eyeballs (glaucoma), headache, nausea, fatigue and dry mouth.
Related article: URISPAS.

Flaxedil (*May & Baker*) is a proprietary SKELETAL MUSCLE RELAXANT, available only on prescription, of the type known as competitive or non-depolarising. It is used during surgical operations, but only after the patient has been rendered unconcscious. Produced in ampoules for injection, Flaxedil's active constituent is gallamine triethiodide.
✚/▲ warning/side-effects: *see* GALLAMINE TRIETHIODIDE.

flecainide acetate is a drug used to slow and regularize the heartbeat. Administration is usually first by slow intravenous injection, followed if necessary by infusion and then orally in the form of tablets. It is not recommended for children.
✚ warning: flecainide acetate should not be administered to patients who suffer from heart disease. Special care must be taken with patients who are pregnant, who use a pacemaker device, or who suffer from impaired kidney function.
▲ side-effects: there may be dizziness and visual disturbances; rarely, there is nausea and vomiting.
Related article: TAMBOCOR.

Fletcher's Arachis Oil (*Pharmax*) is a proprietary non- prescription form of enema, designed to soften and lubricate impacted faeces within the rectum. It comprises a preparation of ARACHIS OIL that should be warmed before use.

Fletcher's Enemette (*Pharmax*) is a proprietary non-prescription form of enema, designed to soften and lubricate impacted faeces within the rectum. Commonly used before and after childbirth, and prior to rectal surgery or examination, it comprises a preparation of DIOCTYL SODIUM SULPHOSUCCINATE (docusate sodium) with GLYCEROL, MACROGOL and SORBIC ACID. It is not recommended for children aged under 3 years.

Fletcher's Magnesium Sulphate (*Pharmax*) is a proprietary non-prescription form of enema, used in hospitals for rapid bowel evacuation to relieve pressure on a patient's cerebrospinal fluid before or during neurosurgery. It comprises an aqueous preparation of MAGNESIUM SULPHATE.

Fletcher's Phosphate (*Pharmax*) is a proprietary non-prescription form of enema, commonly used before and after childbirth, and prior to rectal surgery or examination. It comprises an aqueous preparation of sodium and phosphates, and should not be administered to patients who have increased absorptive capacity in the colon.

Flexical (*Mead Johnson*) is a proprietary, non-prescription, gluten-free powder (for reconstitution) that represents a complete nutritional diet for patients who are severely undernourished (such as with anorexia nervosa) or who are suffering from some problem with the absorption of food (such as following gastrectomy). Also lactose-free, Flexical contains protein, carbohydrate, fats, vitamins and minerals; it is not suitable for children aged under 12 months, and should not constitute the sole source of nourishment for children of any age.

Flolan (*Wellcome*) is a proprietary form of the ANTICOAGULANT epoprostenol (or prostacyclin)

used to prevent blood thickening during or following cardiac surgery. It can also be used as an alternative to HEPARIN in kidney dialysis. Available only on prescription, Flolan is produced in the form of powder for reconstitution in a diluent as a medium for infusion.
✚/▲ warning/side-effects: *see* EPOPROSTENOL.

Florinef (*Squibb*) is a proprietary form of the hormonal substance fludrocortisone acetate, available only on prescription. A mineralocorticoid, it is used to make up a body deficiency in mineralocorticoids (which are essential for the balance of salt and water in the body) resulting from a malfunctioning of the adrenal glands. Florinef is produced in the form of tablets.
✚/▲ warning/side-effects: *see* FLUDROCORTISONE ACETATE.

Floxapen (*Beecham*) is a proprietary ANTIBIOTIC, available only on prescription, used to treat bacterial infections of the skin and of the ear, nose and throat, and especially staphylococcal infections that prove to be resistant to penicillin. Produced in the form of capsules (in two strengths), syrup for dilution (in two strengths; the potency of the dilute syrup is retained for 14 days) and as a powder for reconstitution as injections, Floxapen's active constituent in each case is flucloxacillin or one of its salts.
✚/▲ warning/side-effects: *see* FLUCLOXACILLIN.

Flu-Amp (*Generics*) is a proprietary compound ANTIBIOTIC, available only on prescription, used to treat bacterial infections particularly of the urinary tract, the middle ear and the upper respiratory tract. Produced in the form of capsules, Flu-Amp contains the penicillin-like drug ampicillin together with the antibiotic flucloxacillin (which can treat infections that prove to be resistant to penicillin).
✚/▲ warning/side-effects: *see* AMPICILLIN; FLUCLOXACILLIN.

Fluanxol (*Lundbeck*) is a proprietary ANTIDEPRESSANT, available only on prescription, used to treat depressive illness. Produced in the form of tablets (in two strengths), it represents a preparation of flupenthixol, and is not recommended for children.
✚/▲ warning/side-effects: *see* FLUPENTHIXOL.

fluclorolone acetonide is a powerful CORTICOSTEROID drug, used in very mild solution to treat severe non-infective inflammations of the skin, particularly eczema that is unresponsive to less powerful drugs, and psoriasis. Administration is as a cream or ointment for topical use.
✚ warning: like all topical corticosteroids, fluclorolone acetonide treats symptoms and does not cure underlying disorders.
▲ side-effects: side-effects depend to some extent on the area of the skin treated. If infection is present, it may spread although the symptoms may not be experienced by the patient. Prolonged treatment may cause thinning of the skin, yet increase hair growth; dermatitis or acne may present. These side-effects may be worse in children.
Related article: TOPILAR.

flucloxacillin is a proprietary ANTIBIOTIC used to treat bacterial infections of the skin and of the ear, nose and throat, and especially staphylococcal infections that prove to be resistant to penicillin. Administration is in the form of capsules, dilute syrup and injection.

✚ warning: flucloxacillin should not be administered to patients who have a history of allergy to antibiotic substances, or who suffer from impairment of kidney function.

▲ side-effects: there may be sensitivity reactions, including high temperature; in some patients there is diarrhoea.
Related articles: FLOXAPEN; LADROPEN; STAFOXIL; STAPHCIL.

flucytosine is a synthesized ANTIFUNGAL drug used to treat systemic infections by yeasts – infections such as candidiasis (or thrush). Administration is oral or by intravenous infusion.

✚ warning: flucytosine should be administered only with caution to patients who suffer from impaired function of the kidneys or liver, or from blood disorders; or who are pregnant or lactating. During treatment there should be regular blood counts and liver-function tests.

▲ side-effects: there may be diarrhoea, with nausea and vomiting; rashes may occur. Proportions of various blood cells may decrease.
Related article: ALCOBON.

fludrocortisone acetate is a hormonal substance, a mineralocorticoid used to make up a body deficiency of mineralocorticoids (which are essential to the balance of salt and water in the body) resulting from a malfunctioning of the adrenal glands.

✚ warning: side-effects with fludrocortisone are more marked than with some other mineralocorticoids; in combination with glucocorticoids (the other type of corticosteroids), however, effects are minimal.

▲ side-effects: there may be high blood pressure, sodium and water retention, and potassium deficiency; there may also be muscular weakness.
Related article: FLORINEF.

flunisolide is an ANTI-ALLERGIC drug used to combat hay fever and other forms of nasal allergy. Administration is by nasal spray. It is not recommended for children.

✚ warning: as a CORTICOSTEROID, flunisolide treats only the symptoms and does not treat any underlying disorder. Initially undetected infection may thus spread, its symptoms suppressed by the drug. Prolonged use should be avoided.

▲ side-effects: sneezing may occur immediately after administration.
Related article: SYNTARIS.

flunitrazepam is a BENZODIAZEPINE drug used as a HYPNOTIC to treat insomnia in cases where some degree of sedation during the daytime is acceptable. Doses may have residual effects that make the overall treatment cumulative. Administration is oral, in the form of tablets.

✚ warning: there may be a hangover following prolonged use; abrupt withdrawal is thus to be avoided. Patients should not drink alcohol. Dosage should be reduced for the elderly and the debilitated. Flunitrazepam should be administered with caution to patients who have kidney or liver damage; or who are pregnant or lactating.

▲ side-effects: there may be drowsiness and dry mouth. Hypersensitivity reactions sometimes occur. Prolonged use may result in tolerance and eventual dependence (addiction).
Related article: ROHYPNOL.

fluocinolone acetonide is a powerful CORTICOSTEROID drug, used in very dilute solution to treat severe non-infective inflammations of the skin. Administration is as a cream, gel, or ointment for topical use.
✚ warning: like all topical corticosteroids, fluocinolone acetonide treats symptoms and does not cure underlying disorders.
▲ side-effects: side-effects depend to some extent on the area of the skin treated. If infection is present, it may spread although the symptoms may not be experienced by the patient. Prolonged treatment may cause thinning of the skin, yet increase hair growth; dermatitis or acne may present. These side-effects may be worse in children.
Related article: SYNALAR.

fluocinonide is a powerful CORTICOSTEROID drug, used in very dilute solution to treat severe non-infective inflammations of the skin, particularly eczema that is unresponsive to less powerful drugs, and some allergic skin conditions. Administration is as a cream or ointment for topical use.
✚ warning: like all topical corticosteroids, fluocinonide treats symptoms and does not cure underlying disorders.
▲ side-effects: side-effects depend to some extent on the area of the skin treated. If infection is present, it may spread although the symptoms may not be experienced by the patient. Prolonged treatment may cause thinning of the skin, yet increase hair growth; dermatitis or acne may present. These side-effects may be worse in children.
Related article: METOSYN.

fluocortolone is a powerful CORTICOSTEROID drug, used in very dilute solution to treat severe non-infective inflammations of the skin, particularly eczema that is unresponsive to less powerful drugs. Administration is as a cream or ointment for topical use.
✚ warning: like all topical corticosteroids, fluocortolone treats symptoms and does not cure underlying disorders.
▲ side-effects: side-effects depend to some extent on the area of the skin treated. If infection is present, it may spread although the symptoms may not be experienced by the patient. Prolonged treatment may cause thinning of the skin, yet increase hair growth; dermatitis or acne may present. These side-effects may be worse in children.
Related articles: ULTRADIL; ULTRALANUM.

Fluor-a-day Lac (*Dental Health Promotion*) is a proprietary non-prescription form of fluoride supplement for administration in areas where the water supply is not fluoridated, especially to growing children. Produced in the form of tablets to be dissolved in the mouth, Fluor-a-day Lac's active constituent is SODIUM FLUORIDE.

fluorescein sodium is a proprietary diagnostic medium, a water-soluble dye used to distinguish foreign bodies or injured areas in the surface of an

eyeball. Alternatively, it may be injected into a retinal vein to check the retinal circulation. When light is shone on the dye, it shows up a brilliant green.
Related articles: MINIMS FLUORESCEIN SODIUM; OPULETS.

Fluorigard (*Hoyt*) is a proprietary non-prescription form of fluoride supplement for administration in areas where the water supply is not fluoridated, especially to growing children. Produced in the form of tablets to be dissolved in the mouth (in two strengths, and in assorted flavours and colours), as drops, and as a mouth wash, Fluorigard's active constituent is SODIUM FLUORIDE.

fluorometholone is a CORTICOSTEROID drug used primarily in the treatment of local eye inflammations in cases where the inflammation is not caused by infection. Administration is as eye-drops.
✚ warning: as with all corticosteroids, flurorometholone treats only the symptoms and does not treat any underlying disorder. An undetected or misdiagnosed infection may thus get worse although the symptoms may be suppressed.
▲ side-effects: very rarely, and following weeks of treatment, there may be an acute, temporary form of glaucoma in certain patients who are predisposed to it.
Related articles: FML; FML-NEO.

fluorouracil is an ANTICANCER drug used primarily to treat gastrointestinal cancers or malignant skin lesions, or in combination with other drugs to treat breast cancer. Administration is oral in the form of capsules, by injection, or as a cream.
✚ warning: as with all CYTOTOXIC drugs, fluorouracil causes depression of the bone-marrow's function of providing red blood cells; anaemia and some loss of immunity may result. There should be regular blood counts.
▲ side-effects: gastric upsets with nausea and vomiting are common; there may also be hair loss (even to total baldness).
Related articles: EFUDIX; FLUORO-URACIL.

Fluoro-uracil (*Roche*) is a proprietary ANTICANCER drug, available only on prescription, used primarily to treat gastrointestinal cancers or malignant skin lesions, or in combination with other drugs to treat breast cancer. Produced in the form of capsules or in ampoules for injection, Fluoro-uracil represents a preparation of the cytotoxic drug fluorouracil.
✚/▲ warning/side-effects: *see* FLUOROURACIL.

flupenthixol is a powerful ANTIDEPRESSANT drug used (mainly in the form of its salts) to treat and soothe depressive illness, psychosis (such as schizophrenia), and severe anxiety.
✚ warning: flupenthixol should not be administered to patients who are excitable or overactive, and should be administered only with extreme caution to patients who suffer from heart, vascular, kidney, or liver disease, or parkinsonism, and who are pregnant or lactating. Dosage should be reduced for the elderly; it is not suitable for children.
▲ side-effects: there may be

insomnia with restlessness. *Related articles:* DEPIXOL; DEPIXOL CONC.; FLUANXOL.

fluphenazine is a powerful ANTIPSYCHOTIC drug used (mainly in the form of its salts) to treat and tranquillize psychosis (such as schizophrenia), and to relieve severe anxiety in the short term.

✚ warning: fluphenazine should be administered only with extreme caution to patients who suffer from heart or vascular disease, from kidney or liver disease, from parkinsonism, or from depression; or who are pregnant or lactating. Dosage should be reduced for the elderly; it is not suitable for children.

▲ side-effects: there may be drowsiness, pallor and hypothermia, insomnia, depression and, sometimes, restlessness and nightmares. Rashes and jaundice may occur, and there may be dry mouth, constipation, difficulty in urination, and blurred vision. The heart rate may be raised or lowered on administration by injection. *Related articles:* MODECATE; MODITEN.

flurandrenolone is a powerful CORTICOSTEROID drug, used in very dilute solution to treat severe non-infective inflammations of the skin, particularly eczema that is unresponsive to less powerful drugs. Administration is as a cream or ointment for topical use. One proprietary form combines it with an antibacterial, antifungal agent.

✚ warning: like all topical corticosteroids, flurandrenolone by itself treats symptoms and does not cure underlying disorders.

▲ side-effects: side-effects depend to some extent on the area of the skin treated. If infection is present, it may spread although the symptoms may not be experienced by the patient. Prolonged treatment may cause thinning of the skin, yet increase hair growth; dermatitis or acne may present. These side-effects may be worse in children. *Related article:* HAELAN.

flurazepam is a BENZODIAZEPINE drug used as a HYPNOTIC to treat insomnia in cases where some degree of sedation during the daytime is acceptable. Doses may have residual effects that make the overall treatment cumulative. Administration is oral, in the form of capsules.

✚ warning: there may be a hangover following prolonged use; abrupt withdrawal is thus to be avoided. Patients should not drink alcohol. Dosage should be reduced for the elderly and the debilitated. Flurazepam should be administered with caution to patients who have kidney or liver damage; or who are pregnant or lactating; or who have obstructive lung disease or respiratory depression.

▲ side-effects: there may be drowsiness and dry mouth. Hypersensitivity reactions sometimes occur. Prolonged use may result in tolerance and eventual dependence (addiction). *Related article:* DALMANE.

flurbiprofen is a non-steroidal ANTI-INFLAMMATORY non-narcotic ANALGESIC with effects similar to those of aspirin. It is used particularly in the treatment of pain from rheumatoid arthritis and osteoarthritis, or from ankylosing spondylitis. It is not

recommended for children.
✚ warning: flurbiprofen should not be administered to patients who are suffering from gastric or intestinal bleeding (as with a peptic ulcer); who are pregnant or lactating; who are allergic to aspirin or other anti-inflammatory drugs; who have reduced kidney function; who are asthmatic; or who are already taking aspirin, an anticoagulant or a drug to control the blood level of glucose.
▲ side-effects: there may be a skin rash; rarely, there is an allergic response or gastrointestinal bleeding.
Related article: FROBEN.

fluspirilene is a powerful ANTIPSYCHOTIC drug used to treat and tranquillize psychosis (such as schizophrenia).
✚ warning: fluspirilene should be administered only with extreme caution to patients who suffer from heart or vascular disease, from kidney or liver disease, from parkinsonism, from epilepsy, or from depression; or who are pregnant or lactating. Dosage should be reduced for the elderly; it is not suitable for children.
▲ side-effects: there may be drowsiness, pallor and hypothermia, insomnia, depression and, frequently, restlessness and sweating. Rashes and jaundice may occur, and there may be dry mouth, constipation, difficulty in urination, and blurred vision. Prolonged usage may cause tissue damage (in the form of nodules) at the site of injection.
Related article: REDEPTIN.

Fluvirin (*Evans*) is the name of a series of proprietary flu VACCINES, all comprising inactivated surface antigens of different strains of the influenza virus. None is recommended for children aged under 4 years.
✚ warning: like any flu vaccine, Fluvirin cannot control epidemics and should be used only – in what seems to be the appropriate strain – on people who are at high risk: the elderly, patients with cardiovascular problems, and medical staff. Fluvirin should not be administered to patients who are allergic to egg or chicken protein (in which vaccine viruses are cultured), or who are pregnant.
▲ side-effects: rarely, there is local reaction together with headache and high temperature.

FML (*Allergan*) is a proprietary form of ANTI-INFLAMMATORY eye-drops, available only on prescription, used in cases where the inflammation is not caused by infection. The active constituent of FML is the CORTICOSTEROID fluorometholone.
✚/▲ warning/side-effects: *see* FLUOROMETHOLONE.

FML-Neo (*Allergan*) is a proprietary form of ANTIBIOTIC eye-drops, available only on prescription, used in cases where the inflammation is not caused by infection. The active constituents of FML are the CORTICOSTEROID fluorometholone and the aminoglycoside antibiotic neomycin.
✚/▲ warning/side-effects: *see* FLUOROMETHOLONE; NEOMYCIN.

Folex-350 (*Rybar*) is a proprietary non-prescription mineral-and-VITAMIN compound used primarily as an IRON supplement

prophylactically during pregnancy. Produced in the form of tablets, Folex-350 represents a preparation of ferrous fumarate together with FOLIC ACID (a vitamin of the B complex). It is not recommended for children, and should not be taken simultaneously with tetracycline antibiotics.
✚/▲ warning/side-effects: *see* FERROUS FUMARATE.

folic acid is a VITAMIN of the B complex – also known as pteroylglutamic acid – important in the synthesis of nucleic acids (DNA and RNA). Its importance is parallel with that of CYANOCOBALAMIN (vitamin B_{12}), for both are linked to the processes of cell division. Food sources of folic acid include liver and vegetables; consumption is particularly necessary during pregnancy. Deficiency leads to a form of anaemia, which is usually rapidly remedied by a compensatory injection, although treatment (including supplements of cyanocobalamin) should continue for some months to replenish body stores.
✚ warning: treatment with folic acid generally also indicates parallel treatment with cyanocobalamin (vitamin B_{12}); one without the other may cause various forms of anaemia, and even lead to degeneration of the spinal cord. Folic acid should not be administered to those with malignant disease unless certain forms of anaemia are an important complication.
Related articles: FE-CAP FOLIC; FEFOL; FERROCAP-F 350; FERROCONTIN FOLIC CONTINUS; FERROGRAD FOLIC; FOLEX-350; GALFER F.A.; KELFOLATE; PREGADAY; SLOW-FEFOLIC.

Folicin (*Paines & Byrne*) is a proprietary mineral-and-VITAMIN compound, available only on prescription, used primarily as an IRON supplement during pregnancy. In addition to iron (in the form of dried ferrous sulphate), Folicin contains FOLIC ACID (a vitamin of the B complex), COPPER SULPHATE and MANGANESE SULPHATE. It is not recommended for children, and should not be taken simultaneously with tetracycline antibiotics.
✚/▲ warning/side-effects: *see* FERROUS SULPHATE.

folinic acid is a derivative of FOLIC ACID (a VITAMIN of the B complex), and is used therapeutically to suppress the toxic effects of certain ANTICANCER drugs, especially METHOTREXATE, and to treat some forms of anaemia. Administration is oral in the form of tablets, or by injection or infusion.
✚ warning: treatment with folinic acid may, just as treatment with folic acid, require complementary treatment with CYANOCOBALAMIN (vitamin B_{12}) in order to avoid further deficiency disorders.
Related articles: CALCIUM LEUCOVORIN; RESCUFOLIN.

Forane (*Abbott*) is a proprietary preparation of the general ANAESTHETIC isoflurane, produced as a gas to be used in solution with oxygen or nitrous oxide-oxygen. It is available on prescription only.
✚/▲ warning/side-effects: *see* ISOFLURANE.

Forceval (*Unigreg*) is a proprietary non-prescription mineral-and-VITAMIN compound that is not available from the National Health Service. Used as a supplement to make up body deficiencies, and produced in the form of gelatin capsules in either of two strengths (the weaker one under the trade name Forceval Junior), Forceval contains almost all the vitamins, plus calcium, copper, iodine, phosphorus, potassium and zinc.

Forceval Protein (*Unigreg*) is a proprietary, non-prescription, gluten-free powder (for reconstitution) that represents a complete nutritional diet for patients who are severely undernourished (such as with anorexia nervosa) or who are suffering from some problem with the absorption of food (such as following gastrectomy). Also lactose- and galactose-free, Forceval Protein contains protein, carbohydrate, vitamins and minerals; it is produced in sachets and tins, and in various flavours. Not suitable for children aged under 12 months, it should not constitute the sole source of nourishment for children aged under 5 years.

formaldehyde is a powerful KERATOLYTIC agent, used in mild solution to dissolve away layers of toughened or warty skin, especially in the treatment of verrucas (plantar warts) on the soles of the feet. Treatment of normal skin should be avoided.
✚ warning: effects of treatment are not always predictable. The smell is unpleasantly acrid.
▲ side-effects: formaldehyde solutions may sensitize the skin and become irritant.
Related article: VERACUR.

Formula MCT (1) (*Cow & Gate*) is a proprietary non-prescription powder for reconstitution which is a low-protein high-calorie dietary supplement for patients who suffer from failure of the liver or cystic fibrosis of the pancreas, or following intestinal surgery, when the need is to provide amino acids and protein in a readily available form that does not rely on breakdown by the body. Formula MCT (1) contains triglycerides (fatty acids), protein, carbohydrate, minerals and electrolytes. It does not, however, form a complete diet.

Formula S (*Cow & Gate*) is a proprietary, non-prescription, gluten-free powder for reconstitution which is a complete nutritional diet for patients who for one reason or another cannot tolerate cow's milk; it is lactose-free, and also fructose- and sucrose-free. Formula S contains protein, carbohydrate, fats, vitamins and minerals in appropriate ratios when used in 8 times its own volume of water.

Fortagesic (*Sterling Research*) is a proprietary narcotic ANALGESIC, a controlled drug that is not available from the National Health Service. Produced in the form of tablets containing the OPIATE pentazocine together with paracetamol, Fortagesic is not recommended for children.
✚/▲ warning/side-effects: *see* PARACETAMOL; PENTAZOCINE.

Fortical (*Cow & Gate*) is a proprietary, non-prescription, gluten-free liquid that is not available from the National Health Service, which is a carbohydrate-based supplement for patients with kidney failure, liver cirrhosis, or any other condition that requires a high-calorie, low-electrolyte diet requiring minimum absorption. It is available in six flavours.

F

Fortisip (*Cow & Gate*) is a bland, proprietary, non-prescription, gluten-free liquid that is a complete nutritional diet for patients who are severely undernourished (such as with anorexia nervosa) or who are suffering from some problem with the absorption of food, such as following gastrectomy. Produced in two strengths, Fortisip contains protein, carbohydrate, fats, minerals and vitamins; as the slightly stronger Fortisip Energy Plus, the liquid is produced in three flavours. Neither form is suitable for children aged under 12 months.

Fortison (*Cow & Gate*) is a bland, proprietary, non-prescription, gluten-free liquid that is a complete nutritional diet for patients who are severely undernourished (such as with anorexia nervosa) or who are suffering from some problem with the absorption of food, such as following gastrectomy. Produced in two strengths (Standard, and Energy Plus) and with a choice of protein types, Fortison contains protein, carbohydrate, fats, minerals and vitamins. It is not suitable for children aged under 12 months.

Fortral (*Sterling Research*) is a proprietary narcotic ANALGESIC, a controlled drug that is not available from the National Health Service. Produced in the form of tablets, capsules, ampoules for injection, and anal suppositories, its active constituent is the OPIATE pentazocine. Fortral suppositories are not recommended for children; as tablets and capsules Fortral is not recommended for children aged under 6 years; and as injections Fortral is not recommended for children aged under 12 months.

✚/▲ warning/side-effects: *see* PENTAZOCINE.

Fortum (*Glaxo*) is a proprietary broad-spectrum ANTIBIOTIC, available only on prescription, used to treat bacterial infections, particularly infections of the respiratory tract, the ear, nose or throat, the skin, bones and joints, and more serious infections such as septicaemia and meningitis. Produced in the form of powder for reconstitution as a medium for injection or infusion, Fortum is a preparation of the CEPHALOSPORIN ceftazidime.

✚/▲ warning/side-effects: *see* CEFTAZIDIME.

Fortunan (*Allen & Hanburys*) is a powerful proprietary ANTIPSYCHOTIC drug, available only on prescription, used as a major TRANQUILLIZER to treat patients with behavioural disturbances, or who are psychotic, particularly schizophrenic. More mundanely, it may be used in the short term to treat severe anxiety. Produced in the form of tablets (in five strengths), Fortunan is a preparation of haloperidol.

✚/▲ warning/side-effects: *see* HALOPERIDOL.

fosfestrol tetrasodium is a drug that is converted in the body to the OESTROGEN (female sex HORMONE) STILBOESTROL. It may be used as part of hormone replacement therapy for menopausal women, to treat menstrual difficulties, or be used in men to treat cancer of the prostate gland.

✚ warning: fosfestrol tetrasodium should not be administered to patients who are pregnant, diabetic or epileptic, or who have heart or kidney disease. In men, fosfestrol tetrasodium has a marked feminizing effect, resulting in impotence.

▲ side-effects: there may be fluid retention in the tissues (oedema), high blood pressure (hypertension), a high level of calcium in the bloodstream, and gastrointestinal upsets with nausea and vomiting. There is a greatly increased risk of thrombosis.

Related article: HONVAN.

Fosfor (*Consolidated Chemicals*) is a proprietary nutritional supplement consisting of a phosphoryl compound. It is produced in the form of a syrup (non-prescription, but not available from the National Health Service) and in ampoules for injection (prescription only) or infusion in solution.

framycetin is a relatively toxic aminoglycoside ANTIBIOTIC, used to treat external bacterial infections, or to reduce the quantity of bacteria in the intestines before intestinal surgery. Preparations of framycetin most commonly involve its sulphate form.

✚ warning: oral administration may cause malabsorption of nutrients; application to large areas of the skin may damage the organs of the ears. Framycetin should not be administered to patients who are pregnant, or to those with myasthenia gravis.

▲ side-effects: hypersensitive reactions may occur; there may be temporary kidney malfunction.

Related articles: FRAMYCORT; FRAMYGEN; SOFRADEX; SOFRAMYCIN.

Framycort (*Fisons*) is a proprietary compound, available only on prescription, combining the ANTIBACTERIAL ANTIBIOTIC framycetin sulphate with the fairly potent steroid hydrocortisone acetate. It is used in the form of an ointment to treat skin infections, particularly on the face or in the urogenital area; as eye-drops to treat bacterial infections such as conjunctivitis; and as ear-drops to treat bacterial infections of the outer ear.

✚/▲ warning/side-effects: *see* FRAMYCETIN; HYDROCORTISONE ACETATE.

Framygen (*Fisons*) is a proprietary ANTIBIOTIC, available only on prescription, used in the form of eye ointment and eye-drops to treat infections on and around the eyes; as ear-drops to treat infections of the outer ear; and as a cream to treat bacterial skin infections. In all versions, its active constituent is the aminoglycoside framycetin sulphate in very mild solution.

✚/▲ warning/side-effects: *see* FRAMYCETIN.

Franol (*Winthrop*) is a proprietary BRONCHODILATOR combined with a SEDATIVE and a SMOOTH MUSCLE RELAXANT, and is on the controlled drugs list. This is because the sedative is a barbiturate – phenobarbitone; the bronchodilator is ephedrine hydrochloride, and the muscle relaxant is theophylline. It is produced in the form of tablets, and may be used to treat asthma and chronic bronchitis.

✚/▲ warning/side-effects: *see* BARBITURATE; EPHEDRINE HYDROCHLORIDE; PHENOBARBITONE; THEOPHYLLINE.

Franol Expect (*Winthrop*) is a proprietary EXPECTORANT that also contains a BRONCHODILATOR (ephedrine), a SMOOTH MUSCLE RELAXANT (theophylline) and a

SEDATIVE (phenobarbitone); it is on the controlled drugs list, and is not available from the National Health Service. Produced in the form of a linctus, Franol Expect may be used to treat bronchial asthma, chronic bronchitis, and influenza.
✚/▲ warning/side-effects: *see* EPHEDRINE HYDROCHLORIDE; PHENOBARBITONE; THEOPHYLLINE.

Franol Plus (*Winthrop*) is a proprietary BRONCHODILATOR combined with a SEDATIVE, a SMOOTH MUSCLE RELAXANT and an ANTIHISTAMINE, and is on the controlled drugs list. This is because the sedative is a barbiturate – phenobarbitone; the bronchodilator is ephedrine hydrochloride, and the muscle relaxant is theophylline. It is produced in the form of tablets, and is used to treat asthma and chronic bronchitis.
✚/▲ warning/side-effects: *see* BARBITURATE; EPHEDRINE HYDROCHLORIDE; PHENOBARBITONE; THEOPHYLLINE.

FreAmine II (*Boots*) is a proprietary form of high-calorie nutritional supplement intended for injection or infusion, available only on prescription. Produced in two strengths, it contains amino acids, nitrogen, phosphate and electrolytes.

FreAmine III (*Boots*) is a proprietary form of high-calorie nutritional supplement intended for injection or infusion, available only on prescription. Produced in two strengths, it contains amino acids, nitrogen, phosphate and electrolytes.

Fresubin (*Fresenius Dylade*) is a bland, proprietary, non-prescription, gluten-free liquid that is a complete nutritional diet for patients who are severely undernourished, such as with anorexia nervosa, or who are suffering from some problem with the absorption of food, such as following gastrectomy. Produced in four flavours and three sizes, Fresubin contains protein, carbohydrate, fats, minerals and vitamins. It is not suitable for children aged under 12 months.

Frisium (*Hoechst*) is a proprietary form of the BENZODIAZEPINE clobazam, used primarily as an ANXIOLYTIC to treat anxiety, nervous tension and restlessness. It may also be used to assist in the treatment of epilepsy. Available on prescription only to private patients, Frisium is produced in the form of capsules. It is not recommended for children aged under 3 years.
✚/▲ warning/side-effects: *see* CLOBAZAM.

Froben (*Boots*) is a proprietary, non-steroid, non-narcotic ANALGESIC available only on prescription, used to relieve pain – particularly arthritic and rheumatic pain - and to treat other musculo-skeletal disorders. Its active constituent is flurbiprofen, and it is produced in the form of tablets and as anal suppositories. Not recommended for children, Froben should not be administered to patients with a peptic ulcer or gastrointestinal bleeding; special care is necessary in the treatment of patients who are pregnant or lactating; whose kidneys are not fully functional; or who have asthma.
✚/▲ warning/side-effects: *see* FLURBIPROFEN.

fructose is a simple sugar which with glucose together makes up the carbohydrate sucrose – the usual form of sugar, found in cane sugar and sugar-beet. By itself, fructose is a constituent in honey and in certain fruits (such as figs), and as part of a normal diet is used to create energy in the body through glycolysis in the liver. This is significant particularly for diabetics, for fructose does not require insulin for metabolism – unlike glucose. Fructose is accordingly available, without prescription, for patients who suffer from glucose or galactose intolerance.

Frumil (*Berk*) is a proprietary compound DIURETIC, available only on prescription, used to treat accumulation of fluids within the tissues (oedema) due to heart, kidney or liver disease. Produced in the form of tablets, Frumil combines the potassium-sparing diuretic amiloride hydrochloride with the powerful diuretic frusemide. It is not recommended for children.
✚/▲ warning/side-effects: *see* AMILORIDE; FRUSEMIDE.

frusemide is a powerful DIURETIC which works by inhibiting resorption in part of the kidney known as the loop of Henle. It is used to treat fluid retention in the tissues (oedema) and high blood pressure (*see* ANTIHYPERTENSIVE), and to assist a failing kidney. Administration is oral in the form of tablets, or by injection or infusion.
✚ warning: frusemide should not be administered to patients with kidney damage or who are pregnant, who have gout, diabetes, an enlarged prostate gland, or cirrhosis of the liver. Treatment may cause a deficiency of potassium and sodium in the bloodstream (hypokalaemia, hyponatraemia).
▲ side-effects: the diuretic effect corresponds to dosage; large doses may cause deafness or ringing in the ears (tinnitus). There may be skin rashes.
Related articles: DIUMIDE-K CONTINUS; DIURESAL; FRUMIL; FRUSENE; FRUSETIC; FRUSID; LASIKAL; LASILACTONE; LASIPRESSIN.

Frusene (*Radiol*) is a proprietary compound DIURETIC, available only on prescription, used to treat accumulation of fluids within the tissues (oedema) due to heart or liver disease. Produced in the form of tablets, Frusene combines the potassium-sparing diuretic triamterine with the powerful diuretic frusemide. It is not recommended for children.
✚/▲ warning/side-effects: *see* FRUSEMIDE; TRIAMTERINE.

Frusetic (*Unimed*) is a proprietary DIURETIC, available only on prescription, used to treat accumulation of fluids within the tissues (oedema) due to heart or liver disease. Produced in the form of tablets, Frusetic is a preparation of the powerful diuretic frusemide. It is not recommended for children.
✚/▲ warning/side-effects: *see* FRUSEMIDE.

Frusid (*DDSA Pharmaceuticals*) is a proprietary DIURETIC, available only on prescription, used to treat accumulation of fluids within the tissues (oedema) due to heart or liver disease. Produced in the form of tablets, Frusid is a preparation of the powerful diuretic frusemide. It is not recommended for children.
✚/▲ warning/side-effects: *see* FRUSEMIDE.

FSH is an abbreviation for follicle-stimulating hormone, a HORMONE secreted by the anterior pituitary gland that in women

F

causes the monthly ripening in one ovary of a follicle and stimulates ovulation, and that in men stimulates the production of sperm in the testes. It may be injected therapeutically to make up for a deficiency in the natural hormone, as long as careful biochemical monitoring ensues thereafter.

✚ warning: FSH should be administered to women with care in order to avoid over-stimulation of an ovary which might lead to multiple pregnancy or enlargement and possible rupture. Dosage depends on individual response.

▲ side-effects: there may be local sensitivity reactions.

Related articles: GONADOTROPHIN FSH; METRODIN; PERGONAL.

Fucibet (*Leo*) is a proprietary compound, available only on prescription, combining the potent steroid betamethasone with the ANTIBIOTIC fusidic acid. It is used to treat eczema in which bacterial infection is deemed to be present, and is produced in the form of a cream.

✚/▲ warning/side-effects: *see* BETAMETHASONE; FUSIDIC ACID.

Fucidin (*Leo*) is a proprietary narrow-spectrum ANTIBIOTIC, available only on prescription, used mainly against staphylococcal infections – especially skin infections and abscesses – that prove to be resistant to penicillin. It is produced in many forms: as tablets, as a suspension, as powder for reconstitution as a medium for infusion, as a gel (with or without a special applicator), as a cream, and as an ointment, all for use as indicated by the location of the infection, and all containing as their active constituent either fusidic acid or one of its salts (particularly sodium fusidate).

✚/▲ warning/side-effects: *see* FUSIDIC ACID.

Fucidin H (*Leo*) is a proprietary compound, available only on prescription, combining the ANTIBIOTIC sodium fusidate with the steroid hydrocortisone, and used to treat local skin inflammation deemed to be caused by bacterial infection. It is produced in the form of an ointment, a cream or a gel.

✚/▲ warning/side-effects: *see* FUSIDIC ACID; HYDROCORTISONE.

Fulcin (*ICI*) is a proprietary ANTIFUNGAL ANTIBIOTIC drug, available only on prescription, used to treat fungal infections of the scalp, skin and nails. Produced in the form of tablets (in two strengths) and as a suspension, Fulcin is a preparation of the drug griseofulvin. Treatment may be required to continue over several weeks.

✚/▲ warning/side-effects: *see* GRISEOFULVIN.

fungicidal drugs act to destroy fungal infection, and are also known as an antimycotic or antifungal drugs.
see ANTIFUNGAL drug.

Fungilin (*Squibb*) is a proprietary form of the powerful, but fairly toxic, ANTIFUNGAL ANTIBIOTIC drug amphotericin. Available only on prescription, Fungilin is produced in the form of tablets and as a suspension, as lozenges, as an ointment and as a cream, and used in the appropriate form to treat systemic fungal infections, infections of the urogenital areas (especially

candidiasis, or thrush), and infections of the mouth and nose.
✚/▲ warning/side-effects: *see* AMPHOTERICIN.

Fungizone (*Squibb*) is a proprietary form of the powerful, but fairly toxic, ANTIFUNGAL ANTIOBIOTIC drug amphotericin combined with a sodium salt. Available only on prescription, Fungizone is produced in the form of powder for reconstitution as a medium for intravenous infusion, and used to treat systemic fungal infections.
✚/▲ warning/side-effects: *see* AMPHOTERICIN.

Furacin (*Norwich Eaton*) is a proprietary form of ANTIBACTERIAL ointment in a water-miscible base, available only on prescription, used particularly to treat wounds, burns, ulcers and superficial skin infections. Its active constituent is nitrofurazone.
✚/▲ warning/side-effects: *see* NITROFURAZONE.

Furadantin (*Norwich Eaton*) is a proprietary ANTIMICROBIAL drug, available only on prescription, used to treat infections of the urinary tract. It is produced in the form of tablets (in two strengths) and as a suspension, the active constituent of which is nitrofurantoin.
✚/▲ warning/side-effects: *see* NITROFURANTOIN.

Furamide (*Boots*) is a proprietary form of the AMOEBICIDAL drug diloxanide furoate, available only on prescription, used to treat chronic infection by the organism Entamoeba histolytica where cysts are discernible in the faeces. It is produced in the form of tablets.
✚/▲ warning/side-effects: *see* DILOXANIDE FUROATE.

fusidic acid and its salts are narrow-spectrum ANTIBIOTICS used to treat staphylococcal infections – particularly infections of the skin or of bone – that prove to be resistant to penicillin.
✚ warning: treatment by infusion may require periodic testing of the patients liver function. Keep fusidic acid ointment, cream and gel away from the eyes.
▲ side-effects: local hypersensitivity reactions may occur; rarely, there may be gastric upset, jaundice, and a reversible change in liver function.
Related articles: FUCIBET; FUCIDIN; FUCIDIN H.

Fybogel (*Reckitt & Colman*) is a proprietary form of the type of LAXATIVE known as a bulking agent, which works by increasing the overall mass of faeces within the rectum, so stimulating bowel movement. It is used also to soothe the effects of diverticular disease and irritable colon. In the case of Fybogel, the agent involved is ispaghula husk, presented in the form of effervescent grains in sachets for swallowing with water.
✚/▲ warning/side-effects: *see* ISPAGHULA HUSK.

Fybranta (*Norgine*) is a proprietary form of the type of LAXATIVE known as a bulking agent, which works by increasing the overall mass of faeces within the rectum, so stimulating bowel movement. It is used also to soothe the effects of diverticular disease and irritable colon. In the case of Fybranta, the agent involved is bran, presented in the form of tablets to be chewed and swallowed.
✚/▲ warning/side-effects: *see* BRAN.

Galactomin (*Cow & Gate*) is the name of a proprietary series of powdered formulas representing nutritional supplements for patients whose metabolisms cannot tolerate certain sugars. They contain proteins, fats, carbohydrates, minerals and vitamins but are galactose-free. In the three preparations available (Formulas 17, 18 and 19), Formula 18 may be regarded as standard; Formula 17 has a higher fat content; and Formula 19 has fructose as its carbohydrate.

Galcodine (*Galen*) is a proprietary ANTITUSSIVE, available only on prescription, used to encourage the loosening of a dry, painful cough. Produced in the form of an orange-flavoured sugar-free linctus (in two strengths, the weaker under the name Galcodine Paediatric) for dilution (the potency of the dilute linctus is retained for 14 days), galcodine is a preparation of the OPIATE codeine phosphate. It is not recommended for children aged under 12 months.
✚/▲ warning/side-effects: *see* CODEINE PHOSPHATE.

Galenomycin (*Galen*) is a proprietary ANTIBIOTIC, available only on prescription, used to treat infections of the soft tissues and the repiratory tract. Produced in the form of tablets, Galenomycin is a preparation of the TETRACYCLINE oxytetracycline dihydrate. It is not recommended for children.
✚/▲ warning/side-effects: *see* OXYTETRACYCLINE.

Galenphol (*Galen*) is a proprietary COUGH SUPPRESSANT, available only on prescription, used to encourage the loosening of a dry, painful cough. Produced in the form of an aniseed-flavoured sugar-free linctus (in three strengths, the weakest under the name Galenphol Linctus Paediatric, the strongest under the name Galenphol Linctus Strong) for dilution (the potency of the dilute linctus is retained for 14 days), Galenphol is a preparation of the OPIATE pholcodine.
✚/▲ warning/side-effects: *see* PHOLCODINE.

Galfer (*Galen*) is a proprietary non-prescription IRON supplement, used particularly to treat certain forms of anaemia. Produced in the form of capsules, Galfer is a preparation of ferrous fumarate.
✚/▲ warning/side-effects: *see* FERROUS FUMARATE.

Galfer F.A. (*Galen*) is a proprietary non-prescription IRON-and-VITAMIN supplement, used particularly to prevent iron deficiency or vitamin B deficiency (as sometimes occurs during pregnancy). Produced in the form of capsules, Galfer F.A. is a compound of ferrous fumarate and folic acid.
✚/▲ warning/side-effects: *see* FERROUS FUMARATE; FOLIC ACID.

Galfervit (*Galen*) is a proprietary IRON-and-VITAMIN supplement that is not available from the National Health Service. It is used to treat certain forms of anaemia in which there is simultaneous vitamin deficiency. Produced in the form of capsules, Galfervit is a compound of various forms of vitamin B (THIAMINE, RIBOFLAVINE, PYRIDOXINE and NICOTINAMIDE) and ASCORBIC ACID (vitamin C) with ferrous fumarate.
✚/▲ warning/side-effects: *see* FERROUS FUMARATE.

gallamine triethiodide is a SKELETAL MUSCLE RELAXANT of the type known as competitive or non-depolarizing. It is used during surgical operations to achieve long-duration paralysis. Administration is by injection, but only after the patient has been rendered unconscious.
✚ warning: gallamine triethiodide should not be administered to patients with impaired function of the kidneys. Respiration should be assisted throughout treatment.
▲ side-effects: there may be a precipitate deceleration in the heart rate.
Related article: FLAXEDIL.

Galpseud (*Galen*) is a proprietary non-prescription form of nasal DECONGESTANT administered orally. It is produced as tablets and as an orange-flavoured sugar-free linctus for dilution (the potency of the linctus once dilute is retained for 14 days), and is a preparation of the SYMPATHOMIMETIC ephedrine derivative pseudoephedrine hydrochloride.
✚/▲ warning/side-effects: *see* EPHEDRINE HYDROCHLORIDE.

Gamanil (*Merck*) is a proprietary ANTIDEPRESSANT drug, available only on prescription, used to treat depressive illness and associated symptoms. Produced in the form of tablets, Gamanil represents a preparation of lofepramine hydrochloride. It is not recommended for children.
✚/▲ warning/side-effects: *see* LOFEPRAMINE.

Gamimune-N (*Cutter*) is a proprietary preparation of human normal immunoglobulin (HNIG) as a solution in maltose, used in infusion to confer immediate immunity to such diseases as hepatitis A virus, measles (rubeola) and at least to some degree rubella (German measles), particularly in patients who cannot tolerate the administration of live (though attenuated) viruses in vaccination therapies. Gamimune-N is also used to provide some form of immunity in patients born with immunodeficient conditions. It is available only on prescription, in vials (in three strengths).
✚ warning: *see* HNIG.

Gammabulin (*Immuno*) is a proprietary preparation of human normal immunoglobulin (HNIG) as an aqueous solution, used in infusion to confer immediate immunity to such diseases as hepatitis A virus, measles (rubeola) and at least to some degree rubella (German measles), particularly in patients who cannot tolerate the administration of live (though attenuated) viruses in vaccination therapies. It is available only on prescription, in vials.
✚ warning: *see* HNIG.

Ganda (*Smith & Nephew*) is a proprietary compound of the powerful ANTIHYPERTENSIVE drug guanethidine monosulphate together with the hormone adrenaline, available only on precription, used as eye- drops to treat glaucoma (or occasionally thyrotoxicosis). Both of the drugs contained are effective in relieving intra-ocular pressure, but guanethidine also has the effect of prolonging the action of adrenaline. Ganda drops are produced in four strengths.
✚/▲ warning/side-effects: *see* ADRENALINE; GUANETHIDINE MONOSULPHATE.

Gantrisin (*Roche*) is a proprietary ANTIBACTERIAL drug, available

only on prescription, used primarily to treat infections of the urinary tract, but also to relieve lesser infections of the skin and soft tissues and the respiratory tract, and to treat bacillary dysentery. Produced in the form of tablets and as a syrup, Gantrisin is a preparation of the SULPHONAMIDE sulphafurazole.
✚/▲ warning/side-effects: *see* SULPHAFURAZOLE.

Garamycin (*Kirby-Warrick*) is a proprietary ANTIBIOTIC, available only on prescription, used primarily in the form of drops to treat bacterial infections of the ear or eye, but also in the form of injections for children (under the name Garamycin Paediatric) to treat other bacterial infections, notably those of the urinary tract. In all forms, Garamycin is a preparation of the aminoglycoside gentamicin.
✚/▲ warning/side-effects: *see* GENTAMICIN.

Gardenal sodium (*May & Baker*) is a proprietary form of the ANTICONVULSANT BARBITURATE phenobarbitone, and is on the controlled drugs list. Produced in vials for injection, it is used to treat all forms of epilepsy, although it should be administered with extreme caution to children or the elderly.
✚/▲ warning/side-effects: *see* PHENOBARBITONE.

Gastrils (*Jackson*) is a proprietary non-prescription ANTACID (used for the relief of indigestion and flatulence) that is not available from the National Health Service. Produced in the form of mint- or fruit-flavoured pastilles, Gastrils contain ALUMINIUM HYDROXIDE and magnesium carbonate.
✚/▲ warning/side-effects: *see* MAGNESIUM CARBONATE.

Gastrocote (*MCP Pharmaceuticals*) is a proprietary non-prescription ANTACID (used for the relief of indigestion and flatulence), produced in the form of tablets containing ALUMINIUM HYDROXIDE, SODIUM BICARBONATE and magnesium trisilicate. It is not recommended for children aged under 6 years.
✚ warning: *see* MAGNESIUM TRISILICATE.

Gastron (*Winthrop*) is a proprietary non-prescription ANTACID (used for the relief of indigestion and flatulence), produced in the form of tablets containing ALUMINIUM HYDROXIDE, SODIUM BICARBONATE and magnesium trisilicate. It is not recommended for children.
✚ warning: *see* MAGNESIUM TRISILICATE.

Gastrovite (*MCP Pharmaceuticals*) is a proprietary non- prescription mineral-and-VITAMIN compound that is not available from the National Health Service. The minerals are IRON and CALCIUM, in the form of ferrous glycine sulphate and calcium gluconate, and the vitamins are ASCORBIC ACID (vitamin C) and ERGOCALCIFEROL (vitamin D).
✚/▲ warning/side-effects: *see* CALCIUM GLUCONATE; FERROUS GLYCINE SULPHATE.

Gastrozepin (*Boots*) is a proprietary preparation of the ANTICHOLINERGIC drug pirenzepine, available only on prescription, used to treat gastric and duodenal ulcers. It works by inhibiting the formation and secretion of stomach acids. Produced in the form of tablets, it is not recommended for children.
✚/▲ warning/side-effects: *see* PIRENZEPINE.

Gaviscon (*Reckitt & Colman*) is a proprietary non-prescription ANTACID (used for the relief of indigestion and flatulence), produced in the form of tablets containing alginic acid, ALUMINIUM HYDROXIDE, SODIUM BICARBONATE, magnesium trisilicate and various sugars. There is also a liquid version that contains sodium alginate, sodium bicarbonate and calcium carbonate.
✚ warning: *see* CALCIUM CARBONATE; MAGNESIUM TRISILICATE.

Gee's linctus is a less formal name for the non-proprietary opiate squill cough linctus. *see* OPIATE SQUILL LINCTUS AND PASTILLES.

Gee's pastilles is a less formal name for the non-proprietary opiate squill cough pastilles. *see* OPIATE SQUILL LINCTUS AND PASTILLES.

gelatin is hydrolized animal protein. Therapeutically, gelatin is used as a short-term medium for expanding overall blood volume in patients whose blood volume is dangerously low or whose blood is abnormally liable to clot, as a nutritional supplement in the form of a jelly, and in the form of an absorbent sponge as a HAEMOSTATIC.
✚ warning: gelatin as a medium to expand the blood volume should not be administered to patients with severe congestive heart failure, with disorders of the blood coagulation mechanism, or with severely impaired function of the kidneys.
▲ side-effects: some patients suffer serious hypersensitivity reactions.
Related articles: GELOFUSINE; HAEMACCEL.

Gelcotar (*Quinoderm*) is a proprietary preparation of the ANTISEPTIC COAL TAR, used both to treat skin conditions such as dandruff, dermatitis, eczema and psoriasis, and to remove medicated pastes and dressings following treatment. It is produced in the form of a water-miscible gel (with pine tar) and as a liquid shampoo (with cade oil).

Gelofusine (*Consolidated*) is a proprietary form of gelatin, the hydrolized animal protein. In a special refined (partly degraded) form available only on prescription, it is used in infusion with saline (sodium chloride) as a means of expanding overall blood volume in patients whose blood volume is dangerously low through shock, (particularly in cases of severe burns or septicaemia. It is produced in bottles (flasks) for infusion.
✚/▲ warning/side-effects: *see* GELATIN.

Gelusil (*Warner-Lambert*) is a proprietary non-prescription ANTACID (used for the relief of indigestion and flatulence) that is not available from the National Health Service. It is produced in the form of tablets that can be chewed or sucked, containing ALUMINIUM HYDROXIDE and magnesium trisilicate.
✚ warning: *see* MAGNESIUM TRISILICATE.

gemeprost is a drug used in vaginal inserts (pessaries) to soften and dilate the neck of the womb (cervix) in order to facilitate an operation within the womb – generally an abortion.
✚ warning: gemeprost should not be used by patients with infections of the vagina or uterus, glaucoma, restriction of the upper respiratory tract

(as in asthma) or heart disorders.
▲ side-effects: there may be pain from the uterus and bleeding from the vagina; some patients experience nausea and vomiting, diarrhoea, backache and chest pain, headache, dizziness, flushing and high temperature. The heartbeat may become irregular.
Related article: CERVAGEM.

gemfibrozil is a drug used to reduce high levels of fat in the bloodstream (hyperlipidaemia), particularly cholesterol. Administration is oral in the form of capsules.
✚ warning: gemfibrozil should not be administered to patients with gallstones, impaired function of the liver, alcoholism, or who are pregnant. Before and during treatment there should be blood counts (and specifically to check on the lipid profile), monitoring of kidney function, and an ophthalmic examination.
▲ side-effects: gastrointestinal disturbances are not uncommon. There may also be dizziness, blurred vision and an itching rash. Some patients experience muscle pain, or pain in the fingertips and toes.
Related article: LOPID.

***general anaesthetic**: *see* ANAESTHETIC,

Genexol (*Rendell*) is a proprietary non-prescription form of SPERMICIDAL pessary (vaginal insert) used to reinforce barrier methods of contraception. It is a preparation of two alcohol esters within a base of palm kernel oil.

Genisol (*Fisons*) is a proprietary preparation of the ANTISEPTIC COAL TAR, used to treat skin conditions such as dandruff, dermatitis, eczema and psoriasis. It is produced in the form of a liquid shampoo for weekly application.

gentamicin is a broad-spectrum ANTIBIOTIC drug, an aminoglycoside used to treat many forms of infection, but especially those of the urinary tract, the meninges (meningitis), the prostate gland, the heart (endocarditis), or the blood (septicaemia). It is not capable of being absorbed by the digestive system, so administration is by injection or by topical application in the form of drops, cream or ointment.
✚ warning: gentamicin should not be administered to patients who are pregnant, or who are already taking drugs that affect the neural system. It should be administered with caution to those with parkinsonism or impaired function of the kidneys. Prolonged or high dosage can cause deafness; regular blood counts are essential in such cases.
▲ side-effects: treatment must be discontinued if there are signs of deafness. There may be dysfunction of the kidneys.
Related articles: CIDOMYCIN; GARAMYCIN; GENTICIN; GENTISONE HC; LUGACIN; MINIMS GENTAMICIN.

gentian mixture is a non-proprietary formulation of simple and aromatic constituents intended to stimulate the appetite. (The main active constituent, however, is said to be suggestion.) There are two forms of gentian mixture – an "acid" formulation, and an "alkaline". Both contain a solution of the herb gentian in infusion in chloroform water. The acid mixture additionally contains the stomach acid hydrochloric acid; the alkaline contains SODIUM BICARBONATE.

gentian violet, or crystal violet, is an ANTISEPTIC dye used to treat certain bacterial and fungal skin infections, or abrasions and minor wounds. Administration is mostly in the form of ointment, paint or lotion, but can in dilute solution be oral or in vaginal inserts (pessaries). The dye is also used to stain specimens for examination under a microscope. A non-proprietary antiseptic paint, used particularly to prepare skin for surgery, combines gentian violet with another dye, brilliant green.
✚ warning: gentian violet is a dye: it stains clothes as well as skin.
▲ side-effects: rarely, there may be nausea and vomiting, with diarrhoea.

Genticin (*Nicholas*) is a proprietary ANTIBIOTIC, available only on prescription, used to treat any of a number of serious infections, but especially those of the urinary tract and on the skin. Produced in vials or ampoules for injection (in three strengths, the weakest under the name Genticin Paediatric), as a (water-miscible) cream or an (anhydrous greasy) ointment applied topically to treat skin infections, and as eye- or ear-drops, Genticin is a preparation of the aminoglycoside gentamicin.
✚/▲ warning/side-effects: *see* GENTAMICIN.

Genticin HC (*Nicholas*) is a proprietary compound ANTIBIOTIC, available only on prescription, used in the form of a cream and as an ointment to treat skin infections and to soothe the symptoms of allergic skin conditions. It is a preparation of the aminoglycoside gentamicin sulphate with the CORTICOSTEROID hydrocortisone acetate.
✚/▲ warning/side-effects: *see* GENTAMICIN; HYDROCORTISONE.

G

Gentisone HC (*Nicholas*) is a proprietary compound ANTIBIOTIC, available only on prescription, used in the form of ear-drops to treat bacterial infections of the outer or middle ear. It is a preparation of the aminoglycoside gentamicin sulphate with the CORTICOSTEROID hydrocortisone acetate.
✚/▲ warning/side-effects: *see* GENTAMICIN; HYDROCORTISONE.

Gentran (*Travenol*) is a proprietary form of the plasma substitute dextran, available only on prescription, used in infusion with either saline (sodium chloride) or glucose to make up a deficiency in the overall volume of blood in a patient, or to prevent thrombosis following surgery. Produced in flasks (bottles) for infusion, there is a choice of two concentrations: Gentran 40 and Gentran 70.
✚/▲ warning/side-effects: *see* DEXTRAN.

Gestanin (*Organon*) is a proprietary form of the PROGESTOGEN allyloestrenol, available only on prescription, used to treat recurrent miscarriage or failure of a blastocyst to implant in the uterine wall following conception. It is produced in the form of tablets.
✚/▲ warning/side-effects: *see* ALLYLOESTRENOL.

Gestone (*Paines & Byrne*) is a proprietary form of the PROGESTOGEN progesterone, available only on prescription, used to treat recurrent miscarriage, premenstrual symptoms or abnormal bleeding from the womb. It is produced in ampoules for deep intramuscular injection (in three strengths).

✚/▲ warning/side-effects: *see* PROGESTERONE.

G

gestronol hexanoate is a synthetic PROGESTOGEN used primarily in women to treat cancer of the breast or of the uterine lining (endometrium), but used also in men to treat (malignant) enlargement of the kidneys or (benign) enlargement of the prostate gland.

✚ warning: gestronol hexanoate should not be administered to patients with undiagnosed vaginal bleeding or with thrombosis; it should be administered with caution to those who suffer from heart, liver or kidney disease, from diabetes, or who are lactating.

▲ side-effects: there may be breast tenderness, menstrual irregularity and an alteration in libido; fluid retention and consequent weight gain are not uncommon; there may also be nausea, gastrointestinal disturbances and sensitivity reactions such as acne and urticaria.

Related article: DEPOSTAT.

Gevral (*Lederle*) is a proprietary non-prescription mineral-and-VITAMIN compound that is not available from the National Health Service. Used to make up mineral and vitamin deficiencies, and produced in the form of capsules, Gevral contains IRON (in the form of FERROUS FUMARATE), CALCIUM, copper, iodine, MAGNESIUM, manganese, phosphorus, POTASSIUM and ZINC; and RETINOL (vitamin A), vitamin B in the forms of THIAMINE, RIBOFLAVINE, PYRIDOXINE, CYANOCOBALAMIN, NICOTINAMIDE, INOSITOL and PANTOTHENIC ACID, ASCORBIC ACID (vitamin C), CALCIFEROL (vitamin D) and TOCOPHEROL (vitamin E).

Givitol (*Galen*) is a proprietary non-prescription IRON-and-VITAMIN supplement that is not available from the National Health Service. Produced in the form of capsules, Givitol contains iron in the form of FERROUS FUMARATE, vitamin B in the forms of THIAMINE, RIBOFLAVINE, PYRIDOXINE and NICOTINAMIDE, and ASCORBIC ACID (vitamin C).

Glandosane (*Dylade*) is a proprietary non-prescription form of artificial saliva, produced in an aerosol for spraying on to the membranes of the mouth and throat in conditions that make the mouth abnormally dry. There are neutral and flavoured versions. Constituents include CARMELLOSE SODIUM, SORBITOL, salt (sodium chloride), MAGNESIUM CHLORIDE and POTASSIUM CHLORIDE.

Glauline (*Smith & Nephew*) is a proprietary BETA-BLOCKER, available only on prescription, used in the form of eye-drops to treat glaucoma and other conditions involving pressure within the eyeball. Produced in three strengths, Glauline drops represent a preparation of metipranolol, and are not recommended for children.

✚/▲ warning/side-effects: *see* METIPRANOLOL.

glibenclamide is a drug used to treat (adult-onset) diabetes mellitus, one of the SULPHONYLUREAS which work by augmenting insulin production in the pancreas (as opposed to compensating for its absence).

Administration is oral in the form of tablets.
✚ warning: glibenclamide should not be administered to patients with liver or kidney damage, with endocrine disorders, or who are under stress; who are pregnant or lactating; or who are already taking corticosteroids or oral contraceptives, oral anticoagulants, or aspirin and other antibiotics.
▲ side-effects: there may be some sensitivity reaction (such as a rash).
Related articles: DAONIL; EUGLUCON; LIBANIL; MALIX; SEMI- DAONIL.

Glibenese (*Pfizer*) is a proprietary form of the SULPHONYLUREA glipizide, available only on prescription, used to treat adult-onset diabetes mellitus. It works by augmenting what remains of insulin production in the pancreas, and is produced in the form of tablets.
✚/▲ warning/side-effects: *see* GLIPIZIDE.

glibornuride is a drug used to treat (adult-onset) diabetes mellitus, one of the SULPHONYLUREAS which work by augmenting insulin production in the pancreas (as opposed to compensating for its absence). Administration is oral in the form of tablets.
✚ warning: glibornuride should not be administered to patients with liver or kidney damage, with endocrine disorders, or who are under stress; who are pregnant or lactating; or who are already taking corticosteroids or oral contraceptives, oral anticoagulants, or aspirin and other antibiotics.
▲ side-effects: there may be some sensitivity reaction (such as a rash).
Related article: GLUTRIL.

gliclazide is a drug used to treat (adult-onset) diabetes mellitus, one of the SULPHONYLUREAS which work by augmenting insulin production in the pancreas (as opposed to compensating for its absence). Administration is oral in the form of tablets.
✚ warning: gliclazide should not be administered to patients with liver or kidney damage, with endocrine disorders, or who are under stress; who are pregnant or lactating; or who are already taking corticosteroids or oral contraceptives, oral anticoagulants, or aspirin and other antibiotics.
▲ side-effects: there may be some sensitivity reaction (such as a rash).
Related article: DIAMICRON.

glipizide is a drug used to treat (adult-onset) diabetes mellitus, one of the SULPHONYLUREAS which work by augmenting insulin production in the pancreas (as opposed to compensating for its absence). Administration is oral in the form of tablets.
✚ warning: glipizide should not be administered to patients with liver or kidney damage, with endocrine disorders, or who are under stress; who are pregnant or lactating; or who are already taking corticosteroids or oral contraceptives, oral anticoagulants, or aspirin and other antibiotics.
▲ side-effects: there may be some sensitivity reaction (such as a rash).
Related articles: GLIBENESE; MINODIAB.

gliquidone is a drug used to treat (adult-onset) diabetes mellitus, one of the SULPHONYLUREAS which work by augmenting insulin production in the pancreas (as opposed to compensating for its absence). Administration is oral in the form of tablets.

✚ warning: gliquidone should not be administered to patients with liver or kidney damage, with endocrine disorders, or who are under stress; who are pregnant or lactating; or who are already taking corticosteroids or oral contraceptives, oral anticoagulants, or aspirin and other antibiotics.

▲ side-effects: there may be some sensitivity reaction (such as a rash).

Related article: GLURENORM.

globulin is any of a group of simple proteins that are present in blood and act either as antibodies (immunoglobulins) or as the means of transport for certain minerals and fats (lipids) around the body. Soluble in saline solution, globulins can be coagulated by heat.
Related article: HNIG.

glucagon is a HORMONE produced and secreted by the pancreas to cause an increase in blood sugar levels. In most people it is part of a balancing mechanism complementary to INSULIN, which has the opposite effect. Therapeutically, glucagon is thus administered to patients with low blood sugar levels (hypoglycaemia). Administration is by injection.

Glucophage (*Lipha*) is a proprietary form of the drug metformin hydrochloride, available only on prescription, used to treat adult-onset diabetes. It works by increasing absorption and utilization in the body of glucose, to make up for the reduction in insulin available from the pancreas, and is produced in the form of tablets (in two strengths).

✚/▲ warning/side-effects: *see* METFORMIN HYDROCHLORIDE.

Glucoplex (*Geistlich*) is a proprietary form of high-energy nutritional supplement intended for infusion into patients who are unable to take food via the alimentary tract. Produced in two strengths (under the names Glucoplex 1000 and Glucoplex 1600), its major constituent is the carbohydrate GLUCOSE.

glucose, or dextrose, is a simple sugar that represents an important source of energy for the body – and the sole source of energy for the brain. Following digestion, it is stored in the liver and muscles in the form of glycogen, and its breakdown into glucose again in the muscles produces energy. The level of glucose in the blood is critical: harmful symptoms occur if the level is too high or too low. Therapeutically, it may be administered as a dietary supplement in conditions of low blood sugar level, to treat abnormally high acidity of body fluids (acidosis), or to increase glucose levels in the liver following liver damage. Oral administration of a glucose solution is a good way of making up a deficiency of water or of carbohydrate in the body. The more common form of administration is by infusion.

▲ side-effects: injections of glucose may irritate vascular walls and so tend to promote thrombosis and inflammation.

Glucotard (*MCP Pharmaceuticals*) is a proprietary non-prescription preparation of guar gum, used to assist in the

treatment of patients with too low or too high a blood sugar level (as in diabetes). A high-fibre bulking agent, guar gum has the effect of evening out the peaks and troughs of glucose levels that normally correspond to meals and the intervals between them. Not recommended for children, Glucotard is produced in sachets of mini-tablets for solution.
✚/▲ warning/side-effects: *see* GUAR GUM.

Glucoven (*MCP Pharmaceuticals*) is a proprietary form of high-energy nutritional supplement intended for infusion into patients who are unable to take food via the alimentary tract. Produced in two strengths (under the names Glucoven 1000 and Glucoven 1600), its major constituent is the natural carbohydrate GLUCOSE, although it also contains ions and trace elements.

Glurenorm (*Winthrop*) is a proprietary form of the SULPHONYLUREA gliquidone, available only on prescription, used to treat adult-onset diabetes mellitus. It works by augmenting what remains of insulin production in the pancreas, and is produced in the form of tablets.
✚/▲ warning/side-effects: *see* GLIQUIDONE.

glutaraldehyde is a DISINFECTANT much like FORMALDEHYDE, but stronger and faster-acting. It is used mostly to sterilize medical and surgical equipment, but may alternatively be used therapeutically (in solution) to treat skin conditions such as warts (particularly verrucas on the soles of the feet) and to remove hard, dead skin.
✚ warning: effects of treatment are not always predictable. Skin treated may become sensitized.
Related articles: GLUTAROL; VERUCASEP.

Glutarol (*Dermal*) is a proprietary non-prescription solution for topical application containing the KERATOLYTIC glutaraldehyde, used to treat warts and to remove hard, dead skin.
✚ warning: *see* GLUTARALDEHYDE.

Glutenex (*Cow & Gate*) is the name of a proprietary (non-prescription) brand of gluten-free biscuits made without milk, produced for patients with coeliac disease and similar conditions.

Glutril (*Roche*) is a proprietary form of the SULPHONYLUREA glibornuride, available only on prescription, used to treat adult-onset diabetes mellitus. It works by augmenting what remains of insulin production in the pancreas, and is produced in the form of tablets.
✚/▲ warning/side-effects: *see* GLIBORNURIDE.

glycerol, or glycerin(e), is a mixture of hydrolized fat and oils. A colourless viscous liquid, it is used therapeutically as a constituent in many emollient skin preparations, as a sweetening agent for medications, and as a LAXATIVE in the form of anal suppositories. Taken orally, glycerol has the short-term effect of reducing pressure within the eyeballs (which may be useful for patients with glaucoma).

glyceryl trinitrate is a powerful VASODILATOR that is extremely effective in treating the symptoms of angina pectoris (heart pain). It works by dilating the veins returning blood to the heart, thus reducing the pressure within the heart and and reducing its workload at the same time. Short-acting, glyceryl trinitrate's effect is generally extended through its preparation in sustained-release capsules to be kept under the tongue; administration is in an aerosol as a spray, by intravenous injection, or in ointments and dressings to be placed on the surface of the chest for absorption through the skin.

✚ warning: glyceryl trinitrate should be administered with caution to patients who suffer from low blood pressure (hypotension) and associated conditions.

▲ side-effects: there may be headache and dizziness; some patients experience an increase in heart rate.

Related articles: CORO-NITRO SPRAY; DEPONIT 5; GTN 300 MCG; NITROCINE; NITROCONTIN CONTINUS; NITROLINGUAL SPRAY; NITRONAL; PERCUTOL; SUSCARD BUCCAL; SUSTAC; TRANSIDERM- NITRO; TRIDIL.

Glyconon (*DDSA Pharmaceuticals*) is a proprietary form of the SULPHONYLUREA tolbutamide, available only on prescription, used to treat adult-onset diabetes mellitus. It works by augmenting what remains of insulin production in the pancreas, and is produced in the form of tablets.

✚/▲ warning/side-effects: *see* TOLBUTAMIDE.

glycopyrronium bromide is an ANTICHOLINERGIC drug used to assist in the treatment of gastrointestinal disturbances caused by spasm in the muscles of the intestinal walls. Administration is oral in the form of tablets.

✚ warning: glycopyrronium bromide should not be administered to patients who suffer from glaucoma; it should be administered with caution to those who suffer from heart disease, intestinal bleeding, enlargement of the prostate gland, or urinary retention, those who are lactating, or those who are elderly.

▲ side-effects: dry mouth and difficulty with swallowing is not uncommon; there may also be pressure within the eyeballs, dilation of the pupils and consequent sensitivity to light. The heartbeat may become irregular. Urinating may also become difficult. Rarely, there is high temperature and a state of confusion.

Related article: ROBINUL.

Glykola (*Sinclair*) is a proprietary non-prescription IRON supplement that is not available from the National Health Service. Produced in the form of an elixir for dilution (the potency of the elixir once dilute is retained for 14 days), Glykola contains iron (in the form of ferric chloride), caffeine, calcium and kola extract. There is a version for children (produced under the name Glykola Infans) which instead of the caffeine and calcium contains citric acid and the herb gentian.

Glymese (*DDSA Pharmaceuticals*) is a proprietary form of the SULPHONYLUREA chlorpropamide, available only on prescription, used to treat adult-onset diabetes mellitus. It works by augmenting what remains of insulin production in the pancreas, but because it also has a marked effect in decreasing frequency of urination, it is sometimes also used to treat the condition diabetes insipidus. Glymese is

produced in the form of tablets.
✚/▲ warning/side-effects: *see* CHLORPROPAMIDE.

glymidine is a drug used to treat (adult-onset) diabetes mellitus. Although its effect is that of the SULPHONYLUREAS which work by augmenting insulin production in the pancreas (as opposed to compensating for its absence), it is not actually a sulphonylurea and may be used with caution in patients with known sensitivity to those drugs. Administration is oral in the form of tablets.
✚ warning: glymidine should not be administered to patients with liver or kidney damage, with endocrine disorders, or who are under stress; who are pregnant or lactating; or who are already taking corticosteroids or oral contraceptives, oral anticoagulants, or aspirin and other antibiotics.
▲ side-effects: there may be some sensitivity reaction (such as a rash).
Related article: GONDAFON.

Glypressin (*Ferring*) is a proprietary preparation of the drug terlipressin, a derivative of the HORMONE VASOPRESSIN. Available only on prescription, Glypressin is used to treat the haemorrhaging of varicose veins in the oesophagus (the tubular channel for food between throat and stomach). It is produced in vials for (dilution and) injection.
✚/▲ warning/side-effects: *see* TERLIPRESSIN.

gold, in the form of its salts (in particular sodium aurothiomalate), is used therapeutically in the treatment of rheumatoid arthritis. Not an anti-inflammatory ANALGESIC like other treatments, however, gold works slowly so that full effects are achieved only after four or five months. Improvement then is significant, not only in the reduction of joint inflammation but also in associated inflammations. Administration is by injection. Gold is increasingly rarely also used in dentistry, occasionally for fillings, but more commonly (as alloys) in crowns, inlays and bridges.
✚/▲ warning/side-effects: *see* SODIUM AUROTHIOMALATE.

Goldstar (*Longdon*) is a proprietary form of supportive thigh-length stocking used to give early preventive treatment for varicose veins especially during pregnancy. It is lightweight and elasticated, and available in pairs in different sizes.

gonadorelin is the chemical name of gonadotrophin-releasing hormone.
see GONADOTROPHIN-RELEASING HORMONE.

gonadotrophin is any of a number of HORMONES produced and secreted by the pituitary gland that act on the ovary in women or on the testes in men to promote the production in turn of other sex hormones and of eggs (ova) or sperm. The major gonadotrophins are follicle-stimulating hormone (FSH) and luteinizing hormone (LH). Either may be injected in order to make up hormonal deficiency and so treat infertility.

gonadotrophin-releasing hormone, or gonadorelin, is the HORMONE that acts on the pituitary gland to release the GONADOTROPHINS, which in turn stimulate the production and secretion of sex hormones – such as luteinizing hormone and follicle-stimulating hormone –

G

and sperm and ova. Its therapeutic use is limited mostly to diagnostic purposes (in assessing pituitary function), but it is sometimes injected in women to make up a hormonal deficiency and so treat infertility or absence of menstruation, or in boys to treat undescended testicles.

✚ warning: administration of gonadorelin to treat infertility or absence of menstruation has to be by pulsed subcutaneous infusion, a form of treatment generally available only in a specialist endocrine unit.

▲ side-effects: rarely there may be headache, abdominal pain and nausea; the site of infusion may become painful. *Related articles:* FERTIRAL; HRF; RELEFACT.

Gonadotraphon FSH (*Paines & Byrne*) is a proprietary preparation of follicle-stimulating HORMONE (FSH) in the form of serum GONADOTROPHIN taken from pregnant mares. It is used to treat the absence of menstruation in adolescent girls, and to treat women suffering from specific hormonal deficiency for infertility. Available only on prescription, it is produced in powdered form for reconstitution with solvent as a medium for injection.

Gonadotraphon LH (*Paines & Byrne*) is a proprietary preparation of the HORMONE human chorionic GONADOTROPHIN (HCG), available only on prescription, used to treat undescended testicles in boys, and to treat women suffering from specific hormonal deficiency for infertility. It is produced in powdered form for reconstitution with a solvent as a medium for injection.

✚/▲ warning/side-effects: *see* HCG.

Gondafon (*Schering*) is a proprietary form of the SULPHONYLUREA glymidine, available only on prescription, used to treat adult-onset diabetes mellitus. It works by augmenting what remains of insulin production in the pancreas, and is produced in the form of tablets.

✚/▲ warning/side-effects: *see* GLYMIDINE.

Graneodin (*Squibb*) is a proprietary ANTIBIOTIC, available only on prescription, used to treat bacterial infections of the head and face, and particularly of the eye. Produced in the form of an ointment for topical application, Graneodin contains the aminoglycoside neomycin sulphate.

✚/▲ warning/side-effects: *see* NEOMYCIN.

Gregoderm (*Unigreg*) is a proprietary ANTIBIOTIC, available only on prescription, used to treat inflammation of the skin in which infection is also present. Produced in the form of an ointment for topical application, Gregoderm is a compound of the antibiotics neomycin sulphate, nystatin and polymyxin B sulphate, together with the CORTICOSTEROID hydrocortisone.

✚/▲ warning/side-effects: *see* HYDROCORTISONE; NEOMYCIN; NYSTATIN; POLYMYXIN B SULPHATE.

griseofulvin is a powerful ANTIFUNGAL ANTIBIOTIC drug that during treatment – which may be prolonged – is deposited selectively in the skin, hair and nails, and thus prevents further fungal invasion. It is most commonly used for large-scale infections, or to treat infections that prove intractable to other drugs, but can be used equally successfully on ringworm or localized tinea infections (such as athlete's foot). Administration is oral in the form of tablets or as a suspension.

✚ warning: griseofulvin should not be administered to patients who suffer from liver failure or from porphyria, or who are pregnant or taking oral contraceptives. Avoid alcohol during the period of treatment.

▲ side-effects: there may be headache, with nausea and vomiting; some patients experience a sensitivity to light. Rarely, there may be a rash (which may be mild or serious).

Related articles: FULSIN; GRISOVIN.

Grisovin (*Glaxo*) is a proprietary ANTIFUNGAL ANTIBIOTIC drug, available only on prescription, used to treat infections of the scalp, skin and nails. Produced in the form of tablets (in two strengths), Grisovin is a preparation of the drug griseofulvin. Treatment may be required to continue over several weeks.

✚/▲ warning/side-effects: *see* GRISEOFULVIN.

GTN 300 mcg (*Martindale*) is a proprietary non-prescription preparation of the powerful VASODILATOR glyceryl trinitrate, used to treat angina pectoris (heart pain). It is produced in the form of tablets, of the size specified by its name.

✚/▲ warning/side-effects: *see* GLYCERYL TRINITRATE.

guanethidine monosulphate is an ANTIHYPERTENSIVE drug, used in the treatment of high blood pressure (hypertension), often in combination with a DIURETIC (such as a thiazide) or a beta-blocker. It is also used to relieve pressure within the eyeball in the treatment of glaucoma, for which its effect is often enhanced by the simultaneous administration of the hormone adrenaline.

✚ warning: guanethidine monosulphate should not be administered to patients with Renal failure; it should be administered with caution to those who are elderly or pregnant. In the treatment of low blood pressure, dosage is adjusted according to individual response, and may be high.

▲ side-effects: initial treatment may cause a reduction in heart rate; blood pressure may remain low during periods of rest. There may be muscle weakness and diarrhoea, fluid retention and nasal congestion.

Related articles: GANDA; ISMELIN.

Guanor expectorant (*RP Drugs*) is a proprietary non-prescription EXPECTORANT and ANTITUSSIVE that is not available from the National Health Service. Produced in the form of a syrup, its active constituents include AMMONIUM CHLORIDE, SODIUM CITRATE, diphenhydramine hydrochloride and menthol.

guar gum is a natural, soluble, high-fibre bulking agent which, when consumed in some quantity, has the effect of evening out the peaks and troughs of blood glucose levels that normally correspond to meals and the intervals between them. It is therefore used mainly to assist the treatment of patients with too low or too high blood glucose levels – as happens particularly in diabetes mellitus.

✚ warning: guar gum should not be used in patients who suffer

from intestinal obstruction. An adequately high fluid intake must be maintained. Counselling on this and on dosage is advised.
▲ side-effects: there is commonly flatulence with abdominal distension; occasionally guar gum itself causes intestinal obstruction.
Related articles: GLUCOTARD; GUAREM; GUARINA; LEJGUAR.

G

Guarem (*Rybar*) is a proprietary non-prescription preparation of guar gum, used to assist in the treatment of patients with too low or too high a blood sugar level (as in diabetes). A high-fibre bulking agent, guar gum has the effect of evening out the peaks and troughs of glucose levels that normally correspond to meals and the intervals between them. Not recommended for children, Guarem is produced in sachets of granules for solution.
✚/▲ warning/side-effects: *see* GUAR GUM.

Guarina (*Norgine*) is a proprietary non-prescription preparation of guar gum, used to assist in the treatment of patients with too low or too high a blood sugar level (as in diabetes). A high- fibre bulking agent, guar gum has the effect of evening out the peaks and troughs of glucose levels that normally correspond to meals and the intervals between them. Not recommended for children, Guarina is produced in sachets of granules for solution or for sprinkling over food.
✚/▲ warning/side-effects: *see* GUAR GUM.

Gynatren (*Cabot*) is a proprietary preparation of certain bacilli that ordinarily reside in the alimentary tract and vagina, consisting of a form of VACCINE used to treat recurrent vaginal infections. Available only on prescription, it is produced in ampoules for intramuscular injection, and administered in 3 doses over four weeks.

Gyno-Daktarin (*Janssen*) is a series of proprietary preparations of the ANTIFUNGAL drug miconazole nitrate, used to treat yeast infections of the vagina or vulva (like thrush). All are available only on prescription. There is an intravaginal cream (with its own applicator), vaginal inserts (pessaries), coated tampons, an "ovule" (which is a vaginal capsule, and marketed under the name Gyno-Daktarin 1), and a Combipack combining the cream and the pessaries.
✚/▲ warning/side-effects: *see* MICONAZOLE.

Gynol II (*Ortho-Cilag*) is a proprietary non-prescription form of SPERMICIDAL jelly used to reinforce barrier methods of contraception. It is a preparation of an alcohol ester.

Gyno-Pevaryl (*Ortho-Cilag*) is a series of proprietary preparations of the ANTIFUNGAL drug econazole nitrate, used to treat yeast infections of the vagina or vulva (like thrush). All are available only on prescription. There is a cream for topical application to the anogenital area, vaginal inserts (pessaries, in two formulations, one under the name Gyno-Pevaryl 1), and a Combipack combining the cream and one or other formulation of the pessaries.
▲ side-effects: see ECONAZOLE NITRATE.

Gynovlar (*Schering*) is an combined ORAL CONTRACEPTIVE, available only on prescription, that combines the OESTROGEN ethinyloestradiol with the

PROGESTOGEN norethisterone acetate. It is produced in packs of 21 tablets representing one complete menstrual cycle.

✚/▲ warning/side-effects: *see* ETHINYLOESTRADIOL; NORETHISTERONE.

Gypsona (*Smith & Nephew*) is a proprietary form of bandaging impregnated with plaster of Paris, used primarily for the immobilization of a fracture. Soaking the bandage causes the plaster to set hard.

Haelan (*Dista*) is a proprietary preparation of the CORTICOSTEROID drug flurandrenolone, available only on prescription, used in the form of a water-miscible cream or an anhydrous ointment as a topical application to treat severe non-infective inflammations of the skin. It is particularly used to treat eczema that is unresponsive to less powerful drugs. In both cream and ointment forms, Haelan is produced in two strengths (the stronger under the name Haelan-X), and in another version that additionally contains the antibacterial, antifungal agent CLIOQUINOL (under the name Haelan-C). There is also an impregnated tape for use as a poultice (marketed under the name Haelan Tape, but not available from the National Health Service).
✚/▲ warning/side-effects: *see* FLURANDRENOLONE.

Haemaccel (*Hoechst*) is a proprietary form of gelatin, the hydrolized animal protein. In a special refined (partly degraded) form available only on prescription, it is used in infusion with saline (sodium chloride) as a means of expanding overall blood volume in patients whose blood volume is dangerously low through shock, particularly in cases of severe burns or septicaemia. It is produced in bottles (flasks) for infusion.
✚/▲ warning/side-effects: *see* GELATIN.

haemostatics are agents that prevent or stop bleeding, known also as styptics. Haemostatics are used mostly to treat disorders in which bleeding is prolonged and potentially dangerous, such as haemophilia. Best known and most used are probably PHYTOMENADIONE (of which injections or infusions have to be given very slowly) and the coagulant enzyme-precursor thromboplastin.

Halciderm (*Squibb*) is a proprietary preparation, in the form of a water-miscible cream for topical application, of the extremely powerful CORTICOSTEROID halcinonide. Available only on prescription, it is used to treat severe non-infective inflammation of the skin, particularly eczema that is unresponsive to less powerful drugs.
✚/▲ warning/side-effects: *see* HALCINONIDE.

halcinonide is a powerful CORTICOSTEROID drug, used in very dilute solution to treat severe non-infective inflammations of the skin, particularly eczema that is unresponsive to less powerful drugs. Administration is in the form of a water-miscible cream for topical application.
✚ warning: like all topical corticosteroids, halcinonide by itself treats symptoms and does not cure underlying disorders. If infection is present, it may worsen although the symptoms may be suppressed by the drug.
▲ side-effects: side-effects depend to some extent on the area of skin treated. Prolonged treatment may cause thinning of the skin, yet increase hair growth; there may be acne or dermatitis. These side-effects may be worse in children.
Related article: HALCIDERM.

Halcion (*Upjohn*) is a proprietary TRANQUILLIZER and HYPNOTIC, available only on prescription, used primarily to treat insomnia, particularly in elderly patients. Produced in the form of tablets

(in two strengths), Halcion is a preparation of the BENZODIAZEPINE triazolam. It is not recommended for children.
✚/▲ warning/side-effects: *see* TRIAZOLAM.

Haldol (*Janssen*) is a proprietary form of the powerful ANTIPSYCHOTIC drug haloperidol. Available only on prescription, it is used to treat and tranquillize psychosis (such as schizophrenia), in which it is particularly suitable for treating manic forms of behavioural disturbance. It may be used alternatively to treat anxiety in the short term, as a premedication before surgery, or to control patients in delirium tremens or with alcohol withdrawal problems. Haldol is produced in the form of tablets (in two strengths), as a liquid to take orally (in two strengths, under the name Haldol Oral Liquid), and in ampoules for injection.
✚/▲ warning/side-effects: *see* HALOPERIDOL.

Haldol Decanoate (*Janssen*) is another form of HALDOL, available only on prescription, it is an ANTIPSYCHOTIC to treat and tranquillize forms of psychosis on a long-term maintenance basis. Its active constituent is the decanoate salt of haloperidol. Produced in ampoules (in two strengths) for injection, it is not recommended for children.
✚/▲ warning/side-effects: *see* HALOPERIDOL.

Half-Inderal LA (*ICI*) is a preparation of Inderal-LA at half strength, produced in the form of sustained-release capsules of the BETA-BLOCKER PROPRANOLOL hydrochloride.
see INDERAL-LA.

halibut-liver oil is an excellent source of retinol (vitamin A). A non-proprietary preparation is available in the form of tablets, but should not be taken without initial medical diagnosis; retinol deficiency is very rare, and treatment should be monitored in order to avoid the potentially unpleasant side-effects of excess vitamin A in the body.
✚/▲ warning/side-effects: *see* RETINOL.

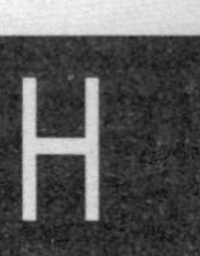

haloperidol is a powerful ANTIPSYCHOTIC drug used to treat and tranquillize psychosis (such as schizophrenia), in which it is particularly suitable for treating manic forms of behavioural disturbance, especially in order to effect emergency control. The drug may also be used to treat severe anxiety in the short term. Administration is oral in the form of capsules, tablets, a liquid or an elixir, or by injection (which may be short-acting or "depot").
✚ warning: haloperidol should not be administered to patients who suffer from a reduction in the bone-marrow's capacity to produce blood cells, or from certain types of glaucoma. It should be administered only with caution to those with heart or vascular disease, kidney or liver disease, parkinsonism, or depression; or who are pregnant or lactating. It is not recommended for children.
▲ side-effects: patients should be warned before treatment that their judgement and powers of concentration may become defective under treatment. There may be restlessness, insomnia and nightmares; rashes and jaundice may occur; and there may be dry mouth, gastrointestinal disturbance, difficulties in urinating, and blurred vision.

Muscles in the neck and back, and sometimes the arms, may undergo spasms. Rarely, there is weight loss and impaired kidney function.
Related articles: DOZIC; FORTUNAN; HALDOL; HALDOL DECANOATE; SERENACE.

H

halothane is a powerful general ANAESTHETIC that is widely used both for induction and for maintenance of anaesthesia during surgical operations. Used in combination with oxygen or nitrous oxide-oxygen mixtures, halothane vapour is non-irritant and even pleasant to inhale, does not induce coughing, and seldom causes post-operative vomiting. Administration is through a calibrated vaporizer in order to control concentration.
✚ warning: halothane causes a slowing of the heart rate and shallowness of breathing; both must be monitored during anaesthesia to prevent high levels of carbon dioxide or dangerously slow pulse and low blood pressure. The vapour is not good as a muscle relaxant, and muscle relaxants may have to be used in addition during specific types of surgery.
▲ side-effects: there may be liver damage. Repetition of anaesthesia by halothane is inadvisable within 3 months.
Related article: FLUOTHANE.

Halycitrol (*L A B*) is a proprietary non-prescription preparation of retinol (vitamin A) and calciferol (vitamin D) that is not available from the National Health Service. Produced in the form of an emulsion, it is used to treat deficiency of either vitamin, or both, but should be taken only under medical supervision because both vitamins in excess can cause unpleasant side-effects.
✚/▲ warning/side-effects: *see* CALCIFEROL; RETINOL.

hamamelis is a natural soothing agent, derived from the witch hazel plant, used mostly to relieve the pain of piles (haemorrhoids). Administration is in the form of anal suppositories; some versions also contain the mild astringent ZINC OXIDE.

Hamarin (*Nicholas*) is a proprietary form of the XANTHINE-OXIDASE INHIBITOR allopurinol, used to treat high levels of uric acid in the bloodstream (which may otherwise cause gout or kidney stones). Available only on prescription, Hamarin is produced in the form of tablets (in two strengths). It is not recommended for children.
✚/▲ warning/side-effects: *see* ALLOPURINOL.

Harmogen (*Abbott*) is a proprietary OESTROGEN, available only on prescription, formerly commonly used to treat symptoms that occur with falling natural levels of oestrogen in women following the menopause. (Now, however, it is far more usual to prescribe an oestrogen-progestogen compound.) Produced in the form of tablets, Harmogen is a preparation of piperazine oestrone sulphate.
✚/▲ warning/side-effects: *see* PIPERAZINE OESTRONE SULPHATE.

Hartmann's solution is another description of sodium lactate in a preparation suitable for intravenous infusion.
see SODIUM LACTATE.

Haymine (*Pharmax*) is a proprietary non-prescription nasal DECONGESTANT that is not available from the National

Health Service. Unlike most nasal decongestants, however, it is produced in the form of tablets (for swallowing) and is a compound of the ANTIHISTAMINE chlorpheniramine maleate together with the BRONCHODILATOR ephedrine hydrochloride.
✚/▲ warning/side-effects: *see* CHLORPHENIRAMINE; EPHEDRINE HYDROCHLORIDE.

Hayphryn (*Winthrop*) is a proprietary non-prescription SYMPATHOMIMETIC nasal DECONGESTANT that is not available from the National Health Service. Produced in the form of a nasal spray, Hayphryn contains phenylephrine hydrochloride.
✚/▲ warning/side-effects: *see* PHENYLEPHRINE.

HBIG, or hepatitis B immunoglobulin, when injected or infused into the body, confers immediate immunity to the potentially dangerous effects of the disease caused by the hepatitis B virus. Prepared from the blood plasma of recent patients, it is used specifically to immunize personnel in medical laboratories and hospitals who may be infected, and to treat babies of mothers infected by the virus during pregnancy. In normal circumstances, however, immunization is with an anti-hepatitis B vaccine.

H-B-Vax (*Merck, Sharp & Dohme*) is a proprietary form of anti-hepatitis B VACCINE, available only on prescription, used on patients with a high risk of infection from the hepatitis B virus mostly through contact with a carrier. Chemically, H-B-Vax consists of an inactivated hepatitis B virus surface antigen derived from the blood plasma of a human carrier and adsorbed on to alum in suspension. It is produced in vials for intramuscular injection; the usual regimen per patient is 3 doses, at intervals of one month and six months.

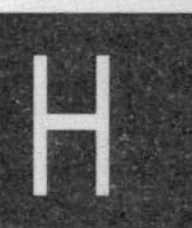

HCG is an abbreviation for human chorionic gonadotrophin, a HORMONE produced by the placenta during pregnancy. Excreted in the urine, its presence there is the basis of most pregnancy tests. Therapeutically, HCG is used in women to treat sterility that is due to lack of ovulation, or to relieve premenstrual tension. In men it is used to treat undescended testes or delayed puberty. Administration is by intramuscular injection.
✚ warning: all treatment with HCG must be under the most rigorously controlled monitoring: in women there is a risk of ovarian rupture, and in men a hormonal balance must be created and maintained. HCG should be administered with caution to patients who suffer from asthma, epilepsy or migraine, or from impairment of heart or liver function.
▲ side-effects: there may be headache and tiredness, mood changes and (especially in male patients) weight gain through the accumulation of fluid in the tissues (oedema).
Related articles: GONADOTRAPHON LH; PROFASI.

Hedex (*Sterling Health*) is a proprietary non-prescription non-narcotic ANALGESIC produced in the form of tablets and as a soluble powder. It contains paracetamol.
✚/▲ warning/side-effects: *see* PARACETAMOL.

Hedex Plus (*Sterling Health*) is a proprietary non-prescription combination ANALGESIC produced in the form of capsules. It contains paracetamol, caffeine and codeine.
✚/▲ warning/side-effects: *see* CAFFEINE; CODEINE; PARACETAMOL.

H

Heminevrin (*Astra*) is a proprietary SEDATIVE, available only on prescription, used to treat insomnia, states of confusion or agitation in the elderly, and (under rigorous monitoring) acute alcohol withdrawal symptoms. Produced in the form of capsules, as a sugar-free syrup for dilution (the potency of the syrup once dilute is retained for 14 days), and in flasks (bottles) for intravenous infusion, Heminevrin is a preparation of chlormethiazole. Not recommended for children.
✚/▲ warning/side-effects: *see* CHLORMETHIAZOLE.

Hepacon (*Consolidated*) is the name of a series of preparations of CYANOCOBALAMIN (vitamin B_{12}) or analogues (including folic acid and/or liver extract), intended to make up body deficiency in the vitamin. Such a deficiency is most commonly caused by malabsorption through disease or surgery (and is now more often remedied through the use of HYDROXOCOBALAMIN than through cyanocobalamin) but may also be caused by extreme forms of vegetarianism. All forms of Hepacon are produced in ampoules for injection, but are available on prescription only to private patients.

Hepacon-Plex (*Consolidated*) is a proprietary VITAMIN B compound, available on prescription only to private patients, used to make up vitamin deficiency. Produced in the form of ampoules for injection, Hepacon-Plex contains many forms of the vitamin: THIAMINE, RIBOFLAVINE, PYRIDOXINE, CYANOCOBALAMIN, NICOTINAMIDE and PANTOTHENIC ACID.

heparin is a natural ANTICOAGULANT in the body, manufactured mostly by the liver and certain leukocytes (white cells). For therapeutic use it is purified after extraction. Administration is generally by injection, to prevent or treat thrombosis and similar conditions, but its effect is short-lived and treatment may have to be repeated at intervals of less than 6 hours, or may have to be by constant infusion.
✚ warning: heparin should not be administered to patients with haemophilia, peptic ulcer, very high blood pressure (hypertension) or severe kidney disease, or who have recently undergone eye surgery. It should be administered with caution to those who are pregnant.
▲ side-effects: should haemorrhage occur, it may be difficult to stop the bleeding for a time – although because heparin is so short-acting, merely discontinuing treatment is usually effective fairly quickly. There may be sensitivity reactions. Prolonged use may cause a loss of calcium from the bones and of hair from the head.
Related articles: CALCIPARINE; MINIHEP; MINIHEP CALCIUM; MONOPARIN; MULTIPARIN; PUMP-HEP; UNIHEP; UNIPARIN; UNIPARIN CALCIUM.

Heparinised Saline (*Paines & Byrne*) is a proprietary solution (available only on prescription) containing the ANTICOAGULANT

HEPARIN sodium, used to wash and rinse the interior surfaces of catheters, cannulas and other medical forms of tubing to ensure that they remain unobstructed while carrying out their functions. The solution has no therapeutic use.

hepatitis B vaccine consists of an inactivated hepatitis B virus surface antigen derived from the blood plasma of a human carrier and adsorbed on to alum in suspension. It is used on patients with a high risk of infection from the hepatitis B virus mostly through contact with a carrier. Administration is by intramuscular injection in the arm or thigh; the usual regimen per patient is 3 doses, at intervals of one month and six months.
✚ warning: vaccination does not guarantee the avoidance of infection: commonsense precautions against infection should still be observed in relation to known carriers.

Hep-Flush (*Burgess*) is a proprietary solution (available only on prescription) containing the ANTICOAGULANT HEPARIN sodium, used to wash and rinse the interior surfaces of catheters, cannulas and other medical forms of tubing to ensure that they remain unobstructed while carrying out their functions. The solution has no therapeutic use.

Hepsal (*CP Pharmaceuticals*) is a proprietary solution (available only on prescription) containing the ANTICOAGULANT HEPARIN sodium, used to wash and rinse the interior surfaces of catheters, cannulas and other medical forms of tubing to ensure that they remain unobstructed while carrying out their functions. The solution has no therapeutic use.

heroin is a more familiar term for the narcotic ANALGESIC drug diamorphine.
see DIAMORPHINE.

Herpid (*WB Pharmaceuticals*) is a proprietary form of the drug idoxuridine, prepared in a solution of dimethyl sulphoxide, used to treat skin infections by the viral organisms Herpes simplex (such as cold sores or genital sores) and Herpes zoster (shingles). Available only on prescription, Herpid is produced as a sort of paint for topical application (with a brush).
✚ warning: *see* IDOXURIDINE.

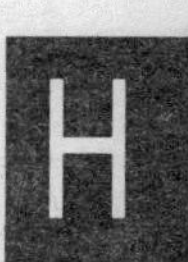

Hespan (*American Hospital Supply*) is a proprietary form of the plasma substitute hetastarch. Available only on prescription, it is used in infusion with saline (sodium chloride) as a means of expanding overall blood volume in patients whose blood volume is dangerously low through shock, particularly in cases of severe burns or septicaemia. It is produced in flexible bags for infusion.
✚/▲ warning/side-effects: *see* HETASTARCH.

hetastarch is a plasma substitute, administered more commonly as an emergency measure until tissue-matched blood is available, that is used in infusion with saline (sodium chloride) as a means of expanding overall blood volume in patients whose blood volume is dangerously low through shock, particularly in cases of severe burns or septicaemia.
✚ warning: hetastarch should not be administered to patients with congestive heart failure, kidney failure, or disorders of the blood that are likely to cause coagulation problems. Ideally, there should

be cross-matching of blood samples before infusion.
▲ side-effects: very rarely, there are sensitivity reactions.
Related article: HESPAN.

Hewletts Antiseptic Cream (*Astra*) is a proprietary ANTISEPTIC cream for topical application on minor abrasions or burns. Available without prescription, it contains boric acid, HYDROUS WOOL FAT and ZINC OXIDE.

hexachlorophane is a powerful DISINFECTANT used on the skin particularly of the face. In the form of a cream it is effective against scabies, and is a good substitute for soap in cases of acne or facial infection. It is also produced as a dusting-powder (which may help prevent bedsores).
✚ warning: hexachlorophane should not be used on areas of raw or abraded skin, and particularly not on raw areas of the skin of infants (in whom neural damage may occur). It is advisable to avoid using hexachlorophane routinely.
▲ side-effects: there are occasionally sensitivity reactions, and even more rarely an increased sensitivity to light.
Related articles: DERMALEX; STER-ZAC.

hexamine is an ANTIBACTERIAL that was formerly used to treat infections of the urinary tract. It is now generally considered to be too limited in its action – it treats only bacterial infection, requires the urine to be measured or made to be acidic, and has many potentially unpleasant side-effects. Administration of its one proprietary form is oral, as tablets.
✚ warning: hexamine should not be administered to patients with impaired function of the kidney or liver, or who are dehydrated. Patients' urine must be measured or made to be acidic.
▲ side-effects: there may be bladder irritation, with frequent and painful urination, and possibly blood in the urine; there may also be gastrointestinal disturbances and rashes.
Related article: HIPREX.

hexetidine is a mouthwash or gargle used for routine oral hygiene, to cleanse and freshen the mouth.
Related article: ORALDENE.

Hexopal (*Winthrop*) is a proprietary non-prescription VASODILATOR, used to treat circulatory disorders of the extremities, chilblains, and arteriosclerosis in the fingers and toes. Should be administered with caution to those with diabetes mellitus. Produced in the form of tablets (in two strengths, the stronger under the name Hexopal Forte) and as a sugar-free syrup for dilution (the resultant suspension retains its potency for 14 days), Hexopal contains two forms of vitamin B, INOSITOL and NICOTINIC ACID.

HGH is an abbreviation for human growth HORMONE, a hormone produced and secreted by the pituitary gland that promotes growth in the long bones of the limbs and increases protein synthesis. (It is also called somatotrophin.) For therapeutic use, however, HGH extracted from the pituitary gland is not viable; genetic engineering has made possible a form of the hormone using sequences of DNA to create what

is known as a growth hormone of human sequence – somatrem – and it is this that can be used in preparations to treat dwarfism and other problems of short stature due to hormone deficiency.
✚/▲ warning/side-effects: *see* SOMATREM.

Hibidil (*ICI*) is a proprietary non-prescription skin DISINFECTANT used to treat wounds and burns, and to provide asepsis during childbirth. Produced in the form of a solution in sachets, for further dilution as required, Hibidil is a preparation of chlorhexidine gluconate.
✚/▲ warning/side-effects: *see* CHLORHEXIDINE.

Hibiscrub (*ICI*) is a proprietary non-prescription DISINFECTANT used instead of soap to wash skin and hands before surgery. Produced in the form of a solution, Hibiscrub is a preparation of chlorhexidine gluconate in a surfactant liquid (a liquid with low surface tension, like a detergent).
✚/▲ warning/side-effects: *see* CHLORHEXIDINE.

Hibisol (*ICI*) is a proprietary non-prescription DISINFECTANT, used to treat minor wounds and burns on the skin and hands. Produced in the form of a solution, Hibisol is a preparation of chlorhexidine gluconate in isopropyl alcohol solvent together with emollients.
✚/▲ warning/side-effects: *see* CHLORHEXIDINE.

Hibitane (*ICI*) is the name of a series of proprietary non-prescription forms of DISINFECTANT, all based on solutions of chlorhexidine gluconate or other chlorhexidine salts. The standard form is that of a powder, used either to prepare solutions of chlorhexidine or to create antiseptic creams or powdered antiseptic compounds. There are two solutions: Hibitane 5% Concentrate (for skin disinfection, following further dilution in water or alcohol) and Hibitane Gluconate 20% (for internal irrigation of body cavities and the bladder, and to treat urethral infections). Hibitane Obstetric is a water-miscible cream used to lubricate the vulva during labour and childbirth. Another cream, Hibitane Antiseptic, is used to treat minor wounds and burns by topical application. Hibitane Lozenges (intended as an oral antiseptic and analgesic) also contain the local ANAESTHETIC BENZOCAINE.
✚/▲ warning/side-effects: *see* CHLORHEXIDINE.

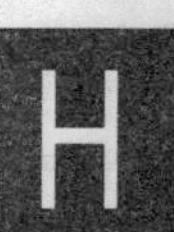

Hioxyl (*Quinoderm*) is a proprietary non-prescription DISINFECTANT used to treat bedsores and leg ulcers, minor wounds and burns. Produced in the form of a cream for topical application, Hioxyl is a preparation of the antiseptic HYDROGEN PEROXIDE.

Hiprex (*Riker*) is a proprietary non-prescription ANTIBACTERIAL used to treat infections of the urinary tract, and to prevent infection following urological surgery. Produced in the form of tablets, Hiprex is a compound of the now less commonly used drug hexamine together with hippuric acid (which renders the urine acidic enough for hexamine to be effective).
✚/▲ warning/side-effects: *see* HEXAMINE.

Hirudoid (*Panpharma*) is a proprietary non-prescription VASODILATOR and ANTICOAGULANT intended to improve the blood circulation in conditions such as varicose veins, chilblains and bruising, and produced in the form of a cream or a gel for topical application. Its active constituent is a derivative of the anticoagulant heparin.

✚/▲ warning/side-effects: *see* HEPARIN.

H

Hismanal (*Janssen*) is a proprietary ANTIHISTAMINE drug used primarily to treat allergic symptoms such as hay fever and urticaria. Produced in the form of tablets and as a fruit- flavoured suspension (under the trade name Hismanal Suspension), it is a preparation of astemizole. Hismanal is not recommended for children aged under 6 years.

✚/▲ warning/side-effects: *see* ASTEMIZOLE.

Histalix (*Wallace*) is a proprietary non-prescription EXPECTORANT and ANTITUSSIVE that is not available from the National Health Service. Produced in the form of a syrup, its active constituents include AMMONIUM CHLORIDE, SODIUM CITRATE, DIPHENHYDRAMINE HYDROCHLORIDE and MENTHOL.

Histryl (*Smith, Kline & French*) is a proprietary ANTIHISTAMINE drug used primarily to treat allergic symptoms such as hay fever and urticaria. Produced in the form of spansules (sustained-release capsules) in two strengths (the weaker under the name Histryl Paediatric Spansule), it is a preparation of diphenylpyraline hydrochloride. Histryl, even in its paediatric form, is not recommended for children aged under 7 years.

✚/▲ warning/side-effects: *see* DIPHENYLPYRALINE HYDROCHLORIDE.

HNIG is an abbreviation for human normal immunoglobulin, an injection of which – incorporating antibodies in serum – confers immediate immunity to such diseases as infective hepatitis (hepatitis A virus), measles (rubeola), and to some degree at least rubella (German measles). Prepared from more than a thousand pooled donations of blood plasma, it is commonly given to patients at risk, such as infants who cannot tolerate vaccines which incorporate live (if attenuated) viruses. Administration is by intramuscular injection or occasionally by intravenous infusion.

✚ warning: HNIG should not be administered within 2 weeks following vaccination with live viruses, or within 3 months before vaccination with live viruses is to be given (except in specific circumstances relating to the likelihood of convulsions in patients known to be at risk from them).

Hollister (*Abbott*) is the name of a series of proprietary non-prescription products for the care, freshening and sanitization of a stoma (an outlet in the skin surface that is the consequence of the surgical curtailment of the intestines). There is a medicated adhesive spray (for retaining an appliance or bag over the stoma) and a corresponding adhesive remover spray; and there are three skin applications for protection and cleanliness: a paste, a powder, and a gel.

Honvan (*WB Pharmaceuticals*) is a proprietary preparation of fosfestrol tetrasodium, a drug that is converted in the body to the OESTROGEN (female sex hormone) STILBOESTROL. Available only on prescription, it may be

used in women as part of hormone replacement therapy during and following the menopause or to treat menstrual difficulties, or used in men to treat cancer of the prostate gland. It is produced in the form of tablets, and in ampoules for injection.
✚/▲ warning/side-effects: *see* FOSFESTROL TETRASODIUM.

Hormofemin (*Medo*) is a proprietary HORMONE containing cream, available only on prescription, used to treat conditions of itching and eroded skin in the vulva caused by hormonal deficiency, generally as a consequence of the menopause. Consisting of a preparation of the OESTROGEN (female sex hormone) dienoestrol, Hormofemin is produced with its own applicator. Treatment should be reduced after about 10 days.
✚/▲ warning/side-effects: *see* DIENOESTROL.

***hormones** are body substances produced and secreted by glands into the bloodstream, where they are carried to specific organs and areas of tissue on which they have a specific effect. Major types of hormone include CORTICOSTEROIDS (produced mainly in the cortex of adrenal glands), ADRENALINE and NORADRENALINE from the medulla of the adrenal gland, thyroid hormones (produced by the thyroid gland), the sex hormones (produced mainly by the ovaries or the testes), the pancreatic hormones (such as INSULIN), and the hormones that cause the secretion or production of these hormones, e.g. GONADOTROPHIN-RELEASING HORMONE. Most hormones can be administered therapeutically to make up hormonal deficiency, sometimes in synthetic form.

Hormonin (*Carnrick*) is a proprietary combination of three natural female sex HORMONES – oestradiol (the main ovarian hormone), oestriol and oestrone – used to make up hormone deficiencies and to treat associated symptoms, especially during or following the menopause. Available only on prescription, Hormonin is produced in the form of tablets.
✚/▲ warning/side-effects: *see* OESTRADIOL; OESTRIOL.

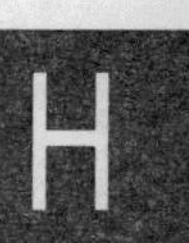

HRF (*Ayerst*) is a proprietary preparation of GONADOTROPHIN-RELEASING HORMONE, available only on prescription, and produced in the form of powder for reconstitution as a medium for injection or infusion. It is used as a diagnostic aid in assessing the functioning of the pituitary gland and its secretions. The administration of HRF in stepped increasing dosages enables the threshold of pituitary response to be indicated through the monitoring of its subsequent effects.

HTIG is an abbreviation for human tetanus immunoglobulin, a specific form of immunoglobulin (antibodies in serum), used mostly as an added precaution to treat patients with contaminated wounds. (It is generally only a precautionary measure because almost everybody today has established immunity through vaccination from an early age, and vaccination is in any case readily available for those at risk.) Administration is by intramuscular injection. It is available only on prescription.

Human Actraphane (*Novo*) is a proprietary preparation of mixed human insulins, available only on prescription, used to treat and maintain diabetic patients. Produced in vials for injection, Human Actraphane contains both isophane and neutral insulins in a ratio of 70% to 30% respectively.

✚/▲ warning/side-effects: *see* INSULIN.

H

Human Actrapid (*Novo*) is a proprietary non-prescription preparation of synthesized neutral human insulin, used to treat and maintain diabetic patients. It is produced in vials for injection, and in cartridges for use with a special injector (under the name Human Actrapid Penfill).

✚/▲ warning/side-effects: *see* INSULIN.

Human Initard 50/50 (*Nordisk Wellcome*) is a proprietary preparation of mixed human insulins, available only on prescription, used to treat and maintain diabetic patients. Produced in vials for injection, Human Initard 50/50 contains both isophane and neutral insulins in equal proportions.

✚/▲ warning/side-effects: *see* INSULIN.

Human Insulatard (*Nordisk Wellcome*) is a proprietary non-prescription preparation of human isophane insulin, used to treat and maintain diabetic patients. It is produced in vials for injection.

✚/▲ warning/side-effects: *see* INSULIN.

Human Mixtard 30/70 (*Nordisk Wellcome*) is a proprietary non-prescription preparation of mixed human insulins, used to treat and maintain diabetic patients. Produced in vials for injection, Human Mixtard contains both isophane and neutral insulins in a ratio of 70% to 30% respectively.

✚/▲ warning/side-effects: *see* INSULIN.

Human Monotard (*Novo*) is a proprietary non-prescription preparation of human insulin zinc suspension, used to treat and maintain diabetic patients. It is produced in vials for injection.

✚/▲ warning/side-effects: *see* INSULIN.

Human Protaphane (*Novo*) is a proprietary non-prescription preparation of human isophane insulin, used to treat and maintain diabetic patients. It is produced in vials for injection.

✚/▲ warning/side-effects: *see* INSULIN.

Human Ultratard (*Novo*) is a proprietary non-prescription preparation of human insulin zinc suspension, used to treat and maintain diabetic patients. It is produced in vials for injection.

✚/▲ warning/side-effects: *see* INSULIN.

Human Velosulin (*Nordisk Wellcome*) is a proprietary non-prescription preparation of synthesized neutral human insulin, used to treat and maintain diabetic patients. It is produced in vials for injection.

✚/▲ warning/side-effects: *see* INSULIN.

Humotet (*Wellcome*) is a proprietary preparation of anti-tetanus immunoglobulin (HTIG), available only on prescription, used mostly as an added precaution to treat patients with contaminated wounds. (It is generally only a precautionary measure because almost everybody today has established immunity through vaccination from an early age, and vaccination is in any case readily available for those at risk.) It is produced in vials for intramuscular injection.

Humulin I (*Lilly*) is a proprietary non-prescription preparation of human isophane insulin, used to treat and maintain diabetic patients. It is produced in vials for injection.
✚/▲ warning/side-effects: *see* INSULIN.

Humulin M1 (*Lilly*) is a proprietary non-prescription preparation of mixed human insulins, used to treat and maintain diabetic patients. Produced in vials for injection, Humulin M1 contains both isophane and neutral insulins in a ratio of 90% to 10% respectively.
✚/▲ warning/side-effects: *see* INSULIN.

Humulin M2 (*Lilly*) is a proprietary non-prescription preparation of mixed human insulins, used to treat and maintain diabetic patients. Produced in vials for injection, Humulin M2 contains both isophane and neutral insulins in a ratio of 80% to 20% respectively.
✚/▲ warning/side-effects: *see* INSULIN.

Humulin S (*Lilly*) is a proprietary non-prescription preparation of synthesized neutral human insulin, used to treat and maintain diabetic patients. It is produced in vials for injection.
✚/▲ warning/side-effects: *see* INSULIN.

Humulin Zn (*Lilly*) is a proprietary non-prescription preparation of human insulin zinc suspension, used to treat and maintain diabetic patients. It is produced in vials for injection.
✚/▲ warning/side-effects: *see* INSULIN.

Hyalase (*CP Pharmaceuticals*) is a proprietary form of the enzyme hyaluronidase, available only on prescription, used to increase the permeability of subcutaneous tissues or muscles into which drugs can be injected. It is produced in the form of a powder for reconstitution as a medium also for injection.
✚/▲ warning/side-effects: *see* HYALURONIDASE.

hyaluronidase is an enzyme that has the power to loosen the chemical bonds between certain structures within connective tissue – and is thus used to increase the permeability of subcutaneous tissues or muscles into which drugs can be injected. In this way, the resorption of excess fluid (such as blood) into the tissues can additionally be promoted. Administration of hyaluronidase is itself by injection or infusion.
✚ warning: hyaluronidase should not be administered to patients who are to receive intravenous injection, who have recently received bites or stings, or who have any kind of infection at or near the site of injection.
▲ side-effects: sometimes there are sensitivity reactions.
Related article: HYALASE.

Hycal (*Beecham*) is a proprietary non-prescription nutritional supplement intended for patients who require a high-energy low-fluid diet low in electrolytes (as with kidney or liver disease). Gluten-free, Hycal contains mostly carbohydrate in the form of corn syrup solids; it is also protein-free and lactose-, fructose- and sucrose-free, and is produced in four flavours.

Hydergine (*Sandoz*) is a proprietary form of the powerful

drug co-dergocrine mesylate, used primarily to assist in the management of elderly patients with mild to moderate dementia. Hydergine works by enhancing the oxidative capacity of cells. Available only on prescription, it is produced in the form of tablets (in two strengths), and is not recommended for children.
✚/▲ warning/side-effects: *see* CO-DERGOCRINE MESYLATE.

H

hydralazine is a VASODILATOR used to treat heart conditions both acute and chronic: acute in the form of a high blood pressure crisis (apoplexy), and chronic in the form of long-term high blood pressure (in which case simultaneous treatment is administered with a BETA-BLOCKER or a DIURETIC). Administration is oral in the form of tablets, and by injection or infusion.
✚ warning: administered by itself, hydralazine over any length of time causes an increase in the heart rate and fluid retention (oedema). Conversely, the reduction of blood pressure may be unexpectedly swift and severe, and require further treatment.
▲ side-effects: there may be nausea and vomiting. Prolonged high-dosage therapy may cause a vivid red rash.
Related article: APRESOLINE.

hydrargaphen is an ANTIMICROBIAL used in vaginal inserts (pessaries) to treat various kinds of infection in the vagina or in the womb. Treatment is usually of two pessaries nightly for a fortnight after menstruation.
✚ warning: hydrargaphen must not be used in patients who have an intrauterine device containing copper.
Related article: PENOTRANE.

Hydrea (*Squibb*) is a proprietary CYTOTOXIC drug, available only on prescription, used to treat certain forms of chronic leukaemia. It works by reacting with cellular DNA. Produced in the form of capsules, Hydrea is a preparation of hydroxyurea.
✚/▲ warning/side-effects: *see* HYDROXYUREA.

Hydrenox (*Boots*) is a proprietary DIURETIC, available only on prescription, used to treat an accumulation of fluid in the tissues (oedema) and high blood pressure (*see* ANTIHYPERTENSIVE). Produced in the form of tablets, Hydrenox is a preparation of the THIAZIDE hydroflumethiazide.
✚/▲ warning/side-effects: *see* HYDROFLUMETHIAZIDE.

hydrochlorothiazide is a THIAZIDE DIURETIC drug used to treat an accumulation of fluid in the tissues (oedema) and high blood pressure (*see* ANTIHYPERTENSIVE). Administration is oral in the form of tablets.
✚ warning: hydrochlorothiazide should not be administered to patients who suffer from urinary retention or kidney failure, or who are lactating. It should be administered with caution to those who are pregnant. It may aggravate conditions of diabetes or gout. (Potassium supplements may be required.)
▲ side-effects: there may be tiredness and a rash. In men, temporary impotence may occur. Rarely, there is a sensitivity to light.
Related articles: DYAZIDE; ESIDREX; HYDROSALURIC.

hydrocortisone is a CORTICOSTEROID hormone, a derivative of cortisone, produced and secreted by the adrenal glands. Sometimes known as cortisol, it is highly important both for the normal metabolism of carbohydrates in the diet and for the neuro-muscular response to stress. Other than to make up hormonal deficiency, hydrocortisone may be administered therapeutically to treat any kind of inflammation (sometimes in combination with ANTIBACTERIAL drugs), including arthritis, and to treat allergic conditions (especially in emergencies). Administration is in many forms.

✚/▲ warning/side-effects: prolonged or high-dosage treatment may lead to peptic ulcers, muscle disorders, bone disorders and (in children) stunting of growth. Another potential result is the onset of adult-type diabetes. In the elderly there may be brittle bones and mental disturbances, particularly depression or euphoria. In addition, treatment with the drug may suppress symptoms of an infection until the infection is far advanced (which may in some cases present its own dangers); treatment should therefore be made as aseptic as possible, and infected areas must not be treated. Withdrawal of treatment must be gradual.
Related articles: ALPHADERM; ALPHOSYL HC; BARQUINOL HC; CALMURID HC; CANESTEN HC; CHLOROMYCETIN HYDROCORTISONE; COBADEX; COLIFOAM; CORLAN; CORTACREAM; CORTENEMA; CORTUCID; DAKTACORT; DIODERM; DOME-CORT; ECONACORT; ECZEDERM WITH HYDROCORTISONE; EFCORTELAN; EFCORTELAN SOLUBLE; EFCORTESOL; EPIFOAM; EURAX-HYDROCORTISONE; FRAMYCORT; FUCIDIN H; GENTICIN HC; GREGODERM; HYDROCORTISTAB; HYDROCORTISYL; HYDROCORTONE; HYDRODERM; NEO-CORTEF; NYBADEX; NYSTAFORM-HC; QUINOCORT; QUINODERM; SENTIAL; SOLU-CORTEF; TERRA-CORTRIL; TIMODINE; VIOFORM-HYDROCORTISONE.

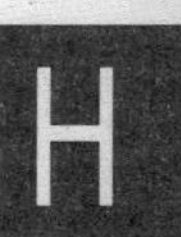

hydrocortisone acetate is a HYDROCORTISONE salt used as an ANTI-INFLAMMATORY to treat local inflammation of the joints or of the soft tissues. Produced in the form of an aqueous suspension, it is administered by injection. In the treatment of inflamed joints, injection may be into the joint itself or into the synovial capsule that acts as a shock-absorber within the joint.

✚/▲ warning/side-effects: *see* HYDROCORTISONE.
Related articles: CHLOROMYCETIN HYDROCORTISONE; CORTUCID; HYDROCORTISTAB; FRAMYCORT; NEO-CORTEF.

hydrocortisone butyrate is a HYDROCORTISONE salt used as an ANTI-INFLAMMATORY to treat severe inflammation of the skin that have failed to respond to treatment with less powerful drugs (as may occur with some forms of eczema). Administration is topical in the form of cream, ointment or lotion.

✚/▲ warning/side-effects: *see* HYDROCORTISONE.
Related article: LOCOID.

hydrocortisone sodium phosphate is a HYDROCORTISONE salt used to treat deficiency of the HORMONE hydrocortisone. Administration is by injection,

optionally diluted.
✚/▲ warning/side-effects: *see* HYDROCORTISONE.
Related article: EFCORTESOL.

hydrocortisone sodium succinate is a HYDROCORTISONE salt used primarily to treat deficiency of the HORMONE hydrocortisone, but also as an ANTI-INFLAMMATORY to treat inflammation and lesions in and around the mouth. Administration is by injection, optionally diluted, or in the form of lozenges.
✚/▲ warning/side-effects: *see* HYDROCORTISONE.
Related articles: CORLAN; EFCORTELAN SOLUBLE; SOLU-CORTEF.

Hydrocortistab (*Boots*) is a proprietary ANTI-INFLAMMATORY drug, available only on prescription, in which the active constituent is the CORTICOSTEROID hormone hydrocortisone. Produced in the form of tablets and in vials for injection, Hydrocortistab is used to treat inflammation in rheumatic or collagen disorders and in allergic conditions. Produced in the form of a cream and an ointment, Hydrocortistab is used to treat severe skin inflammations, such as eczema and various forms of dermatitis.
✚/▲ warning/side-effects: *see* HYDROCORTISONE.

Hydrocortisyl (*Roussel*) is a proprietary ANTI-INFLAMMATORY drug, available only on prescription, in which the active constituent is the corticosteroid hormone hydrocortisone. Produced in the form of a cream and an ointment, Hydrocortisyl is used to treat severe skin inflammations, such as eczema and various forms of dermatitis.
✚/▲ warning/side-effects: *see* HYDROCORTISONE.

Hydrocortone (*Merck, Sharp & Dohme*) is a proprietary form of the CORTICOSTEROID hormone hydrocortisone, used to make up hormonal deficiency and to treat inflammation, shock, and certain allergic conditions. Available only on prescription, Hydrocortone is produced in the form of tablets (in two strengths).
✚/▲ warning/side-effects: *see* HYDROCORTISONE.

Hydroderm (*Merck, Sharp& Dohme*) is a proprietary ANTI-INFLAMMATORY and ANTIBACTERIAL compound, available only on prescription, used to treat skin inflammation in which infection is thought to be present. It is produced in the form of an ointment for topical application, and contains the CORTICOSTEROID hormone hydrocortisone with the powerful ANTIBIOTICS neomycin sulphate and bacitracin zinc, within an emollient base.
✚/▲ warning/side-effects: *see* HYDROCORTISONE; NEOMYCIN.

hydroflumethiazide is a DIURETIC drug used primarily to treat an accumulation of fluid in the tissues (oedema) and high blood pressure (*see* ANTIHYPERTENSIVE). In combination with the weaker diuretic spironolactone (which helps to replace lost potassium), it may be used also to treat congestive heart failure.
✚ warning: hydroflumethiazide should not be administered to patients who suffer from urinary retention or kidney failure, or who are lactating. It should be administered with caution to those who are pregnant. It may aggravate conditions of diabetes or gout. (In treatment with hydroflumethiazide alone, potassium supplements may be required.)
▲ side-effects: there may be

tiredness and a rash. In men, temporary impotence may occur.
Related articles: ALDACTIDE 50; HYDRENOX.

hydrogen peroxide is a general DISINFECTANT used in solution and as a cream to cleanse and deodorize wounds and ulcers, to clean ears in the form of ear-drops, and as a mouth wash and gargle for oral hygiene. Some preparations available require further dilution: a 6% solution is the maximum concentration recommended for use on the skin. Solutions stronger will bleach fabric.
Related article: HIOXYL.

Hydromet (*Merck, Sharp & Dohme*) is a proprietary ANTIHYPERTENSIVE compound, available only on prescription, used to treat moderate to very high blood pressure. Produced in the form of tablets, Hydromet consists of the powerful drug methyldopa (which acts directly on the central nervous system but may cause fluid retention) with the THIAZIDE hydrochlorothiazide (which has complementary DIURETIC properties).
✚/▲ warning/side-effects: *see* HYDROCHLOROTHIAZIDE; METHYLDOPA.

HydroSaluric (*Merck, Sharp & Dohme*) is a proprietary DIURETIC, available only on prescription, used to treat an accumulation of fluid within the tissues (oedema) and high blood pressure (*see* ANTIHYPERTENSIVE). Produced in the form of tablets (in two strengths), HydroSaluric is a preparation of the THIAZIDE hydrochlorothiazide.
✚/▲ warning/side-effects: *see* HYDROCHLOROTHIAZIDE.

hydrotalcite is an ANTACID complex that is readily dissociated internally for rapid relief of dyspepsia, and has deflatulent properties. Administration is oral in the form of tablets that can be chewed, or in suspension. It is not recommended for children aged under 6 years.
Related article: ALTACITE.

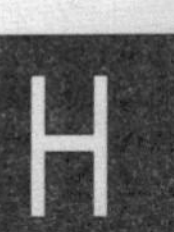

hydrous wool fat ointment, or lanolin, is a greasy preparation of hydrous wool fat in a yellow soft paraffin base. It is used as a protective barrier cream on cracked, dry or thin skin, encourages hydration, and has mild ANTI-INFLAMMATORY properties.
✚ warning: some people are sensitive to wool fat preparations; for them, local reaction may be comparatively severe.

hydroxocobalamin is a form of VITAMIN B_{12} that has recently replaced CYANOCOBALAMIN as the version of the vitamin for therapeutic use. Supplements of vitamin B_{12} are administered only by injection (because vitamin B_{12} deficiency arises most often through malabsorption, which renders oral administration futile), and hydroxocobalamin can be retained in the body for more than 3 months following injection – far longer than the formerly standard preparation. This factor is particularly significant in that treatment, once begun, is usually for life.
Related articles: COBALIN-H; LIPOFLAVONOID; NEO-CYTAMEN.

hydroxychloroquine sulphate is a drug used primarily to treat rheumatoid arthritis and forms of the skin disease lupus erythematosus, but also to prevent and treat malaria. Its treatment of rheumatic disease is effective, but may take up to 6 months to become so; then, the drug improves not only inflammation in the joints but assists circulatory problems and halts erosion of bone surfaces. Because it takes such a time to have such an effect, other forms of treatment are generally tried first – but treatment must be begun before joint damage is irreversible.

✚ warning: hydroxychloroquine sulphate should not be administered to patients who have defects or disease in the retina of the eye (in prolonged courses of treatment the drug may be toxic to the eyes), who are known to be sensitive to quinine, or who are already taking drugs containing gold (for rheumatism). It should be administered with caution to those who are pregnant, elderly, or young; or who suffer from impaired liver or kidney function, psoriasis, porphyria, or severe gastrointestinal disorder.

▲ side-effects: there may be visual disturbances – ophthalmic monitoring is essential throughout treatment to avoid permanent damage. There may also be gastrointestinal disturbances, headache, hair loss, ringing in the ears (tinnitus) and/or skin reactions. Rarely, there are blood disorders, sensitivity to light, or even psychological disturbances.
Related article: PLAQUENIL.

hydroxyprogesterone hexanoate is a PROGESTOGEN used primarily to prevent a miscarriage in a pregnant woman with a history of miscarriages. Administration is by intramuscular injection once a week for the first half of the pregnancy.

✚ warning: hydroxyprogesterone hexanoate should not be administered to patients with vaginal haemorrhage or cancer of the breast, or who have a history of thrombosis; it should be administered with caution to those who are diabetic, who have heart, liver or kidney disease, who suffer from high blood pressure (hypertension), or who are lactating.

▲ side-effects: there may be tenderness of the breasts and menstrual disorders, skin conditions such as acne and urticaria, gastrointestinal disturbances, and weight gain through the accumulation of fluid in the tissues (oedema). Rarely, there is pain at the site of injection.
Related article: PROLUTON DEPOT.

hydroxyurea is a CYTOTOXIC drug used to treat certain forms of chronic leukaemia. It works by reacting with cellular DNA. Administration is oral in the form of capsules.

✚ warning: like all cytotoxic drugs, hydroxyurea may cause life- threatening toxicity: dosage must be the minimum possible still to be effective. The major toxic effect is to suppress the blood-forming function of the bone-marrow.

▲ side-effects: there is commonly nausea and vomiting (which may be separately treated); there may also be skin reactions and hair loss.
Related article: HYDREA.

hydroxyzine hydrochloride is an ANXIOLYTIC drug, an ANTIHISTAMINE used to treat anxiety in association with skin disorders diagnosed to be caused by stress. It can also be used for either purpose singly.

Administration is oral in the form of tablets or as a syrup.

✚ warning: hydroxyzine hydrochloride should not be administered to patients who are pregnant or who are alcoholic; all patients should be warned prior to treatment that their speed of thought and reaction may be impaired by treatment.

▲ side-effects: drowsiness is fairly common; there is sometimes also neural dysfunction and, with high doses, involuntary movements. *Related article*: ATARAX.

Hygroton (*Geigy*) is a proprietary DIURETIC, available only on prescription, used to treat an accumulation of fluid within the tissues (oedema) and high blood pressure (*see* ANTIHYPERTENSIVE). Produced in the form of tablets (in two strengths), Hygroton is a preparation of the THIAZIDE-like drug chlorthalidone.

✚/▲ warning/side-effects: *see* CHLORTHALIDONE.

Hygroton-K (*Geigy*) is a proprietary DIURETIC, available only on prescription, used to treat an accumulation of fluid within the tissues (oedema) and high blood pressure (*see* ANTIHYPERTENSIVE). Produced in the form of sustained-release tablets, Hygroton-K is a compound preparation of the THIAZIDE-like drug chlorthalidone with the potassium supplement POTASSIUM CHLORIDE.

✚/▲ warning/side-effects: *see* CHLORTHALIDONE.

hyoscine, also known as scopolamine (in the USA), is a powerful alkaloid drug derived from plants of the belladonna family. By itself it is an effective SEDATIVE and HYPNOTIC – it is often used together with the OPIATE PAPAVERETUM as a premedication prior to surgery – and an ANTI-EMETIC (in which capacity it is found in travel-sickness medications). In the form of its bromide salts, hyoscine has additional ANTISPASMODIC properties without the side-effects usually associated with other antispasmodic drugs that directly affect the central nervous system (and is thus particularly useful in treating disorders of the muscular walls of the stomach and intestines, or during labour). It is also used (in solution) in ophthalmic treatments to paralyse the muscles of the pupil of the eye either for surgery or to rest the eye following surgery. Administration is oral in the form of tablets, by injection, or as eye-drops.

✚ warning: hyoscine (or its bromide salts) should not be administered to patients with glaucoma; it should be administered with caution to those with heart or intestinal disease, or urinary retention, or who are elderly.

▲ side-effects: there may be drowsiness, dizziness and dry mouth; sometimes there is also blurred vision and difficulty in urinating. *Related articles:* BUSCOPAN; OMNOPON-SCOPOLAMINE.

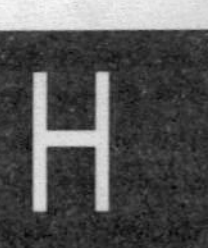

Hypal 2 (*Smith & Nephew*) is a proprietary form of synthetic, permeable, adhesive, surgical tape used to bind up patients known to be sensitive to ordinary types of tape. It is produced in three widths.

Hypercal is an ANTIHYPERTENSIVE drug consisting of Rauwolfia alkaloids – derivatives of the plant Rauwolfia serpentina – which act by depressing certain functions of the central nervous

system. It is used to treat high blood pressure (hypertension). Available only on prescription, Hypercal is produced in the form of tablets.
✚/▲ warning/side-effects: *see* RAUWOLFIA ALKALOIDS.

H

Hypercal-B is an ANTIHYPERTENSIVE drug consisting of Rauwolfia alkaloids – derivatives of the plant Rauwolfia serpentina (which act by depressing certain functions of the central nervous system) – together with the BARBITURATE amylobarbitone. Accordingly, it may be used to treat high blood pressure (hypertension), although because it contains a barbiturate it is on the controlled drugs list and its use is becoming rare. It is produced in the form of tablets.
✚/▲ warning/side-effects: *see* AMYLOBARBITONE; RAUWOLFIA ALKALOIDS.

Hypnomidate (*Janssen*) is a proprietary general ANAESTHETIC used primarily for initial induction of anaesthesia. Available only on prescription, it is produced in ampoules for injection (in two strengths, the stronger for dilution), and is a preparation of etomidate. It should not be allowed to come into contact with plastic equipment.
✚/▲ warning/side-effects: *see* ETOMIDATE.

***hypnotics** are a type of drug that induce sleep by direct action on various centres of the brain. They are used mainly to treat insomnia, and to calm patients who are mentally ill. Best known and most used hynotics are the BENZODIAZEPINES (such as diazepam and nitrazepam), which are for several reasons safer than using derivatives of chloral (such as chloral hydrate) or the BARBITURATES (such as amylobarbitone) which may cause dependence (addiction). Some cause a hangover effect on waking in the mornings.

Hypnovel is a proprietary preparation of the powerful BENZODIAZEPINE midazolam, available only on prescription, used mainly for sedation, particularly as a premedication prior to surgery, for the initial induction of anaesthesia, or for the short-term anaesthesia required for endoscopy or minor surgical examinations. Its effect is often accompanied by a form of amnesia. It is produced in ampoules for infusion (in two strengths).

***hypoglycaemic** drugs reduce the levels of glucose (sugar) in the bloodstream, and are used mainly in the treatment of diabetes mellitus of adult onset, when there is still some residual capacity in the pancreas for the production of INSULIN. The major type of hypoglycaemic drug is provided by the SULPHONYLUREAS (such as CHLORPROPAMIDE and GLIBENCLAMIDE), but the biguanide metformin hydrochloride is effective, as is the administration in quantity of GUAR GUM.

Hypon (*Calmic*) is a proprietary non-prescription compound ANALGESIC preparation that is not available from the National Health Service. Produced in the form of tablets, Hypon is a combination of aspirin, the stimulant caffeine, and the OPIATE codeine phosphate. It is not recommended for children.
✚/▲ warning/side-effects: *see* ASPIRIN; CAFFEINE; CODEINE PHOSPHATE.

Hypotears (*Cooper Vision*) is a

proprietary non-prescription compound of polyethylene glycol with POLYVINYL ALCOHOL, used to supplement the film of tears over the eye when the mucus that normally constitutes that film is intermittent or missing through disease or disorder. It is produced in the form of drops to be used every 3 to 4 hours (or as required).

***hypotensive** is a term used similarly to antihypertensive. *see* ANTIHYPERTENSIVE.

Hypovase (*Pfizer*) is a proprietary ANTIHYPERTENSIVE drug, available only on prescription, used to treat both high blood pressure (hypertension) and congestive heart failure. Produced in the form of tablets (in four strengths), Hypovase is a preparation of prazosin hydrochloride, which acts only on the muscles of the smaller arteries. It is not recommended for children.
✚/▲ warning/side-effects: *see* PRAZOSIN.

Hypurin Isophane (*CP Pharmaceuticals*) is a proprietary non-prescription preparation of highly purified beef isophane insulin, used to treat and maintain diabetic patients. It is produced in vials for injection.
✚/▲ warning/side-effects: *see* INSULIN.

Hypurin Lente (*CP Pharmaceuticals*) is a proprietary non- prescription preparation of highly purified beef INSULIN zinc suspension, used to treat and maintain diabetic patients. It is produced in vials for injection.
✚/▲ warning/side-effects: *see* INSULIN.

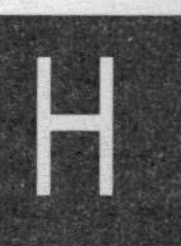

Hypurin Neutral (*CP Pharmaceuticals*) is a proprietary non- prescription preparation of highly purified beef neutral insulin, used to treat and maintain diabetic patients. It is produced in vials for injection.
✚/▲ warning/side-effects: *see* INSULIN.

Hypurin Protamine Zinc (*CP Pharmaceuticals*) is a proprietary non-prescription preparation of highly purified beef protamine zinc insulin, used to treat and maintain diabetic patients. It is produced in vials for injection.
✚/▲ warning/side-effects: *see* INSULIN.

Hypurin Soluble Insulin (*CP Pharmaceuticals*) is a proprietary non-prescription preparation of highly purified beef soluble insulin, used to treat and maintain diabetic patients. It is produced in vials for injection.
✚/▲ warning/side-effects: *see* INSULIN.

Ibular (*Lagap*) is a proprietary ANTI-INFLAMMATORY non-narcotic ANALGESIC, available only on prescription, used to treat the pain of rheumatic and other musculo-skeletal disorders. Produced in the form of tablets, Ibular is a preparation of ibuprofen.
✚/▲ warning/side-effects: *see* IBUPROFEN.

Ibumetin (*Benzon*) is a proprietary ANTI-INFLAMMATORY non-narcotic ANALGESIC, available only on prescription, used to treat the pain of rheumatic and other musculo-skeletal disorders, and menstrual pain (dysmenorrhoea). Produced in the form of tablets (in three strengths), Ibumetin is a preparation of ibuprofen. It is not recommended for children.
✚/▲ warning/side-effects: *see* IBUPROFEN.

ibuprofen is a non-steroid ANTI-INFLAMMATORY non-narcotic ANALGESIC drug used primarily to treat the pain of rheumatism and other musculo-skeletal disorders, but also used sometimes to treat other forms of pain, including menstrual pain (dysmenorrhoea). In its anti-inflammatory capacity it is not as powerful as many other drugs, however, and dosage tends to be high to compensate. Administration is oral in the form of tablets or sustained-release capsules, or as a syrup.
✚ warning: ibuprofen should be administered with caution to patients with impaired liver or kidney function, gastric ulcers, or severe allergies (including asthma), or who are pregnant.
▲ side-effects: administration with or following meals reduces the risk of gastrointestinal disturbance and nausea. But there may be headache, dizziness and ringing in the ears (tinnitus), and some patients experience sensitivity reactions or blood disorders. Occasionally, there is fluid retention.
Related articles: APSIFEN; BRUFEN; EBUFAC; FENBID; IBULAR; IBUMETIN; MOTRIN; PAXOFEN.

Ichthaband (*Seton*) is a proprietary form of bandaging impregnated with ZINC PASTE (15%) and ichthammol (2%), used to treat and dress chronic forms of eczema.
✚/▲ warning/side-effects: *see* ICHTHAMMOL.

ichthammol is a thick, dark brown liquid derived from bituminous oils, used for its mildly ANTISEPTIC properties in ointments or in glycerol solution for the topical treatment of ulcers and inflammation on the skin. Milder than COAL TAR, ichthammol is useful in treating the less severe forms of eczema. A popular mode of administration is in an impregnated bandage with ZINC PASTE.
✚ warning: ichthammol must not be placed in contact with broken skin surfaces.
▲ side-effects: some patients experience skin irritation; the skin may become sensitized.
Related articles: ICHTHABAND; ICHTHOPASTE.

Ichthopaste (*Smith & Nephew*) is a proprietary form of bandaging impregnated with ZINC PASTE (6%) and ichthammol (2%), used to treat and dress chronic forms of eczema.
✚/▲ warning/side-effects: *see* ICHTHAMMOL.

Idoxene (*Spodefell*) is a proprietary ANTIBIOTIC eye ointment, available only on prescription, used to treat local viral infections, particularly of

herpes simplex. It is a solute preparation of idoxuridine.
✚ warning: see IDOXURIDINE.

idoxuridine is an ANTIVIRAL drug used primarily in very mild solution to treat viral infections (such as herpes simplex) in and around the mouth or eye. In a solution of dimethyl sulphoxide, however, it is alternatively used to treat herpes zoster skin infections. It works by inhibiting the growth of the viruses. Administration is as a paint for topical application, as eye-drops or as eye ointment.
✚ warning: because idoxuridine contains iodine, treatment may cause initial irritation and/or stinging.
Related articles: HERPID; IDOXENE; IDURIDIN; KERECID; Ophthalmadine.

Iduridin (*Ferring*) is a proprietary ANTIVIRAL drug, available only on prescription, used to treat infections of the skin by herpes simplex (cold sores, fever sores) or by herpes zoster (shingles). Produced in the form of a lotion or paint, for topical application either with a dropper or its own applicator, Iduridin is a solution of idoxuridine in the organic solvent dimethyl sulphoxide (DMSO).
✚ warning: see IDOXURIDINE.

ifosfamide is a CYTOTOXIC drug used to treat cancers, especially sarcomas, lymphomas, and cancer of the testicles. It works by interfering with cellular DNA, thus inhibiting cell replication. Administration is by injection or infusion, often simultaneously with the synthetic drug MESNA which reduces the toxic side-effects (and particularly prevents cystitis).
✚ warning: prolonged treatment may cause sterility in men and an early menopause in women; prolonged treatment has also been associated with the incidence of leukaemia following simultaneous irradiation treatment. Blood count monitoring is essential. Dosage should be the minimum still to be effective.
▲ side-effects: cystitis, leading to blood in the urine, is not uncommon (unless mesna is administered simultaneously). There may also be nausea and vomiting, and hair loss.
Related article: MITOXANA.

Iliadin-Mini (*Merck*) is a proprietary non-prescription form of nose-drops that is not available from the National Health Service. Used as a nasal DECONGESTANT, Iliadin-Mini is a preparation of the SYMPATHOMIMETIC drug oxymetazoline hydrochloride, and is produced in two strengths (the weaker under the name Iliadin-Mini Paediatric).
✚/▲ warning/side-effects: *see* OXYMETAZOLINE.

Ilonium (*Ilon*) is a proprietary non-prescription OINTMENT made to treat boils and other pus-containing septic sores. In a turpentine, wax and wool fat base, active constituents include the soothing antiseptics phenol and thymol.
✚ warning: keep away from the eyes and from mucous membranes.

Ilosone (*Dista*) is a proprietary macrolide ANTIBIOTIC, available only on prescription, used to treat many serious infections (such as legionnaires' disease and inflammation of the prostate gland) and to prevent others (such as diphtheria or whooping cough), but more commonly used in the treatment of infections of

the upper respiratory tract or of infected wounds, especially in patients who are allergic to penicillin-type antibiotics. Produced in the form of capsules, tablets, and as a suspension (in two strengths, the stronger under the name Ilosone Suspension Forte) for dilution (the potency of the suspension once dilute is retained for 14 days), Ilosone in every form is a preparation of erythromycin estolate.
✚/▲ warning/side-effects: *see* ERYTHROMYCIN.

Ilotycin (*Lilly*) is a proprietary macrolide ANTIBIOTIC, available only on prescription, used to treat many serious infections (such as legionnaires' disease and inflammation of the prostate gland) and to prevent others (such as diphtheria or whooping cough), especially in patients who are allergic to penicillin-type antibiotics. Produced in the form of tablets, Ilotycin is a preparation of erythromycin estolate.
✚/▲ warning/side-effects: *see* ERYTHROMYCIN.

Ilube (*Duncan Flockhart*) is a proprietary preparation of the mucolytic agent acetylcysteine, available only on prescription, used to treat a deficiency of tears in the eyes – a deficiency that can lead to eye dryness and inflammation. It works by breaking down mucus around the eye into a film of tears. Administered as eye-drops, Ilube also contains a small proportion of the synthetic tear fluid hypromellose.
✚/▲ warning/side-effects: *see* ACETYLCYSTEINE.

Imbrilon (*Berk*) is a proprietary ANTI-INFLAMMATORY non-narcotic ANALGESIC, available only on prescription, used to treat the pain of rheumatic and other musculo-skeletal disorders (including gout). Produced in the form of capsules (in two strengths), and as anal suppositories, Imbrilon is a preparation of indomethacin. It is not recommended for children.
✚/▲ warning/side-effects: *see* INDOMETHACIN.

Imferon (*CP Pharmaceuticals*) is a proprietary preparation of IRON and DEXTRAN, a nutritive plasma-and-iron supplement administered in infusion or by injection to patients who are in need of substantial replacement of both, and who, perhaps because of malabsorption, cannot be given iron orally. Administration by infusion is slow – over 6 to 8 hours.
✚ warning: stringent tests must first be carried out to ensure that the patient will not suffer any allergic reaction: if hypersensitivity reactions do occur, they are usually violent. For this reason, treatment by infusion must be supervised throughout and for a time afterwards; there must also be full facilities for emergency cardio-respiratory resuscitation immediately available. Imferon should not be administered to patients with severe disease of the kidneys or liver, and should not be administered by infusion to asthmatic patients.

***imidazoles** are a group of ANTIFUNGAL drugs active against most fungi and yeasts. The most common conditions that they are used to treat are vaginal infections (such as candidiasis, or thrush) and infections of the skin surface and mucous membranes, the hair and the nails. Best known and most used imidazoles include clotrimazole, miconazole,

ketoconazole and econazole.
see CLOTRIMAZOLE; ECONAZOLE; KETOCONAZOLE; MICONAZOLE.

imipramine is an ANTIDEPRESSANT drug of a type that has fewer sedative properties than many others. It is thus suited more to the treatment of withdrawn and apathetic patients than to those who are agitated and restless. As is the case with many such drugs, imipramine can also be used to treat bedwetting at night by children (aged over 7 years). Administration is oral in the form of tablets or as a syrup, or by injection.

✚ warning: imipramine should not be administered to patients with heart disease or liver failure; it should be administered with extreme caution to those who suffer from epilepsy, psychoses or glaucoma, or who are pregnant. Treatment may take up to four weeks to achieve full effect; premature withdrawal of treatment thereafter may cause the return of symptoms.

▲ side-effects: dry mouth, drowsiness, blurred vision, constipation and urinary retention are all fairly common; there may also be heartbeat irregularities accompanying low blood pressure (hypotension). Concentration and speed of reaction are affected. Elderly patients may enter a state of confusion; younger patients may experience behavioural disturbances. There may be alteration in blood sugar levels, and weight gain. Rarely, there is a black tongue, convulsions, or a more serious change in the composition of the blood.
Related articles: PRAMINIL; TOFRANIL.

***immunization** against specific diseases is effected by either of two means. Active immunity is conferred by vaccination, in which live antigens that have been rendered harmless (attenuated) or dead ones (inactivated) are injected into the bloodstream so that the body's own defence mechanisms are required to deal with them (by manufacturing antibodies) and with anything like them that they encounter again. This method gives long-lasting but impermanent protection (and there is a slight risk of allergic reaction or toxic effect). Passive immunity is conferred by the injection of a quantity of blood serum already containing antibodies (immunoglobulins); this method gives immediate and permanent protection.
see IMMUNOGLOBULINS; VACCINES.

***immunoglobulins** are proteins of a specific structure, which act as antibodies in the bloodstream. Created in response to the presence of a specific antigen, immunoglobulins circulate with the blood to give systemic defence and protection as part of the immune system. (A lack of such a response may constitute the basis of an allergy.) Classified according to a differentiation of class and function, immunoglobulins may be administered therapeutically by injection or infusion to confer immediate (passive) immunity.
see IMMUNIZATION.
Related article: HNIG.

***immunostimulants** are used to treat the presence of malignant fluids inside body cavities. A preparation of inactivated bacteria of the species Corynebacterium parvum, for example, may be injected into the lung (pleural) cavity of the chest

or the abdominal (peritoneal) cavity to treat the presence of such fluids (effusions) there. The effect is to increase the local effect of antibacterial activity by the immune system.
Related article: COPARVAX.

I

***immunosuppressants** are drugs used to inhibit the body's resistance to the presence of infection or foreign bodies. In this capacity, such drugs may be used to suppress tissue rejection following donor grafting or transplant surgery (although there is then the risk of unopposed infection). But immunosupressant drugs are even more commonly used in a different capacity – to treat auto-immune disease (when the body's immune system is for some reason triggered into its defence mode against part of the body itself). And in this respect, immunosuppressant drugs may be used to treat cancers or disorders such as rheumatoid arthritis or lupus erythematosus. Best known and most used among immunosuppressants administered both for tissue rejection prevention and to treat auto-immune disease are the non-steroids azathioprine, chlorambucil, cyclophosphamide, methotrexate and cyclosporin, and all the CORTICOSTEROID drugs.
see AZATHIOPRINE; CHLORAMBUCIL; CYCLOPHOSPHAMIDE; CYCLOSPORIN; METHOTREXATE.

Imodium (*Janssen*) is a proprietary ANTIDIARRHOEAL drug, available only on prescription, which works by reducing the speed at which material travels along the intestines. Produced in the form of capsules, and as a syrup, Imodium is a preparation of the OPIATE loperamide hydrochloride. It is not recommended for children aged under 4 years.
✚/▲ warning/side-effects: *see* LOPERAMIDE HYDROCHLORIDE.

Imperacin (*ICI*) is a proprietary broad-spectrum ANTIBIOTIC, available only on prescription, used to treat serious infections by bacteria and other microorganisms (such as chlamydia and rickettsia), and to relieve severe acne. Produced in the form of tablets, Imperacin is a preparation of the tetracycline oxytetracycline dihydrate. It is not recommended for children.
✚/▲ warning/side-effects: *see* OXYTETRACYCLINE.

Imunovir (*Burgess*) is a proprietary preparation of the ANTIVIRAL drug inosine pranobex, available only on prescription, used to treat herpes simplex infections and warts in mucous membranes and adjacent skin, particularly in or on the genitalia. It is produced in the form of tablets.
✚/▲ warning/side-effects: *see* INOSINE PRANOBEX.

Imuran (*Wellcome*) is a proprietary preparation of the CYTOTOXIC drug azathioprine, used to suppress tissue rejection following donor grafting or transplant surgery, particularly in cases where corticosteroids have already been used excessively and/or failed to be fully effective. Available only on prescription, Imuran is produced in the form of tablets (in two strengths), and as a powder for reconstitution as a medium for injection.
✚/▲ warning/side-effects: *see* AZATHIOPRINE.

indapamide is a DIURETIC, a THIAZIDE-like compound used to treat high blood pressure (*see* ANTIHYPERTENSIVE). It works not so much as a vasodilator but as a vasorelaxant, relaxing the walls of blood vessels, and is claimed to be especially beneficial to patients with diabetes mellitus. Administration is oral in the form of tablets.

✚ warning: indapamide should not be administered to patients with impaired kidney or liver function, and should be administered with caution to those who are pregnant. Its proprietary form is not recommended for children.

▲ side-effects: there may be nausea and a headache; slight weight loss is to be expected. *Related article:* NATRILIX.

Inderal (*ICI*) is a proprietary BETA-BLOCKER, available only on prescription, used to prevent the recurrence of a heart attack (myocardial infarction), to promote regularity of the heartbeat, and to treat enlargement of the heart. Produced in the form of tablets (in three strengths), and in ampoules for injection, Inderal is a preparation of propranolol hydrochloride.

✚/▲ warning/side-effects: *see* PROPRANOLOL.

Inderal-LA (*ICI*) is a proprietary BETA-BLOCKER, available only on prescription, used to treat angina pectoris (heart pain), the symptoms of the congenital heart disorder Fallot's tetralogy, high blood pressure (hypertension) and anxiety; to try to prevent migraine attacks; and to assist in the treatment of excess thyroid hormones in the blood (thyrotoxicosis). Produced in the form of sustained-release capsules (in two strengths, the weaker under the name Half-Inderal LA), and as tablets (in four strengths), Inderal-LA is a preparation of propranolol hydrochloride. In the treatment of most of the disorders listed above, Inderal-LA is not recommended for children.

✚ /▲warning/side-effects: *see* PROPRANOLOL.

Inderetic (*ICI*) is a proprietary ANTIHYPERTENSIVE drug, available only on prescription, used to treat mild to moderate high blood pressure (hypertension). Produced in the form of capsules, Inderetic is a preparation that combines the BETA-BLOCKER propranolol hydrochloride with the THIAZIDE DIURETIC bendrofluazide. It is not recommended for children.

✚ /▲warning/side-effects: *see* BENDROFLUAZIDE; PROPRANOLOL.

Inderex (*ICI*) is a proprietary ANTIHYPERTENSIVE drug, available only on prescription, used to treat mild to moderate high blood pressure (hypertension). Produced in the form of sustained- release capsules, Inderex is a preparation that combines the beta-blocker propranolol hydrochloride with the THIAZIDE diuretic bendrofluazide. It is not recommended for children.

✚ /▲warning/side-effects: *see* BENDROFLUAZIDE; PROPRANOLOL.

Indian hemp is the name of the plant from which the psychedelic drug cannabis is prepared. *see* CANNABIS.

Indocid (*Morson*) is a proprietary ANTI-INFLAMMATORY non-narcotic analgesic, available only on prescription, used to treat the pain of rheumatic and other musculo-skeletal disorders (including gout and degenerative bone diseases). Produced in the form of capsules (in two strengths), and as sustained-release capsules (under the name

Indocid-R), as anal suppositories, and as a sugar-free suspension, Indocid is a preparation of indomethacin. It is not recommended for children.
✚/▲ warning/side-effects: *see* INDOMETHACIN.

Indoflex (*Unimed*) is a proprietary anti-inflammatory ANALGESIC, available only on prescription, used to treat the pain of rheumatic and other musculo-skeletal disorders (including gout and degenerative bone diseases). Produced in the form of capsules, Indoflex is a preparation of indomethacin. It is not recommended for children.
✚/▲ warning/side-effects: *see* INDOMETHACIN.

Indolar (*Lagap*) is a proprietary ANTI-INFLAMMATORY non-narcotic ANALGESIC, available only on prescription, used to treat the pain of rheumatic and other musculo-skeletal disorders (including gout and degenerative bone diseases). Produced in the form of capsules (in two strengths), as sustained-release capsules (under the name Indolar SR), and as anal suppositories, Indolar is a preparation of indomethacin.
✚/▲ warning/side-effects: *see* INDOMETHACIN.

indomethacin is a non-steroidal ANTI-INFLAMMATORY non-narcotic ANALGESIC drug used to treat rheumatic and muscular pain caused by inflammation and/or bone degeneration particularly at the joints. Administration is mostly oral in the form of tablets, capsules, sustained-release capsules or as a liquid, but its use in anal suppositories is especially effective for the relief of pain overnight and stiffness in the morning. Some proprietary preparations are not recommended for children.
✚ warning: indomethacin should not be administered to patients who suffer from peptic ulcers or who are sensitive to aspirin. It should be administered with caution to those who suffer from allergic conditions (such as asthma), from epilepsy, from psychological disturbances, or from impaired function of the liver or kidneys, who are elderly, or who are pregnant. Blood counts and ophthalmic checks are advised during prolonged treatment. Suppositories should not be used by patients with anorectal infections or piles (haemorrhoids).
▲ side-effects: all drugs of this type are prone to give gastro-intestinal discomfort. During treatment, concentration and speed of reaction may be affected; there may also be headache and dizziness, although further mental effects (including depression and confusion) are rare. Some patients experience ringing in the ears (tinnitus) blood disorders, and high blood pressure (hypertension). There may be visual disturbances, tingling in the toes and fingertips and (following the use of suppositories) anal itching.
Related articles: ARTRACIN; IMBRILON; INDOCID; INDOFLEX; Indolar; INDOMOD; MOBILAN; RHEUMACIN LA; SLO-INDO.

Indomod (*Benzon*) is a proprietary ANTI-INFLAMMATORY non-narcotic ANALGESIC, available only on prescription, used to treat the pain of rheumatic and other musculo-skeletal disorders (including gout, bursitis and tendonitis). Produced in the form of sustained-release capsules (in

two strengths), Indomod is a preparation of indomethacin. It is not recommended for children.
✚/▲ warning/side-effects: *see* INDOMETHACIN.

indoramin is an ANTIHYPERTENSIVE drug, used usually in combination with a THIAZIDE diuretic or a BETA-BLOCKER to treat high blood pressure (hypertension). It works by selective vasodilation of the arteries. Administration is oral in the form of tablets.
✚ warning: indoramin should not be administered to patients who suffer well-established heart failure; it should be administered with caution to those with impaired kidney or liver function, parkinsonism or epilepsy, or who are elderly. Concentration and speed of reaction may be affected.
▲ side-effects: there is usually drowsiness and dizziness; there may also be dry mouth and nasal congestion. Some patients experience depression.
Related article: BARATOL.

***influenza vaccines** are recommended only for persons at high risk of catching known strains of influenza. This is because the influenza viruses A and B are constantly changing in physical form, and antibodies manufactured in the body to deal with one strain at one time will have no effect at all on the same strain at another time. Consequently, it is only possible to provide vaccine for any single strain once it has already shown itself to be endemic. Moreover, during times when no influenza strain is endemic, vaccination against influenza is positively discouraged. The World Health Organization makes an annual recommendation on the strains of virus for which stocks of vaccine should be prepared.
Administration is by injection of surface-antigen vaccine: a single dose for adults (unless the specific strain is in the process of changing again and two slightly different doses are required), two doses over 5 weeks or so for children.
Related articles: FLUVIRIN; INFLUVAC SUB-UNIT; MFV-JECT.

Influvac Sub-unit (*Duphar*) is the name of a series of proprietary flu vaccines consisting of inactivated surface antigens of the influenza virus. None is recommended for children aged under 4 years.
✚ warning: like any flu vaccine, Influvac Sub-unit cannot control epidemics and should be used only – in what seems to be the appropriate strain – to treat people who are at high risk: the elderly, patients with cardiovascular problems, and medical staff. Influvac Sub-unit should not be administered to patients who are allergic to egg or chicken protein (in which vaccine viruses are cultured), or who are pregnant.
▲ side-effects: rarely, there is local reaction together with headache and high temperature.

***inhalations** of steaming vapours, whether or not they contain volatile substances such as menthol or eucalyptus, are useful in combating nasal congestion (rhinitis, sinusitis) and bronchitis chiefly (if not solely) because they encourage the breathing in of warm, moist air.

Initard 50/50 (*Nordisk Wellcome*) is a proprietary non-prescription preparation of mixed pork insulins used to treat and maintain diabetic patients.

Produced in vials for injection, Initard 50/50 contains both neutral and isophane insulins in equal proportions.

✚/▲ warning/side-effects: *see* INSULIN.

Initard 50/50, Human *see* HUMAN INITARD 50/50.

Innovace (*Merck, Sharp & Dohme*) is a proprietary preparation of the ANTIHYPERTENSIVE drug enalapril maleate, used to treat all forms of high blood pressure (hypertension), and to assist in the treatment of congestive heart failure. Produced in the form of tablets (in four strengths), it is not recommended for children.

✚/▲ warning/side-effects: *see* ENALAPRIL.

inosine pranobex is a drug introduced relatively recently, used primarily to treat herpes simplex infections in mucous membranes and adjacent skin, particularly in or on the genitalia; it is also effective in removing warts in similar areas. Administered in the form of tablets, it works partly by increasing the local activity of the body's own immune system.

✚ warning: inosine pranobex should not be administered to patients with impaired kidney function or high blood levels of uric acid (as with gout).

▲ side-effects: uric acid levels rise in the blood and in the urine.

Related article: IMUNOVIR.

inositol is a compound substance resembling a type of sugar. Present in many foods, particularly in cereals, it is sometimes classified as a member of the vitamin B complex – but unlike true vitamins it can be synthesized in the bodies of most animals, and there is no evidence that it is in any way vital to human life and metabolism. Therapeutically, it is used only in combination with the genuine vitamin B NICOTINIC ACID: inositol nicotinate is a VASODILATOR used mainly to treat circulatory problems of the hands and feet.

✚ warning: inositol nicotinate should be administered with caution to patients with diabetes mellitus.

▲ side-effects: there may be nausea and vomiting, flushing, and dizziness.

Related article: HEXOPAL.

Instant Carobel (*Cow & Gate*) is a proprietary non-prescription powder, used to thicken liquid and semi-liquid diets in the treatment of vomiting. Carobel is a preparation of carob seed flour.

Instillagel (*Rimmer*) is a proprietary compound preparation, available only on prescription, in the form of a water-miscible gel produced in disposable syringes that combines a local ANAESTHETIC with a powerful disinfectant. It is used primarily to treat painful inflammations of the urethra: the compound is instilled into the urethra after external cleansing. But it may also be used to disinfect and lubricate medical equipment following such procedures as catheterization and cystoscopy. The anaesthetic constituent is lignocaine hydrochloride; the major antiseptic constituent is chlorhexidine gluconate.

✚/▲ warning/side-effects: *see* CHLORHEXIDINE; LIGNOCAINE.

Insulatard (*Nordisk Wellcome*) is a proprietary non-prescription preparation of pork isophane insulin, used to treat and

maintain diabetic patients. It is produced in vials for injection.
✚/▲ warning/side-effects: *see* INSULIN.

Insulatard, Human
see HUMAN INSULATARD.

insulin is a protein hormone produced and secreted by the islets of Langerhans within the pancreas. It has the effect of reducing the level of glucose (sugar) in the bloodstream, and is meant as one half of a balancing mechanism with the opposing hormone glycogen (which increases blood sugars). Its absence (in the disorder called diabetes mellitus) therefore results in high levels of blood sugar that can rapidly lead to severe symptoms, and potentially coma and death. Most diabetics therefore take some form of insulin on a regular (daily) basis, generally by injection, although oral administration is becoming popular. Modern genetic engineering has permitted the production of quantities of the human form of insulin that are now replacing the former insulins extracted from oxen (beef insulin) or pigs (pork insulin). There is also a difference in absorption time between insulin with an acid pH (acid insulin injection) and neutral insulin. Other insulin preparations are intermediate-acting (and require administration twice daily, on a "biphasic" basis) or long-acting (and require only once-daily administration). These include insulin zinc suspension (long-acting) and isophane insulin (suitable for the initiation of biphasic regimes). Many diabetic patients use more than one type of insulin in proportions directly related to their own specific needs.

Intal (*Fisons*) is a proprietary preparation of sodium cromoglycate, available only on prescription, used in the form of an inhalant to prevent asthma attacks. The drug is thought to work by effectively inhibiting the release of histamine and other mediators in the membranes of the bronchial passages. Intal is produced in several modes both in liquid form and as a powder: in an aerosol (in two strengths, the stronger under the trade name Intal 5), in an automatic insufflator (under the trade name Halermatic) and in solution for a power-operated nebuliser. Under the trade name Intal Compound, sodium cromoglycate is combined with the BETA-RECEPTOR STIMULANT isoprenaline sulphate, and produced in the form of inhalation cartridges (Spincaps).
✚/▲ warning/side-effects: *see* ISOPRENALINE; SODIUM CROMOGLYCATE.

Integrin (*Sterling Research*) is a powerful drug, available only on prescription, used to treat and tranquillize patients who are undergoing behavioural disturbances (states both of apathetic withdrawal and of hyperactive mania), or who are psychotic (particularly schizophrenic). More mundanely, it is used to treat severe anxiety in the short term. Produced in the form of capsules and tablets, Integrin is a preparation of the antipsychotic drug oxypertine. It is not recommended for children.
✚/▲ warning/side-effects: *see* OXYPERTINE.

***interferons** are proteins produced in tiny quantities by cells infected by a virus; they have the ability to inhibit further growth by the virus. Genetic engineering, including the use of bacteria as host cells, has enabled interferons to be mass-produced – but they have not turned out to be the ultimate weapon against viruses that it was thought they would be. But because they have specific and complex effects on cells, cell function and immunity, interferons are now undergoing trials in the treatment of cancers (particularly lymphomas and certain solid tumours).

✚ warning: regular blood counts are essential during treatment, particularly to check on levels of white blood cells that contribute to the immune system.

▲ side-effects: symptoms of severe fever are common; there may also be lethargy and/or depression. The blood-producing capacity of the bone-marrow may be reduced. Some patients experience high or low blood pressure, and heartbeat irregularities. *Related articles:* INTRON A; ROFERON-A; WELLFERON.

Intraglobin (*Biotest Folex*) is a proprietary preparation of human normal IMMUNOGLOBULIN (HNIG) as a powder for reconstitution in solvent, used in infusion to confer immediate immunity to diseases such as hepatitis A virus, measles (rubeola) and at least to some degree rubella (German measles), particularly in patients who for one reason or another cannot tolerate the administration of live (though attenuated) viruses in vaccination therapies. Intraglobin is also used to provide some form of immunity in patients born with immunodeficient conditions. It is available only on prescription.

✚ warning: *see* HNIG.

Intralgin (*Riker*) is a proprietary COUNTER-IRRITANT and local ANAESTHETIC non-prescription gel which, applied topically, produces an irritation of sensory nerve endings that offsets the pain of underlying muscle or joint ailments. The gel is an alcohol-based preparation of a SALICYLIC ACID-like compound and BENZOCAINE in dilute solution.

Intralipid (*KabiVitrum*) is a proprietary form of high-energy nutritional supplement intended for infusion into patients who are unable to take food via the alimentary canal. Produced in two strengths (under the trade names Intralipid 10% and Intralipid 20%), its major constituent is fat emulsion derived from soya bean oils and from eggs.

Intraval Sodium (*May & Baker*) is a proprietary GENERAL ANAESTHETIC, available only on prescription, used mainly for the induction of anaesthesia or for short-duration effect during minor surgical procedures. Produced in the form of a powder for reconstitution as a medium for injections (in two strengths), and in ampoules and bottles (flasks), Intraval Sodium is a preparation of thiopentone sodium.

✚/▲ warning/side-effects: *see* THIOPENTONE SODIUM.

Intron A (*Kirby-Warrick*) is a proprietary preparation of interferon (in the form of alpha interferon), available only on prescription, and used mainly to treat leukaemia. Administration is by injection. As with virtually all anticancer drugs, some side-effects are inevitable.

✚/▲ warning/side-effects: *see* INTERFERONS.

Intropin (*American Hospital Supply*) is a proprietary

preparation of the powerful SYMPATHOMIMETIC drug dopamine hydrochloride, used to treat cardiogenic shock following a heart attack or during heart surgery. Dosage is critical – too much *or* too little may have harmful effects. It is produced in the form of a liquid (in two strengths) for dilution and infusion.

✚/▲ warning/side-effects: *see* DOPAMINE.

iodine is an element required in small quantities in the diet for healthy growth and development. Good dietary sources are sea food and iodized salt. Internally, iodine is concentrated in the thyroid gland in the neck, because the gland utilizes iodine in the production of the thyroid hormones. The element is thus administered therapeutically to make up for dietary deficiency leading to hypothyroidism, and radioactive isotopes of iodine are used in the diagnosis and treatment of thyroid gland disorders. More mundanely, iodine is still commonly used as an ANTISEPTIC (either as AQUEOUS IODINE SOLUTION or as POVIDONE-IODINE).

✚ warning: in the treatment of thyroid disorders, and particularly to treat thyrotoxicosis before surgery to remove part or all of the thyroid gland, iodine should not be administered to patients who are lactating; it should be administered with caution to those who are pregnant or very young.

▲ side-effects: there may be sensitivity reactions, resulting in symptoms like those of a heavy cold; a rash may also occur. Prolonged treatment with iodine may lead to insomnia and depression, and loss of libido in the patient.

Iodosorb (*Stuart*) is a proprietary antibacterial powder, available only on prescription, and is an absorbent material that cleans, dries and removes dead skin from leg ulcers and open bedsores. Applied to the site, the powder should be covered with a sterile dressing changed daily. Iodosorb powder is based on a form of iodine, and is produced in sachets.

Ionamin (*Lipha*) is a proprietary preparation of the stimulant drug phentermine used, in the short term only, to assist in the medical treatment of obesity. On the controlled drugs list, Ionamin is produced in the form of sustained-release capsules (in two strengths). It is not recommended for children aged under 6 years.

✚/▲ warning/side-effects: *see* PHENTERMINE.

Ionax Scrub (*Alcon*) is a proprietary non-prescription gel and is a preparation of the ANTISEPTIC BENZALKONIUM CHLORIDE together with abrasive polyethylene granules within a foaming aqueous-alcohol base. It is used to treat acne, or to cleanse the skin before the application of further acne treatments.

Ionil T (*Alcon*) is a proprietary preparation of the ANTISEPTICS BENZALKONIUM CHLORIDE and COAL TAR together with the astringent antifungal drug SALICYLIC ACID, all within an alcohol base. It is used to treat seborrhoeic dermatitis of the scalp, and is accordingly produced as a shampoo. If required for strictly medical reasons it is available on prescription.

ipecacuanha is a plant extract that is an irritant to the digestive system. It is a powerful emetic

(used to clear the stomach in some instances of non-corrosive poisoning), but in smaller doses it is also used in non-proprietary mixtures and in proprietary tinctures and syrups as an expectorant.
✚ warning: high dosage can cause severe gastric upset.

Ipral (*Squibb*) is a proprietary ANTIBACTERIAL, available only on prescription, used to treat infections of the upper respiratory tract (particularly bronchitis and bronchial pneumonia) and of the urinary tract. Produced in the form of tablets (in two strengths) and as a sugar-free suspension for children (under the trade name Ipral Paediatric) for dilution (the potency of the suspension once dilute is retained for 14 days), Ipral is a preparation of the antibacterial drug trimethoprim.
✚/▲ warning/side-effects: *see* TRIMETHOPRIM.

ipratropium is an ANTICHOLINERGIC drug that has the properties of a BRONCHODILATOR, and is (in the form of ipratropium bromide) accordingly used to treat restriction of the air passages of the upper respiratory tract, especially in chronic bronchitis. Administration is by inhalation, from an aerosol or from a nebuliser.
✚ warning: ipratropium should be administered with caution to patients with glaucoma or enlargement of the prostate gland. It is advised that treatment should be initiated under hospital supervision; patients on their own should be careful not to exceed the prescribed dose, and should be scrupulous in observing the manufacturer's directions.
▲ side-effects: There may be dryness of mouth. Rarely, there is urinary retention and/or constipation.
Related article: ATROVENT.

iprindole is an ANTIDEPRESSANT drug of a type that has fewer sedative properties than many others. In the treatment of depressive illness it is thus suited more to the treatment of withdrawn and apathetic patients than to those who are agitated and restless. Administration is oral in the form of tablets.
✚ warning: iprindole should not be administered to patients with heart disease or liver failure; it should be administered with extreme caution to those with epilepsy, psychoses or glaucoma, or who are pregnant. Treatment may take up to four weeks to achieve full effect; premature withdrawal of treatment thereafter may cause the return of symptoms.
▲ side-effects: dry mouth, drowsiness, blurred vision, constipation and urinary retention are all fairly common; there may also be minor heartbeat irregularities accompanying low blood pressure (hypotension). Concentration and speed of reaction are likely to be affected.
Related article: PRONDOL.

iproniazid is an ANTIDEPRESSANT drug, an MAO INHIBITOR (mono amine oxidase inhibitor, or MAOI) used accordingly to treat depressive illness. Administration is oral in the form of tablets. It is not suitable for children.
✚ warning: iproniazid should not be administered to patients with disease of the liver or the blood vessels, or epilepsy.

Treatment with this drug requires the strict avoidance of certain foods (particularly cheese, pickled fish or meat extracts), of alcohol, and of certain other medications; professional counselling on this subject is utterly essential. Withdrawal of treatment should be gradual.

▲ side-effects: dizziness is fairly common. There may also be headache, dry mouth, blurred vision and tremor; some patients experience constipation and difficulty in urinating; a rash may break out. Susceptible patients may undergo psychotic episodes. *Related article*: MARSILID.

Irofol C (*Abbott*) is a proprietary non-prescription IRON-and-VITAMIN compound that is not available from the National Health Service. As an iron and a vitamin supplement, it is used particularly during pregnancy. It contains iron (in the form of ferrous sulphate), FOLIC ACID (a vitamin B) and ASCORBIC ACID (vitamin C), and is produced in the form of sustained-release tablets.

iron is a metallic element essential to the body in several ways, and especially important in its role as transporter of oxygen around the body (in the form of the red blood cell constituent oxyhaemoglobin); it is also retained in the muscles. Dietary deficiency of iron leads to any of several forms of anaemia: good food sources include meats, particularly liver. Iron is administered therapeutically mostly to make up a dietary deficiency (and so treat anaemia). Supplements may be administered orally (in the form of FERROUS FUMARATE, FERROUS GLUCONATE, FERROUS GLYCINE SULPHATE, FERROUS SUCCINATE, FERROUS SULPHATE, and other salts) or by injection or infusion (in the form of iron dextran and other preparations). There are also many iron-and-vitamin supplements available to prevent deficiencies of either (particularly during pregnancy).

Ironorm (*Wallace*) is three preparations of a mineral-and-VITAMIN compound. Available without prescription is a tonic (or elixir) containing IRON (in the form of ferric ammonium citrate), calcium, PHOSPHORUS, most forms of vitamin B, and liver extract. Available only on prescription are capsules containing iron (in the form of FERROUS SULPHATE), several forms of vitamin B, ascorbic acid (vitamin C) and fractionated liver. Also available only on prescription are ampoules of the plasma-and-iron infusion fluid, iron dextran complex.

Ismelin (*Ciba/Zyma*) is a proprietary preparation of the antihypertensive drug guanethidine monosulphate, available only on prescription. It is produced in two entirely different forms for two entirely different purposes by two manufacturers – but under the same trade name. In the form of tablets (in two strengths) and in ampoules for injection, Ismelin is used to treat moderate to severe high blood pressure (hypertension) and is administered simultaneously with either a DIURETIC (such as a thiazide) or a BETA-BLOCKER. In the form of eye-drops, Ismelin is used to relieve pressure within the eyeball in the treatment of glaucoma, for which its effect is often enhanced by the simultaneous administration of the hormone ADRENALINE.

✚/▲ warning/side-effects: *see* GUANETHIDINE MONOSULPHATE.

Ismo 20 (*MCP Pharmaceuticals*) is a proprietary VASODILATOR, available only on prescription, used to assist in the treatment of congestive heart failure and to prevent attacks of angina pectoris (heart pain). Produced in the form of tablets (in two strengths only one of which is obtainable independently), it is a preparation of isosorbide mononitrate, and is not recommended for children.
✚/▲ warning/side-effects: *see* ISOSORBIDE MONONITRATE.

isoaminile citrate is a drug that suppresses a cough (ANTITUSSIVE); such drugs are used medically only when absolutely necessary, and when sputum retention is guaranteed to do no harm. Administration is oral in the form of a linctus.
✚ warning: Isoaminile citrate should not be administered to patients with any impairment of airflow in the respiratory passages (as in asthma), or who would find sputum retention a hazard (as in chronic bronchitis).
▲ side-effects: constipation is often associated with treatment.
Related article: DIMYRIL; ISOAMINILE LINCTUS.

isoaminile linctus is a non-proprietary preparation of isoaminile citrate, available only on prescription, used only under specific circumstances to treat a dry or persistent and painful cough (ANTITUSSIVE). It is produced in the form of a syrup for dilution (the potency of the syrup once dilute is retained for 14 days).
✚/▲ warning/side-effects: *see* ISOAMINILE CITRATE.

Iso-Autohaler (*Lewis*) is a proprietary BETA-RECEPTOR STIMULANT, available only on prescription, used in the form of an inhalant to treat bronchial asthma and chronic bronchitis. Produced in an aerosol, Iso-Autohaler is a preparation of isoprenaline sulphate.
✚/▲ warning/side-effects: *see* ISOPRENALINE.

Iso-Brovon (*Napp*) is a proprietary compound BRONCHODILATOR, available only on prescription, used to treat obstruction of the air passages of the respiratory tract (as in asthma). Produced in an aerosol (in two strengths, the stronger under the trade name Iso-Brovon Plus), it is a preparation of atropine methonitrate and isoprenaline hydrochloride.
✚/▲ warning/side-effects: *see* ATROPINE METHONITRATE; ISOPRENALINE.

Isocal (*Mead Johnson*) is a proprietary non-prescription gluten-free liquid that is a complete nutritional diet for patients who are severely undernourished (such as with anorexia nervosa) or who have some problem of absorption of food (such as following gastrectomy). Also lactose-free, Isocal contains protein, carbohydrate and fats, with vitamins and minerals, but is unsuitable as the sole source of nutrition for children, and unsuitable altogether for children aged under 12 months.

isocarboxazid is an ANTIDEPRESSANT drug, an MAO INHIBITOR (mono amine oxidase inhibitor, or MAOI) used accordingly to treat depressive illness. Administration is oral in the form of tablets. It is not suitable for children.
✚ warning: isocarboxazid should not be administered to patients with disease of the

liver or the blood vessels, or epilepsy. Treatment with this drug requires the strict avoidance of certain foods (particularly cheese, pickled fish or meat extracts), of alcohol, and of certain other medications; professional counselling on this subject is utterly essential. Withdrawal of treatment should be gradual.

▲ side-effects: dizziness is fairly common. There may also be headache, dry mouth, blurred vision and tremor; some patients experience constipation and difficulty in urinating; a rash may break out. Susceptible patients may undergo psychotic episodes.
Related article: MARPLAN.

isoconazole is an ANTIFUNGAL drug, one of the IMIDAZOLES used particularly to treat fungal infections of the vagina and anogenital area. Administration is in the form of a cream or as vaginal tablets (pessaries), usually as a single-dose treatment. It is not recommended for children.

▲ side-effects: there may be local irritation, and even a temporary burning sensation.
Related article: TRAVOGYN.

isoetharine is a SYMPATHOMIMETIC drug (and mild VASOCONSTRICTOR) used primarily to treat the bronchospasm of asthma and chronic bronchitis. Administration (in the form of isoetharine hydrochloride or isoetharine mesylate) is oral in the form of sustained-release tablets, or topical (in combination) as an aerosol inhalant.

✚ warning: isoetharine hydrochloride should be administered with caution to patients with heart disease or excessive secretion of thyroid hormones (hyperthyroidism), who are diabetic (in which case regular blood sugar counts are essential during treatment), or who are pregnant or elderly.

▲ side-effects: there may be headache, nervous tension, tremor of the hands, sweating, increased heart rate and heartbeat irregularities, and a decrease in blood potassium levels.
Related article: BRONCHILATOR; NUMOTAC.

isoflurane is a GENERAL ANAESTHETIC related to ENFLURANE, produced as a gas to be used in solution with oxygen or nitrous oxide-oxygen. Administration is through a specially calibrated vaporiser. It is used particularly for the initial induction of anaesthesia.

✚ warning: treatment depresses respiration. The drug also produces muscle relaxation, and/or enhances the effect of muscle-relaxant drugs administered simultaneously.

▲ side-effects: there may be an increase in heart rate accompanied by a fall in blood pressure (especially in younger patients).
Related article: FORANE.

Isogel (*Allen & Hanburys*) is a proprietary form of the type of laxative known as a bulking agent, which works by increasing the overall mass of faeces within the rectum, so stimulating bowel movement. It is thus used both to relieve constipation and to relieve diarrhoea, and also in the control of faecal consistency for patients with a colostomy. Produced in the form of granules for solution in water, Isogel is a preparation of ispaghula husk.

✚/▲ warning/side-effects: *see* ISPAGHULA HUSK.

Isoket (*Schwarz*) is a proprietary non-prescription VASODILATOR used to prevent attacks of angina pectoris (heart pain). Produced in the form of tablets (in three strengths), as sustained-release capsules (under the trade name Isoket Retard), and in ampoules for injection (under the trade name Isoket 0.1%), it is a preparation of isosorbide dinitrate, and is not recommended for children.
✚/▲ warning/side-effects: *see* ISOSORBIDE DINITRATE.

isometheptene mucate is a SYMPATHOMIMETIC drug used in combination with a sedative (such as dichloralphenazone) to treat migraine attacks. Administration is oral in the form of capsules.
✚ warning: the combination should not be administered to patients with glaucoma; it should be administered with caution to those with cardiovascular disease, or those on MAO INHIBITOR therapy.
▲ side-effects: there may be dizziness associated with peripheral disturbances in blood circulation.
Related article: MIDRID.

Isomil (*Abbott*) is a proprietary non-prescription gluten-free powder that when reconstituted is a complete nutritional diet for patients – especially infants – who are unable to tolerate milk or milk sugars. Also therefore milk protein-free and lactose-free, Isomil contains protein, carbohydrate and fats, plus vitamins and minerals.

isoniazid is an ANTITUBERCULAR drug used, as is normal in the treatment of tuberculosis, in combination with other antibacterial drugs to defeat bacterial resistance. It is also administered to prevent the contraction of tuberculosis by close associates of an infected patient. Administration is oral in the form of tablets or as a non-proprietary elixir, or by injection.
✚ warning: isoniazid should not be administered to patients with liver disease induced by drug treatment; it should be administered with caution to those with impaired kidney or liver function, epilepsy or alcoholism, or who are lactating.
▲ side-effects: there may be nausea with vomiting. High dosage may lead to sensitivity reactions, including a rash, and in susceptible patients loss of sensation in the hands and feet, convulsions and/or psychotic episodes.
Related article: RIMIFON.

isoprenaline is a compound substance closely related to the hormone ADRENALINE. In the form of isoprenaline sulphate it is a BETA-RECEPTOR STIMULANT and VASODILATOR produced as an inhalant or in the form of tablets to be held under the tongue, that is used primarily to treat the bronchospasm of asthma and chronic bronchitis. In the form of isoprenaline hydrochloride, however, it is a SYMPATHOMIMETIC administered by injection, that is used to treat extremely slow heart rate and some heart diseases.
✚ warning: isoprenaline should be administered with caution to patients with heart disease or excessive secretion of thyroid hormones (hyperthyroidism), who are diabetic (in which case regular blood sugar counts are essential during treatment), or who are pregnant or elderly.
▲ side-effects: there may be

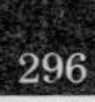

headache, nervous tension, tremor of the hands, sweating, increased heart rate and heartbeat irregularities, and a decrease in blood potassium levels. Administration as an inhalant results in few of these side-effects.
Related articles: ALEUDRIN; DUO-AUTOHALER; ISO-AUTOHALER; Iso-Brovon; ISUPREL; MEDIHALER-ISO; SAVENTRINE.

Isopto (*Alcon*) is a series of proprietary preparations of various drugs, all available only on prescription, each used in the form of eye-drops used variously to treat infections and glaucoma, and to facilitate inspection of the eye. The range comprises Isopto Alkaline (comprising simply the synthetic tear medium hypromellose); Isopto Atropine (comprising ATROPINE SULPHATE); Isopto Carbachol (comprising CARBACHOL and the synthetic tear medium hypromellose); Isopto Carpine (comprising PILOCARPINE hydrochloride, in any of five strengths, and the synthetic tear medium hypromellose); Isopto Cetamide (comprising SULPHACETAMIDE sodium and the synthetic tear medium hypromellose); Isopto Epinal (comprising the hormone ADRENALINE and the synthetic tear medium hypromellose); Isopto Frin (comprising PHENYLEPHRINE hydrochloride and the synthetic tear medium hypromellose); and Isopto Plain (comprising simply the synthetic tear medium hypromellose, at half the strength of Isopto Alkaline).
✚/▲ warning/side-effects: *see primary constituents listed above.*

Isordil (*Ayerst*) is a proprietary non-prescription VASODILATOR used to treat acute congestive heart failure, to assist in the treatment of chronic congestive heart failure, and to prevent attacks of angina pectoris (heart pain). Produced in the form of tablets (in three strengths) and as sustained-release capsules (under the trade name Isordil Tembids), it is a preparation of isosorbide dinitrate, and is not recommended for children.
✚/▲ warning/side-effects: *see* ISOSORBIDE DINITRATE.

isosorbide dinitrate is a VASODILATOR used to treat acute congestive heart failure, to assist in the treatment of chronic congestive heart failure, and to prevent attacks of ANGINA pectoris (heart pain). Administration is oral in the form of tablets (for swallowing, chewing, or holding under the tongue) or as sustained-release capsules, or by infusion.
✚ warning: isosorbide dinitrate should be administered with extreme caution to patients with low blood pressure (hypotension) or severe forms of anaemia. Monitoring of heart function during treatment is advisable.
▲ side-effects: there may be headache, with flushing and dizziness; the heart rate may increase.
Related articles: CEDOCARD; ISOKET; ISORDIL; SONI-SLO; Sorbichew; SORBID SA; SORBITRATE; VASCARDIN.

isosorbide mononitrate is a VASODILATOR used to assist in the treatment of chronic congestive heart failure, and to prevent attacks of angina pectoris (heart pain). Administration is oral in the form of tablets.
✚ warning: isosorbide mononitrate should be

administered with caution to patients who have low blood pressure (hypotension). Monitoring of heart function during treatment is advisable.

▲ side-effects: there may be headache, with flushing and dizziness; the heart rate may increase.
Related articles: ELANTAN; ISMO 20; MONIT; MONO-CEDOCARD.

isotretinoin is a powerful drug of fairly recent provenance, derived from RETINOL (vitamin A), and used for the systemic treatment of severe acne that has failed to respond to more usual therapies. Full medical supervision is required during treatment, which may last for three or four months – during which (from about the second to the fourth week) there may actually be an exacerbation of the acne; if treatment fails, repeat courses should not be given. Administration is oral in the form of capsules (generally from hospitals only).

✚ warning: isotretinoin should not be administered to patients who are pregnant or likely to become so – the drug may cause congenital abnormalities in a foetus; effective contraceptive measures should be continued for at least one month after treatment has ceased. Blood fat levels and liver function should be regularly checked.

▲ side-effects: dry lips and mucous membranes, sore eyes, and joint and muscle pains are not uncommon; there may also be nose-bleeds and temporary hair loss.
Related article: ROACCUTANE.

isoxsuprine hydrochloride is a SYMPATHOMIMETIC VASODILATOR that affects principally the blood vessels of the hands and feet, but also affects the blood supply to the brain. It is therefore used to relieve the symptoms of both cerebral and peripheral vascular disease.The drug also has the effect of inhibiting contractions of the womb, and is thus additionally used to prevent or stall premature labour. Administration is oral in the form of tablets and sustained-release capsules, or by injection or infusion.

✚ warning: isoxsuprine hydrochloride should not be administered to patients who have recently had bleeding from an artery, with heart disease or severe anaemia, or who towards the end of a pregnancy have any infection. Administration to stall or prevent premature labour may cause low blood pressure (hypotension) in the foetus.

▲ side-effects: flushing and an increase in heart rate with some heartbeat irregularity are not uncommon; there may also be nausea and vomiting.
Related articles: DEFENCIN CP; DUVADILAN.

ispaghula husk is a high-fibre substance used as a LAXATIVE because it is an effective bulking agent – it increases the overall mass of faeces within the rectum, so stimulating bowel movement. It is also particularly useful in soothing the symptoms of diverticular disease and irritable colon. Adnministration is oral, generally in the form of granules or a powder for solution in water.

✚ warning: preparations of ispaghula husk should not be administered to patients with obstruction of the intestines, or failure of the muscles of the intestinal wall; it should be administered with caution to those with ulcerative colitis. Fluid intake during treatment

should be higher than usual.
▲ side-effects: there may be flatulence, so much as to distend the abdomen.
Related articles: AGIOLAX; FYBOGEL; ISOGEL; METAMUCIL; Regulan; VI-SIBLIN.

Isuprel (*Winthrop*) is a proprietary SYMPATHOMIMETIC drug, available only on prescription, used to treat extremely slow heart rate and certain heart diseases. Produced in ampoules for injection, it is a preparation of isoprenaline hydrochloride.
✚/▲ warning/side-effects: *see* ISOPRENALINE.

ivermectin is a drug that is not available in the United Kingdom, used to treat the tropical disease onchocerciasis – infestation by the filarial worm-parasite Onchocerca volvulus. The destruction of the worms, however, releases antigens into the bloodstream and causes an allergic response, generally requiring the simultaneous administration of antihistamines or corticosteroids to control it. More than one course of treatment with ivermectin may be necessary to deal with the infestation.
✚ warning: close medical supervision is essential during treatment.
▲ side-effects: headache, with nausea and vomiting, is not uncommon; the dermatitis associated with onchocerciasis may temporarily be aggravated, as may any associated conjunctivitis or other eye inflammation.

J

Jacksons (*Ernest Jackson*) are proprietary non-prescription throat lozenges. They contain acetic acid, camphor, bonzoic acid and menthol.

Jectofer (*Astra*) is a proprietary compound of iron sorbitol and citric acid, available only on prescription, used to replace IRON in patients with iron-deficiency anaemia. It is produced as a dark brown liquid for intramuscular injection.

✚ warning: Jectofer should not be administered to patients with liver or kidney disease.

▲ side-effects: rarely, there are heartbeat irregularities.

Jexin (*Duncan, Flockhart*) is a proprietary SKELETAL MUSCLE RELAXANT, available only on prescription, of the type known as competitive or non-depolarizing. It is used during surgical operations, but only after the patient has been rendered unconscious. Produced in ampoules for injection, Jexin's active constituent is tubocurarine chloride.

✚/▲ warning/side-effects: *see* TUBOCURARINE.

Joy-Rides (*Stafford-Miller*) is a proprietary non-prescription ANTI-CHOLINERGIC formulation for the treatment of MOTION SICKNESS. It contains the atropine-like drug hyoscine.

✚/▲ warning/side-effects: *see* HYOSCINE.

Juvel (*Bencard*) is a proprietary, non-prescription, MULTIVITAMIN compound, used as a vitamin supplement particularly for children and the elderly. Produced in the form of tablets and as an elixir, Juvel contains RETINOL (vitamin A), THIAMINE (vitamin B_1), RIBOFLAVINE (vitamin B_2), PYRIDOXINE (vitamin B_6), NICOTINAMIDE (of the B complex), ASCORBIC ACID (vitamin C) and calciferol (vitamin D).

Juvela (*G F Dietary Supplies*) is a proprietary non-prescription brand of gluten-free bread- and cake-mix, produced for patients with coeliac disease and other forms of gluten sensitivity. There is also a low-protein milk-free version for patients suffering from defects of protein metabolism such as phenylketonuria (PKU).

Kabiglobulin (*KabiVitrum*) is a proprietary preparation of human normal immunoglobulin (HNIG), part of the plasma of the blood that is directly concerned with immunity. Administered by intramuscular injection, Kabiglobulin is used to protect patients at risk from contact with hepatitis A virus, measles (rubeola) or at least to some degree rubella (German measles), or to replace some measure of immunity in patients who have suffered serious shock (as for example with large-scale burns).
✚ warning: see HNIG.

Kabikinase (*KabiVitrum*) is a proprietary form of the effective fibrinolytic drug streptokinase, used to treat and prevent blood clots, particularly in relation to all types of thrombosis. It is produced in the form of powder for reconstitution as a medium for injection.
✚/▲ warning/side-effects: *see* STREPTOKINASE.

Kalspare (*Armour*) is a proprietary compound DIURETIC, available only on prescription, used to treat the accumulation of fluids within the tissues (oedema). Produced in the form of tablets, it combines the THIAZIDE-related diuretic chlorthalidone with a second diuretic triamterene that has the complementary effect of retaining potassium in the body.
✚/▲ warning/side-effects: *see* CHLORTHALIDONE; TRIAMTERENE.

Kalten (*Stuart*) is a proprietary compound BETA-BLOCKER, available only on prescription, used to treat heartbeat irregularities and severe high blood pressure. Produced in the form of capsules, it combines the beta-blocker atenolol with a thiazide DIURETIC (HYDROCHLOROTHIAZIDE) and a complementary potassium-sparing diuretic (AMILORIDE hydrochloride). It is not recommended for children.
✚/▲ warning/side-effects: *see* ATENOLOL.

Kamillosan (*Norgine*) is a proprietary, non-prescription, water-based OINTMENT, used to treat and soothe nappy rash, cracked nipples and chapping on the hands. Its active constituents are various essences of chamomile.

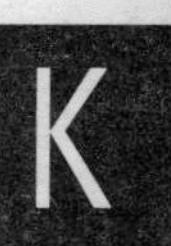

kanamycin is an aminoglycoside ANTIBIOTIC effective in treating a wide range of bacterial infections, especially the more serious ones involving the heart, sensitive tissues or metabolic functions (such as endocarditis, meningitis and septicaemia). Administration is primarily by injection or intravenous infusion.
✚ warning: kanamycin should not be administered to patients who are pregnant (because the drug crosses the placenta) or who suffer from serious muscular disease (because treatment may further impair nuerotransmission). Monitoring of blood count and kidney function is advised.
▲ side-effects: the sense of hearing may be disturbed; there may be temporary kidney dysfunction.
Related article: KANNASYN.

Kannasyn (*Winthrop*) is a proprietary form of the aminoglycoside antibiotic kanamycin sulphate, available only on prescription, used to treat serious bacterial infections. It is produced in the form of solution and as powder for reconstitution, in both cases for injection.

✚/▲ warning/side-effects: *see* KANAMYCIN.

Kaodene (*Boots*) is a proprietary, non-prescription, liquid preparation used to treat diarrhoea, containing the adsorbent kaolin with the opiate codeine phosphate. Not recommended for children aged under 5 years or patients with chronic liver disease (because it may cause sedation), Kaodene should also be used with caution by the elderly (in whom it may cause faecal impaction and constipation). In particular, fluid intake should be increased to more than normal. Prolonged use should be avoided.
✚/▲ warning/side-effects: *see* CODEINE PHOSPHATE.

kaolin is a white clay (china clay) which, when purified (and sometimes powdered), is used as an adsorbent particularly in ANTIDIARRHOEAL preparations (with or without opiates such as CODEINE PHOSPHATE or MORPHINE) but also to treat food poisoning and some digestive disorders. Occasionally used in poultices, it is additionally found in some dusting powders.
Related articles: KAODENE; KAOPECTATE; KLN.

Kaopectate (*Upjohn*) is a proprietary non-prescription suspension of the ANTIDIARRHOEAL adsorbent KAOLIN, in a form suitable for dilution (the potency of the dilute mixture is retained for 14 days) before being taken orally. During treatment, fluid intake should be increased to more than normal.

Karvol (*Crookes*) is a proprietary non-prescription inhalant that is not available from the National Health Service. It may be used to treat symptoms associated with infections of the nose and upper respiratory tract. Containing MENTHOL, THYMOL and several other extracts from plant oils, Karvol capsules may be crushed in a handkerchief or infused in hot water for the essences to be inhaled.

Kay-Cee-L (*Geistlich*) is a proprietary non-prescription form of potassium supplement, used to treat patients with deficiencies and to replace potassium in patients taking potassium-depleting drugs such as CORTICOSTEROIDS. It is produced in the form of a red syrup (not for dilution) containing potassium chloride.

K-Contin Continus (*Napp*) is a proprietary non-prescription form of POTASSIUM supplement, used to treat patients with deficiencies and to replace potassium in patients taking potassium-depleting drugs such as CORTICOSTEROIDS. It is produced in the form of tablets containing potassium chloride.

Kefadol (*Dista*) is a proprietary ANTIBIOTIC, available only on prescription, used to treat bacterial infections, but also to provide freedom from infection during surgery. Produced in the form of a powder for reconstitution as injections, Kefadol is a compound of the cephalosporin cephamandole with sodium carbonate.
✚/▲ warning/side-effects: *see* CEPHAMANDOLE.

Keflex (*Lilly*) is a proprietary ANTIBIOTIC, available only on prescription, used to treat bacterial infections. Produced in the form of capsules (in two strengths), tablets (in two strengths), a suspension (for dilution, in two strengths), and

(under the name Keflex-C) chewy tablets (in two strengths), Keflex is a preparation of the cephalosporin cephalexin.
✚/▲ warning/side-effects: *see* CEPHALEXIN.

Keflin (*Lilly*) is a proprietary ANTIBIOTIC, available only on prescription, used to treat bacterial infections, but also to provide freedom from infection during surgery. Produced in the form of powder for reconstitution as injections, Keflin is a preparation of the cephalosporin cephalothin.
✚/▲ warning/side-effects: *see* CEPHALOTHIN.

Kefzol (*Lilly*) is a proprietary ANTIBIOTIC, available only on prescription, used to treat bacterial infections, but also to provide freedom from infection during surgery. Produced in the form of powder for reconstitution as injections, Kefzol is a preparation of the cephalosporin cephazolin.
✚/▲ warning/side-effects: *see* CEPHAZOLIN.

Kelferon (*MCP Pharmaceuticals*) is a proprietary non-prescription preparation of the drug ferrous glycine sulphate, used as an IRON supplement in the treatment of iron-deficiency anaemia, and produced in the form of tablets.
✚/▲ warning/side-effects: *see* FERROUS GLYCINE SULPHATE.

Kelfizine W (*Farmitalia Carlo Erba*) is a proprietary antibacterial, available only on prescription, used primarily to treat chronic bronchitis and infections of the urinary tract. Produced in the form of tablets, Kelfizine W is a preparation of the SULPHONAMIDE sulfametopyrazine.
✚/▲ warning/side-effects: *see* SULFAMETOPYRAZINE.

Kelfolate (*MCP Pharmaceuticals*) is a proprietary non-prescription compound of iron-rich FERROUS GLYCINE SULPHATE and FOLIC ACID (a vitamin of the B complex), used to prevent iron and vitamin deficiency during pregnancy.
✚ warning: prolonged administration may cause constipation.
▲ side-effects: there may be gastrointestinal upsets with diarrhoea following large doses.

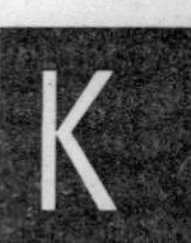

Kelocyanor (*Lipha*) is a proprietary CHELATING AGENT, available only on prescription, that is an emergency antidote to cyanide poisoning. It is produced in the form of ampoules for injection, containing dicobalt edetate in glucose solution.
▲ side-effects: see DICOBALT EDETATE.

Kemadrin (*Wellcome*) is a proprietary preparation of the ANTICHOLINERGIC procyclidine hydrochloride, available only on prescription, used in the treatment of parkinsonism and to control tremors within drug-induced states involving involuntary movement (*see* ANTIPARKINSONISM). Produced in the form of tablets and in ampoules for injection, Kemadrin is not recommended for children.
✚/▲ warning/side-effects: *see* PROCYCLIDINE HYDROCHLORIDE.

Kemicetine (*Farmitalia Carlo Erba*) is a proprietary broad-spectrum ANTIBIOTIC, available only on prescription. Produced in the form of powder for reconstitution as injections, Kemicetine is a preparation of the powerful drug chloramphenicol which, because of its potential toxicity, is generally used only to treat life-

threatening infections.
✚/▲ warning/side-effects: *see* CHLORAMPHENICOL.

Kenalog (*Squibb*) is a proprietary form of the anti-inflammatory glucocorticoid (corticosteroid) drug triamcinolone acetonide, available only on prescription. Produced in the form of pre-filled hypodermics, Kenalog is used in two different ways in order to achieve either of two distinct purposes: intramuscular injection relieves allergic states (such as hay fever or pollen induced asthma) and some collagen disorders, and can reduce severe dermatitis; injection directly into a joint relieves pain, swelling and stiffness (such as with rheumatoid arthritis, bursitis and tenosynovitis). It is not recommended for children aged under 6 years.
✚/▲ warning/side-effects: *see* TRIAMCINOLONE ACETONIDE.

Keralyt (*Westwood*) is a proprietary non-prescription gel containing salicylic acid, used to treat thickened patches of skin (hyperkeratoses), as occur in some forms of eczema, in ichthyosis and in psoriasis. Each evening the gel is smoothed on to cleansed skin and held by bandaging overnight; it is washed off each morning.
✚/▲ warning/side-effects: *see* SALICYLIC ACID.

keratolytics are drugs and preparations intended to clear the skin of thickened, horny patches (hyperkeratoses) and scaly areas, as occur in some forms of eczema, ichthyosis and psoriasis, and in the treatment of acne. The standard, classic keratolytic is salicylic acid, generally used in very mild solution. Others include ichthammol, coal tar, etretinate and dithranol (which is the most powerful), several of which can usefully be applied in the form of paste inside an impregnated bandage.
Related articles: COAL TAR; DITHRANOL; ETRETINATE; ichthammol; SALICYLIC ACID; ZINC PASTE.

Kerecid (*Smith, Kline & French*) is a proprietary preparation, available only on prescription, used to treat herpes simplex infections of the eye. Containing a mild solution of the antiviral agent IDOXURIDINE, it is produced in the form of eye- drops (with polyvinyl alcohol) for use during the day, and eye ointment for use overnight.

Keri (*Westwood*) is a proprietary non-prescription lotion used to soften dry skin and to relieve itching. Active constituents include liquid paraffin and lanolin oil. It is produced in a pump pack, and is intended to be massaged into the skin.

Kerlone (*Lorex*) is a proprietary BETA-BLOCKER, available only on prescription, used to treat high blood pressure (*see* ANTIHYPERTENSIVE). It is produced in the form of tablets consisting (as an antihypertensive) of a preparation of betaxolol hydrochloride. Kerlone is not recommended for children; dosage should be reduced for the elderly (at least initially), and in patients with kidney impairment.
✚/▲ warning/side-effects: *see* BETAXOLOL HYDROCHLORIDE.

Keromask (*Innoxa*) is the name of a proprietary non-prescription camouflage CREAM, in two shades, designed for use in masking scars and other skin disfigurements; there is an additional finishing powder. It may be obtained on prescription if the skin disfigurement is the result of surgery or is giving rise to emotional disturbance.

Kest (*Berk*) is a proprietary non-prescription LAXATIVE that is not available from the National Health Service. Produced in the form of tablets containing MAGNESIUM SULPHATE and phenolphthalein, Kest is not recommended for children.
▲ side-effects: laxative effects may continue for several days; there may be dysfunction of the kidneys, leading possibly to discoloration of the urine. A mild skin rash may appear.

Ketalar (*Parke-Davis*) is a proprietary preparation of the general ANAESTHETIC ketamine, in the form of ketamine chloride. Available only on prescription, Ketalar is produced as vials for injection (in three strengths).
✚/▲ warning/side-effects: *see* KETAMINE.

ketamine is a general ANAESTHETIC that is used mainly for surgery on children, in whom hallucinogenic side-effects seem to appear less often than in adults. Ketamine has a good reputation for increasing muscle tone, maintaining good air passage, and having fair analgesic qualities in doses too low for actual anaesthesia (and the hallucinations can be avoided through the simultaneous use of other drugs). Administration is either by intramuscular injection or by intravenous infusion.
✚ warning: ketamine should not be administered to patients who suffer from high blood pressure (hypertension) or who are mentally ill.
▲ side-effects: transient hallucinations may occur. Recovery is relatively slow.
Related article: KETALAR.

ketazolam is an ANXIOLYTIC drug, one of the BENZODIAZEPINES, used to treat chronic states of anxiety. Dosage must be measured to each patient's individual response. It is also sometimes used to relieve muscle spasm and as a muscle relaxant.
✚ warning: sedative effects may inhibit intricate movement or rapid reaction, and may increase the effect of alcohol. Dosage should be reduced for the elderly and for patients with impaired functioning of the kidneys or liver.
▲ side-effects: drowsiness and lethargy are common, with or without dizziness; there may be a dry mouth and headache. Occasionally there is a hypersensitivity reaction.
Related article: ANXON.

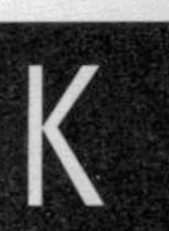

ketoconazole is a broad-spectrum ANTIFUNGAL agent, an IMIDAZOLE that is surprisingly effective when taken orally, used to treat deep-seated fungal infections (mycoses) or superficial ones that have not responded to other treatment. In particular, ketoconazole is used to treat resistant candidiasis (thrush, or moniliasis) and dermatophytic infections of the skin or fingernails.
✚ warning: ketoconazole should not be administered to patients who have impaired function of the liver, or who are pregnant.
▲ side-effects: liver damage may occur – and to a serious extent; rarely, there may be an itching skin rash, or nausea.
Related article: NIZORAL.

ketoprofen is a non-steroid ANTI-INFLAMMATORY non-narcotic ANALGESIC drug, used to treat rheumatic and muscular pain caused by inflammation, and to treat gout. It is produced in the

form of capsules and anal suppositories. In all forms, the drug should be taken with food in order to avoid possible gastrointestinal upset.
✚ warning: use with caution in the presence of gastric ulceration, liver or kidney damage, allergic disorders or pregnancy. It tends to enhance the effect of anticoagulant drugs. Dosage should be closely monitored.
▲ side-effects: there may be gastrointestinal upset; suppositories may cause irritation.
Related articles: ALRHEUMAT; ORUDIS; ORUVAIL.

ketotifen is an effective ANTIHISTAMINE used primarily to prevent asthmatic attacks, although it may alternatively be used to treat other allergic disorders. Taken orally, it may require up to a month to become fully operational, and may in the meantime cause some minor but inconvenient side-effects. Administration should be simultaneous with a meal.
✚ warning: consumption of alcohol should be avoided during treatment.
▲ side-effects: ketotifen may cause drowsiness and dryness in the mouth; the ability to drive a vehicle or operate machinery may be affected.
Related article: ZADITEN.

Ketovite (*Paines & Byrne*) is a proprietary MULTIVITAMIN supplement, available only on prescription, used as an adjunct in synthetic diets. Produced in the form of tablets and a liquid, both forms are intended to be taken daily following a specified regimen. The tablets contain THIAMINE (vitamin B_1), RIBOFLAVINE (vitamin B_2), PYRIDOXINE (vitamin B_6), CYANOCOBALAMIN (vitamin B_{12}), NICOTINAMIDE (of the vitamin B complex), FOLIC ACID (of the B complex), ASCORBIC ACID (vitamin C) and other useful factors; the sugar-free liquid contains RETINOL (vitamin A), CYANOCOBALAMIN (vitamin B_{12}), and a form of CALCIFEROL (vitamin D) in a purified water base.

Kiditard (*Delandale*) is a proprietary ANTIARRHYTHMIC drug, available only on prescription, used to treat heartbeat irregularities and to prevent speeding up of the heart rate. Produced in the form of capsules – the interval between doses being the regulating factor to suit each individual patient – Kiditard is a preparation of quinidine bisulphate. It is not recommended for children.
✚/▲ warning/side-effects: *see* QUINIDINE.

Kinidin Durules (*Astra*) is a proprietary ANTIARRHYTHMIC drug, available only on prescription, used to treat heartbeat irregularities and to prevent speeding up of the heart rate. Produced in the form of tablets – the interval between doses being the regulating factor to suit each individual patient – Kinidin Durules is a preparation of quinidine bisulphate. It is not recommended for children.
✚/▲ warning/side-effects: *see* QUINIDINE.

KLN (*Ashe*) is a proprietary non-prescription mixture of the mineral adsorbent KAOLIN with the gelatinous adsorbent pectin and the alkaline diuretic SODIUM CITRATE. Prepared as a liquid for oral intake, KLN is used to treat diarrhoea. During the course of treatment with KLN, fluid intake by the patient should be increased to more than normal.

Kloref (*Cox*) is a proprietary non-prescription form of POTASSIUM supplement, used to treat patients with deficiencies and to replace potassium in patients taking potassium-depleting drugs such as CORTICOSTEROIDS. It is produced in the form of effervescent tablets and (under the name Kloref-S) sachets of granules containing potassium chloride, potassium bicarbonate and betaine hydrochloride.

Klyx (*Ferring*) is a proprietary non-prescription form of enema administered rectally to promote bowel movement, especially before labour or endoscopy. Produced in single-dose disposable packs with a plastic sleeve, Klyx's active constituent is the softening agent DIOCTYL SODIUM SULPHOSUCCINATE (also called docusate sodium).

Kolanticon (*Merrell Dow*) is a proprietary non-prescription anticholinergic drug that is not available from the National Health Service. An ANTACID, it is used to treat hyperacidity in the stomach and intestines, peptic ulcer, flatulence, and gastrointestinal spasm: Produced in the form of a gel, Kolanticon is a sugar-free compound of dicyclomine hydrochloride, dimethicone, ALUMINIUM HYDROXIDE and MAGNESIUM oxide, for dilution with purified water (the potency of the dilute gel is retained for 14 days).

✚/▲ warning/side-effects: *see* DICYCLOMINE HYDROCHLORIDE.

Kolantyl (*Merrell Dow*) is a proprietary non-prescription anticholinergic drug that is not available from the National Health Service. An ANTACID, it is used to treat hyperacidity in the stomach and intestines, and peptic ulcers. Produced in the form of a gel, Kolantyl is a sugar-free compound of dicyclomine hydrochloride, ALUMINIUM HYDROXIDE and MAGNESIUM oxide, for dilution with purified water (the potency of the dilute gel is retained for 14 days).

✚/▲ warning/side-effects: *see* DICYCLOMINE HYDROCHLORIDE.

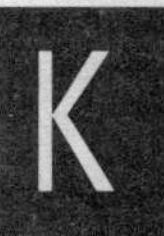

Konakion (*Roche*) is a proprietary form of VITAMIN K – or phytomenadione – used to treat newborn infants in need of the vitamin, and to treat patients deficient in the vitamin because of fat malabsorption. It is produced in the form of (non-prescription) tablets, and ampoules for injection (available in two strengths, only on prescription).

Kwells (*Nicholas-Kiwi*) is a proprietary ANTCHOLINERGIC non-prescription anti-motion sickness preparation containing hyoscine.

✚/▲ warning/side-effects: *see* HYOSCINE.

labetalol hydrochloride is a mixed BETA-BLOCKER and ALPHA-BLOCKER used to treat high blood pressure (hypertension) and to control blood pressure during surgery. Administration is oral in the form of tablets, and by injection. It is not recommended for children.

✚ warning: labetalol hydrochloride should be administered with caution to patients who have heart failure, who are already taking drugs to control the heart rate, or who have a history of bronchospasm.

▲ side-effects: there may be lethargy and debility, headache and/or tingling of the scalp; rashes may break out. Higher dosages may lead to low blood pressure (hypotension).

Related article: LABROCOL; TRANDATE.

Labiton (*L A B*) is a proprietary non-prescription tonic that is not available from the National Health Service. Used primarily to stimulate the appetite, Labiton contains the stimulant CAFFEINE, vitamin B in the form of THIAMINE, extract of kola nut, and ethyl alcohol. It is not recommended for children.

✚ warning: labiton should not be taken by patients who are already taking drugs that directly affect the central nervous system, or who have liver disease.

Laboprin (*L A B*) is a proprietary non-prescription preparation of the non-narcotic ANALGESIC aspirin that is not available from the National Health Service. Produced in the form of tablets, Laboprin also contains the essential amino acid LYSINE. It is not recommended for children.

✚/▲ warning/side-effects: *see* ASPIRIN.

Labosept (*L A B*) is a proprietary non-prescription form of pastilles used to treat mild fungal or bacterial infections of the mouth. The pastilles, to be sucked slowly, are not available from the National Health Service; their active constituent is the ANTISEPTIC drug DEQUALINIUM CHLORIDE.

Labrocol (*Lagap*) is a proprietary form of the mixed BETA-BLOCKER and ALPHA-BLOCKER labetalol hydrochloride, available only on prescription, used to treat high blood pressure (*see* ANTIHYPERTENSIVE) and to control the heart rate during surgery. Produced in the form of tablets (in three strengths), Labrocol is not recommended for children.

✚/▲ warning/side-effects: *see* LABETALOL HYDROCHLORIDE.

lachesine chloride is an ANTICHOLINERGIC drug used to dilate the pupil of the eye, generally in order that the eye may be examined by an ophthalmologist, but sometimes to treat an inflammation in the eye or the eye muscle. It is useful in treating patients who are hypersensitive to other mydriatic drugs. Administration is in the form of eye-drops.

✚ warning: its dilating action is persistent, and prolonged treatment risks the precipitation of glaucoma. Driving may be difficult following mydriatic treatment.

Lacri-Lube (*Allergan*) is a proprietary non-prescription form of liquid paraffin used as a lubricant for the eyes in patients whose tear glands are not functioning effectively. Produced in the form of an ointment, Lacri-Lube also contains HYDROUS WOOL FAT.

✚/▲ warning/side-effects: *see* LIQUID PARAFFIN.

Lacticare (*Stiefel*) is a proprietary non-prescription skin emollient (softener and soother), used to treat chronic conditions of dry skin. Produced in the form of a lotion for topical application, Lacticare contains the simple sugar lactic acid and a moisturizer.

lactulose is a LAXATIVE that works by causing a volume of fluid to be retained in the colon through osmosis. Its action also discourages the increase of ammonia-producing microbes – although it may take up to 48 hours to have full effect.
✚ warning: lactulose should not be administered to patients with any form of intestinal obstruction. Because lactulose is itself a form of sugar, patients who have blood sugar level abnormalities should be checked before being treated.
▲ side-effects: rarely, there is nausea and vomiting.
Related article: DUPHALAC.

Ladropen (*Berk*) is a proprietary ANTIBIOTIC, available only on prescription, used to treat bacterial infections of the skin and of the ear, nose and throat, and especially staphylococcal infections that prove to be resistant to penicillin. Produced in the form of capsules (in two strengths), Ladropen is a preparation of flucloxacillin. It is not suitable for children.
✚/▲ warning/side-effects: *see* FLUCLOXACILLIN.

Laevuflex 20 (*Geistlich*) is a proprietary form of the simple sugar laevulose, prepared in a form for infusion. It may be administered as an alternative to DEXTROSE (glucose) – especially to diabetics, because laevulose is not only easy to absorb but can be converted to glycogen (producing energy) in the absence of insulin.

Lamprene (*Geigy*) is a proprietary preparation of the phenazine drug clofamizine, used to halt the progress of leprosy. Available only on prescription and produced in the form of gelatin capsules, Lamprene is not recommended for children.
✚/▲ warning/side-effects: *see* CLOFAMIZINE.

lanatoside C is a CARDIAC GLUYCOSIDE drug that acts as a heart stimulant, used to treat heart failure and severe heartbeat irregularity. Administration is oral in the form of tablets; ingestion into the body causes the conversion of lanatoside C into another glycoside, digoxin.
✚/▲ warning/side-effects: *see* DIGOXIN.
Related article: CEDILANID.

Lanitop (*Roussel*) is a proprietary form of the CARDIAC GLYCOSIDE heart stimulant medigoxin, available only on prescription, used to treat congestive heart failure and severe heartbeat irregularity. It is produced in the form of tablets.
✚/▲ warning/side-effects: *see* MEDIGOXIN.

lanolin (hydrous wool fat) is a non-proprietary skin emollient (softener and soother) commonly used also as a base for other medications. It has some antibacterial properties, but in some patients can cause a sensitivity reaction (in the form usually of an eczematous rash).

Lanoxin (*Wellcome*) is a proprietary form of the powerful heart stimulant digoxin (a CARDIAC GLYCOSIDE), available only on prescription, used to treat

heart failure and severe heartbeat irregularity. It is produced in the form of tablets (in several strengths, under the names Lanoxin, Lanoxin 125 and Lanoxin PG), as an elixir (under the name Lanoxin PG Elixir) and in ampoules for injection (under the name Lanoxin Injection).
✚/▲ warning/side-effects: *see* DIGOXIN.

Lanvis (*Calmic*) is a proprietary CYTOTOXIC drug, available only on prescription, used to treat acute forms of leukaemia. An antimetabolite, it works by incorporating itself into new-forming cells or by combining with intracellular enzymes. Produced in the form of tablets, Lanvis is a preparation of thioguanine.
✚/▲ warning/side-effects: *see* THIOGUANINE.

Laracor (*Lagap*) is a proprietary form of the BETA-BLOCKER oxprenolol hydrochloride, available only on prescription, used to control and regulate the heart rate and to treat high blood pressure (hypertension). It is produced in the form of tablets (in four strengths).
✚/▲ warning/side-effects: *see* OXPRENOLOL.

Laractone (*Lagap*) is a proprietary DIURETIC drug, available only on prescription, used to treat accumulation of fluids within the tissues (oedema), particularly when due to cirrhosis of the liver. Produced in the form of tablets (in two strengths), Laractone is a preparation of the weak potassium-sparing diuretic spironolactone.
✚/▲ warning/side-effects: *see* SPIRONOLACTONE.

Laraflex (*Lagap*) is a proprietary, non-steroidal, ANTI-INFLAMMATORY non-narcotic ANALGESIC, available only on prescription, used to relieve pain – particularly rheumatic and arthritic pain – and to treat other musculo-skeletal disorders. Its active constituent is naproxen, and it is produced in the form of tablets (in two strengths). Not recommended for children, Laraflex should not be administered to patients with a peptic ulcer, gastrointestinal haemorrhage or asthma, or who are pregnant or lactating.
✚/▲ warning/side-effects: *see* NAPROXEN.

Larapam (*Lagap*) is a proprietary, non-steroidal, ANTI-INFLAMMATORY non-narcotic ANALGESIC, available only on prescription, used to relieve pain – particularly rheumatic and arthritic pain – and to treat other musculo-skeletal disorders. Its active constituent is piroxicam, and it is produced in the form of tablets (in two strengths). Not recommended for children, Larapam should not be administered to patients with a peptic ulcer, gastrointestinal haemorrhage or asthma, or who are pregnant or lactating.
✚/▲ warning/side-effects: *see* PIROXICAM.

Laratrim (*Lagap*) is a proprietary broad-spectrum ANTIBACTERIAL, available only on prescription, used to treat infections of the urinary tract, the sinuses or the middle ear, an inflamed prostate gland, or exacerbated chronic bronchitis. Produced in the form of tablets (in two strengths, the stronger under the name Laratrim Forte) and as a suspension (in two strengths, Laratrim Paediatric Suspension and Laratrim Adult Suspension), Laratrim is a compound

combination of the SULPHONAMIDES trimethoprim and sulphamethoxazole – a compound itself known as co-trimoxazole.
✚/▲ warning/side-effects: *see* CO-TRIMOXAZOLE.

Largactil (*May & Baker*) is a proprietary preparation of the powerful PHENOTHIAZINE drug chlorpromazine hydrochloride, used primarily to treat patients who are undergoing behavioural disturbances (as a major TRANQUILLIZER), or who are psychotic (as an ANTIPSYCHOTIC), particularly schizophrenic. It is also used to treat severe anxiety, or as an anti-emetic sedative prior to surgery. Available only on prescription, Largactil is produced in the form of tablets (in three strengths), as a syrup (under the name Largactil Syrup), as a suspension (under the name Largactil Forte Suspension), as anal suppositories (under the name Largactil Suppositories), and in ampoules for injection (under the name Largactil Injection). In the form of the suppositories and the ampoules for injection Largactil is not recommended for use with children.
✚/▲ warning/side-effects: *see* CHLORPROMAZINE HYDROCHLORIDE.

Larodopa (*Roche*) is a proprietary form of the powerful drug levodopa, used in ANTIPARKINSONISM treatment. It is particularly good at relieving the rigidity and slowness of movement associated with the disease, although it does not always improve the tremor. Produced in the form of tablets, Larodopa is not recommended for children.
✚/▲ warning/side-effects: *see* LEVODOPA.

Lasikal (*Hoechst*) is a proprietary compound DIURETIC drug, available only on prescription, used to treat accumulation of fluids in the tissues (oedema) in cases where extra potassium is also required. Produced in the form of two-layered tablets (consisting of a sustained-release matrix), Lasikal combines the diuretic frusemide with POTASSIUM CHLORIDE. It is not suitable for children.
✚/▲ warning/side-effects: *see* FRUSEMIDE.

Lasilactone (*Hoechst*) is a proprietary compound DIURETIC, available only on prescription, used to treat accumulation of fluids within the tissues (oedema) in cases that have failed to respond to other forms of treatment. Produced in the form of capsules, Lasilactone combines the weak diuretic spironolactone with the powerful diuretic frusemide. It is not recommended for children.
✚/▲ warning/side-effects: *see* FRUSEMIDE; SPIRONOLACTONE.

Lasipressin (*Hoechst*) is a proprietary ANTIHYPERTENSIVE compound, available only on prescription, used to treat mild to moderate high blood pressure (hypertension). Produced in the form of tablets, Lasipressin contains the BETA-BLOCKER penbutolol sulphate with the DIURETIC frusemide.
✚/▲ warning/side-effects: *see* FRUSEMIDE; PENBUTOLOL.

Lasix (*Hoechst*) is a proprietary DIURETIC drug, available only on prescription, used to treat accumulation of fluids within the tissues (oedema), particularly when due to heart, kidney or liver disease, or associated with high blood pressure (hypertension). Produced in the

form of tablets (in three strengths, the third under the name Lasix 500 for use in hospitals only), as a syrup for children (under the name Lasix Paediatric Liquid), and in ampoules for injection (under the name Lasix Injection, and intended particularly to treat conditions associated with cirrhosis of the liver).
✚/▲ warning/side-effects: *see* FRUSEMIDE.

Lasix + K (*Hoechst*) is a proprietary compound DIURETIC drug, available only on prescription, used to treat accumulation of fluids in the tissues (oedema) in cases where extra potassium is also required. Produced in the form of pairs of tablets (the one being the potassium supplement within a sustained-release matrix), Lasix + K combines the diuretic frusemide with POTASSIUM CHLORIDE. It is not suitable for children.
✚/▲ warning/side-effects: *see* FRUSEMIDE.

Lasma (*Pharmax*) is a proprietary non-prescription BRONCHODILATOR, used to treat asthmatic bronchospasm, emphysema and chronic bronchitis. Produced in the form of sustained-release tablets, Lasma is a preparation of the xanthine drug theophylline. It is not recommended for children.
✚/▲ warning/side-effects: *see* THEOPHYLLINE.

Lasonil (*Bayer*) is a proprietary non-prescription ointment used to soothe and treat piles (haemorrhoids) and anal itching. It contains heparinoids (which promote the resorption of fluids accumulating in the tissues) together with the absorptive agent hyaluronidase.

Lassar's paste is a non-proprietary formulation of ZINC OXIDE, salicylic acid and starch in white soft paraffin. Applied topically, it is used to treat hard, layered, dead skin. The compound must not be put on broken or inflamed skin.

latamoxef disodium is a broad-spectrum cephalosporin ANTIBIOTIC used to treat many bacterial infections. Administration is by injection.
✚ warning: latamoxef should not be administered to patients who are already taking aspirin or non-steroid anti-inflammatory drugs; it should be administered with caution to those known to have penicillin sensitivity. Dosage should be reduced in patients with impaired kidney function.
▲ side-effects: there may be hypersensitivity reactions, including effects on the composition of the blood (on which it may have an anticoagulating influence). Rarely, there is diarrhoea.
Related article: MOXALACTAM.

***laxatives** are preparations that promote defecation and so relieve constipation. There are several types. One major type is represented by faecal softeners (which soften the faeces for easier evacuation): they include LIQUID PARAFFIN. Another type is the bulking agent (which increases the overall volume of the faeces in the rectum and thus stimulates bowel movement): bulking agents are mostly what is also called fibre, and include BRAN, ispaghula husk, METHYLCELLULOSE and STERCULIA. A third type is the stimulant laxative, which acts on the intestinal muscles to increase motility: many old-fashioned remedies are stimulants of this kind, including CASCARA, CASTOR OIL, FIGS, and SENNA – but there are modern variants too, such as BISACODYL, DANTHRON, DIOCTYL SODIUM SULPHOSUCCINATE (docusate sodium) and SODIUM PICOSULPHATE. Some laxatives work by bringing in water from surrounding tissues, so increasing overall liquidity: such osmotic laxatives include MAGNESIUM HYDROXIDE, MAGNESIUM SULPHATE and LACTULOSE. Suppositories and enemas also aid in promoting defecation.

Laxoberal (*Windsor*) is a proprietary non-prescription LAXATIVE that is not available from the National Health. A stimulant laxative, Laxoberal is produced in the form of a liquid containing sodium picosulphate.
✚/▲ warning/side-effects: *see* SODIUM PICOSULPHATE.

Ledclair (*Sinclair*) is a proprietary CHELATING AGENT, an antidote to poisoning by heavy metals, especially by lead, available only on prescription. Produced in liquid form in ampoules for injection, and as a cream for topical use on areas of skin that have become broken or sensitive through contact with the metals, Ledclair's active constituent is sodium calciumedetate.
✚/▲ warning/side-effects: *see* SODIUM CALCIUMEDETATE.

Ledercort (*Lederle*) is a proprietary form of the anti-inflammatory glucocorticoid (CORTICOSTEROID) drug triamcinolone, available only on prescription. Produced in the form of tablets (in two strengths) and, as triamcinolone acetonide, as a water-based cream and an anhydrous ointment, Ledercort treats inflammations of the skin (such as severe eczema), and particularly inflammations arising as a result of allergy.
✚/▲ warning/side-effects: *see* TRIAMCINOLONE; TRIAMCINOLONE ACETONIDE.

Lederfen (*Lederle*) is a proprietary, non-steroid, ANTI-INFLAMMATORY non-narcotic ANALGESIC, available only on prescription, used to relieve pain – particularly rheumatic and arthritic pain – and to treat other musculo-skeletal disorders. Its active constituent is fenbufen, and it is produced in the form of tablets (in two strengths) and capsules (under the name Lederfen Capsules). Not recommended for children, Lederfen should not be administered to patients with a peptic ulcer, gastrointestinal haemorrhage or asthma, or who are pregnant or lactating.
✚/▲ warning/side-effects: *see* FENBUFEN.

Ledermycin (*Lederle*) is a proprietary ANTIBIOTIC, available only on prescription, used to treat infections of soft tissues, particularly of the upper respiratory tract. Produced in the form of tablets (in two strengths, the stronger under the name Ledermycin Tablets), Ledermycin is a preparation of the TETRACYCLINE demeclocycline hydrochloride.
✚/▲ warning/side-effects: *see* DEMECLOCYCLINE HYDROCHLORIDE.

Lederspan (*Lederle*) is a proprietary CORTICOSTEROID drug, available only on prescription, used to treat INFLAMMATION of the joints and the soft tissues. Produced in the form of a suspension in vials for injection (in two concentrations), Lederspan's active constituent is

the corticosteroid triamcinolone hexacetonide.
✚/▲ warning/side-effects: *see* TRIAMCINOLONE HEXACETONIDE.

Lejfibre (*Britannia*) is a proprietary non-prescription LAXATIVE that is not available from the National Health Service. A bulking agent – which works by increasing the overall mass of faeces within the rectum, so stimulating bowel movement – Lejfibre is produced in the form of biscuits containing oat BRAN meal. It is not recommended for children.

Lejguar (*Britannia*) is a proprietary non-prescription preparation of guar gum, used to assist in the treatment of patients with uneven blood sugar level (as in diabetes). A high-fibre bulking agent, guar gum has the effect of evening out the peaks and troughs of glucose levels that normally correspond to meals and the intervals between them. Produced in the form of soluble (dispersible) granules, Lejguar is not recommended for children.
✚/▲ warning/side-effects: *see* GUAR GUM.

Lem-sip (*Nicholas-Kiwi*) is a proprietary non-prescription cold relief preparation containing the non-narcotic ANALGESIC paracetamol, the SYMPATHOMIMETIC phenylephrine, sodium citrate and ascorbic acid.
✚/▲ warning/side-effects: *see* ASCORBIC ACID; PARACETAMOL; PHENYLEPHRINE; SODIUM CITRATE.

Lenium (*Winthrop*) is a proprietary non-prescription cream shampoo containing SELENIUM SULPHIDE, a salt thought to act as an antidandruff agent. Lenium should not be used within 48 hours of a hair colorant or a permanent wave.

Lentard MC is a proprietary non-prescription preparation of the protein hormone insulin, in the form of insulin zinc suspension, used to treat diabetic patients. Containing highly purified bovine and porcine insulin, Lentard MC's effect is of intermediate duration, intended to maintain background residual levels of the hormone. It is produced in vials for injection.
✚/▲ warning/side-effects: *see* INSULIN.

Lentizol (*Parke-Davis*) is a proprietary ANTIDEPRESSANT, available only on prescription, used to treat depressive illness, and particularly in cases where some degree of sedation is called for. Produced in the form of capsules (in two strengths), Lentizol is a preparation of the TRICYCLIC amitriptyline hydrochloride, and is not recommended for children.
✚/▲ warning/side-effects: *see* AMITRIPTYLINE.

Leo K (*Leo*) is a proprietary non-prescription form of POTASSIUM supplement, used to treat patients with deficiencies and to replace potassium in patients taking potassium-depleting drugs such as CORTICOSTEROIDS. It is produced in the form of tablets containing potassium chloride.
✚/▲ warning/side-effects: *see* POTASSIUM CHLORIDE.

Lergoban (*Riker*) is a proprietary non-prescription ANTIHISTAMINE drug used to treat various allergic conditions, particularly conditions of the nose (hay fever) and skin (urticaria). Produced in the form of tablets, Lergoban is a preparation of diphenylpyraline

hydrochloride. It is not recommended for children.
✚/▲ warning/side-effects: *see* DIPHENYLPYRALINE HYDROCHLORIDE.

Leukeran (*Calmic*) is a proprietary CYTOTOXIC drug, available only on prescription, used to treat various forms of cancer, particularly leukaemia, ovarian cancer and certain lymphomas. Produced in the form of tablets (in two strengths), Leukeran is a preparation of chlorambucil.
✚/▲ warning/side-effects: *see* CHLORAMBUCIL.

levamisole is an ANTHELMINTIC drug used specifically to treat infestation by roundworms. Effective, it is also well tolerated and side-effects are rare. Occasionally there may be mild nausea.

Levius (*Farmitalia Carlo Erba*) is a proprietary, non-prescription non-steroid, ANTI-INFLAMMATORY non-narcotic ANALGESIC, used to relieve pain – particularly rheumatic and arthritic pain – and to treat other musculo-skeletal disorders. Its active constituent is aspirin, and it is produced in the form of tablets. Not recommended for children aged under 10 years, Levius should not be administered to patients with a peptic ulcer, gastrointestinal haemorrhage, asthma, renal or hepatic disfunction, or to those who are pregnant or lactating.
✚/▲ warning/side-effects: *see* ASPIRIN.

levodopa is an immensely powerful ANTIPARKINSONISM drug used to treat parkinsonism (but not the symptoms of parkinsonism induced by drugs). Effective in reducing the slowness of movement and rigidity associated with parkinsonism, levodopa is not so successful in controlling the tremor. Administration is in the form of capsules or tablets, often combined with another form of drug that inhibits the conversion of levodopa to dopamine outside the brain. It is the presence of such an inhibitor that may produce involuntary movements. Initial dosage should be minimal and increase gradually; intervals between doses may be critical to each individual patient. Treated with levodopa a patient may be expected to improve quality of life for 6 to 18 months, and for that improvement to obtain for up to another 2 years; thereafter a slow decline is to be expected.

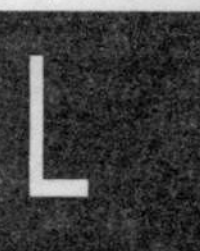

✚ warning: levodopa should not be administered to patients with a specific form of glaucoma; it should be administered with caution to those with heart disease, psychiatric illness, diabetes or peptic ulcers. Monitoring of heart, blood, liver and kidney functions is advisable during prolonged treatment; some check on psychological disposition should also be made.
▲ side-effects: there may be nausea, dizziness, irregularity of the heart rate, insomnia and restlessness, and discoloration of the urine. Psychiatric symptoms and involuntary movements may direct dosage quantities.
Related articles: BROCADOPA; LARODOPA; MADOPAR; SINEMET.

levonorgestrel is a female sex hormone, a PROGESTOGEN used especially in ORAL CONTRACEPTIVES – in which it may or may not be combined with an OESTROGEN. It is occasionally alternatively used, also in combination with oestrogens, in hormone replacement therapy in menopausal women. The hormone NORGESTREL is a weaker form of levonorgestrel.

✚ warning: levonorgestrel should not be administered to patients who are pregnant, or with vascular or liver disease, cancer of the liver or of the breast, or vaginal bleeding. It should be administered with caution to those with heart disease or high blood pressure (hypertension), diabetes, or migraine.

▲ side-effects: there may be nausea and vomiting, with a headache; menstrual irregularities and breast tenderness are common, but there may also be weight gain and depression. Some patients experience skin disorders. *Related articles:* EUGYNON; LOGYNON; MICROGYNON 30; MICROVAL; Norgeston; OVRAN; OVRANETTE; SCHERING PC4; TRINORDIOL.

Levophed (*Winthrop*) is a proprietary VASOCONSTRICTOR, a sympathomimetic used in emergencies to raise the blood pressure in cases of dangerously low blood pressure or even cardiac arrest. Available only on prescription, Levophed is produced in ampoules (in two strengths) for injection or infusion following dilution, and is a preparation of noradrenaline acid tartrate.

✚/▲ warning/side-effects: *see* NORADRENALINE.

levorphanol is a narcotic ANALGESIC used to treat severe pain. Because it is a narcotic, its prolonged use may lead to dependence (addiction) and the proprietary form of the drug is therefore on the controlled drugs list. Nevertheless it causes fewer sedative effects than many other narcotics, and is administered (as levorphanol tartrate) orally in the form of tablets, or by injection.

✚ warning: levorphanol should not be administered to patients who suffer from respiratory difficulties (such as asthma), from head injury or from pressure within the skull; it should be administered with extreme caution to patients with low blood pressure (hypotension), thyroid problems, or impaired kidney or liver function. Dosage should be reduced for elderly or debilitated patients.

▲ side-effects: breathing may become shallow, and coughing be suppressed. Commonly there is also constipation and urine retention, with or without nausea. There may be pain at the site of injection. *Related article:* DROMORAN.

Lexotan (*Roche*) is a proprietary ANXIOLYTIC drug, available on prescription only to private patients, used to treat anxiety in the short term. Produced in the form of tablets (in two strengths), Lexotan is a preparation of the BENZODIAZEPINE bromazepam. It is not recommended for children.

✚/▲ warning/side-effects: *see* BROMAZEPAM.

Lexpec (*RP Drugs*) is a proprietary preparation of the VITAMIN B folic acid, available only on prescription, used to treat body deficiency of the vitamin (as occurs in certain types of anaemia). It is produced in the form of a syrup. Two further versions are also available, both including iron (in the form of ferric ammonium citrate), under the names Lexpec with Iron and Lexpec with Iron-M, and intended

as mineral-and-vitamin supplements for use in treating anaemia during pregnancy.
✚ warning: the iron preparations should not be taken by patients who are already being treated with tetracycline antibiotics.
▲ side-effects: the iron preparations may cause nausea or constipation, and should be drunk through a straw because the syrup can cause a discoloration of the teeth.

Libanil (*Approved Prescription Services*) is a proprietary preparation of the SULPHONYLUREA glibenclamide, used to treat adult-onset diabetes; it works by promoting the formation of insulin in whatever remains of the capacity of the pancreas for it, and increasing the number of insulin receptors. Available only on prescription, Libanil is produced in the form of tablets (in two strengths).
✚/▲ warning/side-effects: *see* GLIBENCLAMIDE.

Libraxin (*Roche*) is a proprietary compound, available on prescription only to private patients, now less commonly used to treat peptic ulcers, gastrointestinal disturbance caused by anxiety, or muscle spasm. Produced in the form of tablets, Libraxin's major active constituent is the BENZODIAZEPINE chlordiazepoxide. It is not recommended for children, and all use is now not recommended.
✚/▲ warning/side-effects: *see* CHLORDIAZEPOXIDE.

Librium (*Roche*) is a proprietary form of the BENZODIAZEPINE chlordiazepoxide, used to treat anxiety, insomnia in the short term, and symptoms of acute alcohol withdrawal. Available on prescription only to private patients, Librium is produced in the form of tablets (in three strengths), capsules (in two strengths) and powder for reconstitution as a medium for injection. It is not recommended for children.
✚/▲ warning/side-effects: *see* CHLORDIAZEPOXIDE.

Lidocaton is a proprietary preparation of the local ANAESTHETIC lignocaine, used in cartridges for dental surgery.
✚/▲ warning/side-effects: *see* LIGNOCAINE.

lidoflazine is a CALCIUM ANTAGONIST and VASODILATOR used to reduce blood pressure and prevent recurrent attacks of angina pectoris (heart pain). Administration is oral in the form of tablets.
✚ warning: lidoflazine should not be administered to patients who are pregnant.
▲ side-effects: the heart rate is increased. There may be headache, dizziness and ringing in the ears (tinnitus); some patients have nightmares. Gastrointestinal disturbance may occur.
Related article: CLINIUM.

lignocaine is primarily a local ANAESTHETIC, the medium of choice for very many topical or minor surgical procedures, especially in dentistry (because it is absorbed directly through mucous membranes). It is, for example, used on the throat to prepare a patient for bronchoscopy. For general anaesthesia it may be combined with adrenaline. But it is also administered in the treatment of heart conditions involving heartbeat irregularities, and is effective in safely slowing the heart rate (particularly after a heart attack). Administration is (in the form of a solution of lignocaine hydrochloride) by infiltration, injection or infusion, or topically as a gel, an ointment, a spray, a lotion, or as eye-drops.

✚ warning: lignocaine should not be administered to patients with the neuromuscular disease myasthenia gravis; it should be administered with caution to those with heart or liver failure (in order not to cause depression of the central nervous system and convulsions), or from epilepsy. Dosage should be reduced for the elderly and the debilitated. Full facilities for emergency cardio-respiratory resuscitation should be on hand during anaesthetic treatment.

▲ side-effects: there is generally a slowing of the heart rate and a fall in blood pressure. Some patients under anaesthetic become agitated, others enter a state of euphoria.

Related articles: DEPO-MEDRONE WITH LIDOCAINE; INSTILLAGEL; LIDOCATON; LIGNOSTAB; MINIMS; NEO-LIDOCATON; XYLOCAINE; XYLOCARD; XYLODASE; XYLOPROCT; XYLOTOX.

Lignostab is a proprietary preparation of the local ANAESTHETIC lignocaine, used in cartridges for dental surgery.

✚/▲ warning/side-effects: *see* LIGNOCAINE.

Limbitrol (*Roche*) is a proprietary compound ANTIDEPRESSANT, available on prescription only to private patients, used to treat depressive illness and associated anxiety. Produced in capsules (in two strengths, under the names Limbitrol 5 and Limbitrol 10), Limbitrol's active constituents are amitriptyline and chlordiazepoxide. It is not recommended for the elderly or for children.

✚/▲ warning/side-effects: *see* AMITRIPTYLINE; CHLORDIAZEPOXIDE.

Limclair (*Sinclair*) is a proprietary preparation of trisodium edetate, available only on prescription, used to treat the symptoms of an excess of calcium in the blood (hypercalcaemia). It is produced in ampoules for injection.

✚/▲ warning/side-effects: *see* TRISODIUM EDETATE.

Lincocin (*Upjohn*) is a proprietary ANTIBIOTIC, available only on prescription, used to treat serious infections of the tissues and bones (particularly infections that prove to be resistant to penicillin). Produced in the form of capsules, as a syrup for dilution (the potency of the syrup once dilute is retained for 14 days) and in ampoules for injection, Lincocin is a preparation of lincomycin.

✚/▲ warning/side-effects: *see* LINCOMYCIN.

lincomycin is an ANTIBIOTIC that is now used less commonly than it once was (because of side-effects) to treat infections of bones and joints, and peritonitis (inflammation of the peritoneal lining of the abdominal cavity). Administration is oral in the form of capsules and as a dilute syrup, or by injection or infusion.

✚ warning: lincomycin should not be administered to patients suffering from diarrhoea; if diarrhoea or other symptoms of colitis appear during treatment, administration must be halted at once. This is because lincomycin's comparatively high toxicity is especially disposed towards promoting colitis (particularly in mature or elderly women), causing potentially severe symptoms. It should be administered with caution to patients impaired liver or kidney function.

▲ side-effects: if diarrhoea or other symptoms of colitis appear during treatment, administration must be halted at once (see above). There may be nausea and vomiting.
Related article: LINCOCIN.

***linctuses** are medicated syrups, thick and soothing enough to relieve sore throats or loosen a cough. (A linctus is not the same as an expectorant, however, which is intended to increase the viscosity of sputum and so make it easier to cough up. Nor is it necessarily an elixir, which disguises a potentially horrible taste with a sweetening substance like glycerol or alcohol.)

lindane, or gamma benzene hexachloride, is a drug used to treat parasitic infestation by lice (pediculosis) or by itch-mites (scabies) on the skin surface, particularly under the hair. However, strains of head-lice resistant to lindane have recently emerged, and the drug is now not recommended for use on the scalp. Administration is topical in the form of a lotion or a shampoo, to be left wet as long as possible.

✚ warning: keep lindane away from the eyes.

▲ side-effects: side-effects are rare, but a few patients suffer minor skin irritation.
Related articles: ESODERM; LOREXANE; QUELLADA.

Lingraine (*Winthrop*) is a proprietary anti-migraine drug, available only on prescription. Produced in the form of tablets, Lingraine is a preparation of the ergot-derived alkaloid ergotamine tartrate. It is not recommended for children.

✚/▲ warning/side-effects: *see* ERGOTAMINE TARTRATE.

liniments are medicated lotions for rubbing into the skin; many contain alcohol and/or camphor, and are intended to relieve minor muscle indispositions. Some liniments are alternatively produced for application on a surgical dressing.

Lioresal (*Ciba*) is a proprietary SKELETAL MUSCLE RELAXANT, available only on prescription, used to treat muscle spasm caused by injury or disease in the central nervous system. Produced in the form of tablets and as a sugar-free liquid for dilution (the potency of the diluted liquid is retained for 14 days), Lioresal is a preparation of baclofen.

✚/▲ warning/side-effects: *see* BACLOFEN.

liothyronine sodium is a form of the natural thyroid HORMONE triiodothyronine, used to make up a hormonal deficiency (hypothyroidism) and to treat the associated symptoms (myxoedema). It may also be used in the treatment of goitre and of thyroid cancer. Liothyronine sodium is rapidly absorbed by the body and is administered by intravenous injection in emergency treatment of hypothyroid coma. In other circumstances, administration is oral in the form of tablets, or by injection.

✚ warning: liothyronine sodium should not be administered to patients with cardiovascular disease or angina pectoris (heart pain), or impaired secretion from the adrenal glands.

▲ side-effects: there may be an increase in the heart rate, heartbeat irregularities and angina; some patients experience headache, muscle cramp, flushing and sweating; there may also be diarrhoea. Dramatic weight loss occurs in some patients.
Related article: TERTROXIN.

L

Lipobase (*Brocades*) is a proprietary non-prescription skin emollient (softener and soother), used to treat dry conditions of the skin (especially in alternation with corticosteroid preparations). Produced in the form of cream, Lipobase contains stearyl alcohol in a paraffin base, and is a base in which other medications can be applied topically.

Lipoflavonoid (*Lewis*) is a proprietary non-prescription MULTIVITAMIN compound that is not available from the National Health Service. Produced in the form of capsules, Lipoflavonoid contains THIAMINE (vitamin B_1), RIBOFLAVINE (vitamin B_2), PYRIDOXINE (vitamin B_6), HYDROXOCOBALAMIN (vitamin B_{12}), NICOTINAMIDE and INOSITOL (both of the B complex), in addition to ASCORBIC ACID (vitamin C) and other metabolic constituents. It is not recommended for children.

Lipotriad (*Lewis*) is a proprietary non-prescription MULTIVITAMIN compound that is not available from the National Health Service. Produced in the form of capsules and as an elixir, Lipotriad contains THIAMINE (vitamin B_1), RIBOFLAVINE (vitamin B_2), PYRIDOXINE (vitamin B_6), HYDROXOCOBALAMIN (vitamin B_{12}), NICOTINAMIDE, INOSITOL (both of the B complex) and other metabolic constituents. It is not recommended for children.

liquid paraffin is an old-fashioned but effective LAXATIVE, used in many households to relieve constipation. It is a constituent of a number of proprietary laxatives and some non-proprietary formulations. But it can also be used as a tear-substitute, administered as an eye ointment for patients whose lachrymal apparatus is dysfunctioning.

✚ warning: prolonged or continuous use of liquid paraffin as a laxative is to be avoided.

▲ side-effects: little is absorbed in the intestines: seepage of the paraffin may thus occur from the anus, causing local irritation. Prolonged use may interfere with the internal absorption of fat- soluble vitamins.
Related articles: AGAROL; LACRI-LUBE; PETROLAGAR.

Liquifilm Tears (*Allergan*) is a proprietary non-prescription tear-substitute, used to lubricate the eyes of patients whose lachrymal apparatus is not working properly. Produced in the form of eye drops, Liquifilm Tears is a solution of POLYVINYL ALCOHOL.

Liquigen (*Scientific Hospital Supplies*) is a proprietary non-prescription gluten-free milk substitute, produced for patients recovering from intestinal surgery or with chronic disease of the liver or of the pancreas; it may also be used for patients on the special diet associated with epilepsy. Produced in the form of an emulsion, Liquigen is a preparation of neutral lipids.

liquorice, deglycyrrhizinized, is a constituent of some compound drugs used to treat peptic ulcers particularly in the stomach, but also in the duodenum.

Liskonum (*Smith, Kline & French*) is a proprietary drug, available only on prescription, used to treat mania and to prevent manic-depressive illnesses. Produced in the form of sustained-release tablets, Liskonum is a preparation of lithium carbonate. It is not recommended for children.

✚/▲ warning/side-effects: *see* LITHIUM.

Litarex (*CP Pharmaceuticals*) is a proprietary drug, available only on prescription, used to treat acute mania and to prevent manic-depressive illnesses. Produced in the form of sustained- release tablets, Litarex is a preparation of lithium citrate. It is not recommended for children.

✚/▲ warning/side-effects: *see* LITHIUM.

lithium, in the form of lithium carbonate or lithium citrate, is effective in preventing the euphoric or hyperactive form of psychosis that is mania, and in preventing manic-depressive illness. How it works remains imperfectly understood, but its use is so successful that the side-effects caused by its toxicity are deemed to be justified. Administration is oral in the form of tablets and sustained-release tablets.

✚ warning: lithium should not be administered to patients with heart disease, impaired kidney function or imperfect sodium balance in the bloodstream. It should be administered with caution to those who are pregnant or lactating, or who are elderly. Prolonged treatment may cause kidney and thyroid gland dysfunction; prolonged overdosage causes eventual brain disease, convulsions, coma, and finally death. Consequently, blood levels of lithium must be regularly checked for toxicity; thyroid function must be monitored; and there must be adequate intake of fluids and sodium.

▲ side-effects: many long-term patients experience nausea, thirst and excessive urination, gastrointestinal disturbance, weakness and tremor. There may be fluid retention and consequent weight gain. Visual disturbances and increasing gastric problems indicate lithium intoxication.

Related articles: CAMCOLIT; LISKONUM; LITAREX; PHASAL; Priadel.

LoAsid (*Calmic*) is a proprietary, non-prescription, compound ANTACID that is not available from the National Health Service. Used to treat severe indigestion, heartburn, gastric or peptic ulcers, and hiatus hernia, it is produced in the form of tablets to be chewed, and represents a preparation of ALUMINIUM HYDROXIDE together with MAGNESIUM HYDROXIDE and the antifoaming agent dimethicone. It is not recommended for children.

Lobak (*Sterling Research*) is a proprietary non-narcotic ANALGESIC, available on prescription only to private patients, used to treat painful muscle spasm. Produced in the form of tablets, Lobak represents a preparation of paracetamol together with the SKELETAL MUSCLE RELAXANT chlormezanone. It is not recommended for children.

✚/▲ warning/side-effects: *see* CHLORMEZANONE; PARACETAMOL.

Locabiotal (*Servier*) is a proprietary ANTIBIOTIC, available only on prescription, used to treat infection and inflammation in the nose and throat. Produced in an aerosol with a nose and mouth adaptor, Locabiotal is a preparation of the minor anti-inflammatory agent fusafungine. It is not recommended for children aged under 3 years.

***local anaesthetic:** *see* ANAESTHETIC.

Locan (*Duncan Flockhart*) is a proprietary non-prescription local ANAESTHETIC, used to treat painful skin conditions and itching. Produced in the form of cream, Locan is a compound of amethocaine and two other local anaesthetics.
✚/▲ warning/side-effects: *see* AMETHOCAINE.

Locasol New Formula (*Cow & Gate*) is a proprietary non-prescription nutritional formulation, used instead of milk in diets for people who suffer from calcium intolerance. Produced in the form of powder, Locasol New Formula is a preparation of protein, carbohydrate, fat, lactose, vitamins and minerals.

Lockets (*Mars*) are a proprietary non-prescription cold relief preparation containing honey, GLYCEROL, citric acid, menthol and eucalyptus.
✚/▲ warning/side-effects: *see* MENTHOL.

Locobase (*Brocades*) is a proprietary non-prescription skin emollient (softener and soother), used to treat dry conditions of the skin (especially in alternation with corticosteroid preparations). Produced in the form of a water-miscible cream and an anhydrous ointment, Locobase is a base in which other medications can be applied topically to the skin.

Locoid (*Brocades*) is a proprietary CORTICOSTEROID, available only on prescription, used to treat serious non-infective inflammatory skin conditions, such as eczema. Produced in the form of a water-miscible cream, in a fatty cream base (under the name Lipocream), ointment and a scalp lotion, Locoid is a preparation of the steroid hydrocortisone butyrate. Another version of Locoid additionally containing the broad-spectrum ANTIBIOTIC CHLORQUINALDOL is also available (under the name Locoid C), produced in the form of a cream and an ointment.
✚/▲ warning/side-effects: *see* HYDROCORTISONE BUTYRATE.

Locorten-Vioform (*Ciba*) is a proprietary ANTIBACTERIAL and ANTIFUNGAL, available only on prescription, used to treat infections in the ear. Produced in the form of ear-drops, Locorten-Vioform is a compound of CLIOQUINOL and the minor CORTICOSTEROID FLUMETHASONE PIVALATE.
✚/▲ warning/side-effects: *see* CLIOQUINOL.

Lodine (*Ayerst*) is a proprietary ANTI-INFLAMMATORY, non-narcotic ANALGESIC, available only on prescription, used to treat the pain of rheumatism and of other musculo-skeletal disorders. Produced in the form of capsules, Lodine is a preparation of etodolac. It is not recommended for children.
✚/▲ warning/side-effects: *see* ETODOLAC.

Loestrin (*Parke-Davis*) is an ORAL CONTRACEPTIVE, available only on prescription, that combines the OESTROGEN ethinyloestradiol with the PROGESTOGEN norethisterone acetate. It is produced in packs of 21 tablets (in two strengths, under the names Loestrin 20 and Loestrin 30) representing one complete menstrual cycle.
✚/▲ warning/side-effects: *see* ETHINYLOESTRADIOL; NORETHISTERONE.

Lofenalac (*Bristol-Myers*) is a proprietary non-prescription nutritional supplement, used to nourish patients with amino-acid abnormalities (such as phenylketonuria). Produced in the form of a powder, Lofenalac contains protein, carbohydrate, fats, vitamins and minerals. It is gluten-, sucrose- and lactose-free.

lofepramine is an ANTIDEPRESSANT drug of a type that has fewer sedative properties than many others. Used to treat depressive illness, it is thus suited more to the treatment of withdrawn and apathetic patients than to those who are agitated and restless. Administration is oral in the form of tablets.
✚ warning: lofepramine should not be administered to patients with heart disease or liver failure; it should be administered with extreme caution to those with epilepsy, psychoses or glaucoma, or who are pregnant. Treatment may take up to four weeks to achieve full effect; premature withdrawal of treatment thereafter may cause the return of symptoms.
▲ side-effects: dry mouth, drowsiness, blurred vision, constipation and urinary retention are all fairly common; there may also be heartbeat irregularities accompanying low blood pressure (hypotension). Concentration and speed of reaction are affected. Elderly patients may enter a state of confusion; younger patients may experience behavioural disturbances. There may be alteration in blood sugar levels, and weight gain.
Related article: GAMANIL.

Logynon (*Schering*) is an ORAL CONTRACEPTIVE, available only on prescription, that combines the OESTROGEN ethinyloestradiol with the PROGESTOGEN levonorgestrel. It is produced in packs either of 21 tablets or (under the name Logynon ED) of 28 tablets, both representing one complete menstrual cycle.
✚/▲ warning/side-effects: *see* ETHINYLOESTRADIOL; LEVONORGESTREL.

Lomodex (*CP Pharmaceuticals*) is a proprietary form of the plasma substitute dextran, available only on prescription, used in infusion with either saline (sodium chloride) or glucose to make up a deficiency in the overall volume of blood in a patient, or to prevent thrombosis following surgery. Produced in flasks (bottles) for infusion, there is a choice of two concentrations: Lomodex 40 and Lomodex 70.
✚/▲ warning/side-effects: *see* DEXTRAN.

Lomotil (*Gold Cross*) is a proprietary ANTIDIARRHOEAL drug, available only on prescription, which works by reducing the speed at which material travels along the intestines. Produced in the form of tablets and as a sugar-free liquid for dilution (with glycerol: the potency of the diluted liquid is retained for 14 days), Lomotil is a preparation of the OPIATE diphenoxylate

hydrochloride and the ANTICHOLINERGIC belladonna alkaloid, atropine sulphate. It is not recommended for children aged under 2 years.
✚/▲ warning/side-effects: *see* ATROPINE SULPHATE; DIPHENOXYLATE HYDROCHLORIDE.

lomustine is a CYTOTOXIC drug that is used particularly to treat Hodgkin's disease (cancer of the lymphatic tissues) and some solid tumours. It works by disrupting cellular DNA, so inhibiting cell replication, and is administered orally in the form of capsules at intervals of between 4 and 6 weeks.
✚ warning: prolonged use may cause sterility in men and an early menopause in women; in both sexes it may lead to permanent bone- marrow damage. Prolonged treatment has also been associated with the incidence of leukaemia following simultaneous irradiation treatment. Blood count monitoring is essential. Dosage should be the minimum still to be effective.
▲ side-effects: there is commonly nausea and vomiting. The blood-producing capacity of the bone-marrow is impaired (although the effect is delayed – which is why there should be a good interval between doses). There may be hair loss.
Related article: CCNU.

Loniten (*Upjohn*) is a proprietary VASODILATOR, available only on prescription, used – in combination with a DIURETIC (such as a thiazide) and a BETA-BLOCKER – to treat severe high blood pressure (hypertension). Produced in the form of tablets (in three strengths), Loniten is a preparation of minoxidil.
✚/▲ warning/side-effects: *see* MINOXIDIL.

loperamide hydrochloride is an ANTIDIARRHOEAL drug which acts on the sympathetic nervous system to inhibit peristalsis – the waves of muscular activity that force along the intestinal contents – so reducing motility. Although loperamide is an OPIATE, even prolonged treatment is unlikely to cause dependence; it also has fewer sedative effects on patients than other opiates used to treat chronic diarrhoea. Administration is oral in the form of capsules or as a dilute syrup.
✚ warning: loperamide hydrochloride should be administered with caution to patients who are elderly, in whom it may cause faecal impaction. Prolonged use should be avoided in order not to wear out the muscles on which the drug has its effect, causing irritable bowel syndrome. Adequate fluid intake must be maintained.
▲ side-effects: there may be a rash.
Related articles: ARRET; IMODIUM.

Lopid (*Parke-Davis*) is a proprietary preparation of the drug gemfibrozil, available only on prescription, used to treat high levels of cholesterol or other lipids (fats) in the blood (hyperlipidaemia). Lopid works by inhibiting the uptake of fats by the liver. Produced for oral adminstration in the form of capsules, Lopid is not recommended for children.
✚/▲ warning/side-effects: *see* GEMFIBROZIL.

loprazolam is a HYPNOTIC drug, one of the BENZODIAZEPINES, used as a tranquillizer to treat insomnia. Administration is oral in the form of tablets.
✚ warning: loprazolam should

not be administered to patients with acute pulmonary insufficiency (lung disease or shallow breathing) or with myasthenia gravis; it should be administered with caution to those with impaired liver or kidney function, who are pregnant or lactating, or who are elderly and debilitated.

▲ side-effects: concentration and speed of reaction are affected. There may also be drowsiness, dry mouth and dizziness; elderly patients may enter a state of confusion. Some patients experience sensitivity reactions. Prolonged use may eventually result in tolerance, and finally dependence.
Related article: DORMONOCT.

Lopresor (*Geigy*) is a proprietary preparation of the BETA-BLOCKER metoprolol tartrate, available only on prescription, used to control and regulate the heart rate and to treat high blood pressure (hypertension), angina pectoris (heart pain), or an excess of thyroid hormones in the blood (thyrotoxicosis). It is produced in the form of tablets (in two strengths) and in ampoules for injection. A stronger form is also produced (under the name Lopresor SR). None of these is recommended for children.

✚/▲ warning/side-effects: *see* METOPROLOL.

Lopresoretic (*Geigy*) is a proprietary ANTIHYPERTENSIVE compound, available only on prescription, used to treat mild to moderate high blood pressure (hypertension). Produced in the form of tablets, Lopresoretic is a preparation of the BETA-BLOCKER metoprolol tartrate together with the THIAZIDE DIURETIC chlorthalidone. It is not recommended for children.

✚/▲ warning/side-effects: *see* CHLORTHALIDONE; METOPROLOL.

lorazepam is an ANXIOLYTIC and ANTIDEPRESSANT drug, one of the BENZODIAZEPINES, used to treat mental stress ranging from anxiety to severe panic, including depressive illness. It may also be used to treat insomnia. Administration is oral in the form of tablets, or by injection.

✚ warning: lorazepam should be administered with caution to patients with repiratory difficulties, glaucoma, or kidney or liver damage; who are in the last stages of pregnancy or are lactating; or who are elderly or debilitated. Prolonged use or abrupt withdrawal of the drug should be avoided.

▲ side-effects: concentration and speed of reaction are affected. Drowsiness, dizziness, headache, dry mouth and shallow breathing are all fairly common. Elderly patients may enter a state of confusion. Sensitivity reactions may occur. The drug may enhance the effects of alcohol consumption.
Related articles: ALMAZINE; ATIVAN.

Lorexane (*Care*) is a proprietary non-prescription preparation of the parasiticidal drug lindane, used to treat infestation of the skin of the trunk and limbs by itch-mites (scabies) or by lice (pediculosis). It is produced in the form of a water-miscible cream and (under the name Lorexane No.3) as a shampoo.

✚/▲ warning/side-effects: *see* LINDANE.

lormetazepam is a HYPNOTIC drug, one of the BENZODIAZEPINES, used as a TRANQUILLIZER to treat

insomnia (especially in the elderly). Administration is oral in the form of tablets.
✚ warning: lormetazepam should be administered with caution to patients with lung disease or shallow breathing, or impaired liver or kidney function, who are pregnant or lactating, or who are elderly and debilitated.
▲ side-effects: concentration and speed of reaction are affected. There may also be drowsiness, dry mouth and dizziness. Some patients experience sensitivity reactions. Prolonged use may eventually result in tolerance, and finally dependence.
Related article: NOCTAMID.

lotio rubra is a non-proprietary formulation of ZINC SULPHATE in solution with amaranth, used as a lotion to clean and dress ulcers.

***lotions** are medicated liquids used to bathe or wash skin conditions, the hair or the eyes. In many cases lotions should be left wet after application for as long as possible.

Lotussin (*Searle*) is a proprietary non-prescription ANTIHISTAMINE EXPECTORANT and cough mixture that is not available from the National Health Service. Produced in the form of a syrup for dilution (the potency of the mixture once dilute is retained for 14 days), Lotussin is a compound of the cough suppressant dextromethorphan hydrobromine, the antihistamine diphenhydramine hydrochloride, the SYMPATHOMIMETIC ephedrine hydrochloride and the EXPECTORANT guaiphenesin. It is not recommended for children aged under 12 months.
✚/▲ warning/side-effects: *see* DEXTROMETHORPHAN; DIPHENHYDRAMINE HYDROCHLORIDE; EPHEDRINE HYDROCHLORIDE.

LSD, or lysergic acid diethylamide, is a powerful hallucinogenic drug that was occasionally used therapeutically to assist in the treatment of psychological disorders. Although the drug expands awareness and perception, and creates a false world at the same time, there are many toxic side-effects and its use – apart from being illegal – can lead to severely psychotic conditions in which life itself may be at risk.
✚ warning: LSD should be used only to treat cases for which it is deemed essential. Alteration in the experience of all the senses occurs; psychotic affects are common; confusion and depression may follow. Tolerance of the drug develops rapidly; for the same effect, dosages therefore tend to increase equally rapidly.
▲ side-effects: usage may cause dizziness and sweating, tingling and dilated pupils, gastrointestinal disturbance and anxiety, tremor and loss of delicate control of the muscles.

Ludiomil (*Ciba*) is a proprietary ANTIDEPRESSANT, available only on prescription, used to treat depressive illness especially in cases where sedation is deemed additionally to be necessary. Produced in the form of tablets (in four strengths), Ludiomil is a preparation of maprotiline hydrochloride. It is not recommended for children.
✚/▲ warning/side-effects: *see* MAPROTILINE HYDROCHLORIDE.

Lugacin (*Lagap*) is a proprietary ANTIBIOTIC, available only on prescription, used to treat serious infections in specific body organs, such as meningitis. Produced in

ampoules for injection, Lugacin is a preparation of the aminoglycoside gentamicin.
✚/▲ warning/side-effects: *see* GENTAMICIN.

Lugol's solution is a non-proprietary solution of iodine and potassium iodide in water (and is also known as aqueous iodine solution). It is used as an iodine supplement for patients suffering from an excess of thyroid hormones in the bloodstream (thyrotoxicosis), especially prior to thyroid surgery.
✚/▲ warning/side-effects: *see* IODINE.

Luminal (*Winthrop*) is a proprietary form of the BARBITURATE phenobarbitone, and is on the controlled drugs list. Produced in the form of tablets (in three strengths), Luminal is used to treat all forms of epilepsy, although it should be administered with extreme caution to children or to the elderly.
✚/▲ warning/side-effects: *see* PHENOBARBITONE.

Lurselle (*Merrell Dow*) is a proprietary form of the drug probucol, available only on prescription, used to treat high levels of cholesterol or other lipids (fats) in the blood. Produced in the form of tablets, Lurselle is not recommended for children.
✚/▲ warning/side-effects: *see* PROBUCOL.

lymecycline is a broad-spectrum ANTIBIOTIC, one of the tetracyclines, used to treat infections of many kinds. Administration is oral in the form of capsules.
✚ warning: lymecycline should not be administered to patients with kidney failure, who are pregnant, or who are aged under 12 years. It should be administered with caution to those who are lactating, or who have impaired liver function.
▲ side-effects: there may be nausea and vomiting, with diarrhoea. Some patients experience a sensitivity to light. Rarely, there are allergic reactions.
Related article: TETRALYSAL.

lynoestrenol is a PROGESTOGEN used in combination ORAL CONTRACEPTIVES that contain both a progestogen and an OESTROGEN. Administration is oral in the form of tablets.
✚ warning: lynoestrenol in combination with an oestrogen should not be administered to patients with thrombosis, liver disease, sickle- cell anaemia, cancer of the womb or of the breast, an excess of lipids (fats) in the blood, or severe migraine; who are pregnant; or who are bleeding from the vagina for an undiagnosed reason. It should be administered with caution to those with epilepsy, diabetes, heart or kidney disease, high blood pressure (hypertension), asthma, varicose veins and/or obesity, or depression. Many doctors will not prescribe a combined oral contraceptive for women aged over 35 years or who smoke cigarettes.
▲ side-effects: the combined oral contraceptive may cause nausea and vomiting, with headache; there may be breast tenderness, slight weight gain and a change in libido. Some women experience high blood pressure (hypertension), a tendency to thrombosis, and/or reduced menstrual flow. Rarely, there is impaired

liver function or a sensitivity to light.
Related article: MINILYN.

lypressin, or 8-lysine vasopressin, is one of two major forms of the ANTIDIURETIC HORMONE vasopressin, used to treat pituitary-originated diabetes insipidus. Administration of lypressin is topical in the form of a nasal spray.

L

✚/▲ warning/side-effects: *see* VASOPRESSIN.
Related article: SYNTOPRESSIN.

lysergide is another chemical name for lysergic acid diethylamide, or LSD.
see LSD.

8-lysine vasopressin is a chemical name for lypressin.
see LYPRESSIN.

Maalox (*Rorer*) is a proprietary, non-prescription, compound ANTACID used to treat severe indigestion, heartburn, and gastric or duodenal ulcers. Produced in the form of tablets to be chewed (in two strengths, the stronger under the name Maalox Concentrated Tablets, not available from the National Health Service) and as a suspension (under the name Maalox Suspension), Maalox is a preparation of ALUMINIUM HYDROXIDE together with magnesium hydroxide – both known antacids in their own right. There is also a version of Maalox that incorporates the additional constituent DIMETHICONE, an antifoaming agent; this is produced in the form of a syrup (under the name Maalox Plus Suspension) and as tablets (under the name Maalox Plus Tablets, not available from the National Health Service). None of these preparations is recommended for children.

Mac (*Beecham Health Care*) are proprietory non-prescription throat sweets containing sucrose and glucose syrups, menthol and amylmetacresol.

Macrodantin (*Norwich Eaton*) is a proprietary ANTIBACTERIAL drug, available only on prescription, used to treat infections of the urinary tract. It works by interfering with the DNA of specific bacteria. Produced in the form of capsules (in two strengths), Macrodantin is a preparation of the powerful antibacterial nitrofurantoin. It is not recommended for children aged under 30 months.
✚/▲ warning/side-effects: *see* NITROFURANTOIN.

Macrodex (*Pharacia*) is a proprietary form of DEXTRAN 70 intravenous infusion, available only on prescription, used to make up a deficiency in the overall volume of blood in a patient, or to prevent thrombosis following surgery. It is produced in flasks, and prepared in a glucose or a saline matrix.
✚/▲ warning/side-effects: *see* DEXTRAN.

Macrofix (*Macarthy*) is a proprietary brand of elasticated tubular stockinette bandaging, produced in various diameters corresponding to average thicknesses of parts of the body.

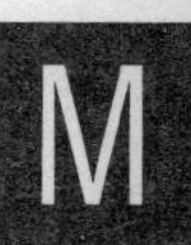

macrogol ointment is a skin emollient (softener and soother) consisting of a compound of two water-soluble constituent macrogols; unlike most emollient ointments, therefore, it is readily washed off – a property that is sometimes useful.

Madopar (*Roche*) is a proprietary preparation of the powerful drug levodopa in combination with the enzyme inhibitor BENSERAZIDE; it is available only on prescription. Madopar is used to treat parkinsonism, but not the parkinsonian symptoms induced by drugs (*see* ANTIPARKINSONISM). The benserazide prevents too rapid a breakdown of the levodopa (into dopamine), thus allowing more levodopa to reach the brain to make up the deficiency (of dopamine) that is the cause of parkinsonian symptoms. Madopar is produced in the form of capsules (in three strengths).
✚/▲ warning/side-effects: *see* LEVODOPA.

Madribon (*Roche*) is a proprietary ANTIBACTERIAL, available only on prescription, used to treat any of a number of bacterial infections – of the upper respiratory tract, of the ear, nose or throat, the skin, but particularly of the urinary tract. Produced in the form of tablets, Madribon is a preparation of the sulphonamide sulphadimethoxine. It is not recommended for children aged under 2 years.

✚/▲ warning/side-effects: *see* SULPHADIMETHOXINE.

mafenide is an ANTIBACTERIAL, a SULPHONAMIDE used (as mafenide propionate) to treat infections in and around the eye, and (as mafenide acetate) to treat infectious burns. Administration is thus both in solution as eye-drops, and as a cream.

✚ warning: mafenide acetate should be administered with caution to patients with respiratory problems.

▲ side-effects: acid levels in the body may become high.

Related articles: SULFAMYLON; SULFOMYL.

magaldrate is an ANTACID complex, used to treat severe indigestion; it may be administered after meals and before going to sleep at night. The complex is not recommended for children aged under 6 years.

Related article: DYNESE.

Magnapen (*Beecham*) is a proprietary compound ANTIBIOTIC, available only on prescription, used to treat severe infection where the causative organism has not been identified or where penicillin-resistant bacterial infection is probable. Produced in the form of capsules, as a syrup (under the name Magnapen Syrup), as a powder for reconstitution as a syrup, and in vials for injections (under the name Magnapen Injection), Magnapen is a preparation of the broad-spectrum penicillin-like antibiotic ampicillin together with the anti-staphylococcal antibiotic flucloxacillin. It should not be used for blind treatment of infections because many organisms are now resistant.

✚/▲ warning/side-effects: *see* AMPICILLIN; FLUCLOXACILLIN.

magnesium is a metallic element necessary to the body; ingested as a trace element in the diet, it is essential to the bones and important to the functioning of the nerves and muscles. Good dietary sources include green vegetables. Therapeutically, magnesium is used in the form of its salts. Magnesium carbonate, hydroxide, oxide ("magnesia") and trisilicate are ANTACIDS; magnesium sulphate (Epsom salt/salts) is a saline LAXATIVE; magnesium deficiency is usually treated with supplements of magnesium chloride.

✚/▲ warning/side-effects: *see* MAGNESIUM CARBONATE; MAGNESIUM CHLORIDE; MAGNESIUM HYDROXIDE; MAGNESIUM SULPHATE; MAGNESIUM TRISILICATE.

magnesium carbonate is a natural ANTACID that also has LAXATIVE properties. As an antacid it is actually comparatively weak, but fairly long-acting. Used to relieve indigestion and to soothe duodenal ulcer pain, it is commonly combined with other antacids. Administration is oral, most commonly in the form of a non-proprietary water-based mixture that also includes sodium bicarbonate.

✚ warning: magnesium carbonate should be administered with caution to patients with impaired function of the kidney, or who are taking any other form of drug.

▲ side-effects: there may be

belching – due to the internal liberation of carbon dioxide – and diarrhoea.
Related articles: ACTONORM; ALGICON; ALUDROX; ANDURSIL; APP; Bellocarb; CAVED-S; DIJEX; DIOVOL; GASTRILS; NULACIN; POLYCROL; PRODEXIN; ROTER; SIMECO; TOPAL.

magnesium chloride is the form of MAGNESIUM most commonly used to make up a deficiency of the metallic element in the body (as may occur through prolonged diarrhoea or vomiting, or through alcoholism).

magnesium hydroxide, or hydrated magnesium oxide ("magnesia"), is a natural ANTACID that also has LAXATIVE properties. As an antacid it is actually comparatively weak, but fairly long- acting. Used to relieve indigestion and to soothe duodenal ulcer pain, it is sometimes combined with other antacids. Administration is oral in the form of tablets or as an aqueous suspension.
✚ warning: magnesium hydroxide should be administered with caution to patients with impaired function of the kidney, or who are taking any other form of drug.
▲ side-effects: there may be diarrhoea.
Related articles: ACTONORM; ANDURSIL; ANTASIL; CARBELLON; Diovol; LOASID; MAALOX; MUCAINE; MUCOGEL; POLYCROL; SIMECO.

magnesium sulphate, or Epsom salt(s), is a LAXATIVE that works by preventing the resorption of water within the intestines. It is sometimes also used as a MAGNESIUM supplement administered to patients whose bodies are deficient in the mineral. And as a paste with glycerol, it is used topically to treat boils and carbuncles.

magnesium trisilicate is a natural ANTACID that also has absorbent properties. As an antacid it is long-acting. Used to relieve indigestion and to soothe peptic ulcer pain, it is sometimes combined with other antacids. Administration is oral in the form of tablets or as an aqueous suspension.
✚ warning: magnesium trisilicate should be administered with caution to patients with impaired function of the kidney, or who are taking any other form of drug.
Related articles: BELLOCARB; DROXALIN; GASTROCOTE; GASTRON; Gaviscon; GELUSIL; NULACIN; PYROGASTRONE.

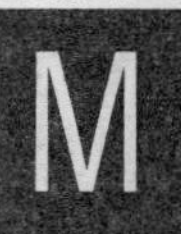

***major tranquillizer:** *see* TRANQUILLIZER.

Malarivon (*Wallace*) is a proprietary ANTIMALARIAL drug, available only on prescription, used both to prevent and to treat malaria. It is sometimes used to treat some forms of amoebiasis (particularly in the liver). Produced in the form of an elixir, Malarivon is a preparation of the powerful drug chloroquine.
✚/▲ warning/side-effects: *see* CHLOROQUINE.

Malatex (*Norton*) is a proprietary non-prescription agent for sloughing off dead skin or old clots in wounds or ulcers. Produced in the forms of both a cream and a solution, Malatex's active constituents are SALICYLIC ACID and various other natural acids (including benzoic acid and malic acid).

malathion is a powerful drug used to treat infestations by lice (pediculosis) or by itch-mites (scabies). Administration is topical in the form of a lotion or a shampoo, but treatment should not take place more than once a week for more than three weeks in succession. Some of the proprietary forms are highly inflammable.

✚ warning: avoid contact with the eyes.
Related articles: DERBAC-M; PRIODERM; SULEO-M.

M

Malinal (*Robins*) is a proprietary non-prescription ANTACID that is not available from the National Health Service. Produced in the form of tablets and as a syrup (under the name Malinal Suspension), it is used to treat acid stomach, inflammation of the stomach lining and gastric ulcers, but is not recommended for children. It is a preparation of ALMASILATE SUSPENSION.

Malix (*Lagap*) is a proprietary form of the SULPHONYLUREA drug glibenclamide, used to treat adult-onset diabetes; it works by promoting the formation of insulin in whatever remains of the capacity of the pancreas for it, and increasing the number of insulin receptors. Available only on prescription, Malix is produced in the form of tablets (in two strengths).

✚/▲ warning/side-effects: *see* GLIBENCLAMIDE.

Maloprim (*Wellcome*) is a proprietary ANTIMALARIAL drug, available only on prescription, used to prevent travellers to tropical areas from contracting the disease. Produced in the form of tablets, Maloprim is a compound of the SULPHONE dapsone together with the catalytic enzyme-inhibitor pyrimethamine (which is particularly useful in relation to malarial strains resistant to chloroquine). Treatment is weekly, not daily, but must be continued for at least 4 weeks after the patient leaves the tropical area.

✚/▲ warning/side-effects: *see* DAPSONE; PYRIMETHAMINE.

mannitol is a form of sugar that cannot be metabolized. Therapeutically, it is used primarily as a powerful DIURETIC – to treat the accumulation of fluids in the body (oedema), especially in emergency situations (such as drug overdose) – but it may also be used to decrease pressure within the eyeball in acute attacks of glaucoma. Administration is by intravenous infusion.

✚ warning: treatment may in the short term expand the overall blood volume, and should not be administered to patients with heart complaints or fluid on the lungs (pulmonary oedema). An escape of mannitol into the tissues from the site of infusion or from a blood vessel causes inflammation and forms of thrombosis.

▲ side-effects: there may be high body temperature with chills.
Related article: OSMITROL.

Mansil is a proprietary form of the ANTHELMINTIC drug oxamniquine, used to treat schistosomiasis (bilharziasis). *see* OXAMINIQUINE.

Manusept (*Hough/Hoseason*) is a proprietary non-prescription ANTIBACTERIAL, used particularly as an ANTISEPTIC hand cleanser prior to surgery, but also to moisturize dry skin. It consists of a preparation of the alcohol-based disinfectant TRICLOSAN in very mild solution.

***MAO inhibitors** are one of the two main classes of ANTIDEPRESSANT. Chemically, they are (usually) hydrazine derivatives. They are used less often than members of the TRICYCLIC group of antidepressants.

maprotiline hydrochloride is an ANTIDEPRESSANT drug used to treat depressive illness, particularly in cases where some degree of sedation is called for. Administration is oral in the form of tablets, or by intramuscular or intravenous injection.

✚ warning: maprotiline hydrochloride should not be administered to patients who have serious heart complaints or have recently had a heart attack, or to those who have manic episodes. It should be administered with caution to patients with epilepsy, diabetes, impaired liver function, heartbeat irregularities, thyroid disorders, glaucoma, or urinary retention; who are pregnant; or who are mentally unstable. Withdrawal of treatment should be gradual.

▲ side-effects: concentration and intricacy in thought and movement may be reduced. There may be an increased heart rate, sweating and tremor; constipation and difficulty in urinating; blurred vision and rashes; and weight changes and loss of libido. The composition of the blood may alter, especially in blood sugars.

Related article: LUDIOMIL.

Marcain (*Astra*) is a proprietary form of the local ANAESTHETIC drug bupivacaine, used particularly when duration of treatment is to be prolonged. Administration is thus most commonly as a nerve block injection, or as a lumbar puncture or epidural. Available only on prescription, Marcain is produced in ampoules by itself (in four strengths, the strongest under the name Marcain Heavy) and with additional adrenaline (in two strengths, under the name Marcain with Adrenaline).

✚/▲ warning/side-effects: *see* ADRENALINE; BUPIVACAINE HYDROCHLORIDE.

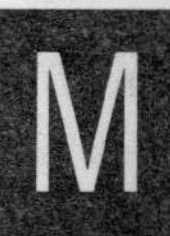

Marevan (*Duncan, Flockhart*) is a proprietary ANTICOAGULANT, available only on prescription, used to prevent or treat thrombosis. Produced in the form of tablets (in three strengths), Marevan is a preparation of warfarin; it is not recommended for children.

✚/▲ warning/side-effects: *see* WARFARIN.

Marplan (*Roche*) is a proprietary ANTIDEPRESSANT drug, available only on prescription, used to treat depressive illness. Produced in the form of tablets, Marplan is a preparation of the potentially dangerous drug isocarboxazid (which requires a careful dietary regimen to accompany treatment). It is not suitable for children.

✚/▲ warning/side-effects: *see* ISOCARBOXAZID.

Marsilid (*Roche*) is a proprietary ANTIDEPRESSANT drug, available only on prescription, used to treat depressive illness. Produced in the form of tablets (in two strengths), Marsilid is a preparation of the potentially dangerous drug iproniazid (which requires a careful dietary regimen to accompany

treatment). It is not suitable for children.
✚/▲ warning/side-effects: *see* IPRONIAZID.

Marvelon (*Organon*) is a proprietary ORAL CONTRACEPTIVE pill, available only on prescription, of the type that combines an OESTROGEN and a PROGESTOGEN. In this case the oestrogen is ethinyloestradiol, and the progestogen is DESOGESTREL.
✚/▲ warning/side-effects: *see* ETHINYLOESTRADIOL.

Massé Cream (*Ortho-Cilag*) is a proprietary non-prescription cream used as an emollient (softener and soother) for the nipples of women about to give birth and during lactation. Water-miscible, it contains many constituents, including arachis oil, wool fat, stearic acid and potassium hydroxide.

Masteril (*Syntex*) is a proprietary preparation of the STEROID drostanolone propionate, available only on prescription, used as a rather desperate measure against breast cancer that is spreading around the body. It is produced in ampoules for injection.
✚/▲ warning/side-effects: *see* DROSTANOLONE PROPIONATE.

Maxamaid XP (*Scientific Hospital Supplies*) is a proprietary, non- prescription, orange-flavoured powder consisting of a virtually complete nutritional supplement for patients with amino-acid abnormalities (such as phenylketonuria). It thus contains amino acids (except phenylalanine), carbohydrate, vitamins and trace elements; it is also gluten-free. Maxamaid XP is not recommended for children aged under 2 years.

Maxidex (*Alcon*) is a proprietary compound, available only on prescription, used to treat inflammation of the surface of the eye. Produced in the form of eye-drops, Maxidex is a combination of the CORTICOSTEROID dexamethasone with the water-soluble cellulose derivative hypromellose (the basis of "artificial tears", a spreading agent).
✚/▲ warning/side-effects: *see* DEXAMETHASONE.

Maxijul (*Scientific Hospital Supplies*) is the name of a proprietary non-prescription series of preparations consisting of nutritional supplements for patients who require a high-energy low-fluid diet. Consisting mostly of polyglucose polymer, sodium and potassium, the standard form of Maxijul is produced as a gluten-, sucrose-, lactose-, galactose- and fructose-free powder. There is also a liquid form (in three flavours, under the name Maxijul Liquid), and a form with less sodium and potassium (under the name Maxijul LE).

Maxipro HBV (*Scientific Hospital Supplies*) is a proprietary non-prescription protein supplement used to treat patients who are undernourished through lack of food or poor internal absorption (particularly those who have undergone gastrectomy). It may, in patients aged over 5 years, be used as the sole source of nutrition. Its major constituent is whey protein.

Maxitrol (*Alcon*) is a proprietary compound, available only on prescription, used to treat inflammation of the surface of the eye. Produced in the form of eye-drops for daytime use, and as an ointment for use overnight, Maxitrol is a combination of the corticosteroid dexamethasone and the ANTIBIOTICS neomycin and polymyxin B sulphate; the eye-drops also contain the water-soluble cellulose derivative hypromellose (the basis of "artificial tears", a spreading agent).

✚/▲ warning/side-effects: *see* DEXAMETHASONE; NEOMYCIN; POLYMYXIN B SULPHATE.

Maxolon (*Beecham*) is a proprietary ANTINAUSEANT, used to treat severe indigestion, flatulence, peptic, gastric or duodenal ulcer, hiatus hernia or gallstones. Available only on prescription, Maxolon's primary constituent – metoclopramide hydrochloride – works by encouraging the flow of absorbable nutrients in food in the stomach down into the intestines. It is produced in the form of tablets, in liquid form (under the name Maxolon Paediatric Liquid), as a syrup (under the name Maxolon Syrup) and in ampoules for injection (under the names Maxolon Injection and Maxolon High Dose).

✚/▲ warning/side-effects: *see* METOCLOPRAMIDE.

Maxtrex (*Farmitalia Carlo Erba*) is a proprietary preparation of the ANTICANCER drug methotrexate, available only on prescription, used to treat some forms of leukaemia, certain solid tumours, and other conditions in which abnormal cell replication is occurring. For this reason it may also be used to treat severe psoriasis. It is produced in the form of a solution (in two strengths) in vials, and as tablets (in two strengths, under the name Maxtrex Tablets).

✚/▲ warning/side-effects: *see* METHOTREXATE.

mazindol is a drug used to aid slimming regimes because it acts as an appetite suppressant. It also has stimulant properties, however, and there is a slight risk of dependence (addiction). Administration is oral in the form of tablets. The drug should be used only in cases where there is genuine medical need for weight loss, and is not recommended for children.

✚ warning: mazindol is merely an aid to a slimming regime, not a treatment for obesity. Its use should be short-term only. Prolonged treatment may result in dependence (addiction). It should not be administered to patients with glaucoma or from disorders of the thyroid gland, and should be administered with caution to those with epilepsy, diabetes, heart disease or peptic ulcer, or who are unstable psychologically.

▲ side-effects: there may be agitation, insomnia and restlessness, and a increased heart rate; headache and dizziness may occur; there may also be gastrointestinal disturbances. In predisposed patients there may be manic episodes.

Related article: TERONAC.

MCT Oil (*Bristol-Myers*) is a proprietary non-prescription form of fats (lipids) used as a nutritional supplement for patients whose metabolism finds fat absorption difficult or impossible (for instance following intestinal surgery, with cirrhosis of the liver, or with cystic fibrosis of the pancreas). MCT Oil is a preparation of triglycerides from fatty acids.

MCT (1) (*Cow & Gate*) is a proprietary non-prescription nutritional supplement for patients whose capacity for food absorption has been reduced (for instance following intestinal surgery, with chronic liver disease, or with cystic fibrosis of the pancreas). In the form of a powder for reconstitution, MCT (1) contains protein, carbohydrate, and fats (triglycerides); it is also low in lactose and sucrose-free.

M

mebendazole is an ANTHELMINTIC drug used in the treatment of infections by roundworm, threadworm, whipworm and hookworm. A powerful drug generally well tolerated, it is the treatment of choice for patients of all ages over 2 years. Administration is oral in the form of tablets or a suspension.

✚ warning: mebendazole should not be administered to patients who are aged under 2 years; it should be administered with caution to those who are pregnant.

▲ side-effects: side-effects are uncommon, but there may be diarrhoea and abdominal pain.
Related article: VERMOX.

mebeverine hydrochloride is an ANTISPASMODIC drug used to treat muscle spasm in both the gastrointestinal tract (leading to abdominal pain and constipation) and the uterus or vagina (leading to menstrual problems). Administration is oral in the form of tablets, as a sugar-free liquid concentrate, and as soluble (dispersible) granules, to be taken before food. It is not recommended for children.

✚ warning: Mebeverine hydrochloride should not be administered to patients with paralytic ileus.
Related articles: COLOFAC; COLVEN.

mebhydrolin is an ANTIHISTAMINE used to treat allergic conditions such as hay fever and urticaria, some forms of dermatitis, and some sensitivity reactions to drugs. Its additional sedative properties are useful in the treatment of some allergic conditions. Administration is oral in the form of tablets or a dilute suspension (mixture).

✚ warning: mebhydrolin should not be administered to patients with glaucoma, urinary retention, intestinal obstruction, enlargement of the prostate gland, or peptic ulcer, or who are pregnant; it should be administered with caution to those with epilepsy or liver disease.

▲ side-effects: sedation may affect patients' capacity for speed of thought and movement; there may be nausea, headache and/or weight gain, dry mouth, gastrointestinal disturbances and visual problems.
Related article: FABAHISTIN.

mecillinam is a penicillin-type ANTIBIOTIC used primarily to treat infections caused by bacteria in the intestines. Administration is in the form of injection.

✚ warning: mecillinam should not be administered to patients known to be allergic to penicillins; it should be administered with caution to those with impaired kidney function. Prolonged treatment requires regular checks on liver and kidney function.

▲ side-effects: there may be sensitivity reactions ranging from a minor rash to urticaria and joint pains, and (occasionally) to high temperature or anaphylactic shock. High doses may in any case cause convulsions.
Related article: SELEXIDIN.

meclozine is an ANTIHISTAMINE used primarily as an ANTI-EMETIC in the treatment or prevention of motion sickness and vomiting. Administration (as meclozine hydrochloride, generally with a form of vitamin B) is oral in the form of tablets.

✚ warning: meclazine should be administered with caution to patients with epilepsy, liver disease, glaucoma or enlargement of the prostate gland. Drowsiness may be increased by alcohol consumption.

▲ side-effects: concentration and speed of thought and movement may be affected. There is commonly dry mouth and drowsiness; there may also be headache, blurred vision and gastrointestinal disturbances.

Related article: ANCOLOXIN.

medazepam is an ANXIOLYTIC drug, one of the BENZODIAZEPINES, used primarily to treat chronic anxiety, and less commonly, insomnia. It may also be used to relieve acute alcohol withdrawal symptoms. But it also has the properties of a SKELETAL MUSCLE RELAXANT, and may also be administered to relieve conditions of skeletal muscle spasticity. Administration is oral in the form of capsules.

✚ warning: medazepam should be administered with caution to patients with respiratory difficulties, glaucoma, or kidney or liver disease; who are in the last stages of pregnancy or are lactating; or who are elderly or debilitated. Prolonged use or abrupt withdrawal of the drug should be avoided.

▲ side-effects: concentration and speed of reaction are affected. Drowsiness, dizziness, headache, dry mouth and shallow breathing are all fairly common. Elderly patients may enter a state of confusion. Sensitivity reactions may occur.

Related article: NOBRIUM.

Medicoal (*Lundbeck*) is a proprietary non-prescription adsorbent preparation for oral administration, used to treat patients suffering from poisoning or a drug overdose. It works by binding the toxic material to itself before being excreted in the normal way. Produced in the form of granules for effervescent solution in water, Medicoal is a preparation of CHARCOAL.

medigoxin is a derivative of DIGOXIN, a CARDIAC GLYCOSIDE that acts as a strong heart stimulant, and is thus used to treat heart failure and severe heartbeat irregularity. Administration is oral in the form of tablets.

✚ warning: medigoxin should be administered with caution to patients who have undergone a recent heart attack, or who have disorders of the thyroid gland. Dosage should be reduced for the elderly.

▲ side-effects: there may be serious effects on the heart rate. Sometimes there is nausea and vomiting, visual disturbances and weight loss.

Related article: LANITOP.

Medihaler-Duo (*Riker*) is a proprietary BRONCHOLDILATOR, available only on prescription, used in the form of an inhalant to treat bronchial asthma and chronic bronchitis. Produced in a metered-dosage aerosol, Medihaler-Duo is a compound preparation of the SYMPATHOMIMETICS isoprenaline hydrochloride and phenylephrine bitartrate.

✚/▲ warning/side-effects: *see* ISOPRENALINE; PHENYLEPHRINE.

Medihaler-epi (*Riker*) is a proprietary BRONCHODILATOR, available only on prescription, used in the form of an inhalant to treat bronchial asthma and chronic bronchitis. Produced in a metered- dosage aerosol, Medihaler-epi is a preparation of the SYMPATHOMIMETIC adrenaline acid tartrate.
✚/▲ warning/side-effects: *see* ADRENALINE.

Medihaler-Ergotamine (*Riker*) is a proprietary anti-migraine treatment, available only on prescription, used in the form of an inhalant to treat migraine and recurrent vascular headache. Produced in a metered-dosage aerosol, Medihaler-Ergotamine is a preparation of the vegetable alkaloid ergotamine tartrate.
✚/▲ warning/side-effects: *see* ERGOTAMINE TARTRATE.

Medihaler-iso (*Riker*) is a proprietary BRONCHODILATOR, available only on prescription, used in the form of an inhalant to treat bronchial asthma and chronic bronchitis. Produced in a metered- dosage aerosol (in two strengths, the stronger under the trade name Medihaler-iso Forte), it is a preparation of the SYMPATHOMIMETIC isoprenaline sulphate.
✚/▲ warning/side-effects: *see* ISOPRENALINE.

Medilave (*Martindale*) is a proprietary non-prescription preparation for topical application, used to relieve pain in sores and ulcers in the mouth. Produced in the form of a gel, Medilave is a preparation of the local ANAESTHETIC benzocaine and the ANTISEPTIC CETYLPYRIDINIUM CHLORIDE, and is not recommended for children aged under 6 months.
✚/▲ warning/side-effects: *see* BENZOCAINE.

Medised (*Martindale/Panpharma*) is a proprietary non-prescription compound non-narcotic ANALGESIC that is not available from the National Health Service. Used to treat pain, especially that associated with fever and respiratory congestion, and to relieve the symptoms of chickenpox, Medised is produced in the form of tablets (which are not recommended for children) and as a suspension (which is not recommended for children aged under 3 months). Medised is a combination of the analgesic paracetamol and the ANTIHISTAMINE promethazine hydrochloride.
✚/▲ warning/side-effects: *see* PARACETAMOL; PROMETHAZINE HYDROCHLORIDE.

Meditar (*Brocades*) is a proprietary non-prescription preparation used to treat eczema and psoriasis. Produced in the form of a wax stick for topical application, Meditar is a specialized form of COAL TAR.

Medocodene (*Medo*) is a proprietary non-prescription compound ANALGESIC that is not available from the National Health Service. Used to treat pain anywhere in the body, and produced in the form of tablets, Medocodene is a combination of the analgesic paracetamol and the OPIATE codeine phosphate (a combination itself known as co-codamol). It is not recommended for children aged under 6 years.
✚/▲ warning/side-effects: *see* CODEINE PHOSPHATE; PARACETAMOL.

Medomet (*DDSA Pharmaceuticals*)

is a proprietary form of the powerful ANTIHYPERTENSIVE drug methyldopa, which works by direct action on the central nervous system. Available only on prescription, Medomet is used – usually in combination with a DIURETIC drug – to treat moderate to very high blood pressure (hypertension), and is produced in the form of tablets (in two strengths) and capsules.

✚/▲ warning/side-effects: *see* METHYLDOPA.

Medrone (*Upjohn*) is a proprietary preparation of the anti-inflammatory CORTICOSTEROID drug methylprednisolone, available only on prescription, used to treat arthritis, joint pain and allergies, and to relieve the symptoms of severe acne. It is produced in the form of tablets (in three strengths) and as a lotion (which additionally contains the KERATOLYTIC aluminium chlorhydroxide).

✚/▲ warning/side-effects: *see* METHYLPREDNISOLONE.

medroxyprogesterone acetate is a long-acting female sex hormone, a PROGESTOGEN most commonly administered by intramuscular injection. One of its uses is as an ORAL CONTRACEPTIVE of a type that is particularly useful in being effective for a short period of time (as for example during the time a partner's vasectomy takes to become effective). Prolonged use in contraception may be accompanied by potentially uncomfortable side-effects, however, although for some women it may be the only tolerable method. The drug can also be used to make up hormonal deficiency in such conditions as an absence of menstruation (amenorrhoea), or to treat the relatively common condition in which some womb-lining tissue that is located outside the womb in the abdominal cavity continues to go through the menstrual cycle (endometriosis). Medroxyprogesterone acetate can also be used in the treatment of cancers of the breast that are related to the presence of OESTROGENS.

✚ warning: medroxyprogesterone acetate should not be administered to patients with liver disease, undiagnosed vaginal haemorrhage or sex-hormone-linked cancer; who are pregnant; or who have a history of ectopic pregnancy, of arterial disease or of jaundice. It should be administered with caution to those who suffer from diabetes, heart disease, ovarian cysts, or high blood pressure (hypertension); who have recently given birth; or who have started suffering from migraine since beginning to use oral contraceptive methods.

▲ side-effects: there may be nausea and vomiting, with headache; there may also be weight gain, breast tenderness, depression and skin disorders. Withdrawal of long-term treatment may cause temporary infertility and the onset of some irregular menstrual cycles.

Related articles: DEPO-PROVERA; FARLUTAL; PROVERA.

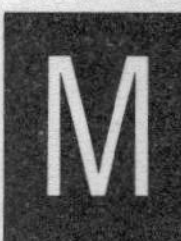

mefenamic acid is a non-steroidal ANTI-INFLAMMATORY non-narcotic ANALGESIC. It is primarily used to treat mild to moderate pain in rheumatic disease and other musculo-skeletal disorders, although it may also be used either to reduce high body temperature (especially in

children) or to lessen the pain of menstrual problems.
✚ warning: mefenamic acid should not be administered to patients with inflammations in the intestines, peptic ulcers, or impaired liver or kidney function; or who are pregnant. It should be administered with caution to those with any allergic condition (including asthma). Prolonged treatment requires regular blood counts.
▲ side-effects: there may be drowsiness and dizziness; some patients experience nausea; gastrointestinal disturbances may eventually result in ulceration. Treatment should be withdrawn if diarrhoea, jaundice, anaemia or sensitivity reactions such as asthma-like symptoms occur.
Related article: PONSTAN.

Mefoxin (*Merck, Sharp & Dohme*) is a proprietary broad-spectrum antibiotic, available only on prescription, used to treat bacterial infections and to ensure asepsis during surgery. Produced in the form of a powder for reconstitution as a medium for injection, Mefoxin is a preparation of the CEPHALOSPORIN cefoxitin.
✚/▲ warning/side-effects: *see* CEFOXITIN.

mefruside is a DIURETIC, one of the THIAZIDES, used to treat fluid retention in the tissues (oedema) and high blood pressure (hypertension). Because all thiazides tend to deplete body reserves of potassium, mefruside may be administered in combination either with potassium supplements or with diuretics that are complementarily potassium-sparing. Administration is oral in the form of tablets.
✚ warning: mefruside should not be administered to patients with kidney failure or urinary retention, or who are lactating. It should be administered with caution to those who are pregnant. It may aggravate conditions of diabetes or gout.
▲ side-effects: there may be tiredness and a rash. In men, temporary impotence may occur.
Related article: BAYCARON.

Megace (*Bristol-Myers*) is a proprietary preparation of the PROGESTOGEN megestrol acetate, available only on prescription, used to treat sex-hormone-linked cancers (such as cancer of the breast or of the womb-lining). It is produced in the form of tablets (in two strengths).
✚/▲ warning/side-effects: *see* MEGESTROL ACETATE.

Megaclor (*Pharmax*) is a proprietary ANTIBIOTIC, available only on prescription, used to treat infections of soft tissues, particularly of the upper respiratory tract, and to relieve the symptoms of acne. Produced in the form of capsules, Megaclor is a preparation of the TETRACYCLINE clomocycline sodium. It is not recommended for children.
✚/▲ warning/side-effects: *see* CLOMOCYCLINE SODIUM.

megestrol acetate is a female sex hormone, a PROGESTOGEN used primarily to treat forms of cancer in which the presence of OESTROGENS is significant (such as breast cancer or cancer of the womb-lining). Administration is oral in the form of tablets.
✚ warning: megestrol acetate should not be administered to patients with breast cancer that is not sex-hormone-linked, or who have undiagnosed

vaginal haemorrhage; or who have a history of thrombosis. It should be administered with caution to those with diabetes, heart, liver or kidney disease, or high blood pressure (hypertension); or who are lactating.

▲ side-effects: side-effects are generally mild, but there may be nausea, fluid retention, and weight gain. Some patients experience irregular menstrual cycles and/or gastrointestinal disturbances. *Related article:* MEGACE.

Megozzones (*Kirby-Warrick Pharmaceuticals*) are proprietary non-prescription throat pastilles containing MENTHOL, benzoin and liquorice.

Melleril (*Sandoz*) is a proprietary form of the powerful ANTIPSYCHOTIC drug thioridazine. Available only on prescription, it is used to treat and tranquillize psychosis (such as schizophrenia) in which it is particularly suitable for treating manic forms of behavioural disturbance. It may also be used to treat anxiety in the short term. Melleril is produced in the form of tablets (in four strengths), as a suspension (in two strengths) and as a syrup for dilution (the potency of the syrup once dilute is retained for 14 days).

✚/▲ warning/side-effects: *see* THIORIDAZINE.

melphalan is a CYTOTOXIC drug used in the treatment of various forms of cancers, especially cancer of the bone-marrow. It works by direct action on the DNA of new-forming cells, so preventing normal cell replication. Administration is oral in the form of tablets, or by injection.

✚ warning: prolonged treatment may cause sterility in men and an early menopause in women. Regular and frequent blood counts are essential. Dosage should be reduced for patients with impaired kidney function. Because the effect of the drug on the bone marrow is delayed, treatment may be required only at intervals of between 4 and 6 weeks.

▲ side-effects: there is commonly nausea and vomiting; there is often also hair loss. *Related article:* ALKERAN.

menadiol sodium phosphate is an analogue of VITAMIN K (phytomenadione) which because it is water-soluble – whereas other forms are only fat-soluble – is primarily used in oral application to treat vitamin deficiency caused by the malabsorption of fats in the diet (perhaps through obstruction of the bile ducts or liver disease). The vitamin is necessary on a regular basis to maintain the presence in the blood of clotting factors and other factors that are responsible for the calcification of bone. Administration is both oral in the form of tablets, and by injection.

✚ warning: menadiol sodium phosphate should be administered with caution to patients who are pregnant. *Related article:* SYNKAVIT.

Menophase (*Syntex*) is a proprietary compound sex-HORMONE preparation, available only on prescription, used to treat menopausal symptoms. Produced in the form of a calendar pack corresponding to one complete menstrual cycle, Menophase is a preparation of the PROGESTOGEN norethisterone and the OESTROGEN mestranol.

✚/▲ warning/side-effects: *see* MESTRANOL; NORETHISTERONE.

menthol is a white, crystalline substance derived from peppermint oil (an essential oil in turn derived from a plant of the mint family). It is used, with or without the volatile substance eucalyptus oil, mostly in inhalations meant to clear nasal or catarrhal congestion in conditions such as rhinitis or sinusitis.
Related articles: ARADOLENE; ASPELLIN; BALMOSA; BENGUÉ'S BALSAM; BENYLIN DECONGESTANT; COPHOLCO; EXPULIN; EXPURHIN; GUANOR EXPECTORANT; HISTALIX; PHYTOCIL; ROWACHOL; SALONAIR; Tercoda; TERPOIN.

M

Mentholatum (*Mentholatum*) is a proprietary non-prescription preparation for the relief of cold symptoms produced in the form of ANTISEPTIC lozenges, balm, deep heat lotion, and spray. These preparations contain MENTHOL, CAMPHOR, EUCALYPTUS OIL, METHYL SALYCILATE and AMYLMETACERSOL.

mepacrine hydrochloride is a synthetic drug used primarily to treat infection by the intestinal protozoan Giardia lamblia: giardiasis occurs throughout the world, particularly in children, and is contracted by eating contaminated food. The drug more commonly used to treat it, however, is METRONIDAZOLE. Mepacrine can also be used to assist in the treatment of most forms of malaria.

mepenzolate bromide is an ANTICHOLINERGIC drug used to assist in the treatment of gastrointestinal disorders that involve muscle spasm of the intestinal wall. Administration is oral in the form of tablets or an elixir.
✚ warning: mepenzolate bromide should not be administered to patients with glaucoma; it should be administered with caution to those with heart problems and rapid heart rate, ulcerative colitis, urinary retention or enlargement of the prostate gland; who are elderly; or who are lactating.
▲ side-effects: there is commonly dry mouth and thirst; there may also be visual disturbances, flushing, irregular heartbeat and constipation. Rarely, there may be high temperature accompanied by delirium.
Related articles: CANTIL; CANTIL WITH PHENOBARBITONE.

Meprate (*DDSA Pharmaceuticals*) is a proprietary ANXIOLYTIC drug that is on the controlled drugs list. Used in the short-term treatment of nervous anxiety and associated muscular tension, and produced in the form of tablets, Meprate is a preparation of the (potentially addictive) tranquillizer meprobamate. It is not recommended for children.
✚/▲ warning/side-effects: *see* MEPROBAMATE.

meprobamate is a minor TRANQUILLIZER and ANXIOLYTIC used to relieve nervous tension and anxiety, particularly that associated with premenstrual syndrome. It may also be used to assist in the treatment of minor forms of neurosis. Prolonged treatment, however, may lead to tolerance and dependence (addiction). Administration is oral in the form of tablets.
✚ warning: meprobamate should not be administered to patients with porphyria, or who are lactating. It should be administered with caution to those with respiratory difficulties, glaucoma, epilepsy, or impaired liver or kidney function, who are in

the last stages of pregnancy, or who are elderly or debilitated. Withdrawal of treatment must be gradual (abrupt withdrawal may cause convulsions).

▲ side-effects: concentration and speed of thought and movement are affected; the degree of sedation may be marked. There may also be low blood pressure (hypotension), debility, gastrointestinal disturbances, headache, blurred vision and rashes. The effect of alcohol consumption may be enhanced.
Related articles: EQUAGESIC; EQUANIL; MEPRATE; TENAVOID.

meptazinol is a powerful synthetic narcotic ANALGESIC, an OPIATE that is used to treat moderate to severe pain, including pain in childbirth or following surgery. The onset of its effect is said to take place within 15 minutes of injection, and the duration is said to be between 2 and 7 hours; however, there are some post-operative side-effects. Administration is also oral in the form of tablets.

✚ warning: meptazinol should not be administered to patients with head injury or intracranial pressure; it should be administered with caution to those with impaired kidney or liver function, asthma, depressed respiration, insufficient secretion of thyroid hormones (hypothyroidism) or low blood pressure (hypotension), or who are pregnant or lactating. Dosage should be decreased for the elderly or debilitated.

▲ side-effects: nausea, vomiting, dizziness, sweating and drowsiness are fairly common. However, unlike most drugs of its type, meptazinol is said not to cause shallow breathing.
Related article: MEPTID.

Meptid (*Wyeth*) is a proprietary narcotic ANALGESIC, available only on prescription, used to treat moderate to severe pain, particularly during or following surgical procedures (including childbirth). Produced in the form of tablets and in ampoules for injection, Meptid is a preparation of the OPIATE meptazinol, and is not recommended for children.

✚/▲ warning/side-effects: *see* MEPTAZINOL.

mepyramine is an ANTIHISTAMINE used to treat the symptoms of allergic conditions such as hay fever and urticaria, and – as an anti-emetic – to treat or prevent nausea and vomiting, especially in connection with motion sickness or the vertigo caused by infection of the middle or inner ear. Administration (as mepyramine maleate) is oral in the form of tablets.

✚ warning: mepyramine should not be administered to patients with glaucoma, urinary retention, intestinal obstruction, enlargement of the prostate gland, or peptic ulcer, or who are pregnant; it should be administered with caution to those with epilepsy or liver disease.

▲ side-effects: sedation may affect patients' capacity for speed of thought and movement; there may be headache and/or weight gain, dry mouth, gastrointestinal disturbances and visual problems.
Related article: ANTHISAN.

mequitazine is an ANTIHISTAMINE, used to treat the symptoms of allergic conditions such as hay fever and urticaria. Administration is oral in the form of tablets.

✚ warning: mequitazine should not be administered to patients who are pregnant, or who have glaucoma, urinary retention, intestinal obstruction, enlargement of the prostate gland, or peptic ulcer; it should be administered with caution to those with epilepsy or liver disease.

▲ side-effects: concentration and speed of thought and movement may be affected. There may be nausea, headache, and/or weight gain, dry mouth, gastrointestinal disturbances and visual problems.

Related article: PRIMALAN.

Merbentyl (*Merrell*) is a proprietary ANTICHOLINERGIC drug, available only on prescription, used to treat gastrointestinal disorders that result from muscle spasm in the stomach or intestinal walls. Produced in the form of tablets (in two strengths, the stronger under the name Merbentyl 20) and as a syrup for dilution (the potency of the syrup once dilute is retained for 14 days), Merbentyl is a preparation of dicyclomine hydrochloride and is not recommended for children aged under 6 months.

✚/▲ warning/side-effects: *see* DICYCLOMINE HYDROCHLORIDE.

mercaptopurine is a CYTOTOXIC drug used in the treatment of acute leukaemia. It works by combining with new-forming cells in a way that prevents normal cell replication. Administration is oral in the form of tablets.

✚ warning: prolonged treatment may cause sterility in men and an early menopause in women. Regular blood counts are essential during treatment. Mercaptopurine should be administered with caution to patients who are already taking the drug allopurinol for gout or similar conditions.

▲ side-effects: there is commonly nausea and vomiting; there is often also hair loss.

Related article: PURI-NETHOL.

mercuric oxide is a substance used as the basis for an eye ointment intended for topical application to treat infections in and around the eye. It is not now recommended as a form of treatment.

Merieux Inactivated Rabies Vaccine is a proprietary preparation of rabies vaccine for administration to medical personnel and relatives who may come into contact with patients who have been bitten by an animal that might or might not have been rabid. Available only on prescription, the vaccine is of a type known as human diploid cell vaccine and has no known contra-indications. It is freeze-dried and produced in vials with a diluent for injection.

see RABIES VACCINE.

Merieux Tetavax (*Merieux*) is a proprietary preparation of tetanus vaccine, adsorbed on to a mineral carrier (in the form of aluminium hydroxide) and produced in syringes and in vials for injection.

see TETANUS VACCINE.

Merocaine (*Merrell*) is a proprietary non-prescription local anaesthetic, used to treat painful mouth and throat infections. Produced in the form of lozenges, Merocaine is a preparation of the local anaesthetic benzocaine together with the minor ANTISEPTIC CETYLPYRIDINIUM

CHLORIDE. It is not recommended for children.
✚/▲ warning/side-effects: *see* BENZOCAINE.

Merocet (*Merrell*) is a proprietary non-prescription mouth-wash which is a preparation of the ANTISEPTIC CETYLPYRIDINIUM CHLORIDE. Although it can (but need not) be used in dilute form, it is not recommended for children aged under 6 years.

Merocets (*Merrell*) are proprietary non-prescription lozenges that are a preparation of the ANTISEPTIC CETYLPYRIDINIUM CHLORIDE, used in general oral hygiene.

mersalyl is a powerful DIURETIC that is used only when all other methods of treating fluid retention have failed or are not tolerated. The drug is so toxic that it can be administered only by intramuscular injection: an intravenous injection may cause a fatal fall in blood pressure.
✚ warning: mersalyl should not be administered to patients with impaired kidney function; it should be administered with caution to those who are pregnant, who have recently had a heart attack, who suffer from heartbeat irregularities, or who are taking drugs that stimulate the heart's action.
▲ side-effects: there may be gastrointestinal disturbances; some patients experience allergic reactions.

Meruvax II (*Morson*) is a proprietary VACCINE against German measles (rubella) in the form of a solution containing live but attenuated viruses of the Wistar RA27/3 strain. Available only on prescription, it is administered in the form of an injection.
see RUBELLA VACCINE.

mesalazine is an ANTIBACTERIAL used in the long-term treatment of diarrhoea caused by ulcerative colitis in patients who are sensitive to the commonly-prescribed sulphonamide antibacterials. Administration is oral in the form of tablets.
✚ warning: mesalazine should not be administered to patients who are allergic to aspirin or other salicylates; it should be administered with caution to those with impaired kidney function.
▲ side-effects: there may be nausea, with diarrhoea and abdominal pain; some patients experience a headache.
Related article: ASACOL.

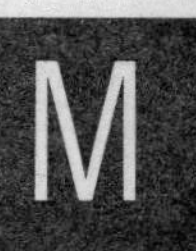

mesna is a synthetic drug that has the remarkable property of reducing the incidence of the serious form of cystitis (inflammation of the bladder) that is a toxic complication of the use of the CYTOTOXIC drugs CYCLOPHOSPHAMIDE and ifosfamide, without inhibiting the cytotoxic effects of the drugs. Used therefore as an adjunct in the treatment of certain forms of cancer, mesna is administered by injection.
▲ side-effects: overdosage may cause gastrointestinal disturbances and headache, with tiredness.
Related article: UROMITEXAN.

mesterolone is an ANDROGEN, a male sex HORMONE produced mainly in the testes that, with other androgens, promotes the development of the secondary male sexual characteristics. Therapeutically, it may be administered to treat hormonal deficiency (but only following careful investigation and under strict medical supervision), particularly in cases of delayed puberty and underdevelopment in boys. Administration is oral in the form of tablets.

✚ warning: mesterolone should not be administered to male patients with kidney disease, cancer of the prostate gland or cancer of the breast, or to female patients who are pregnant or lactating; it should be administered with caution to those with impaired function of the heart, liver or kidney, circulatory disorders and/or high blood pressure, epilepsy or diabetes, thyroid disorders, or migraine.

▲ side-effects: there may be fluid retention in the tissues (oedema) leading to weight gain. Increased levels of calcium in the body may cause bone growth (and in younger patients may fuse bones before fully grown) and the symptoms of hypercalcaemia. In elderly patients there may be (increased) enlargement of the prostate gland. High doses halt the production of sperm in men and cause the visible masculinization of women.
Related article: PRO-VIRON.

Mestinon (*Roche*) is a proprietary form of the drug pyridostigmine bromide, which has the effect of increasing the activity of the neurotransmitter acetylcholine that transmits the neural instructions of the brain to the muscles. It is thus used primarily to treat the neuromuscular disease myasthenia gravis, but may also be used to stimulate intestinal motility and so promote defecation. Available only on prescription, Mestinon is produced in the form of tablets and in ampoules for injection.

✚/▲ warning/side-effects: *see* PYRIDOSTIGMINE.

mestranol is a female sex hormone, a synthetic OESTROGEN that is a constituent in several ORAL CONTRACEPTIVES that contain relatively high oestrogen levels in comparison with the PROGESTOGEN content. It is also used in some similarly combined preparations to assist in hormone replacement therapy for women experiencing menopausal problems. Administration is on a regular, calendar basis corresponding to menstrual cycles.

✚ warning: mestranol should not be taken by patients who have cancers proved to be sex-hormone-linked, who have a history of thrombosis or of inflammation of the womb, or who suffer from porphyria or impaired liver function. It should be taken with caution by patients who are diabetic or epileptic, who have heart or kidney disease, who are lactating, or who have high blood pressure (hypertension) or recurrent severe migraine. Prolonged treatment increases the risk of cancer of the endometrium (the lining of the womb).

▲ side-effects: there may be nausea and vomiting. Fluid and sodium retention in the tissues may result in overall weight gain. The breasts may become tender and enlarge slightly. The patient may also suffer from a headache and/or depression; sometimes a rash breaks out.
Related articles: NORINYL-1; ORTHO-NOVIN 1/50.

Metabolic Mineral Mixture (*Scientific Hospital Supplies*) is a proprietary non-prescription mineral supplement, used to supplement special diets. Produced in the form of a powder, it contains various mineral salts.

Metamucil (*Searle*) is a

proprietary non-prescription LAXATIVE of the type known as a bulking agent, which works by increasing the overall mass of faeces within the rectum, so stimulating bowel movement. It is also used to soothe the effects of diverticular disease and irritable colon, and to control the consistency of faecal material in patients who have had a colostomy. Produced in the form of a gluten-free powder, Metamucil is a preparation of ispaghula husk.
✚/▲ warning/side-effects: *see* ISPAGHULA HUSK.

Metanium (*Bengué*) is a proprietary non-prescription astringent, used to relieve nappy rash and other macerated skin conditions. Produced in the form of an ointment, Metanium is a preparation of titanium salts in a silicone base.

metaraminol is a SYMPATHOMIMETIC drug and as such also has the properties of a VASOCONSTRICTOR. It is used to treat cases of acute low blood pressure (particularly in emergency situations as a temporary measure while preparations are made for blood transfusion). Administration is by injection or infusion.
✚ warning: metaraminol should not be administered to patients who are pregnant, or who are undergoing a heart attack. Leakage of the drug at the site of injection or infusion may cause local tissue death.
▲ side-effects: there is a reduction in the flow of blood through the kidneys; there is also an increase in the heart rate and there may be heartbeat irregularities.
Related article: ARAMINE.

Metatone (*Parke-Davis*) is a proprietary non-prescription tonic that is not available from the National Health Service: it is used to remedy loss of appetite. Metatone is a preparation of THIAMINE (vitamin B_1) and minerals such as calcium, manganese, potassium and sodium in a diluent (the potency of the preparation is retained for 14 days). It is not recommended for children aged under 6 years.

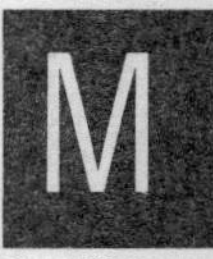

Metenix (*Hoechst*) is a proprietary DIURETIC, available only on prescription, used to treat an accumulation of fluid within the tissues (oedema) and high blood pressure (*see* ANTIHYPERTENSIVE). Produced in the form of tablets, Metenix is a preparation of the thiazide- like diuretic metolazone. It is not recommended for children.
✚/▲ warning/side-effects: *see* METOLAZONE.

Meterfer (*Sinclair*) is a proprietary non-prescription IRON supplement, used particularly to treat certain forms of anaemia. Produced in the form of tablets, Meterfer is a preparation of ferrous fumarate. It is not recommended for children.
✚/▲ warning/side-effects: *see* FERROUS FUMARATE.

Meterfolic (*Sinclair*) is a proprietary non-prescription IRON-and-VITAMIN supplement, used particularly to prevent iron deficiency or vitamin B deficiency (as sometimes occurs during pregnancy). Produced in the form of tablets, Meterfolic is a compound of ferrous fumarate and folic acid.
✚/▲ warning/side-effects: *see* FERROUS FUMARATE; FOLIC ACID.

metformin hydrochloride is a drug used to treat adult-onset

diabetes, particularly in patients who are not totally dependent on additional supplies of INSULIN. It works by increasing the absorption and utilization in the body of glucose, to make up for the reduction in insulin available from the pancreas.
Administration is oral in the form of tablets.

✚ warning: metformin hydrochloride should not be administered to patients with heart, liver or kidney failure, dehydration, alcoholism, or severe infection or trauma; it should be administered with caution to those who are lactating.

▲ side-effects: there may be nausea and vomiting, with diarrhoea and weight loss. Body uptake of CYANOCOBALAMIN (vitamin B_{12}) or its analogues may be reduced.
Related articles: GLUCOPHAGE; ORABET.

methadone is a powerful and long-acting narcotic ANALGESIC used both to relieve severe pain and – like several narcotic analgesics – to suppress coughs. One of its principal uses is in the treatment of heroin addicts. Ironically, prolonged use of methadone can also lead to dependence (addiction). Administration (in the form of methadone hydrochloride) is oral in the form of tablets, as a linctus, or by injection.

✚ warning: methadone should not be administered to patients with liver disease, raised intracranial pressure, or head injury. It should be administered with caution to those with asthma, low blood pressure (hypotension), underactivity of the thyroid gland (hypothyroidism) or impaired liver or kidney function; who are pregnant or lactating; who are taking monoamine oxidase inhibitors; or have a history of drug abuse. Its effect is cumulative. Dosage should be reduced for elderly or debilitated patients.

▲ side-effects: there is commonly constipation, drowsiness and dizziness. High dosage may result in respiratory depression.
Related article: PHYSEPTONE.

methenamine is another name for the somewhat toxic ANTIBACTERIAL ANTISEPTIC hexamine.
see HEXAMINE.

methicillin is a PENICILLIN derivative used primarily to treat forms of infection which other penicillins are incapable of countering. This is because methicillin is not inactivated by the enzymes produced, for example, by certain Staphylococci. However, because administration is only by injection or infusion, other similar penicillin derivatives that can be administered orally have rather superseded methicillin.

✚ warning: methicillin should not be administered to patients known to be allergic to penicillins; it should be administered with caution to those with impaired kidney function.

▲ side-effects: there may be sensitivity reactions ranging from a minor rash to urticaria and joint pains, and (occasionally) to high body temperature or anaphylactic shock. High dosage may in any case cause convulsions.
Related article: CELBENIN.

methionine is an antidote to poisoning by the analgesic paracetamol (which has the greatest toxic effect on the liver). Administration is oral in the form of tablets; dosage depends on the results of blood counts every 4 hours.

methixene hydrochloride is a powerful ANTIPARKINSONISM drug, used to relieve some of the symptoms of parkinsonism, specifically the tremor of the hands, the overall rigidity of the posture, and the tendency to produce an excess of saliva. (The drug also has the capacity to treat these conditions in some cases where they are produced by drugs.) It is thought to work by compensating for the lack of dopamine in the brain that is the major cause of such parkinsonian symptoms. Administration – which may be in parallel with the administration of LEVODOPA – is oral in the form of tablets.

✚ warning: methixene hydrochloride should not be administered to patients with not merely tremor but with distinct involuntary movements; it should be administered with caution to those with impaired kidney or liver function, cardiovascular disease, glaucoma, or urinary retention. Withdrawal of treatment must be gradual.

▲ side-effects: there may be dry mouth, dizziness and blurred vision, and/or gastrointestinal disturbances. Some patients experience sensitivity reactions and anxiety. Rarely, and in susceptible patients, there may be confusion, agitation and psychological disturbance (at which point treatment must be withdrawn).
Related article: TREMONIL.

methocarbamol is a SKELETAL MUSCLE RELAXANT used primarily to relieve muscle spasm in the limbs caused by injury, but also is a constituent in several compound analgesic preparations. It works by direct action on the central nervous system. Administration is oral in the form of tablets, or by injection.

✚ warning: methocarbamol should not be administered to patients with glaucoma, epilepsy, enlargement of the prostate gland, rapid heart rate or defective bladder sphincter muscles, who have brain damage, or who are in a comatose state. It should be administered only orally to those with impaired kidney function. The drug may increase the effects of alcohol consumption.

▲ side-effects: concentration and speed of thought and movement is affected. There may be light-headedness, dizziness, drowsiness and/or nausea; or there may be restlessness, anxiety and mild confusion. Some patients experience sensitivity reactions such as a rash. Rarely, there are convulsions.
Related articles: ROBAXIN 750; ROBAXISAL FORTE.

methohexitone sodium is a general ANAESTHETIC used for both the induction and the maintenance of general anaesthesia in surgical operations; administration is intravenous (generally in 1% solution). It is less irritant to tissues than some other anaesthetics, and recovery afterwards is quick, but the induction of anaesthesia is not particularly smooth.

✚ warning: maintenance of anaesthesia is usually in combination with other anaesthetics. Induction may take up to 60 seconds.

▲ side-effects: induction may cause hiccups and involuntary movements. The patient may feel pain on the initial injection.
Related article: BRIETAL SODIUM.

methotrexate is a CYTOTOXIC drug used primarily in the treatment of lymphoblastic leukaemia, but also to treat other lymphomas and the lymphatic cancer Hodgkin's disease, as well as some solid tumours. It works by inhibiting the activity of an enzyme essential to the DNA metabolism in cells, and is administered orally or by injection.

✚ warning: methotrexate should not be administered to patients with severely impaired kidney function, or who have fluid within the pleural cavity. Leakage of the drug into the tissues at the site of injection may cause tissue damage. Regular blood counts are essential during treatment.

▲ side-effects: there is commonly nausea and vomiting; there may also be hair loss. The capacity of the bone-marrow to produce blood cells is reduced. The drug may also cause inflammation in various body tissues.
Related articles: EMTEXATE; MAXTREX.

methotrimeprazine is an ANTIPSYCHOTIC drug used to tranquillize patients suffering from schizophrenia and other psychoses, and to calm and soothe patients who are dying. Administration is oral in the form of tablets or by injection.

✚ warning: methotrimeprazine should not be administered to patients with certain forms of glaucoma, whose blood-cell formation by the bone-marrow is reduced, or who are taking drugs that depress certain centres of the brain and spinal cord. It should be administered with caution to those with lung disease, cardiovascular disease, epilepsy, parkinsonism, abnormal secretion by the adrenal glands, impaired liver or kidney function, undersecretion of thyroid hormones (hypothyroidism), enlargement of the prostate gland or any form of acute infection; who are pregnant or lactating; or who are elderly. Prolonged use requires regular physical checks. Withdrawal of treatment should be gradual.

▲ side-effects: concentration and speed of thought and movement are affected; the effects of alcohol consumption are enhanced. There may be dry mouth and blocked nose, constipation and difficulty in urinating, and blurred vision; menstrual disturbances in women or impotence in men may occur, with weight gain; there may be sensitivity reactions. Some patients feel cold and depressed, and tend to suffer from poor sleep patterns. Blood pressure may be low and the heartbeat irregular. Prolonged high dosage may cause opacity in the cornea and lens of the eyes, and a purple pigmentation of the skin. Treatment by intramuscular injection may be painful.
Related articles: NOZINAN; VERACTIL.

methoxamine hydrochloride is a SYMPATHOMIMETIC drug that as such has the properties of a VASOCONSTRICTOR. It is used primarily to raise the blood pressure of a patient whose blood pressure has dropped because of the induction of anaesthesia. Administration is by injection.

✚ warning: methoxamine hydrochloride should not be administered to patients with severe heart disease of any kind; it should be administered with caution to those who suffer from overactivity of the thyroid gland (hyperthyroidism), or who are pregnant.

▲ side-effects: there may be headache and a slow heartbeat; the blood pressure may be raised too high.

Related article: VASOXINE.

methyclothiazide is a DIURETIC, one of the THIAZIDES, used to treat fluid retention in the tissues (oedema), and high blood pressure (hypertension). Because all thiazides tend to deplete body reserves of potassium, methyclothiazide may be administered in combination either with potassium supplements or with diuretics that are complementarily potassium-sparing.
Administration is oral in the form of tablets.

✚ warning: methyclothiazide should not be administered to patients with liver or kidney impairment or urinary retention, or who are lactating. It should be administered with caution to those who are pregnant. It may aggravate conditions of diabetes or gout.

▲ side-effects: there may be tiredness and a rash. In men, temporary impotence may occur.

Related article: ENDURON.

methyl salicylate is an non-narcotic ANALGESIC for topical application in solution. It works by producing an irritation of sensory nerve endings within the skin that offsets the pain of underlying muscle or joint pains, and is produced in the form of a non-proprietary liniment and ointment, in addition to several proprietary preparations in the form of a cream or a balsam, for gently massaging in.

✚ warning: preparations of methyl salicylate in the form of an ointment may contain wool fat, which can cause sensitivity reactions in some patients.

Related articles: ASPELLIN; BALMOSA; BENGUÉ'S BALSAM; DUBAM; Phytex; SALONAIR.

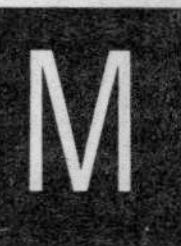

methylcellulose is a high-fibre substance used as a LAXATIVE because it is an effective bulking agent – it increases the overall mass of faeces within the rectum, so stimulating bowel movement. It is also particularly useful in soothing the symptoms of diverticular disease and irritable colon. Moreover, it can additionally be used to treat diarrhoea (as well as constipation) and to assist in the medical treatment of obesity because it reduces the intake of food by producing the sensation of satiety. Administration is oral, generally in the form of tablets, granules for solution, or a mixture.

✚ warning: preparations of methylcellulose should not be administered to patients with obstruction of the intestines, or failure of the muscles of the intestinal wall; it should be administered with caution to those with ulcerative colitis. Fluid intake during treatment should be higher than usual.

▲ side-effects: there may be flatulence, so much as to distend the abdomen.

Related articles: CELEVAC; CELLUCON; COLOGEL; NILSTIM.

methylcysteine is a mucolytic drug, used to reduce the viscosity of sputum and thus facilitate expectoration (the coughing up of sputum) in patients with disorders of the upper respiratory tract such as asthma and bronchitis. Administration is oral in the form of tablets or, rarely, aerosol spray.

✚ warning: methylcysteine should not be administered to patients with a peptic ulcer; it should be administered with caution to those who are pregnant.

▲ side-effects: side-effects are uncommon, but there may be gastrointestinal disturbance, with nausea, or a rash.

Related article: VISCLAIR.

M

methyldopa is a powerful ANTIHYPERTENSIVE drug used, in combination with a diuretic drug, to treat moderate to severe high blood pressure (hypertension). With other antihypertensives that work by direct action on the brain, however, methyldopa is becoming ever more rarely used, although triple combinations involving a diuretic and a beta-blocker in addition to methyldopa remain fairly popular. Administration is oral in the form of capsules, tablets and a suspension, or by injection.

✚ warning: methyldopa should not be administered to patients with abnormal secretion of corticosteroids by the adrenal glands or chronic liver disease, or who have a history of depression. It should be administered with caution to those with impaired kidney function. Regular blood counts and tests on liver function are essential during treatment.

▲ side-effects: there is dry mouth, drowsiness, fluid retention and diarrhoea; there may also be sedation, depression, impaired liver function, and skin and blood disorders.

Related articles: ALDOMET; DOPAMET; HYDROMET; MEDOMET.

methyldopate hydrochloride is the form of the ANTIHYPERTENSIVE drug methyldopa that is used for injection.

see METHYLDOPA.

methylphenobarbitone is a drug used to treat grand mal (tonic-clonic) and focal (partial) seizures of epilepsy. Administered orally in the form of tablets, it is converted in the liver to the powerful SEDATIVE and ANTICONVULSANT BARBITURATE phenobarbitone, with which it shares action and effects.

see PHENOBARBITONE.

methylprednisolone is a CORTICOSTEROID used primarily to treat the symptoms of inflammation or allergic reaction, but useful also in the treatment of fluid retention in the brain or of shock. Administration (as methylprednisolone, methylprednisolone acetate or methylprednisolone sodium succinate) is oral in the form of tablets, or by injection or infusion.

✚ warning: methylprednisolone should not be administered to patients with psoriasis; it should be administered with caution to the elderly (in whom overdosage can cause osteoporosis, "brittle bones"). In children, administration of methylprednisolone may lead to stunting of growth. The effects of potentially serious infections may be masked by the drug during treatment. Withdrawal of treatment must be gradual.

▲ side-effects: treatment of

susceptible patients may engender a euphoria, or a state of confusion or depression. Rarely, the patient suffers from a peptic ulcer.
Related articles: DEPO-MEDRONE; DEPO-MEDRONE WITH LIDOCAINE; MEDRONE; MIN-I-MIX METHYLPREDNISOLONE; SOLU-MEDRONE.

methyltestosterone is an ANDROGEN, a male sex HORMONE that with other androgens promotes the development of the secondary male sexual characteristics. Therapeutically it is administered to make up a hormonal deficiency (but only following careful investigation and under strict medical supervision), particularly in cases of delayed puberty and underdevelopment in boys. Administration is oral in the form of tablets.

✚ warning: methyltestosterone should not be administered to male patients with kidney disease, cancer of the prostate gland or cancer of the breast (or to female patients who are pregnant or lactating); it should be administered with caution to those with impaired function of the heart, liver or kidney, or those suffering from circulatory disorders and/or high blood pressure (hypertension), epilepsy, diabetes, thyroid disorders, or from migraine.

▲ side-effects: there may be fluid retention in the tissues (oedema) leading to weight gain. Increased levels of calcium in the body may cause bone growth (and in younger patients may fuse bones before fully grown) and the symptoms of hypercalcaemia. In elderly patients there may be (increased) enlargement of the prostate gland. High doses halt the production of sperm in men (and cause the visible masculinization of women); in both sexes it may also cause jaundice.
Related articles: MIXOGEN; PLEX-HORMONE; VIRORMONE-ORAL.

methyprylone is a BARBITURATE used as a HYPNOTIC to treat severe and intractable insomnia. Repeated doses are cumulative in effect and result in tolerance and dependence (addiction). Administration is oral in the form of tablets. The proprietary preparation is on the controlled drugs list.

✚ warning: methyprylone should not be administered to patients whose insomnia is caused by pain, who have porphyria, who are children or elderly or debilitated, who are pregnant or lactating, or who have a history of drug abuse. It should be administered with caution to those with respiratory depression for any reason, or who have impaired liver or kidney function. Dosage should be the least still to be effective; prolonged treatment should be avoided. Withdrawal of treatment should nevertheless be gradual.

▲ side-effects: there is a marked degree of sedation that may affect concentration and speed of thought and movement. There may also be dizziness and respiratory depression, headache and sensitivity reactions (particularly in the elderly).
Related article: NOLUDAR.

methysergide is a potentially dangerous drug used, generally under strict medical supervision in a hospital, to prevent severe

M

recurrent migraine and similar headaches in patients for whom other forms of treatment have failed. But the drug may also be used to treat patients with tumours of the intestinal glands that have spread to the liver: the liver then produces excess serotonin in the bloodstream – and it is the symptoms of that excess that methysergide treats. Administration is oral in the form of tablets.

✚ warning: methysergide should not be administered to patients with heart, lung, liver or kidney disease, or who suffer from collagen disorders, or who are pregnant or lactating. It should be administered with caution to those with peptic ulcer. Withdrawal of treatment should be gradual, although no course of treatment should last for more than 6 months at a time.

▲ side-effects: there is initial nausea, drowsiness and dizziness; there may also be fluid retention and consequent weight gain, spasm of the arteries, numbness of the fingers and toes, increased heart rate and even psychological changes.

Related article: DESERIL.

metipranolol is a BETA-BLOCKER used in the form of eye-drops to treat glaucoma. It is thought to work by slowing the rate of production of the aqueous humour in the eyeball, but it may be absorbed and have systemic effects as well.

✚ warning: because systemic absorption may occur, metipranolol should be administered with caution to patients with slow heart rate, heart failure or asthma. It should not be administered to patients who have a history of asthmatic symptoms.

▲ side-effects: there may be periods in which the eyes temporarily become dry; at such times there may be infections such as conjunctivitis or blepharitis.

Related article: GLAULINE.

metirosine is an ANTIHYPERTENSIVE drug used, generally under strict medical supervision in a hospital, primarily to treat the symptoms of high blood pressure associated with conditions that result in abnormal secretion of CORTICOSTEROIDS by the adrenal glands due to phaeochromocytoma, or in patients for whom surgery is not possible. It works by inhibiting an enzyme that contributes to the secretion of catecholamines such as adrenaline and noradrenaline (as occurs in situations of stress). Administration is oral in the form of capsules.

✚ warning: increased fluid intake during treatment is essential. Regular checks on overall blood volume are advisable.

▲ side-effects: there is a degree of sedation such that concentration and speed of thought and movement may be affected. There is commonly also severe diarrhoea. Some patients experience sensitivity reactions – which may also be severe.

Related article: DEMSER.

metoclopramide is an effective ANTI-EMETIC drug used to prevent vomiting caused by gastrointestinal disorders or by chemotherapy or radiotherapy in the treatment of cancer. It works both by direct action on the vomiting centre of the brain and by inhibiting the motility of the intestinal walls, and has fewer side-effects than many other anti-emetics (such as the phenothiazine derivatives). Administration (as metoclopramide hydrochloride) is oral in the form of tablets and syrups, or by injection.

✚ warning: metoclopramide should not be administered to patients who have had gastrointestinal surgery within the previous 4 days; it should be administered with caution to those with impaired kidney function, or who are chilren or elderly. Dosage should begin low and gradually increase. The effects of the drug may mask underlying disorders.

▲ side-effects: side-effects are relatively uncommon, especially in male patients. There may, however, be mild neuromuscular symptoms, drowsiness and constipation.

Related articles: MAXOLON; METOX; METRAMID; MIGRAVESS; Mygdalon; PARAMAX; PARMID; PRIMPERAN.

metolazone is a DIURETIC, one of the THIAZIDES, used to treat fluid retention in the tissues (oedema), high blood pressure (hypertension) and mild to moderate heart failure. Because all thiazides tend to deplete body reserves of potassium, metolazone may be administered in combination either with potassium supplements or with diuretics that are complementarily potassium-sparing. Administration is oral in the form of tablets.

✚ warning: metolazone should not be administered to patients with kidney failure or urinary retention, or who are lactating. It should be administered with caution to those who are pregnant. It may aggravate conditions of diabetes or gout.

▲ side-effects: there may be tiredness and a rash. In men, temporary impotence may occur.

Related article: METENIX.

Metopirone (*Ciba*) is a proprietary form of metyrapone, available only on prescription, used with corticosteroids (glucocorticoids) to treat resistant accumulation of fluid within the tissues (oedema) caused by increased secretion of the mineralocorticoid aldosterone. It may also be used to test the functioning of the pituitary gland. Produced in the form of capsules, Metopirone is not recommended for children.

✚/▲ warning/side-effects: *see* METYRAPONE.

metoprolol is a BETA-BLOCKER used to treat high blood pressure (*see* ANTIHYPERTENSIVE), heartbeat irregularities, angina pectoris (heart pain), and the effects of an excess of thyroid hormones in the bloodstream (thyrotoxicosis), to provide emergency relief in a heart attack, and to prevent recurrent attacks of migraine. Administration (as metoprolol tartrate) is oral in the form of tablets and sustained-release tablets, or by injection.

✚ warning: as a hypertensive drug, metoprolol tartrate should not be administered to patients with heart disease or asthmatic symptoms; it should be administered with caution to those with impaired kidney function, or who are nearing the end of pregnancy or lactating. Withdrawal of treatment should be gradual.

▲ side-effects: there may be some gastrointestinal or slight respiratory disturbance following oral administration. Some patients experience sensitivity reactions.

Related articles: BETALOC; CO-BETALOC; Lopresor; LOPRESORETIC.

Metosyn (*Stuart*) is a proprietary CORTICOSTEROID preparation, available only on prescription, used to treat inflammations of the skin (such as severe eczema) in patients not responding to less potent corticosteroids. Produced in the form of a water- miscible cream, as a paraffin-based ointment, and as a scalp lotion, Metosyn is a preparation of the potent steroid fluocinonide.
✚/▲ warning/side-effects: *see* FLUOCINONIDE.

Metox (*Steinhard*) is a proprietary preparation of the ANTI-EMETIC drug metoclopramide hydrochloride, available only on prescription, used to relieve symptoms of nausea and vomiting caused by gastrointestinal disorders, or by chemotherapy or radiotherapy in the treatment of cancer. It is produced in the form of tablets.
✚/▲ warning/side-effects: *see* METOCLOPRAMIDE.

Metramid (*Nicholas*) is a proprietary preparation of the ANTI-EMETIC drug metoclopramide hydrochloride, available only on prescription, used to relieve symptoms of nausea and vomiting caused by gastrointestinal disorders, or by chemotherapy or radiotherapy in the treatment of cancer. It is produced in the form of tablets, and is not recommended for children aged under 15 years.
✚/▲ warning/side-effects: *see* METOCLOPRAMIDE.

metriphonate is a drug that destroys the blood fluke Schistosoma haematobium, which causes a form of bilharzia that is quite common in Africa and the Middle East. The disease is contracted by bathing in water contaminated with the larvae of the flukes; adult flukes of this species infest the blood vessels of the liver, bladder and organs, causing severe inflammation that may eventually lead to cancers. Administration is oral in three doses over four weeks.

Metrodin (*Serono*) is a proprietary preparation of the pituitary HORMONE follicle-stimulating hormone (FSH), available only on prescription, used primarily to treat women suffering from specific hormonal deficiencies resulting in infertility. The treatment is ordinarily undertaken in specialist centres because monitoring is essential. Produced in the form of a powder for reconstitution as a medium for injection, Metrodin is a form of the hormone prepared from human menopausal urine.
✚/▲ warning/side-effects: *see* FSH.

Metrolyl (*Lagap*) is a proprietary ANTIMICROBIAL and anti-parasitic, available only on prescription, used to treat many forms of infection including those caused by bacteria (such as non-specific vaginitis), by protozoa, or by amoebae. Produced in the form of tablets (in two strengths), as anal suppositories (in two strengths), and in solution for intravenous infusion, Metrolyl is a preparation of metronidazole.
✚/▲ warning/side-effects: *see* METRONIDAZOLE.

metronidazole is a broad-spectrum ANTIMICROBIAL and anti-parasitic used to treat a wide range of infections including those caused by bacteria (particularly infections of the urinary, intestinal and genital tracts), by protozoa (such as Giardia and Trichomonas) and by amoebae (such as Entamoeba histolytica). It is also effective in treating infestation by guinea worms. Administration is oral in the form of tablets or a suspension, topical in the form of anal suppositories, or by injection or infusion.

✚ warning: metronidazole should not be taken regularly on a high-dosage basis. It should be administered with caution to patients with impaired liver function, or who are pregnant or lactating. During treatment patients must avoid alcohol consumption (the presence of alcohol in the body during treatment gives rise to most unpleasant side-effects).

▲ side-effects: these are uncommon – but there may be nausea and vomiting, with drowsiness, headache and gastrointestinal disturbances; gastrointestinal effects may be reduced by taking the drug during or after food. Some patients experience a discoloration of the urine. Prolonged treatment may eventually give rise to neuromuscular disorders or even seizures reminiscent of epilepsy with high doses.
Related articles: ELYZOL; FLAGYL; FLAGYL COMPAK; FLAGYL S; Flagyl 400; METROLYL; NIDAZOL; VAGINYL; ZADSTAT.

metronidazole benzoate is the form in which the broad-spectrum antibiotic metronidazole is administered in a suspension.
see METRONIDAZOLE.

metyrapone is a substance that has the effect of inhibiting the production of mineralocorticoids by the adrenal glands. It can thus be used with glucocorticoids to treat resistant fluid retention within the tissues (oedema) caused by increased secretion of the mineralocorticoid aldosterone, and to treat other conditions that result from the abnormal secretion of adrenal hormones (such as Cushing's syndrome). It may also be used to test the functioning of the pituitary gland.

✚ warning: metyrapone should be administered with caution to patients with severe under-secretion of pituitary hormones.

▲ side-effects: there may be nausea and vomiting; in some patients, the overall production and secretion of adrenal hormones is drastically reduced, causing further symptoms.
Related article: METOPIRONE.

Mevillin-L (*Evans*) is a proprietary VACCINE against measles (rubeola), available only on prescription. It is a powdered preparation of live but attenuated measles viruses for administration within a diluent by injection.

✚ warning: mevillin-L should not be administered to patients with any infection, particularly tuberculosis; who are allergic to eggs (the viruses are cultured in chick embryo tissue); who have known immune-system abnormalities; who are pregnant; hypersensitive to neomycin or polymyxin; or who are already taking corticosteroid drugs, cytotoxic drugs or are undergoing radiating treatment. It should be administered with caution to those with epilepsy or any other condition potentially involving convulsive fits.

▲ side-effects: there may be inflammation at the site of

injection. Rarely, there may be high temperature, cough and sore throat, a rash, swelling of the lymph glands and/or pain in the joints.

mexiletine is an ANTIARRHYTHMIC drug used to reduce the rate of the heartbeat, especially following a heart attack, and especially when the more commonly-used local ANAESTHETIC lignocaine has proved to be ineffective. Administration (in the form of mexiletine hydrochloride) is by injection followed by infusion as necessary. Overdosage is, however, dangerous.

✚ warning: mexiletine should not be administered to patients who have a slow heart rate, who have heart block, who are taking diuretic drugs, or who suffer from PARKINSOMISM.

▲ side-effects: there may be slow heart rate and low blood pressure; some patients have neuromuscular reactions such as tremor or nystagmus (eye-twitch) and gastrointestinal disturbances. Rarely, there is a state of confusion.
Related article: MEXITIL.

Mexitil (*Boehringer Ingelheim*) is a proprietary ANTIARRHYTHMIC drug, available only on prescription. It is a preparation of mexiletine hydrochloride and is produced in the form of capsules (in two strengths), as sustained-release capsules ("Perlongets", under the name Mexitil PL), and in ampoules for injection. It is not recommended for children.

✚/▲ warning/side-effects: *see* MEXILETINE.

mezlocillin is a derivative of the broad-spectrum penicillin-type ANTIBIOTIC ampicillin that is additionally effective in treating some infections by bacteria resistant to ampicillin. Administration is by injection or infusion.

✚ warning: mezlocillin should not be administered to pregnant women or to patients known to be allergic to penicillins; it should be administered with caution to those with impaired kidney function.

▲ side-effects: there may be sensitivity reactions ranging from a minor rash to urticaria and joint pains, and (occasionally) to high temperature and anaphylactic shock. High doses may in any case cause convulsions.
Related article: BAYPEN.

MFV-Ject (*Merieux*) is the name of a series of proprietary flu VACCINES consisting of suspensions containing inactivated viral material derived from influenza viruses. It is not recommended for children.

✚ warning: like any flu vaccine, MFV-Ject cannot control epidemics and should be used only against what seems to be the appropriate viral strain – on people who are at high risk: the elderly, patients with cardiovascular problems, and medical staff. MFV-Ject should not be administered to patients who are allergic to egg or chicken protein (in which vaccine viruses are cultured), or who are pregnant.

▲ side-effects: rarely, there is local reaction together with headache and high temperature.

mianserin is an ANTIDEPRESSANT drug used to treat depressive illness, especially in cases in which a degree of sedation may be useful. Administration is oral in the form of tablets.

✚ warning: mianserin should not be administered to patients with heart disease or psychosis, or who are already taking other types of antidepressants, barbiturates, anti-hypertensives or alcohol; it should be administered with caution to those with diabetes, epilepsy, liver or thyroid disease, glaucoma or urinary retention; or who are pregnant or lactating. Withdrawal of treatment must be gradual.

▲ side-effects: concentration and speed of thought and movement may be affected; there may also be dry mouth, blurred vision, difficulty in urinating, sweating, and irregular heartbeat; some patients experience a rash, behavioural disturbances, a state of confusion and/or a loss of libido. Treatment must be withdrawn if blood disorders occur: regular blood counts are essential in connection with the use of this drug.
Related article: LUDIOMIL.

Micolette (*Ayerst*) is a proprietary non-prescription form of small enema administered rectally to promote defecation, especially pre- or post-operatively or before labour or rectal examination by endoscope. Produced in single-dose disposable packs with a nozzle, Micolette is a preparation that includes sodium citrate, sodium laurylsulphoacetate and GLYCEROL in a viscous solution. It is not recommended for children aged under 3 years.

✚/▲ warning/side-effects: *see* SODIUM CITRATE.

miconazole is an ANTIFUNGAL drug used in the treatment of many forms of fungal infection, generally by topical application (for instance, as an oral gel, as a spray powder, or as a water-miscible cream), although tablets are also available for use in recurrent or resistant infection and as an injection for systemic infections. In solution, the drug may be used for irrigation of the bladder.

✚ warning: topical treatment should be continued for more than a week after lesions or other symptoms have healed.

▲ side-effects: Rarely, there is irritation of the skin or minor sensitivity reaction. Miconazole may cause nausea and vomiting.
Related articles: DAKTARIN; DERMONISTAT.

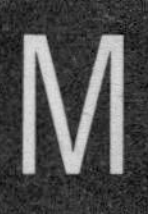

Micralax (*Smith, Kline & French*) is a proprietary non- prescription form of small enema administered rectally to promote defecation, especially before labour or rectal examination by endoscope. Produced in single-dose disposable packs with a nozzle, Micralax is a preparation that includes sodium citrate, sodium alkylsulphoacetate and sorbic acid in a viscous solution. It is not recommended for children aged under 3 years.

✚/▲ warning/side-effects: *see* SODIUM CITRATE.

Microgynon 30 (*Schering*) is a proprietary combined ORAL CONTRACEPTIVE, available only on prescription, used also (because it is a combination of female sex hormones) to treat menstrual problems. Produced in the form of tablets in a calendar pack, Microgynon 30 is a preparation of the OESTROGEN ethinyloestradiol and the PROGESTOGEN levonorgestrel.

✚/▲ warning/side-effects: *see* ETHINYLOESTRADIOL; LEVONORGESTREL.

Micro-K (*Merck*) is a proprietary non-prescription form of potassium supplement, used to treat patients with deficiencies and to replace potassium in patients taking potassium-depleting drugs such as CORTICOSTEROIDS or the THIAZIDE diuretics. Produced in the form of sustained-release capsules, Micro-K is a preparation of POTASSIUM CHLORIDE.

✚ warning: should not be used in patients with advanced renal failure. Should be discontinued if it produces ulceration or obstruction of the small bowel.

Micronor (*Ortho-Cilag*) is a proprietary progesterone-only ORAL CONTRACEPTIVE, available only on prescription. Produced in the form of tablets in a calendar pack corresponding to one complete menstrual cycle, Micronor is a preparation of the PROGESTOGEN norethisterone.

✚/▲ warning/side-effects: *see* NORETHISTERONE.

Microval (*Wyeth*) is a proprietary progesterone-only ORAL CONTRACEPTIVE, available only on prescription. Produced in the form of tablets in a calendar pack corresponding to one complete menstrual cycle, Microval is a preparation of the PROGESTOGEN levonorgestrel.

✚/▲ warning/side-effects: *see* LEVONORGESTREL.

Mictral (*Winthrop*) is a proprietary ANTIBIOTIC, available only on prescription, used primarily to treat infections of the urinary tract, including cystisis. Produced in the form of granules in a sachet for solution in water, Mictral's major active constituents are the ANTIBACTERIAL drug nalidixic acid and SODIUM CITRATE. It is not recommended for infants under 3 months.

✚/▲ warning/side-effects: *see* NALIDIXIC ACID.

Midamor (*Morson*) is a proprietary DIURETIC, available only on prescription, used to treat fluid retention in the tissues (oedema), and to conserve potassium when administered in combination with other diuretics. Produced in the form of tablets, Midamor is a preparation of the potassium-sparing diuretic amiloride hydrochloride; it is not recommended for children.

✚/▲ warning/side-effects: *see* AMILORIDE.

midazolam is an ANXIOLYTIC drug, one of the BENZODIAZEPINES, used primarily to provide sedation for minor surgery such as dental operations or as a premedication prior to surgical procedures and, because it also has some SKELETAL MUSCLE RELAXANT properties, to treat some forms of spasm. Prolonged use results in tolerance and may lead to dependence (addiction), especially in patients with a history of drug (including alcohol) abuse. Administration is by injection.

✚ warning: concentration and speed of thought and movement are often affected. Midazolam should be administered with caution to patients with respiratory difficulties (it sometimes causes a sharp fall in blood pressure), glaucoma, or kidney or liver disease; who are in especially the last stages of pregnancy; or who are elderly or debilitated. Abrupt withdrawal of treatment should be avoided.

▲ side-effects: there may be drowsiness, dizziness, headache, dry mouth and shallow breathing; hypersensitivity reactions may occur.

Related article: HYPNOVEL. DIAZEPAM

Midrid (*Carnrick*) is a proprietary compound non-narcotic ANALGESIC, available only on prescription, used to treat migraine and other headaches caused by tension.. Produced in the form of capsules, Midrid is a preparation of the SYMPATHOMIMETIC isometheptene mucate, the SEDATIVE dichloralphenazone and the analgesic paracetamol; it is not recommended for prescription to children.
✚/▲ warning/side-effects: *see* DICHLORALPHENAZONE; ISOMETHEPTENE MUCATE; PARACETAMOL.

Migen (*Bencard*) is a proprietary suspension containing extracts of the house dust mite, for use in desensitizing patients who are allergic to it. It is available only on prescription and administered by injection.
✚ warning: injections should be administered under close medical supervision and in locations where emergency facilities for full cardio-respiratory resuscitation are immediately available.

Migraleve (*International Labs*) is a proprietary non-prescription compound ANALGESIC and ANTIHISTAMINE, used to treat migraine. Produced in the form of tablets, Migraleve is a preparation of the antihistamine buclizine hydrochloride, the analgesic paracetamol and the OPIATE codeine phosphate; tablets without buclizine hydrochloride are also available separately or in a duo-pack. These preparations are not recommended for children aged under 10 years. They should never be prescribed prophylactically.
✚/▲ warning/side-effects: *see* CODEINE PHOSPHATE; PARACETAMOL.

Migravess (*Bayer*) is a proprietary compound non-narcotic ANALGESIC, available only on prescription, used to treat migraine. Produced in the form of tablets (in two strengths, the stronger under the name Migravess Forte), Migravess is a preparation of the analgesic aspirin together with the ANTI-EMETIC metoclopramide hydrochloride. It is not recommended for children aged under 10 years.
✚/▲ warning/side-effects: *see* ASPIRIN; METOCLOPRAMIDE.

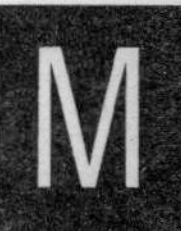

Migril (*Wellcome*) is a proprietary compound non-narcotic ANALGESIC, available only on prescription, used to treat migraine and some other vascular headaches. Produced in the form of tablets, Migril is a preparation of the vegetable alkaloid ergotamine tartrate, the ANTIHISTAMINE cyclizine hydrochloride and the mild stimulant caffeine hydrate. It is not recommended for children.
✚/▲ warning/side-effects: *see* CYCLIZINE; ERGOTAMINE TARTRATE.

Minafen (*Cow & Gate*) is a proprietary non-prescription nutritional preparation, used to feed infants and young children who have the amino acid metabolic abnormality phenylketonuria (PKU). Produced in the form of a powder, Minafen is a preparation of protein, fat, carbohydrate, vitamins and minerals, and is low in the amino acid phenylalanine. It is not, however, usable as a complete diet.

Minamino (*Consolidated*) is a proprietary non-prescription VITAMIN-and-mineral preparation that is not available from the National Health Service.

Produced in the form of a syrup, Minamino is a preparation of essential and non-essential amino acids, B-group vitamins and minerals, together with liver, spleen and gastric mucosa extracts. It is used as a vitamin and mineral supplement in the elderly, and during pregnancy and lactation.

Minihep (*Leo*) is a proprietary ANTICOAGULANT, available only on prescription, used to treat and prevent various forms of thrombosis. Produced in the form of "darts" and in ampoules for subcutaneous injection, Minihep is a preparation of the natural anticoagulant heparin sodium, and is also available as Minihep Calcium.
✚/▲ warning/side-effects: *see* HEPARIN.

Min-i-Jet Adrenaline (*International Medication Systems*) is a proprietary form of the natural catecholamine adrenaline, available only on prescription, used as a SYMPATHOMIMETIC drug to treat bronchial asthma, in the emergency treatment of acute allergic reactions, and to relieve the symptoms of heart failure. Produced in disposable syringes for injection (straight into the heart muscle if necessary), Min-i-Jet Adrenaline is a preparation of adrenaline hydrochloride.
✚/▲ warning/side-effects: *see* ADRENALINE.

Minilyn (*Organon*) is a proprietary combined ORAL CONTRACEPTIVE, available only on prescription. Produced in the form of tablets in a calendar pack corresponding to one complete menstrual cycle, Minilyn is a preparation of the OESTROGEN ethinyloestradiol and the PROGESTOGEN lynoestrenol.
✚/▲ warning/side-effects: *see* ETHINYLOESTRADIOL; LYNOESTRENOL.

Min-I-Mix Methylprednisolone (*International Medication Systems*) is a proprietary CORTICOSTEROID, available only on prescription, used to suppress inflammation or allergic symptoms, to relieve fluid retention around the brain, or to treat shock. Produced in the form of powder for reconstitution as a solution for injection, it is a preparation of methylprednisolone sodium succinate.
✚/▲ warning/side-effects: *see* METHYLPREDNISOLONE.

Minims Amethocaine (*Smith & Nephew*) is a proprietary local ANAESTHETIC for topical application, and ophthalmic procedures available only on prescription. Produced in the form of single-dose eye-drops, Minims Amethocaine is a preparation of amethocaine hydrochloride.
✚/▲ warning/side-effects: *see* AMETHOCAINE.

Minims Atropine Sulphate (*Smith & Nephew*) is a proprietary ANTICHOLINERGIC mydriatic drug, available only on prescription, used to dilate the pupils and paralyse certain eye muscles for the purpose of ophthalmic examination especially in young children (or occasionally to assist in antibiotic treatment). It is produced in the form of single-dose eye-drops (and indeed is a preparation of the ANTICHOLINERGIC drug atropine sulphate).
✚/▲ warning/side-effects: *see* ATROPINE SULPHATE.

Minims Benoxinate (*Smith & Nephew*) is a proprietary local

ANAESTHETIC, available only on prescription, used to relieve pain in the eyes especially during minor surgery or ophthalmic examination. Produced in the form of single-dose eye-drops, Minims Benoxinate is a preparation of oxybuprocaine hydrochloride.
✚/▲ warning/side-effects: *see* OXYBUPROCAINE.

Minims Castor Oil (*Smith & Nephew*) is a proprietary non-prescription form of eye-drops consisting of castor oil, for use as a lubricant in removing foreign bodies from the eye.

Minims Chloramphenicol (*Smith & Nephew*) is a proprietary ANTIBIOTIC for topical application, available only on prescription, used to treat bacterial infections in the eye. Produced in the form of single-dose eye-drops, Minims Chloramphenicol is a preparation of chloramphenicol.
✚/▲ warning/side-effects: *see* CHLORAMPHENICOL.

Minims Cyclopentolate (*Smith & Nephew*) is a proprietary ANTI-CHOLINERGIC mydriatic drug, available only on prescription, used to dilate the pupils and paralyse certain eye muscles for the purpose of ophthalmic examination (or occasionally to assist in antibiotic treatment). Produced in the form of single-dose eye- drops, it is a preparation of drug cyclopentolate hydrochloride.
✚/▲ warning/side-effects: *see* CYCLOPENTOLATE.

Minims Fluorescein Sodium (*Smith & Nephew*) is a proprietary non-prescription dye used in the diagnosis of certain disorders of the eye – for instance, to locate abrasions and foreign bodies. Produced in the form of single-dose eye-drops, it is a preparation of FLUORESCEIN SODIUM.

Minims Gentamicin (*Smith & Nephew*) is a proprietary ANTIBIOTIC, available only on prescription, used to treat bacterial infections in the eye. Produced in the form of single-dose eye- drops, Minims Gentamicin is a preparation of the aminoglycoside gentamicin sulphate.
✚/▲ warning/side-effects: *see* GENTAMICIN.

Minims Homatropine (*Smith & Nephew*) is a proprietary ANTI-CHOLINERGIC, mydriatic drug, available only on prescription, used to dilate the pupils and paralyse certain eye muscles for the purpose of ophthalmic examination (or occasionally to assist in antibiotic treatment). Produced in the form of single-dose eye-drops, it is a preparation of the ATROPINE derivative homatropine hydrobromide.

Minims Lignocaine and Fluorescein (*Smith & Nephew*) is a proprietary local ANAESTHETIC, available only on prescription. Produced in the form of single-dose eye-drops, Minims Lignocaine and Fluorescein is a preparation of lignocaine hydrochloride together with the diagnostic dye FLUORESCEIN SODIUM.
✚/▲ warning/side-effects: *see* LIGNOCAINE.

Minims Neomycin (Smith & Nephew) is a proprietary ANTIBIOTIC, available only on prescription, used to treat bacterial infections in the eye. Produced in the form of single-dose eye-drops.
✚/▲ warning/side-effects: *see* NEOMYCIN.

Minims Phenylephrine (*Smith & Nephew*) is a proprietary non-prescription SYMPATHOMIMETIC, used to dilate the pupils and paralyse certain eye muscles for the purpose of ophthalmic examination (or occasionally to assist in antibiotic treatment). Produced in the form of single-dose eye-drops, it is a preparation of the SYMPATHOMIMETIC phenylephrine hydrochloride.
✚/▲ warning/side-effects: *see* PHENLYEPHRINE.

M

Minims Pilocarpine (*Smith & Nephew*) is a proprietary PARASYMPATHOMIMETIC miotic drug, available only on prescription, used in the treatment of glaucoma. It works by improving drainage in the trabecular meshwork of the eyeball. Produced in the form of eye- drops (in three strengths), it is a preparation of pilocarpine nitrate.
✚/▲ warning/side-effects: *see* PILOCARPINE.

Minims Prednisolone (*Smith & Nephew*) is a proprietary corticosteroid, available only on prescription, used to treat non-infective inflammatory conditions in and around the eye. Produced in the form of eye-drops, it contains prednisolone sodium phosphate.
✚/▲ warning/side-effects: *see* PREDNISOLONE SODIUM PHOSPHATE.

Minims Rose Bengal (*Smith & Nephew*) is a proprietary non-prescription dye used in the diagnosis of certain conditions in the eye, such as the presence of degenerated cells in dry eye syndrome or pressure marks from contact lenses. Produced in the form of single-dose eye-drops, it is a preparation of ROSE BENGAL. It is not recommended for children.

Minims Sodium Chloride (*Smith & Nephew*) is a proprietary non-prescription preparation of saline solution used for the irrigation of the eyes, and to facilitate the first-aid removal of harmful substances. It is produced in the form of single-dose eye-drops.
✚/▲ warning/side-effects: *see* SODIUM CHLORIDE.

Minims Sulphacetamide Sodium (*Smith & Nephew*) is a proprietary ANTIBACTERIAL, available only on prescription, used to treat local infections in the eye. Produced in the form of single-dose eye-drops, it is a preparation of the SULPHONAMIDE sulphacetamide sodium.
✚/▲ warning/side-effects: *see* SULPHACETAMIDE.

Minims Thymoxamine (*Smith & Nephew*) is a proprietary miotic drug, available only on prescription, used to constrict the pupil after dilation caused by the administration of a SYMPATHOMIMETIC drug (for the purpose usually of ophthalmic examination). Produced in the form of single-dose eye-drops, it is a preparation of thymoxamine hydrochloride.
✚/▲ warning/side-effects: *see* THYMOXAMINE.

Minims Tropicamide (*Smith & Nephew*) is a proprietary mydriatic drug, available only on prescription, used to dilate the pupils and paralyse certain eye muscles for the purpose of ophthalmic examination (or occasionally to assist in antibiotic treatment). Produced in the form of single-dose eye-drops, it is a preparation of the short-acting ANTICHOLINERGIC drug tropicamide.
✚/▲ warning/side-effects: *see* TROPICAMIDE.

Minocin (*Lederle*) is a proprietary broad-spectrum ANTIBIOTIC, available only on prescription, used to treat many forms of infection but particularly those of the urinary tract, the respiratory tract, skin and soft tissue (including acne), and to prevent meningococcal infections. Produced in the form of tablets (in two strengths), Minocin is a preparation of the TETRACYCLINE minocycline hydrochloride. It should not be given to children under 12 years or to pregnant women.
✚/▲ warning/side-effects: *see* MINOCYCLINE.

minocycline is a broad-spectrum ANTIBIOTIC, a TETRACYCLINE with a wider range of action than any other tetracycline in that it is effective also in treating and preventing certain forms of meningitis. As if to compensate, however, it also causes more side-effects than most. Administration is oral in the form of tablets.
✚ warning: minocycline should not be administered to patients who are aged under 12 years, or who are pregnant. It should be administered with caution to those who are lactating or who have impaired liver or kidney function.
▲ side-effects: there may be nausea and vomiting, with diarrhoea; dizziness and vertigo are not uncommon, especially in female patients. Rarely, there are sensitivity reactions.
Related article: MINOCIN.

Minodiab (*Farmitalia Carlo Erba*) is a proprietary SULPHONYLUREA, available only on prescription, used to treat adult-onset diabetes mellitus. It works by augmenting what remains of insulin production in the pancreas. Produced in the form of tablets (in two strengths), Minodiab is a preparation of glipizide and is not recommended for children.
✚/▲ warning/side-effects: *see* GLIPIZIDE.

***minor tranquillizer:** *see* TRANQUILLIZER; ANXIOLYTIC.

Minovlar (*Schering*) is a proprietary combined ORAL CONTRACEPTIVE, available only on prescription. Produced in the form of tablets in a calendar pack corresponding to one complete menstrual cycle (in two forms, one requiring the administration of a tablet daily per month, the other requiring a week's rest after every three weeks), Minovlar is a compound preparation of the OESTROGEN ethinyloestradiol and the PROGESTOGEN norethisterone acetate.
✚/▲ warning/side-effects: *see* ETHINYLOESTRADIOL; NORETHISTERONE ACETATE.

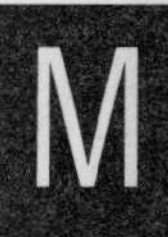

minoxidil is a powerful ANTIHYPERTENSIVE drug that works primarily by being a VASODILATOR – and that has many side-effects. Useful as it is in treating severe high blood pressure (hypertension), particularly when administered simultaneously with a diuretic and a beta-blocker, the drug has come to be employed really only when other vasodilators have failed. Administration is oral in the form of tablets.
✚ warning: minoxidil should not be administered to patients with adrenal disorders that cause abnormal secretion of corticosteroid hormones; it should be administered with caution to patients who undergo renal dialysis. The drug may aggravate conditions of heart failure and angina

pectoris (heart pain).
▲ side-effects: there are commonly gastrointestinal disturbances and weight gain; there may also be fluid retention, a rise in the heart rate and, in women, breast tenderness.
Related article: LONITEN.

Mintec (*Smith, Kline & French*) is a proprietary non-prescription ANTISPASMODIC drug, used to treat the discomfort and sensation of distension associated with irritable bowel syndrome. Produced in the form of capsules, Mintec is a preparation of PEPPERMINT OIL; it is not recommended for children.

Mintezol (*Merck Sharp & Dohme*) is a proprietary non-prescription ANTHELMINTIC drug, used to treat intestinal infestations by threadworm and guinea worm, and to assist in the treatment of resistant infections by hookworm, whipworm and roundworm. Produced in the form of tablets, Mintezol is a preparation of thiabendazole.
✚/▲ warning/side-effects: *see* THIABENDAZOLE.

Miochol (*CooperVision*) is a proprietary preparation of the PARASYMPATHOMIMETIC drug acetylcholine chloride, available only on prescription, used mainly to contract the pupil of the eye for the purpose of surgery on the iris, the cornea, or other sections of the exterior of the eye. It is produced in the form of a solution for intra-ocular irrigation.
✚/▲ warning/side-effects: see ACETYLCHOLINE CHLORIDE.

Miol (Formula M1) (*Brit Cair*) is a proprietary ANTISEPTIC, available only on prescription, used in topical application to treat inflammatory and ulcerative skin conditions. Produced in the form of a cream and a lotion, Miol is a preparation of various antiseptic and antifungal agents.

Miraxid (*Leo*) is a proprietary compound ANTIBIOTIC preparation, available only on prescription, used to treat infections in the respiratory tract, the ear and the urinary tract. Produced in the form of tablets (in two strengths, the stronger under the name Miraxid 450, which is not recommended for children) and as a suspension for children, Miraxid is a compound preparation of the penicillins pivampicillin and pivmecillinam hydrochloride.
✚/▲ warning/side-effects: *see* PIVAMPICILLIN; PIVMECILLINAM.

Mithracin (*Pfizer*) is a proprietary form of the drug plicamycin, formerly used as a CYTOTOXIC drug in the treatment of cancers but now used mainly in the emergency treatment of hypercalcaemia (excessive levels of calcium in the bloodstream) caused by malignant disease. It is produced in the form of powder for reconstitution as a medium for injection (in combination with other constituents, such as the diuretic mannitol).
✚/▲ warning/side-effects: *see* PLICAMYCIN.

mithramycin is the name formerly used for the drug plicamycin.
see PLICAMYCIN.

mitobronitol is a CYTOTOXIC drug used primarily to treat leukaemia, particularly the type that involves the bone marrow. It works by interfering with the DNA of new-forming cells, thus preventing normal cell replication. Administration is oral in the form of tablets (generally only in hospitals).

✚ warning: prolonged treatment may cause sterility in men and an early menopause in women; in both sexes it may lead to permanent bone marrow damage. Blood count monitoring is essential. Dosage should be the minimum still to be effective.

▲ side-effects: there may be nausea and vomiting; there may also be hair loss. The blood-cell producing capacity of the bone-marrow is impaired.

Related article: MYELOBROMOL.

mitomycin is a CYTOTOXIC drug that also has ANTIBIOTIC properties, and is used to treat cancers of the stomach, duodenum or jejunum, or of the breast. It is a comparatively toxic drug, and may cause severe side-effects such as permanent bone marrow damage. Administration is by injection.

✚ warning: prolonged treatment may cause sterility in men and an early menopause in women; in both sexes it may lead to permanent bone marrow, lung and kidney damage. Blood count monitoring is essential. Dosage should be the minimum still to be effective. If spilled, the drug is an irritant to tissues.

▲ side-effects: there may be nausea and vomiting; there may also be hair loss. The blood-cell producing capacity of the bone marrow is impaired.

Related article: MITOMYCIN C KYOWA.

Mitomycin C Kyowa (*Martindale*) is a proprietary preparation of the CYTOTOXIC drug mitomycin, available generally for hospital use only, used to treat upper gastrointestinal and breast cancers. Produced in the form of powder for reconstitution as a medium for injection, it is a preparation of mitomycin.

✚/▲ warning/side-effects: *see* MITOMYCIN.

Mitoxana (*Boehringer Ingelheim*) is a proprietary preparation of the CYTOTOXIC drug ifosamide, available for hospital use only, and used pretty well always in combination with MESNA to reduce some of the toxic effects. It is produced in the form of powder for reconstitution as a medium for injection.

✚/▲ warning/side-effects: *see* IFOSFAMIDE.

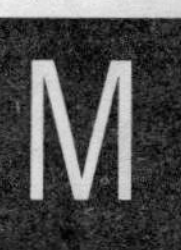

mitozantrone is a CYTOTOXIC drug that is chemically related to doxorubicin. It is used principally to treat breast cancer, although it tends to suppress the blood-cell forming capacity of the bone marrow and to have toxic effects on the heart. Administration is by intravenous infusion.

✚ warning: prolonged treatment may cause an early menopause in women; in both sexes it may lead to permanent bone-marrow, lung and kidney damage. Blood count monitoring is essential. Dosage should be the minimum still to be effective.

▲ side-effects: there may be nausea and vomiting; there may also be hair loss. The blood-cell producing capacity of the bone marrow is impaired.

Related article: NOVANTRONE.

Mixogen (*Organon*) is a proprietary compound HORMONE preparation, available only on prescription, used as part of hormone replacement therapy to relieve menopausal symptoms. Produced in the form of tablets,

Mixogen is a preparation of the OESTROGEN ethinyloestradiol and the ANDROGEN methyltestosterone.
✚/▲ warning/side-effects: *see* ETHINYLOESTRADIOL; METHYLTESTOSTERONE.

Mixtard 30/70 (*Nordisk Wellcome*) is a proprietary non-prescription preparation of mixed pork insulins used to treat and maintain diabetic patients. Produced in vials for injection, Mixtard 30/70 is a preparation of both neutral (30%) and isophane (70%) insulins. HUMAN MIXTARD 30/70 is also available.
✚/▲ warning/side-effects: *see* INSULIN.

Mobilan (*Galen*) is a proprietary ANTI-INFLAMMATORY non-narcotic ANALGESIC, available only on prescription, used to treat the pain of rheumatic and other musculo-skeletal disorders (including gout, bursitis and tendonitis). Produced in the form of capsules (in two strengths), Mobilan is a preparation of indomethacin.
✚/▲ warning/side-effects: *see* INDOMETHACIN.

Modecate (*Squibb*) is a proprietary ANTIPSYCHOTIC drug, available only on prescription, used in the long-term maintenance of tranquillization for patients suffering from psychoses (including schizophrenia). Produced in ampoules for injection (in two strengths, the stronger under the trade name Modecate Concentrate), Modecate is a preparation of fluphenazine decanoate. It is not recommended for children.
✚/▲ warning/side-effects: *see* FLUPHENAZINE.

Moditen (*Squibb*) is a proprietary ANTIPSYCHOTIC drug, available only on prescription, used in the long-term maintenance, as a major TRANQUILLIZER, for patients suffering from psychoses (including schizophrenia) and patients with behavioural disturbances. It may also be used in the short term to treat severe anxiety. Produced in the form of tablets (in three strengths), Moditen is a preparation of fluphenazine hydrochloride. Ampoules for depot injection are also available (under the name Moditen Enanthate) containing fluphenazine enanthate. Neither of these preparations is recommended for children.
✚/▲ warning/side-effects: *see* FLUPHENAZINE.

Modrasone (*Kirby-Warrick*) is a proprietary ANTI-INFLAMMATORY CORTICOSTEROID drug, available only on prescription, used in topical application to treat severe skin inflammation, such as eczema and various forms of dermatitis. Produced in the form of a cream and as an ointment, Modrasone is a preparation of the corticosteroid alclometasone dipropionate.
✚/▲ warning/side-effects: *see* ALCLOMETASONE DIPROPIONATE.

Modrenal (*Sterling Research*) is a proprietary preparation, available only on prescription, of the unusual drug trilostane, which inhibits the production of corticosteroids by the adrenal glands. It is thus used to treat conditions that result from the excessive secretion of adrenal hormones into the bloodstream (such as Cushing's disease). It is produced in the form of capsules, and is not recommended for children.
✚/▲ warning/side-effects: *see* TRILOSTANE.

Moducren (*Morson*) is a proprietary ANTIHYPERTENSIVE DIURETIC compound, available only on prescription, used to treat mild to moderate high blood pressure (hypertension). Produced in the form of tablets, Moducren is a preparation of the THIAZIDE hydrochlorothiazide, the weak but potassium-sparing diuretic amiloride hydrochloride and the BETA-BLOCKER timolol maleate. It is not recommended for children.
✚/▲ warning/side-effects: *see* AMILORIDE; HYDROCHLOROTHIAZIDE; TIMOLOL MALEATE.

Moduret 25 (*Morson*) is a proprietary DIURETIC, available only on prescription, used to treat congestive heart failure, high blood pressure (*see* ANTIHYPERTENSIVE) and cirrhosis of the liver. Produced in the form of tablets, it is a compound of the weak but potassium-sparing diuretic amiloride hydrochloride together with the THIAZIDE hydrochlorothiazide. It is not recommended for children.
✚/▲ warning/side-effects: *see* AMILORIDE; HYDROCHLOROTHIAZIDE.

Moduretic (*Merck, Sharp & Dohme*) is a proprietary DIURETIC, available only on prescription, used to treat congestive heart failure, high blood pressure (*see* ANTIHYPERTENSIVE) and cirrhosis of the liver. Produced in the form of tablets and as an oral solution, it is a compound of the weak but potassium-sparing diuretic amiloride hydrochloride together with the THIAZIDE hydrochlorothiazide. It is not recommended for children.
✚/▲ warning/side-effects: *see* AMILORIDE; HYDROCHLOROTHIAZIDE.

Mogadon (*Roche*) is a proprietary HYPNOTIC, available on prescription only to private patients, used to treat insomnia in cases where some degree of daytime sedation is acceptable. Produced in the form of tablets and as capsules, Mogadon is a preparation of the long-acting BENZODIAZEPINE nitrazepam, and is not recommended for children.
✚/▲ warning/side-effects: *see* NITRAZEPAM.

Molcer (*Wallace*) is a proprietary non-prescription form of ear-drops designed to soften and dissolve ear-wax (cerumen), and commonly prescribed for use at home two nights consecutively before syringing of the ears in a doctor's surgery. Its solvent constituent is DIOCTYL SODIUM SULPHOSUCCINATE (also called docusate sodium).
✚ warning: molcer should not be used if there is inflammation in the ear, or where there is any chance that eardrum has been perforated.

Molipaxin (*Roussel*) is a proprietary ANTIDEPRESSANT, available only on prescription, used to treat depressive illness (especially in cases where there is anxiety). It causes sedation. Produced in the form of capsules (in two strengths) and as a sugar-free liquid, Molipaxin is a preparation of the drug trazodone hydrochloride; it is not recommended for children.
✚/▲ warning/side-effects: *see* TRAZODONE HYDROCHLORIDE.

Monaspor (*Ciba*) is a proprietary ANTIBIOTIC, available only on prescription, used to treat many forms of infection, especially those of the respiratory tract, certain bone and soft tissue infections, and those caused by the organism Pseudomonas aeruginosa. It is also sometimes

used to ensure asepsis during surgery. Produced in the form of a powder for reconstitution as a medium for injection, Monaspor is a preparation of the cephalosporin cefsulodin sodium.
✚/▲ warning/side-effects: *see* CEFSULODIN.

Monistat (*Ortho-Cilag*) is a proprietary ANTIFUNGAL preparation for topical application, available only on prescription, used to treat yeast infections (such as thrush) of the vagina or vulva. Produced in the form of a vaginal cream and vaginal inserts (pessaries), Monistat is a preparation of miconazole nitrate. Not for use in children.
✚/▲ warning/side-effects: *see* MICONAZOLE.

Monit (*Stuart*) is a proprietary VASODILATOR, available only on prescription, used to prevent attacks of angina pectoris (heart pain). Produced in the form of tablets (in two strengths, the weaker under the name Monit LS), Monit is a preparation of isosorbide mononitrate. It is not recommended for children.
✚/▲ warning/side-effects: *see* ISOSORBIDE MONONITRATE.

***monoamine oxidase inhibitor:** *see* MAO INHIBITOR.

Mono-Cedocard 20 (*Tillotts*) is a proprietary VASODILATOR, available only on prescription, used to prevent attacks of angina pectoris (heart pain). Produced in the form of tablets (in two strengths, the stronger under the name Mono-Cedocard 40), Mono-Cedocard is a preparation of isosorbide mononitrate. It is not recommended for children.
✚/▲ warning/side-effects: *see* ISOSORBIDE MONONITRATE.

Monoparin (*CP Pharmaceuticals*) is a proprietary ANTICOAGULANT, available only on prescription, used to treat or prevent various forms of thrombosis, such as post-operatively. Produced in ampoules for subcutaneous and intravenous injection, Monoparin is a preparation of the anticoagulant heparin sodium.
✚/▲ warning/side-effects: *see* HEPARIN.

Monophane (*Boots*) is a proprietary non-prescription preparation of highly purified beef isophane insulin, used to treat and maintain diabetic patients. It is produced in vials for injection.
✚/▲ warning/side-effects: *see* INSULIN.

monosulfiram is a parasitocidal drug used mainly in topical application to treat skin surface infestation by the itch-mite (scabies). In this it is particularly valuable in treating children. Administration is in the form of a dilute spiritous solution (generally applied topically after a hot bath).
✚ warning: keep the solution away from the eyes. During treatment, patients should avoid alcohol consumption (if absorbed, the drug may give rise to a severe reaction – as does the closely-related drug DISULFIRAM – in the presence of alcohol).
▲ side-effects: rarely, there are sensitivity reactions.
Related article: TETMOSOL.

Monotard MC (*Nova*) is a proprietary, non-prescription, highly purified pork insulin zinc suspension, used to treat and maintain diabetic patients. It is produced in vials for injection.
✚/▲ warning/side-effects: *see* INSULIN.

Monotrim (*Duphar*) is a proprietary ANTIBIOTIC, available only on prescription, used to treat infections of the upper respiratory tract (particularly bronchitis and bronchial pneumonia) and of the urinary tract. Produced in the form of tablets (in two strengths), as a sugar-free suspension for dilution (the potency of the suspension once dilute is retained for 14 days), and in ampoules for injection, Monotrim is a preparation of the antibacterial drug trimethoprim. It is not recommended for children aged under 6 weeks.
✚/▲ warning/side-effects: *see* TRIMETHOPRIM.

Monovent (*Lagap*) is a proprietary BETA-RECEPTOR STIMULANT BRONCHODILATOR, available only on prescription, used to relieve the bronchial spasm associated with such conditions as asthma and bronchitis. Produced in the form of tablets, as sustained-release tablets (under the name Monovent SA), and as a syrup for dilution (the potency of the syrup once dilute is retained for 14 days), Monovent is a preparation of terbutaline sulphate.
✚/▲ warning/side-effects: *see* TERBUTALINE.

Monphytol (*LAB*) is a proprietary non-prescription ANTIFUNGAL liquid used in topical application to treat skin infections (particularly nail) caused by fungi of the genus Tinea (such as athlete's foot). Produced in the form of a paint, Monphytol is a preparation of various acids and antibacterial agents, including SALICYLIC ACID and CHLORBUTOL.

Morhulin (*Napp*) is a proprietary non-prescription skin emollient (softener and soother), used to treat nappy rash and bedsores. Produced in the form of an ointment, Morhulin is a preparation of cod-liver oil and ZINC OXIDE in a wool fat and paraffin base.
✚ warning: wool fat causes sensitivity reactions in some patients.

morphine is a powerful narcotic ANALGESIC that is the principal alkaloid of opium. It is widely used to treat severe pain and to soothe the associated stress and anxiety; it may be used in treating shock (with care since it lowers blood pressure), in suppressing coughs (although it may cause nausea and vomiting), and in reducing peristalsis (the muscular waves that urge material along the intestines) as a constituent in some antidiarrhoeal mixtures. It is also sometimes used as a premedication prior to surgery, or to supplement anaesthesia during an operation. Tolerance occurs extremely readily; dependence (addiction) may follow. Administration is oral and by injection; given by injection, morphine is more active. Proprietary preparations that contain morphine (in the form of morphine, morphine tartrate, morphine hydrochloride or morphine sulphate) are all on the controlled drugs list.
✚ warning: morphine should not be administered to patients with depressed breathing (the drug may itself cause a degree of respiratory depression), or who have intracranial pressure or head injury. It should be administered with caution to those with low blood pressure (hypotension), impaired liver or kidney function, or underactivity of the thyroid gland (hypothyroidism); or who are

pregnant or lactating. Dosage should be reduced for the elderly or debilitated. Treatment by injection may cause pain and tissue damage at the site of the injection. Prolonged treatment should be avoided.

▲ side-effects: there may be nausea and vomiting, loss of appetite, urinary retention and constipation. There is generally a degree of sedation, and euphoria which may lead to a state of mental detachment or confusion.
Related articles: CYCLIMORPH; DUROMORPH; MST CONTINUS; NEPENTHE.

Morsep (*Napp*) is a proprietary non-prescription skin emollient (softener and soother), used to treat urinary dermitis and nappy rash. Produced in the form of a cream, Morsep is a preparation of the ANTISEPTIC CETRIMIDE, RETINOL (vitamin A) and CALCIFEROL (vitamin D).

Motilium (*Janssen*) is a proprietary preparation of the ANTINAUSEANT and ANTI-EMETIC drug domperidone, available only on prescription. It works by inhibiting the action of the natural substance dopamine on the vomiting centre of the brain, and may be used to treat nausea and vomiting in gastrointestinal disorders, or during treatment with cytotoxic drugs or radiotherapy. It is produced in the form of tablets, as a sugar-free suspension and as anal suppositories.

✚/▲ warning/side-effects: *see* DOMPERIDONE.

Motipress (*Squibb*) is a proprietary mixed ANTIDEPRESSANT-ANTIPSYCHOTIC compound, available only on prescription, used to treat depressive illness and associated anxiety. Produced in the form of tablets, Motipress is a preparation of the antipsychotic drug fluphenazine hydrochloride and the antidepressant nortriptyline hydrochloride in the ratio 1:20. It is not recommended for children.

✚/▲ warning/side-effects: *see* FLUPHENAZINE; NORTRIPTYLINE.

Motival (*Squibb*) is a proprietary mixed ANTIDEPRESSANT-ANTIPSYCHOTIC compound, available only on prescription, used to treat depressive illness and associated anxiety. Produced in the form of tablets, Motival is a preparation of the antipsychotic drug fluphenazine hydrochloride and the antidepressant nortriptyline hydrochloride in the ratio 50:1. It is not recommended for children.

✚/▲ warning/side-effects: *see* FLUPHENAZINE; NORTRIPTYLINE.

Motrin (*Upjohn*) is a proprietary ANTI-INFLAMMATORY non-narcotic ANALGESIC, available only on prescription, used to treat the pain of rheumatic and other musculo-skeletal disorders. Produced in the form of tablets (in four strengths), Motrin is a preparation of ibuprofen.

✚/▲ warning/side-effects: *see* IBUPROFEN.

Movelat (*Panpharma*) is a proprietary CORTICOSTEROID COUNTER-IRRITANT preparation that has some ANALGESIC properties, available only on prescription, used in topical application to treat the inflammatory symptoms of arthritis and to relieve muscular back pain and soft tissue pain. Produced in the form of a cream and a gel in an alcohol base,

Movelat is a compound that includes corticosteroids and SALICYLIC ACID.

Moxalactam (*Lilly*) is a proprietary broad-spectrum ANTIBIOTIC, available only on prescription, used to treat many forms of bacterial infection. Produced in the form of a powder for reconstitution as a medium for injection, Moxalactam is a preparation of the CEPHALOSPORIN latamoxef disodium.
✚/▲ warning/side-effects: *see* LATAMOXEF.

MST Continus (*Napp*) is a proprietary narcotic ANALGESIC that is on the controlled drugs list. It is used primarily to relieve pain following surgery, or the pain experienced during the final stages of terminal malignant disease. Produced in the form of sustained-release tablets (in four strengths), MST Continus is a preparation of the OPIATE and NARCOTIC morphine sulphate; it is not recommended for children.
✚/▲ warning/side-effects: *see* MORPHINE.

MSUD Aid (*Scientific Hospital Supplies*) is a proprietary essential and non-essential amino acid mixture, used as a nutritional supplement for patients with the congenital abnormality maple syrup urine disease. Produced in the form of a powder containing vitamins, minerals and trace elements, it is isoleucine-, leucine- and valine-free, but does not consist of a complete diet.

Mucaine (*Wyeth*) is a proprietary ANTACID that also has local anaesthetic properties, available only on prescription, used to treat inflammation of the oesophagus and hiatus hernia. Produced in the form of a sugar-free suspension for dilution (the potency of the suspension once dilute is retained for 14 days), Mucaine is a preparation of ALUMINIUM HYDROXIDE mixture and magnesium hydroxide with the ANAESTHETIC oxethazaine. It is not recommended for children.
✚/▲ warning/side-effects: *see* OXETHAZAINE.

Mucodyne (*Berk*) is a proprietary MUCOLYTIC drug, available on prescription only to private patients, used to reduce the viscosity of sputum and thus facilitate expectoration in patients with asthma or bronchitis. Produced in the form of capsules, as a syrup (in two strengths, the stronger labelled Forte) for dilution (the potency of the syrup once dilute is retained for 14 days), and as another syrup for children (which is not recommended for children aged under 2 years), Mucodyne is a preparation of carbocisteine.
✚/▲ warning/side-effects: *see* CARBOCISTEINE.

Mucogel (*Pharmax*) is a proprietary non-prescription ANTACID used to treat severe indigestion and heartburn and to relieve the symptoms of gastric and duodenal ulcers. Produced in the form of tablets and as a sugar-free suspension, Mucogel is a preparation of ALUMINIUM HYDROXIDE and MAGNESIUM HYDROXIDE. It is not recommended for children.

Mucolex (*Parke-Davis*) is a proprietary MUCOLYTIC drug, available on prescription only to private patients, used to reduce the viscosity of sputum and thus facilitate expectoration in patients with asthma or bronchitis. Produced in the form of tablets (which are not recommended for children) and as

a syrup for dilution (the potency of the syrup once dilute is retained for 14 days; it is not recommended for children aged under 2 years), Mucolex is a preparation of carbocisteine.
✚/▲ warning/side-effects: *see* CARBOCISTEINE.

***mucolytic** describes an agent that dissolves or otherwise breaks down mucus. Mucolytic drugs are generally used in an endeavour to reduce the viscosity of sputum in the upper respiratory tract, and thus facilitate expectoration (coughing up sputum). Not all authorities agree that they work, although mucolytic agents are commonly prescribed to treat such conditions as asthma and chronic bronchitis. Best known and most used mucolytic agents are CARBOCISTEINE, TYLOXAPOL, BROMHEXINE HYDROCHLORIDE, ACETYLCYSTEINE and METHYLCYSTEINE HYDROCHLORIDE. Many proprietary preparations are available on prescription only to private patients.

Multibionta (*Merck*) is a proprietary MULTIVITAMIN solution, available only on prescription, for addition to infusion solutions to feed patients who for one reason or another cannot be fed via the alimentary canal such as during severe disorders of the gastrointestinal tract, and coma. Produced in ampoules, Multibionta represents a preparation of RETINOL (vitamin A), THIAMINE (vitamin B_1), RIBOFLAVINE (vitamin B_2), PYRIDOXINE (vitamin B_6), NICOTINAMIDE (of the B complex), DEXPANTHENOL (of the B complex), ASCORBIC ACID (vitamin C) and TOCOPHERYL ACETATE (vitamin E).

Multilind (*Squibb*) is a proprietary ANTIBIOTIC preparation, available only on prescription, used in topical application to treat fungal infections, especially forms of candidiasis (such as thrush), and to relieve the symptoms of nappy rash. Produced in the form of an ointment, Multilind is a preparation of the ANTIFUNGAL agent nystatin together with ZINC OXIDE.
✚/▲ warning/side-effects: *see* NYSTATIN.

Multiparin (*CP Pharmaceuticals*) is a proprietary ANTICOAGULANT, available only on prescription, used to treat and prevent various forms of thrombosis. Produced in ampoules for intravenous injection, Multiparin is a preparation of the natural anticoagulant heparin sodium.
✚/▲ warning/side-effects: *see* HEPARIN.

***multivitamin** preparations contain selections of various VITAMINS. There are a large number of such preparations available, and are mostly used as dietary supplements and for making up vitamin deficiencies. Choice of a particular multivitamin depends on its content; they are not usually available on the National Health.

Multivitamins (*Evans*) is a proprietary non-prescription MULTIVITAMIN preparation that is not available from the National Health Service. Produced in the form of tablets, Multivitamins is a preparation of RETINOL (vitamin A), THIAMINE (vitamin B_1), RIBOFLAVINE (vitamin B_2), NICOTINAMIDE (of the B complex), ASCORBIC ACID (vitamin C) and CALCIFEROL (vitamin D).

Multivite (*Duncan, Flockhart*) is a proprietary non-prescription MULTIVITAMIN preparation for use in vitamin deficiency states that is not available from the National Health Service. Produced in the form of pellets, Multivite is a preparation of RETINOL (vitamin A), THIAMINE (vitamin B_1), ASCORBIC ACID (vitamin C) and CALCIFEROL (vitamin D).

mumps vaccine is a suspension of live but attentuated mumps viruses cultured in chick embryo tissue. It is a VACCINE not recommended for routine use in the United Kingdom, although it is readily available for patients at risk. Administration is by injection.

Mumpsvax (*Morson*) is a proprietary MUMPS VACCINE, available only on prescription. Produced in the form of powder in a single-dose vial with diluent, Mumpsvax is a preparation of live but attenuated viruses that when injected cause the body to provide itself with antibodies against the virus. It is not recommended for children aged under 1 year.

mupirocin, or pseudomonic acid, is an ANTIBACTERIAL drug unrelated to any other ANTIBIOTIC, used in topical application to treat many forms of skin infection. Administration is in the form of a water-miscible cream.

✚ warning: mupirocin should be administered with caution to patients with impaired kidney function.

▲ side-effects: topical application may sting.

Related article: BACTROBAN.

Muripsin (*Norgine*) is a proprietary non-prescription compound used to make up a deficiency of hydrochloric acid and other digestive juices in the stomach. Produced in the form of tablets, Muripsin is a preparation of glutamic acid hydrochloride and the gastric enzyme pepsin.

***muscle relaxants** are agents that reduce tension in or paralyse muscles. They include ANTISPASMODIC drugs or SMOOTH MUSCLE RELAXANTS, which relieve spasm (rigidity) in smooth muscles that are not under voluntary control (such as the muscles of the respiratory tract or of the intestinal walls – or of blood vessels). They also include those drugs that are used in surgical operations to paralyse skeletal muscles that are normally under voluntary control (neuromuscular blocking drugs): such drugs work either by competing with the neurotransmitter acetylcholine at receptor sites between nerve and muscle (non-depolarizing) or by imitating the action of acetylcholine and so blocking the receptor sites (depolarizing). Non-depolarizing muscle relaxants include TUBOCURARINE CHLORIDE, GALLAMINE TRIETHIODIDE, ALCURONIUM CHLORIDE and VECURONIUM BROMIDE; depolarizing muscle relaxants include SUXAMETHONIUM CHLORIDE. Antagonists used to reverse the effects of one of these two drug types once surgery has finished prolong the effect of the other drug type. Patients receiving a muscle relaxant during surgery must have their respiration assisted or controlled. Other drugs again relax skeletal muscle spasm by an action on the spinal cord and these SKELETAL MUSCLE RELAXANTS iniclude mephanesin, baclophen and certain benzodiazepines.

mustine hydrochloride is a CYTOTOXIC drug used principally to treat the lymphatic cancer

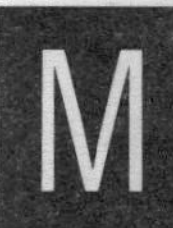

Hodgkin's disease. Because it is so toxic, however, mustine is now much less commonly used. Administration is by fast-running infusion.

✚ warning: prolonged treatment may cause sterility in men and an early menopause in women. Regular and frequent blood counts are essential. Leakage of the drug into the tissues at the site of infusion may cause severe tissue damage. The drug must be handled with care: it is caustic to the skin and irritating to the nose.

▲ side-effects: there is severe nausea and vomiting; there is commonly also hair loss. The formation of red blood cells by the bone marrow is reduced.

Myambutol (*Lederle*) is a proprietary ANTITUBERCULAR drug, available only on prescription, used for the prevention and treatment of tuberculosis in conjunction with other drugs. Produced in the form of tablets (in two strengths) and as an oral powder, Myambutol is a preparation of ethambutol hydrochloride.

✚/▲ warning/side-effects: *see* ETHAMBUTOL HYDROCHLORIDE.

Mycardol (*Winthrop*) is a proprietary non-prescription VASODILATOR, used as an ANTIHYPERTENSIVE drug in the prevention or treatment of angina pectoris (heart pain). Produced in the form of tablets, Mycardol is a preparation of pentaerythritol tetranitrate; it is not recommended for children.

✚/▲ warning/side-effects: *see* PENTAERYTHRITOL TETRANITRATE, GLYCERYL TRINITRATE

Mycifradin (*Upjohn*) is a proprietary ANTIBIOTIC, available only on prescription, used to treat infections of skin and mucous membranes, or to reduce bacterial levels in the intestines before surgery. Produced in the form of a powder in vials, Mycifradin is a preparation of the aminoglycoside neomycin sulphate; it is not recommended for children.

✚/▲ warning/side-effects: *see* NEOMYCIN.

Myciguent (*Upjohn*) is a proprietary ANTIBIOTIC, available only on prescription, used to treat infections of the skin and the eye. Produced in the form of an ointment and an eye ointment, Myciguent is a preparation of the aminoglycoside neomycin sulphate.

✚/▲ warning/side-effects: *see* NEOMYCIN.

Mycota (*Crookes Products*) is a proprietary non-prescription ANTIFUNGAL preparation, used in topical application to treat skin infections caused by Tinea organisms (such as athlete's foot). Produced in the form of a cream, as a dusting powder, and as an aerosol spray, Mycota is a preparation of undecenoic acid and its salts.

Mydriacyl (*Alcon*) is a proprietary ANTICHOLINERGIC mydriatic drug, available only on prescription, used to dilate the pupils and paralyse certain eye muscles generally for the purpose of ophthalmic examination (but occasionally to assist in antibiotic treatment). Produced in the form of eye-drops (in two strengths), Mydriacyl is a preparation of tropicamide.

✚/▲ warning/side-effects: *see* TROPICAMIDE.

Mydrilate (*Boehringer Ingelheim*) is a proprietary ANTICHOLINERIC

MYDRIATIC drug, available only on prescription, used to dilate the pupils and paralyse certain eye muscles generally for the purpose of ophthalmic examination (but occasionally to assist in antibiotic treatment). Produced in the form of eye-drops (in two strengths), Mydrilate is a preparation of cyclopentolate hydrochloride.
✚/▲ warning/side-effects: *see* CYCLOPENTOLATE HYDROCHLORIDE.

Myelobromol (*Sinclair*) is a proprietary CYTOTOXIC drug, available only on prescription (and generally only in hospital), used to treat chronic myeloid leukaemia. Produced in the form of tablets, Myelobromol is a preparation of the drug mitobronitol – which has some severe side-effects.
✚/▲ warning/side-effects: *see* MITOBRONITOL.

Mygdalon (*DDSA Pharmaceuticals*) is a proprietary ANTINAUSEANT, available only on prescription, used to treat nausea and vomiting especially when associated with gastrointestinal disorders, during radiotherapy, or accompanying treatment with CYTOTOXIC drugs. Produced in the form of tablets, Mygdalon is a preparation of metoclopramide hydrochloride.
✚/▲ warning/side-effects: *see* METOCLOPRAMIDE.

Myleran (*Wellcome*) is a proprietary CYTOTOXIC drug, available only on prescription, used to treat chronic myeloid leukaemia. It works by interfering with the DNA of new-forming cells, so preventing normal cell replication. Produced in the form of tablets (in two strengths), Myleran is a preparation of busulphan.
✚/▲ warning/side-effects: *see* BUSULPHAN.

Mynah (*Lederle*) is a proprietary ANTITUBERCULAR drug, available only on prescription, used for the prevention and treatment of tuberculosis in conjunction with other drugs. Produced in the form of tablets (in four strengths, under the names Mynah 200, Mynah 250, Mynah 300 and Mynah 365), it is a compound preparation of ethambutol hydrochloride and isoniazid. It is not recommended for children.
✚/▲ warning/side-effects: *see* ETHAMBUTOL HYDROCHLORIDE; ISONIAZID.

Myocrisin (*May & Baker*) is a proprietary preparation of one of the salts of gold, available only on prescription, used to treat rheumatoid arthritis. Produced in ampoules (in five strengths) for injection, Myocrisin is a preparation of sodium aurothiomalate.
✚/▲ warning/side-effects: *see* SODIUM AUROTHIOMALATE.

Myolgin (*Cox*) is a proprietary non-prescription COMPOUND ANALGESIC that is not available from the National Health Service. Used to treat mild to moderate pain, and produced in the form of soluble (dispersible) tablets, Myolgin is a preparation of paracetamol, ASPIRIN, CODEINE PHOSPHATE and CAFFEINE citrate; it is not recommended for children.

Myotonine Chloride (*Glenwood*) is a proprietary preparation of the parasympathomimetic drug bethanechol chloride, available only on prescription, used to treat urinary retention. It works by increasing the contraction of the muscle that retains urine within the bladder. It is produced in the form of tablets (in two strengths).
✚/▲ warning/side-effects: *see* BETHANECHOL CHLORIDE.

Mysoline (*ICI*) is a proprietary ANTICONVULSANT, available only on prescription, used to treat and prevent epileptic attacks, especially grand mal (tonic-clonic) and partial (focal) seizures (but not petit mal epilepsy). Produced in the form of tablets and an oral suspension, Mysoline is a preparation of primidone.
✚/▲ warning/side-effects: *see* PRIMIDONE.

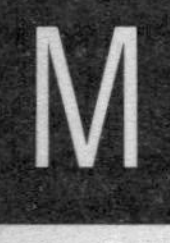

Mysteclin (*Squibb*) is a proprietary ANTIBIOTIC compound preparation, available only on prescription, used to treat infections anywhere in the body, but especially of mucous membranes. Produced in the form of capsules and as tablets, Mysteclin is a preparation of the broad-spectrum TETRACYCLINE tetracycline hydrochloride with the ANTIFUNGAL agent nystatin. Under the same name, a syrup is also available containing tetracycline and the antifungal agent amphotericin. These preparations are not recommended for children.
✚/▲ warning/side-effects: *see* AMPHOTERICIN; NYSTATIN; TETRACYCLINE.

nabilone is a synthetic cannabinoid (a drug derived from CANNABIS) used to relieve some of the toxic side-effects, particularly the nausea and vomiting, associated with chemotherapy in the treatment of cancer. However, it too has significant side-effects. Administration is oral in the form of capsules.

✚ warning: nabilone should be administered with caution to patients with severely impaired liver function or unstable personality. Concentration and speed of reaction is affected, and the effects of alcohol may be increased.

▲ side-effects: drowsiness, dry mouth and decreased appetite are common; there may also be an increase in the heart rate, dizziness on rising from a sitting or lying position (indicating low blood pressure), and abdominal cramps. Some patients experience psychological effects such as euphoria, confusion, depression, hallucinations and general disorientation. There may be headache, blurred vision and tremors.
Related article: CESAMET.

Nacton (*Bencard*) is a proprietary ANTICHOLINERGIC ANTISPASMODIC drug, available only on prescription, used to assist in the treatment of gastrointestinal disorders, such as peptic ulceration and hyperacidity, arising from muscular spasm of the intestinal walls. As a SMOOTH MUSCLE RELAXANT, it is also sometimes used to treat children for nocturnal bedwetting (because the bladder sphincter muscles have to contract to let urine through). Produced in the form of tablets (in two strengths), Nacton is a preparation of poldine methylsulphate. Other than for reasons stated it is not recommended for children.

✚/▲ warning/side-effects: *see* POLDINE METHYLSULPHATE.

nadolol is a BETA-BLOCKER used to treat high blood pressure (*see* ANTIHYPERTENSIVE), angina pectoris (heart pain) and heartbeat irregularities. It is sometimes also used to treat the effects of an excess of thyroid hormones in the bloodstream (thyrotoxicosis), or to prevent attacks of migraine. Administration is oral in the form of tablets.

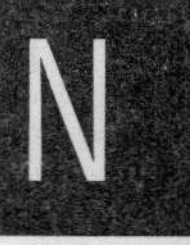

✚ warning: nadolol should not be administered to patients who suffer from heart disease or asthma, and should be administered with caution to those who are nearing the end of pregnancy or who are lactating. Withdrawal of treatment should be gradual.

▲ side-effects: the heartbeat may slow more than intended; there may be some gastrointestinal or respiratory disturbance. Fingers and toes may turn cold.
Related article: CORGARD.

naftidrofuryl oxalate is a VASODILATOR that affects the blood vessels of the brain and of the extremities. Because it improves blood circulation in the brain, it is thought by some also to improve memory in the elderly. Administration is oral in the form of capsules (in a course of treatment that lasts for at least 3 months), or by injection or infusion.

✚ warning: naftidrofuryl oxalate should not be administered to patients with heart block.

▲ side-effects: there may be nausea and pain in the small intestine.
Related article: PRAXILENE.

nalbuphine hydrochloride is a narcotic ANALGESIC that is very similar to morphine (although it has fewer side-effects and possibly less addictive potential). Like morphine, it is used primarily to relieve moderate to severe pain, especially during or after surgery. Administration is by injection.

✚ warning: nalbuphine should not be administered to patients who suffer from head injury or intracranial pressure; it should be administered with caution to those with impaired kidney or liver function, asthma, depressed respiration, insufficient secretion of thyroid hormones (hypothyroidism) or low blood pressure (hypotension), or who are pregnant or lactating. Dosage should be reduced for the elderly or debilitated.

▲ side-effects: shallow breathing, urinary retention, constipation, and nausea are all common; tolerance and dependence (addiction) are possible. There may also be drowsiness and pain at the site of injection (where there may also be tissue damage).

Related article: NUBAIN.

Nalcrom (*Fisons*) is a proprietary compound mast cell stabiliser, available only on prescription, used to assist in the treatment of allergy to specific foods. Produced in the form of capsules, Nalcrom is a preparation of sodium cromoglycate, a drug that prevents some cellular allergic response. It is not recommended for children aged under 2 years.

✚/▲ warning/side-effects: *see* SODIUM CROMOGLYCATE.

nalidixic acid is an ANTIBACTERIAL used primarily to treat infection of the urinary tract. Administration is oral in the form of tablets, as a dilute suspension, and as an effervescent solution.

✚ warning: nalidixic acid should not be administered to patients who suffer from epilepsy, or who are aged under 3 months. It should be administered with caution to those with kidney or liver dysfunction or who are lactating. During treatment it is advisable for patients to avoid strong sunlight.

▲ side-effects: nausea, vomiting, diarrhoea and gastrointestinal disturbance are fairly common, but there may also be sensitivity reactions (such as urticaria or a rash). A very few patients experience visual disturbances and convulsions.

Related articles: MICTRAL; NEGRAM; URIBEN.

naloxone is a powerful OPIATE antagonist drug used primarily (in the form of naloxone hydrochloride) as an antidote to an overdose of narcotic ANALGESICS. Quick but short-acting, it effectively reverses the respiratory depression, coma and convulsions that follow overdosage of opiates. Administration is by intramuscular or intravenous injection, and may be repeated at intervals of 2 minutes (up to a maximum dose of 10mg) until there is some response. Also used at the end of operations to reverse respiratory depression caused by narcotic analgesics.

✚ warning: naloxone should not be administered to patients who are physically dependent on (addicted to) narcotics.

Related article: NARCAN.

nandrolone is an anabolic STEROID related to the male sex hormone testosterone (although it has far fewer masculinizing properties), used to assist the metabolic synthesis of protein in the body following major surgery or long- term debilitating disease, or to treat osteoporosis ("brittle bones"). Sometimes also used to treat sex-hormone-linked cancers in women, particularly cancer of the breast, it is additionally used in the treatment of certain forms of anaemia, although how it works in this respect – and even whether it works – remains the subject of some debate: variations in patient response are wide. Administration (in the form of nandrolone decanoate or nandrolone phenylpropionate) is by injection.

✚ warning: nandrolone should not be administered to patients with impaired liver function, or cancer of the prostate gland (in men) or of the breast, or who are pregnant; it should be administered with caution to those with impaired heart or kidney function, circulatory disorders, high blood pressure (hypertension), diabetes, epilepsy, or recurrent attacks of migraine. Treatment of young patients may affect bone growth.

▲ side-effects: there may be fluid retention in the tissues, leading to weight gain; blood levels of calcium generally rise. High dosage in women may cause menstrual irregularity and eventual signs of masculinization.
Related articles: DECA-DURABOLIN; DECA-DURABOLIN 100; Durabolin.

Naprosyn (*Syntex*) is a proprietary, non-steroidal ANTI-INFLAMMATORY non-narcotic ANALGESIC, available only on prescription, used to relieve pain – particularly rheumatic and arthritic pain, and that of acute gout – and to treat other musculo-skeletal disorders. Produced in the form of tablets (in two strengths), as a suspension (the potency of the suspension once dilute is retained for 14 days), and as anal suppositories, Naprosyn is a preparation of naproxen. In the form of tablets or suspension it is not recommended for children aged under 5 years; the suppositories are not suitable for children.

✚/▲ warning/side-effects: *see* NAPROXEN.

naproxen is a non-steroidal ANTI-INFLAMMATORY non-narcotic ANALGESIC used to relieve pain – particularly rheumatic and arthritic pain, and that of acute gout – and to treat other musculo-skeletal disorders. It is also effective in relieving the pain of menstrual disorders and difficulties, in preventing recurrent attacks of migraine, and in reducing high body temperature. Administration (in the form of naproxen or naproxen sodium) is oral in the form of tablets or as a dilute suspension, or by anal suppositories.

✚ warning: naproxen should be administered with caution to patients with allergic disorders (such as asthma), impaired liver or kidney function, or gastric ulcers, or who are pregnant.

▲ side-effects: side-effects are relatively uncommon, but may include gastrointestinal disturbance with nausea; patients may be advised to take the drug with food or milk. Some patients experience sensitivity reactions or fluid retention in the tissues (oedema).
Related articles: LARAFLEX; NAPROSYN; SYNFLEX.

Narcan (*Du Pont*) is a proprietary drug, available only on prescription, that is most often used to treat the symptoms of acute overdosage of OPIATES such as morphine. Produced in ampoules for injection, Narcan is a preparation of naloxone hydrochloride. A weaker form is available (under the name Narcan Neonatal) for the treatment of respiratory depression in babies born to mothers on whom narcotic analgesics have been used during the birth, or who are drug addicts.
✚/▲ warning/side-effects: *see* NALOXONE.

N

***narcotic** is a description that applies to drugs that induce stupor and insensibility. Commonly the term is applied to the opiates (such as MORPHINE and DIAMORPHINE), but it can also be used to describe SEDATIVES and HYPNOTIC drugs and alcohol that act directly on the brain centres to depress their functioning. In law, however, the term describes an addictive drug that is the subject of abuse (especially in the USA).

***narcotic analgesic** *see* ANALGESIC.

Nardil (*Parke-Davis*) is a proprietary ANTIDEPRESSANT drug, available only on prescription, used to treat depressive illness. Produced in the form of tablets, Nardil is a preparation of the potentially dangerous drug phenelzine (which requires a careful dietary regimen to accompany treatment because of complex interactions with various foods such as cheese, yeast extract, chocolate etc). It is not recommended for children.
✚/▲ warning/side-effects: *see* PHENELZINE

Narphen (*Smith & Nephew Pharmaceuticals*) is a proprietary narcotic ANALGESIC, a controlled OPIATE consisting of a preparation of phenazocine hydrobromide, used to relieve severe pain and pancreatic or biliary pain. Produced in the form of tablets, Narphen is not recommended for children.
✚/▲ warning/side-effects: *see* PHENAZOCINE.

Naseptin (*ICI*) is a proprietary ANTIBIOTIC, available only on prescription, used to treat staphylococcal infections in and around the nostrils. Produced in the form of a cream for topical application, Naseptin is a preparation of the ANTISEPTIC antibiotic drugs chlorhexidine hydrochloride and neomycin sulphate.
✚/▲ warning/side-effects: *see* CHLORHEXIDINE; NEOMYCIN.

natamycin is an ANTIBIOTIC, an ANTIFUNGAL drug used specifically to treat candidiasis (thrush) and trichomoniasis. Administration is in many forms, depending on the site of infection: oral as a sugar-free suspension (sometimes in drops), topical as an aerosol inhalant and as a water-miscible cream, and also as vaginal tablets (pessaries).
✚ warning: diagnosis should preferably be confirmed (through analysis of tissue from the site of infection) before administration.
Related article: PIMAFUCIN.

Natirose (*Lewis*) is a proprietary VASODILATOR, available only on prescription, used to prevent and treat angina pectoris (heart pain). Produced in the form of tablets, Natirose is a compound preparation of the vasodilator glyceryl trinitrate, the ANALGESIC ethylmorphine hydrochloride,

and the MUSCLE RELAXANT hyoscyamine hydrobromide.
✚/▲ warning/side-effects: *see* GLYCERYL TRINITRATE.

Natrilix (*Servier*) is a proprietary DIURETIC, available only on prescription, used to treat an accumulation of fluid within the tissues (oedema) and high blood pressure (*see* ANTIHYPERTENSIVE), particularly in cases of DIABETES mellitus. Produced in the form of tablets, Natrilix is a preparation of the THIAZIDE-like drug indapamide. It is not recommended for children.
✚/▲ warning/side-effects: *see* INDAPAMIDE.

Natuderm (*Burgess*) is a proprietary non-prescription skin emollient (softener and soother), used to treat dry conditions of the skin. Produced in the form of a cream, Natuderm is a preparation of glycerides, sterols and other lipids, water, waxes and GLYCEROL.

Natulan (*Roche*) is a proprietary preparation of the CYTOTOXIC drug procarbazine, available only on prescription, used primarily to treat the lymphatic cancer Hodgkin's disease, but also to assist in the treatment of solid tumours resistant to other therapy. Advice and counselling on diet during treatment is recommended (eating foods such as cheese or meat extracts, or drinking alcohol, for example, is inadvisable). Natulan is produced in the form of capsules.
✚/▲ warning/side-effects: *see* PROCARBAZINE.

Navidrex (*Ciba*) is a proprietary DIURETIC, available only on prescription, used to treat high blood pressure (*see* ANTIHYPERTENSIVE) and the accumulation of fluid within the tissues (oedema). Produced in the form of tablets, it is a preparation of the THIAZIDE cyclopenthiazide.
✚/▲ warning/side-effects: *see* CYCLOPENTHIAZIDE.

Navidrex-K (*Ciba*) is a proprietary DIURETIC, available only on prescription, used to treat high blood pressure (*see* ANTIHYPERTENSIVE) and the accumulation of fluid within the tissues (oedema). Produced in the form of tablets, it is a preparation of the thiazide cyclopenthiazide (which is potassium-depleting) together with POTASSIUM in a form for sustained release.
✚/▲ warning/side-effects: *see* CYCLOPENTHIAZIDE.

Naxogin 500 (*Farmitalia Carlo Erba*) is a proprietary non-prescription ANTIPROTOZOAL, used to treat protozoan infections particularly of the urogenital areas or of the gums (ulcerative gingivitis). Produced in the form of tablets, Naxogin 500 is a preparation of nimorazole. Alcohol consumption should be avoided during treatment.
✚/▲ warning/side-effects: *see* NIMORAZOLE.

Nebcin (*Lilly*) is a proprietary ANTIBIOTIC, available only on prescription, used to treat serious infections in specific body organs, such as meningitis and gastrointestinal infections. Produced in ampoules (in two strengths) for injection, Nebcin is a preparation of the aminoglycoside tobramycin.
✚/▲ warning/side-effects: *see* TOBRAMYCIN.

nedocromil is used to prevent recurrent attacks of asthma; it is not useful in treating an acute attack, but is particularly effective in forestalling attacks in patients whose asthma is allergy related, and especially when administered before exercise. Patient response varies, however: dosage should be adjusted for individually optimal results, and should be regular whether symptoms are present or not. Administration is topical by inhalation from an aerosol.

✚ warning: some patients may find that the administration of a bronchodilator (such as salbutamol) some 10 minutes before taking nedocromil may enhance the effects. Should not be taken by pregnant women.

▲ side-effects: the taste is rather bitter. There may be a tendency to mild nausea and/or headache.

Related article: TILADE.

N

nefopam is an non-narcotic ANALGESIC used to treat moderate to severe pain, such as that following surgery, or in cancer or toothache. Administration is oral in the form of tablets, or by injection.

✚ warning: nefopam should not be administered to patients who suffer from convulsive disorders, or who are undergoing a heart attack. It should be administered with caution to those with glaucoma, liver disease or urinary retention. Not recommended for children.

▲ side-effects: there may be nausea, dry mouth, nervous agitation and insomnia. A few patients experience blurred vision, drowsiness, headache, an increase in the heart rate and sweating. Rarely, there is discoloration of the urine.

Related article: ACUPAN.

Negram (*Sterling Research*) is a proprietary ANTIBACTERIAL agent, available only on prescription, used to treat gastrointestinal infections and infections of the urinary tract. Produced in the form of tablets and as a sugar-free suspension for dilution (the potency of the suspension once dilute is retained for 14 days), Negram is a preparation of the antimicrobial drug nalidixic acid.

✚/▲ warning/side-effects: *see* NALIDIXIC ACID.

Neocon-1/35 (*Ortho-Cilag*) is a combined ORAL CONTRACEPTIVE, available only on prescription, that combines the OESTROGEN ethinyloestradiol with the PROGESTOGEN norethisterone. It is produced in packs of 21 tablets corresponding to one complete menstrual cycle.

✚/▲ warning/side-effects: *see* ETHINYLOESTRADIOL; NORETHISTERONE.

Neo-Cortef (*Upjohn*) is a proprietary compound ANTIBIOTIC, available only on prescription, used to treat bacterial infections in the outer ear and inflammation in the eye. Produced in the form of ear- or eye-drops and as an ointment, Neo-Cortef is a compound preparation of the antibiotic aminoglycoside neomycin sulphate with the CORTICOSTEROID hydrocortisone acetate.

✚/▲ warning/side-effects: *see* HYDROCORTISONE; NEOMYCIN.

Neo-Cytamen (*Duncan, Flockhart*) is a proprietary VITAMIN B_{12} preparation, available on prescription only to private patients, used to make up vitamin B_{12} deficiency in the body (pernicious anaemia). Produced in ampoules (in two strengths) for injection, Neo-Cytamen is a preparation of hydroxocobalamin.

✚/▲ warning/side-effects: *see* HYDROXOCOBALAMIN.

Neogest (*Schering*) is a

proprietary progesterone-only ORAL CONTRACEPTIVE, available only on prescription, that is a preparation of the PROGESTOGEN norgestrel. On first using Neogest, an additional form of contraception is advisable for the initial fortnight.

✚/▲ warning/side-effects: *see* NORGESTREL.

Neo-Lidocaton is a proprietary preparation of the local ANAESTHETIC lignocaine, used in cartridges for dental surgery.

✚/▲ warning/side-effects: *see* LIGNOCAINE.

Neo-Medrone (*Upjohn*) is a proprietary CORTICOSTEROID preparation, available only on prescription, used for topical application to treat inflammatory skin conditions, particularly those resulting from allergy. Produced in the form of a cream, Neo-Medrone is a preparation of the steroid methylprednisolone acetate and the antibacterial ANTIBIOTIC neomycin sulphate. Neo-Medrone Lotion is also available for the treatment of acne, and additionally contains SULPHUR and aluminium chlorhydroxide.

✚/▲ warning/side-effects: *see* METHYLPREDNISOLONE; NEOMYCIN.

Neo-Mercazole (*Nicholas*) is a proprietary preparation of the drug carbimazole, available only on prescription, used to treat the effects of an excess of thyroid hormones in the bloodstream (thyrotoxicosis). It works by inhibiting the formation of the hormone thyroxine in the thyroid gland, and is produced in the form of tablets (in two strengths, under the names Neo-Mercazole 5 and Neo-Mercazole 20).

✚/▲ warning/side-effects: *see* CARBIMAZOLE.

neomycin is a broad-spectrum ANTIBIOTIC drug that is effective in treating topical bacterial infections. Too toxic to be used in intravenous or intramuscular administration, it is nevertheless sometimes also used to reduce the levels of bacteria in the colon prior to intestinal surgery or examination, or in the case of liver failure. Even prolonged or widespread topical application may eventually lead to sensitivity reactions. Administration (most often in the form of neomycin sulphate) is oral as tablets or in solution, or topical as nose-drops, ear-drops, eye-drops, ear ointment, eye ointment or nasal spray.

✚ warning: neomycin should not be administered to patients with the neuromuscular disease myasthenia gravis, or who are pregnant. Intervals between doses should be increased for patients with impaired kidney function.

▲ side-effects: prolonged use may eventually lead to temporarily impaired kidney function, malabsorption from the intestines, or to deafness. Prolonged use to treat infection in the outer ear may lead to fungal invasion.

Related articles: AUDICORT; BETNESOL-N; DERMOVATE-NN; DEXA- RHINASPRAY; GRANEODIN; GREGODERM; HYDRODERM; MINIMS; Mycifradin; MYCIGUENT; NEO-CORTEF; NEOSPORIN; NIVEMYCIN; Predsol-N; SILDERM; STIEDEX; VIBROCIL; VISTA-METHASONE N.

Neo-NaClex (*Duncan, Flockhart*) is a proprietary DIURETIC, available only on prescription, used to treat high blood pressure (*see* ANTIHYPERTENSIVE) and the accumulation of fluid within the tissues (oedema). Produced in the

N

form of tablets, Neo-NaClex is a preparation of the THIAZIDE bendrofluazide.
✚/▲ warning/side-effects: *see* BENDROFLUAZIDE.

Neo-NaClex-K (*Duncan, Flockhart*) is a proprietary DIURETIC, available only on prescription, used to treat high blood pressure (*see* ANTIHYPERTENSIVE) and the accumulation of fluid within the tissues (oedema). Produced in the form of sustained-release tablets, Neo-NaClex-K is a preparation of the THIAZIDE bendrofluazide (which is potassium-depleting) with a POTASSIUM CHLORIDE supplement.
✚/▲ warning/side-effects: *see* BENDROFLUAZIDE.

Neophryn (*Winthrop*) is a proprietary non-prescription SYMPATHOMIMETIC nasal DECONGESTANT available as nose-drops, that is not available from the National Health Service. Neophryn is a preparation of the drug phenylephrine hydrochloride, and is also produced as a nasal spray.
✚/▲ warning/side-effects: *see* PHENYLEPHRINE.

Neoplatin (*Bristol-Myers*) is a proprietary CYTOTOXIC drug, available only on prescription, used to treat certain solid tumours (such as cancer of the ovary or of the testes). Produced in the form of powder for reconstitution as a medium for injection, Neoplatin is a preparation of cisplatin.
✚/▲ warning/side-effects: *see* CISPLATIN.

Neosporin (*Calmic*) is a proprietary ANTIBIOTIC, available only on prescription, used to treat bacterial infections in the eye. Produced in the form of eye-drops, Neosporin is a compound preparation of the antiseptic antibiotics neomycin sulphate, polymyxin B sulphate and gramicidin.
✚/▲ warning/side-effects: *see* NEOMYCIN; POLYMYXIN B.

neostigmine is an anticholinesterase drug that has the effect of increasing the activity of the neurotransmitter (acetylcholine) which transmits the neural instructions of the brain to the skeletal muscles. It works by inhibiting the "switching-off" of the neural impulses by the breakdown of acetylcholine by enzymes. Its main use is therefore in the treatment of the neuromuscular disease myasthenia gravis (which causes extreme muscle weakness amounting even to paralysis); it is also commonly used to counter the effects of muscle relaxants administered during surgical operations. Occasionally the drug is alternatively used as a PARASYMPATHOMIMETIC to stimulate intestinal motility and so promote defecation. Administration is oral in the form of tablets, or by injection.
✚ warning: neostigmine should not be administered to patients with intestinal or urinary blockage; it should be administered with caution to those with epilepsy, asthma, parkinsonism, low blood pressure (hypotension) or a slow heart rate, who have recently suffered a heart attack, or who are pregnant.
▲ side-effects: there may be nausea and vomiting, diarrhoea and abdominal cramps, and an excess of saliva in the mouth. Overdosage may cause gastrointestinal disturbance, an excess of bronchial mucus, sweating, faecal and urinary

incontinence, vision disorders, nervous agitation and muscular weakness.
Related article: PROSTIGMIN.

Nepenthe (*Evans*) is a proprietary narcotic ANALGESIC which, because it is a preparation of the OPIATES anhydrous morphine and opium tincture, is on the controlled drugs list. Used to relieve severe pain, especially during the final stages of terminal malignant disease, it is produced in the form of a syrup for dilution (the potency of the syrup once dilute is 4 retained for weeks) and in ampoules for injection. Nepenthe solution is not recommended for children aged under 12 months; the injection is not recommended for children aged under 6 years.
✚/▲ warning/side-effects: *see* MORPHINE.

Nephramine (*Boots*) is a proprietary nutritional supplement for patients unable to feed or be fed via the alimentary canal. Not a complete diet, however, Nephramine is a selection of essential amino acids in a form suitable for intravenous infusion. 6

Nephril (*Pfizer*) is a proprietary DIURETIC, available only on prescription, used to treat high blood pressure (*see* ANTIHYPERTENSIVE) and the accumulation of fluid within the tissues (oedema). Produced in the form of tablets, Nephril is a preparation of the THIAZIDE polythiazide. It is not recommended for children.
✚/▲ warning/side-effects: *see* POLYTHIAZIDE.

Nericur (*Schering*) is a proprietary, non-prescription, topical preparation for the treatment of acne. Produced in the form of a gel (in two strengths), Nericur is a solute preparation of the KERATOLYTIC benzoyl peroxide. It is not recommended for children.
✚/▲ warning/side-effects: *see* BENZOYL PEROXIDE.

Nerisone (*Schering*) is a proprietary CORTICOSTEROID preparation, available only on prescription, used to treat serious non- infective inflammatory skin conditions, such as eczema. Produced in the form of a cream, as an oily cream and as an ointment, Nerisone is a preparation of the steroid diflucortolone valerate. A stronger form is also available in the form of an oily cream and an ointment (under the name Nerisone Forte), which is not recommended for children aged under 4 years.
✚/▲ warning/side-effects: *see* DIFLUCORTOLONE VALERATE.

Nestargel (*Nestlé*) is a proprietary non-prescription nutritional preparation, used to thicken foods for patients who suffer from vomiting and regurgitation. Produced in the form of a powder, Nestargel contains CALCIUM LACTATE and carob seed flour.

Nestosyl (*Bengué*) is a proprietary non-prescription local ANAESTHETIC used in topical application to treat local pain and skin irritation. Produced in the form of an ointment, Nestosyl contains the anaesthetic BENZOCAINE, the antiseptic hexachlorophane, the keratolytic RESORCINOL and the astringent zinc oxide. It is not recommended for infants or longterm use.

Nethaprin Dospan (*Merrell Dow*) is a proprietary compound SYMPATHOMIMETIC BRONCHODILATOR, available only

on prescription, used to treat conditions such as chronic bronchitis and asthma. Produced in the form of tablets, Nethaprin Dospan's major active constituent is phenylephrine hydrochloride. It is not recommended for children aged under 6 years.
✚/▲ warning/side-effects: *see* PHENYLEPHRINE.

Nethaprin Expectorant (*Merrell Dow*) is a proprietary EXPECTORANT, available on prescription only to private patients, used to treat coughing and wheezing. Produced in the form of a syrup, Nethaprin Expectorant's major active constituent is the expectorant agent guaiphenesin. It is not recommended for children aged under 6 years.

Netillin (*Kirby-Warrick*) is a proprietary form of the aminoglycoside ANTIBIOTIC netilmicin sulphate, available only on prescription. Used to treat any of many serious bacterial infections, it is produced in ampoules (in three strengths) for injection.
✚/▲ warning/side-effects: *see* NETILMICIN.

netilmicin is a broad-spectrum ANTIBIOTIC, one of the aminoglycosides used (singly or in combination with other types of antibiotic) to treat any of many serious bacterial infections, especially those that prove to be resistant to the more commonly used aminoglycoside gentamicin. Administration is by injection.
✚ warning: netilmicin should not be administered to patients with the neuromuscular disease myasthenia gravis, or who are pregnant. Intervals between doses should be increased for patients with impaired kidney function.
▲ side-effects: there may be temporary kidney dysfunction; some patients experience deafness.
Related article: NETILLIN.

Neulactil (*May & Baker*) is a powerful ANTIPSYCHOTIC drug, available only on prescription, used to treat and tranquillize patients who are undergoing behavioural disturbances, or who are psychotic (particularly schizophrenic); it may also be used to treat severe anxiety in the short term. Produced in the form of tablets (in three strengths) and as a strong syrup for dilution (the potency of the syrup once dilute is retained for 14 days), Neulactil is a preparation of the antipsychotic drug pericyazine.
✚/▲ warning/side-effects: *see* PERICYAZINE.

Neulente (*Wellcome*) is a proprietary non-prescription preparation of highly purified beef insulin zinc suspension, used to treat and maintain diabetic patients. It is produced in vials for injection.
✚/▲ warning/side-effects: *see* INSULIN.

Neuphane (*Wellcome*) is a proprietary non-prescription preparation of highly purified beef isophane insulin, used to treat and maintain DIABETIC patients. It is produced in vials for injection.
✚/▲ warning/side-effects: *see* INSULIN.

Neurodyne (*Radiol*) is a proprietary, non-prescription, compound ANALGESIC that is not available from the National Health Service. Used to treat pain anywhere in the body, Neurodyne is a preparation of paracetamol and the OPIATE codeine phosphate. Produced in the form of capsules, it is not recommended for children.

✚/▲ warning/side-effects: *see* CODEINE PHOSPHATE; PARACETAMOL.

Neusulin (*Wellcome*) is a proprietary non-prescription preparation of highly purified beef neutral insulin, used to treat and maintain diabetic patients. It is produced in vials for injection.

✚/▲ warning/side-effects: *see* INSULIN.

Neutradonna (*Nicholas*) is a proprietary, non-prescription, ANTACID and ANTISPASMODIC compound that is not available from the National Health Service. It is used to treat muscle spasm (rigidity) of the intestinal and stomach walls and the resulting gastrointestinal discomfort, and to relieve acid stomach and indigestion. Produced in the form of tablets and as a powder, Neutradonna is a preparation of the ANTICHOLINERGIC belladonna alkaloids and the mild antacid aluminium sodium silicate. It is not recommended for children.

✚/▲ warning/side-effects: *see* BELLADONNA.

niacin is another name for the B VITAMIN nicotinic acid.
see NICOTINIC ACID.

nicardipine is a CALCIUM ANTAGONIST drug used as an ANTIHYPERTENSIVE to prevent or treat chronic angina pectoris (heart pain) and high blood pressure (hypertension) by means of its VASODILATOR properties. Administration (in the form of nicardipine hydrochloride) is oral, as capsules.

✚ warning: nicardipine should not be administered to patients with advanced disease of the aorta; it should be administered with caution to those with impaired liver or kidney function. Treatment should be stopped if heart pain occurs.

▲ side-effects: there may be nausea, headache, dizziness, flushing and fluid retention in the fingers and toes; some patients experience gastrointestinal disturbances, palpitations, low blood pressure (hypotension), an excess of saliva in the mouth, a rash, and a frequent urge to urinate.
Related article: CARDENE.

niclosamide is a synthetic ANTHELMINTIC drug used to rid the body of an infestation of tapeworms. Administration is oral in the form of tablets.

✚ warning: side-effects are minimal, but in case the tapeworms are multiplying some doctors prefer to prescribe an additional ANTI-EMETIC for patients to take on waking. The dose should be administered on a relatively empty stomach, and be followed by a purgative after about 2 hours.

▲ side-effects: there may be gastrointestinal disturbance.
Related article: YOMESAN.

nicofuranose is a derivative of the B vitamin NICOTINIC ACID, used therapeutically primarily to reduce the level of fats (lipids) in the blood, and therefore to slow the progression of premature arteriosclerosis and to treat vascular disease in the limbs. Administration is oral in the form of tablets.

✚/▲ warning/side-effects: *see* NICOTINIC ACID.
Related article: BRADILAN.

nicotinamide is a compound derived from the B vitamin

N

NICOTINIC ACID that is used primarily as a constituent in vitamin supplements, especially in cases when a large dose is required (for nicotinamide does not have as great a VASODILATOR effect as does nicotinic acid).

nicotinic acid, or niacin, is a VITAMIN of the B complex, a derivative of pyridine that is required in the diet but that is also synthesized in the body to a small degree from the amino acid tryptophan. Dietary deficiency results in the disease pellagra (the symptoms of which are dermatitis, diarrhoea and depression), but deficiency is comparatively rare. Good food sources include meat, cereals and yeast extract. Nicotinic acid may be administered therapeutically as a vitamin supplement (in the form of tablets), but its effect as a VASODILATOR prevents high dosage. It is, indeed, more commonly used as a vasodilator, especially in relieving circulatory disorders in the limbs, which it also does by reducing blood levels of fats (lipids) such as cholesterol.

✚ warning: nicotinic acid should not be administered to patients who are pregnant or lactating; it should be administered with caution to those with diabetes, liver disease, peptic ulcers or gout.

▲ side-effects: there may be nausea and vomiting, flushing and sweating, dizziness and heartbeat irregularities: taking the drug initially in low dosage and with food may reduce these effects – some doctors, however, prescribe aspirin to be taken half an hour before the dose. Sensitivity reactions may occur.

nicotinyl alcohol is a derivative of the B vitamin NICOTINIC ACID, used therapeutically primarily to reduce the level of fats (lipids) in the blood, and so to treat vascular disease in the limbs. In this it is similar to nicotinic acid, but its effect has longer duration. Administration is oral in the form of tablets and sustained-release tablets.

✚/▲ warning/side-effects: *see* NICOTINIC ACID.
Related article: RONICOL.

nicoumalone is a synthetic ANTICOAGULANT, used to treat deep-vein thrombosis and conditions in which the blood supply to the brain is reduced; it is also used to assist heart function following heart surgery, and especially following the implantation of prosthetic heart valves. Administration is oral in the form of tablets.

✚ warning: nicoumalone should not be administered to patients with peptic ulcer (or any other potential source of haemorrhage), bacterial heart disease, or severe high blood pressure (hypertension), or who are pregnant or lactating. It should be administered with caution to those with liver or kidney disease.

▲ side-effects: if bleeding starts, it may be difficult to stop.
Related article: SINTHROME.

Nidazol (*Steinhard*) is a proprietary ANTIBIOTIC, available only on prescription, used to treat infections by anaerobic bacteria and protozoa (particularly in the vagina or on the gums), and to provide asepsis during surgery. Produced in the form of tablets, Nidazol is a preparation of the amoebicidal drug metronidazole.

✚/▲ warning/side-effects: *see* METRONIDAZOLE.

nifedipine is a CALCIUM ANTAGONIST VASODILATOR that is

primarily used to assist in the treatment of angina pectoris (heart pain), coldness and numbness of the arteries of the fingers (Raynaud's phenomenon), and high blood pressure (*see* ANTIHYPERTENSIVE). Administration is oral in the form of capsules or sustained-release tablets.

✚ warning: treatment should be halted if heart pain occurs. In late pregnancy the drug may inhibit the onset or stages of labour.

▲ side-effects: headache, flushing and swelling of the ankles (through fluid retention) are not uncommon; there may also be lethargy or swelling of the gums.

Related article: ADALAT.

Niferex (*Tillotts*) is a proprietary, non-prescription IRON preparation, used to treat iron-deficiency anaemia. Produced in the form of tablets and as an elixir for dilution (the potency of the elixir once dilute is retained for 14 days), Niferex is a polysaccharide-iron complex. An additional preparation in the form of capsules is available (under the name Niferex-150) which is not recommended for children.

✚/▲ warning/side-effects: *see* POLYSACCHARIDE-IRON COMPLEX.

Night Nurse (*Beecham Health Care*) is a proprietary non-prescription cold relief preparation produced in the form of capsules. It contains the ANALGESIC paracetamol, ALCOHOL, the ANTITUSSIVE dextromethorphan and the ANTIHISTAMINE promethazine, which has a marked sedative activity.

✚/▲ warning/side-effects: *see* DEXTROMETHORPHAN; PARACETAMOL; PROMETHAZINE HYDROCHLORIDE.

nikethamide is a respiratory stimulant drug, used to relieve severe respiratory difficulties in patients who have been suffocated (particularly with carbon dioxide), who suffer from chronic disease of the respiratory tract, or who undergo respiratory depression following major surgery – particularly in cases where ventilatory support is not applicable. As a respiratory stimulant, however, nikethamide is now less commonly used (and nikethamide or doxapram is generally the drug of first choice). Administration is by slow intravenous injection, and may be repeated at intervals of between 15 and 30 minutes. It should only be given under expert supervision in a hospital.

✚ warning: nikethamide should not be administered to patients with respiratory failure resulting from drug overdose or neurological disease, or with coronary artery disease, severe asthma, or an excess of thyroid hormones in the blood (thyrotoxicosis). It should be administered with caution to those with severe high blood pressure (hypertension) or a reduced supply of blood to the heart. Effective dosage is unfortunately close to the level that causes toxic effects, especially convulsions.

▲ side-effects: there may be nausea, restlessness and tremor, leading possibly to convulsions and heartbeat irregularities.

Nilodor (*Loxley*) is a proprietary, non-prescription deodorant solution, used to freshen and sanitize the appliance or bag that is attached to a stoma (an outlet on the skin surface) following ileostomy or colostomy (surgical curtailment of the intestines).

Nilstim (*De Witt*) is a proprietary, non-prescription absorbent agent used, perhaps controversially, to assist in the medical treatment of obesity. The intention is that food consumed is bulked up internally and thus satisfies the patient. Produced in the form of tablets, Nilstim is a preparation in which the active constituent is methylcellulose. It is not recommended for children.

✚/▲ warning/side-effects: *see* METHYLCELLULOSE.

nimorazole is a powerful ANTIPROTOZOAL used to treat protozoan infections (such as candidiasis or trichomoniasis), particularly of the urogenital areas and of the gums (ulcerative gingivitis), and especially in cases when the major alternative drug metronidazole has failed. Administration is oral in the form of tablets.

✚ warning: nimorazole should not be administered to patients with severe kidney failure or disease of the central nervous system. In cases of sexually transmitted disease, both partners should be treated even if one presents no symptoms. Alcohol consumption should be avoided during treatment.

▲ side-effects: there may be nausea and vomiting, drowsiness and vertigo; a rash may appear.

Related article: NAXOGIN 500.

Nipride (*Roche*) is a proprietary ANTIHYPERTENSIVE drug, available only on prescription (and generally only in hospitals), used to treat high blood pressure (hypertension) or acute or chronic heart failure. Produced in the form of a powder for reconstitution as a medium for infusion, Nipride is a preparation of the VASODILATOR sodium nitroprusside.

✚/▲ warning/side-effects: *see* SODIUM NITROPRUSSIDE.

niridazole is an ANTIAMOEBAL drug used to treat infestations of guinea worms (dracontiasis), of amoebae (amoebiasis) or of blood fluke schistosomes (bilharziasis). In treating guinea worm infestation the drug kills the worms and facilitates their removal from the tissues – but they do still have to be removed physically from the ulcers they cause, and the ulcers require dressing.

✚ warning: niridazole should not be administered to patients with epilepsy; it should be administered with caution to those with impaired liver function.

▲ side-effects: there may be nausea and anxiety; some patients enter a state of confusion.

Nitoman (*Roche*) is a proprietary preparation of the powerful drug tetrabenazine, available only on prescription, used to assist a patient to regain voluntary control of movement in Huntington's chorea and related disorders. It is thought to work by reducing the amount of dopamine in the nerve endings of the brain. Produced in the form of tablets, Nitoman is not recommended for children.

✚/▲ warning/side-effects: *see* TETRABENAZINE.

Nitrados (*Berk*) is a proprietary HYPNOTIC drug, available on prescription only to private patients, used in the short term to treat insomnia in patients for whom a degree of sedation during

the daytime is acceptable. Produced in the form of tablets, Nitrados is a preparation of the BENZODIAZEPINE nitrazepam. It is not recommended for children.
✚/▲ warning/side-effects: *see* NITRAZEPAM.

nitrates are VASODILATORS that work by relaxing the walls of blood vessels. They are therefore used mainly in the treatment or prevention of angina pectoris (heart pain), heart failure, and high blood pressure (hypertension). Best known and most used nitrates include GLYCERYL TRINITRATE, ISOSORBIDE DINITRATE and isosorbide MONONITRATE. Administration is commonly in the form of tablets to be held under the tongue until dissolved, but aerosol sprays are also numerous; other presentations are as sustained-release tablets, as impregnated dressings, as ointment for topical application on the chest, and in ampoules for injection.

nitrazepam is a comparatively mild HYPNOTIC drug, one of the benzodiazepines used primarily as a TRANQUILLIZER for patients with insomnia, and in whom a degree of sedation during the daytime is acceptable. However, nitrazepam is thought to be potentially habituating (addictive), and continuous use may in any case have cumulative effects, so many doctors now prefer to prescribe other shorter-acting benzodiazepines instead. Administration is oral in the form of tablets, as capsules, or as a suspension (mixture).
✚ warning: nitrazepam should be administered with caution to patients with diseases of the lungs, particularly if respiratory depression is a symptom, who are elderly or debilitated, who have impaired liver or kidney function, or who are pregnant or lactating. The consumption of alcohol enhances the hypnotic effect of the drug. Withdrawal of treatment should be gradual (abrupt withdrawal after prolonged use may give rise to withdrawal symptoms).
▲ side-effects: concentration and speed of reaction are affected. There is commonly drowsiness and dry mouth; there may also be sensitivity reactions and, in the elderly, a mild state of confusion. Prolonged use may lead to tolerance and a form of dependence (in which there may be insomnia that is worse than before).
Related articles: MOGADON; NITRADOS; NOCTESED; REMNOS; SOMNITE; SUREM; UNISOMNIA.

Nitrocine (*Schwarz*) is a proprietary VASODILATOR, available only on prescription, used to treat congestive heart failure and angina pectoris (heart pain). Produced in the form of ampoules for injection (to be administered diluted or undiluted), Nitrocine is a preparation of glyceryl trinitrate.
✚/▲ warning/side-effects: *see* GLYCERYL TRINITRATE; NITRATES.

Nitrocontin Continus (*Degussa*) is a proprietary, non-prescription VASODILATOR, used to treat angina pectoris (heart pain). Produced in the form of sustained-release tablets (in two strengths), Nitrocontin Continus is a preparation of glyceryl trinitrate. It is not recommended for children.
✚/▲ warning/side-effects: *see* GLYCERYL TRINITRATE; NITRATES.

nitrofurantoin is an

N

ANTIBACTERIAL that is used particularly to treat inflammation and infections of the urinary tract. It is especially useful in treating kidney infections that prove to be resistant to other forms of therapy. Administration is oral in the form of tablets, as capsules, or as a suspension.

✚ warning: nitrofurantoin should not be administered to patients with impaired kidney function, or who are aged under 1 month. The drug is ineffective in patients whose urine is alkaline.

▲ side-effects: there may be nausea and vomiting. Some patients experience tingling in the fingers and toes, or a rash. Rarely, there is allergic liver damage, pulmonary infiltration, peripheral neuropathy.

Related articles: FURADANTIN; MACRODANTIN; URANTOIN.

N

nitrofurazone is an ANTIBACTERIAL drug used primarily in the treatment or prevention of infection on the skin surface, and to prepare skin for grafting, and for some bladder infections. (Occasionally an oral preparation is used to treat the protozoan infection trypanosomiasis.) Administration is thus ordinarily topical, in the form of an ointment.

✚ warning: nitrofurazone should be administered with caution to patients with impaired kidney function.

▲ side-effects: there may be local sensitivity reactions, especially following prolonged use.

Related article: FURACIN.

Nitrolingual Spray (*Lipha*) is a proprietary, non-prescription VASODILATOR, used for the treatment and prevention of angina pectoris (heart pain). Produced in the form of an aerosol spray, Nitrolingual Spray is a preparation of glyceryl trinitrate. It is not recommended for children.

✚/▲ warning/side-effects: *see* GLYCERYL TRINITRATE.

Nitronal (*Lipha*) is a proprietary VASODILATOR, available only on prescription, used to treat congestive heart failure and angina pectoris (heart pain). Produced in ampoules for injection (to be administered diluted or undiluted), Nitronal is a preparation of glyceryl trinitrate.

✚/▲ warning/side-effects: *see* GLYCERYL TRINITRATE.

nitrophenol is an ANTIFUNGAL drug used in topical application to treat skin infections (such as athlete's foot). Administration is as an alcohol-based paint, using a special applicator.

Related article: PHORTINEA.

Nivaquine (*May & Baker*) is a proprietary ANTIMALARIAL drug, available only on prescription, used primarily in combination with other drugs (such as tetracycline) for the prevention and treatment of malaria, although it can be used to counter the symptoms of amoebic infections. Produced in the form of tablets, as a syrup for dilution (the potency of the elixir once diluted is retained for 14 days), and in ampoules for injection (during emergency treatment only), Nivaquine is a preparation of chloroquine sulphate.

✚/▲ warning/side-effects: *see* CHLOROQUINE.

Nivemycin (*Boots*) is a proprietary form of the aminoglycoside ANTIBIOTIC neomycin sulphate, available

only on prescription, used to reduce bacterial levels in the intestines before surgery. Nivemycin is produced in the form of tablets and as an elixir.
✚/▲ warning/side-effects: *see* NEOMYCIN.

Nizoral (*Janssen*) is a proprietary ANTIFUNGAL drug, available only on prescription, used to treat both systemic and skin-surface fungal infections. Produced in the form of tablets, as a suspension, and as a water-miscible cream for topical application, Nizoral is a preparation of the IMIDAZOLE ketoconazole.
✚/▲ warning/side-effects: *see* KETOCONAZOLE.

Nobrium (*Roche*) is a proprietary TRANQUILLIZER, available on prescription only to private patients, used in the short-term treatment of anxiety. Produced in the form of capsules (in two strengths), Nobrium is a preparation of the long-acting benzodiazepine medazepam. It is not recommended for children.
✚/▲ warning/side-effects: *see* MEDAZEPAM.

Noctamid (*Schering*) is a proprietary HYPNOTIC drug, available on prescription only to private patients, used in the short-term treatment of insomnia. Produced in the form of tablets (in two strengths), Noctamid is a preparation of the BENZODIAZEPINE lormetazepam. It is not recommended for children.
✚/▲ warning/side-effects: *see* LORMETAZEPAM.

Noctec (*Squibb*) is a proprietary HYPNOTIC drug, available only on prescription, used to treat insomnia and for sedation in the elderly. Produced in the form of capsules, Noctec is a preparation of the powerful SEDATIVE chloral hydrate, and is not recommended for children.
✚/▲ warning/side-effects: *see* CHLORAL HYDRATE.

Noctesed (*Unimed*) is a proprietary TRANQUILLIZER, available on prescription only to private patients, used to treat insomnia in cases where some degree of daytime sedation is acceptable. Produced in the form of tablets, Noctesed is a preparation of the long-acting BENZODIAZEPINE nitrazepam.
✚/▲ warning/side-effects: *see* NITRAZEPAM.

Noltam (*Lederle*) is a proprietary preparation of the powerful drug tamoxifen, available only on prescription, which because it inhibits or blocks the effect of OESTROGENS, is used primarily to treat cancers that depend on the presence of oestrogen in women, particularly breast cancer. But it may also be used (under strict medical supervision) to treat certain conditions of infertility in which the presence of oestrogens may be preventing other hormonal activity. It is produced in the form of tablets (in two strengths).
✚/▲ warning/side-effects: *see* TAMOXIFEN.

Noludar (*Roche*) is a proprietary HYPNOTIC, a BARBITURATE on the controlled drugs list, used to treat intractable insomnia. Use should be only when essential. Produced in the form of tablets, it is a preparation of methyprylone. It is not recommended for children.
✚/▲ warning/side-effects: *see* METHYPRYLONE.

Nolvadex (*ICI*) is a proprietary preparation of the powerful drug tamoxifen, available only on prescription, which because it

inhibits or blocks the effect of OESTROGENS, is used primarily to treat cancers that depend on the presence of oestrogen in women, particularly breast cancer. But it may also be used (under strict medical supervision) to treat certain conditions of infertility in which the presence of oestrogens may be preventing other hormonal activity. It is produced in the form of tablets (in three strengths, the stronger ones under the trade names Nolvadex-D and Nolvadex-Forte).
✚/▲ warning/side-effects: *see* TAMOXIFEN.

nomifensine is an ANXIOLYTIC and ANTIDEPRESSANT drug formerly used in the treatment of depressive illness, and in combination with other drugs to treat the symptoms of parkinsonism. Unfortunately, however, it also had a stimulant action upon the central nervous system and an inhibitory action on the heart, for which reasons it is no longer used.

***non-narcotic analgesic:** *see* ANALGESIC.

***non-steroidal anti-inflammatory drug** is usually abbreviated to NSAID. *see* ANALGESIC; ANTI-INFLAMMATORY; ANTIRHEUMATIC.

Noradran (*Norma*) is a proprietary non-prescription ANTIHISTAMINE expectorant and cough mixture that is not available from the National Health Service. Produced in the form of a syrup, Noradran is a compound that includes the antihistamine diphenhydramine hydrochloride, the SYMPATHOMIMETIC ephedrine hydrochloride and the EXPECTORANT guaiphenesin. It is not recommended for children aged under 5 years.
✚/▲ warning/side-effects: *see* DIPHENHYDRAMINE HYDROCHLORIDE; EPHEDRINE HYDROCHLORIDE.

noradrenaline is a catecholamine – a HORMONE – produced and secreted by the central core (medulla) of the adrenal glands. Like the closely-related ADRENALINE, it represents one contributory element of the sympathetic nervous system in that, as a NEUROTRANSMITTER (transmitting neural impulses between nerves, and between nerves and muscles), it relays a response to stress. In the face of stress, the body thus uses noradrenaline (and adrenaline) to organize constriction of the small blood vessels (vasoconstriction, so increasing blood pressure), increased blood flow through the heart while the heart rate falls or rises, dilatation of the muscles of the airways, and relaxation of the muscles of the intestinal walls. And it is to effect one or more of these responses that noradrenaline, as a sympathomimetic, may be administered therapeutically. In an emergency, for example, noradrenaline (in the form of noradrenaline acid tartrate) may be injected to raise depressed blood pressure.
✚ warning: noradrenaline should not be administered to patients who are undergoing a heart attack, or who are pregnant. Leakage of the hormone into the tissues at the site of injection may cause tissue damage.
▲ side-effects: there may be headache, with reduced heart rate and uneven heartbeat.
Related article: LEVOPHED.

Noratex (*Norton*) is a proprietary non-prescription skin emollient (softener and soother), used to treat nappy rash and bedsores. Produced in the form of a cream, it contains WOOL FAT, ZINC OXIDE, KAOLIN and talc.

✚ warning: wool fat causes sensitivity reactions in some patients.

Norcuron (*Organon-Teknika*) is a proprietary SKELETAL MUSCLE RELAXANT of the type known as competitive or non-depolarizing; it is used during surgical operations, but only after the patient has been rendered unconscious. Available only on prescription, and produced in ampoules for injection, Norcuron is a preparation of vecuronium bromide.

✚ warning: see VECURONIUM BROMIDE.

Nordox (*Norton*) is a proprietary broad-spectrum ANTIBIOTIC, available only on prescription, used to treat infections of many kinds such as acne, chronic prostatitis. Produced in the form of capsules, Nordox is a preparation of the TETRACYCLINE doxycycline.

✚/▲ warning/side-effects: *see* DOXYCYCLINE.

norethisterone is a PROGESTOGEN (a sex HORMONE) that is an analogue of testosterone (the major male sex hormone). Like all progestogens, norethisterone opposes or modifies some of the effects of OESTROGENS (female sex hormones), and may be used therapeutically to treat several forms of menstrual disorder, endometriosis, dysfunctional uterine bleeding, and to assist in the treatment of sex-hormone-linked cancer. It is also a constituent in many ORAL CONTRACEPTIVES that combine an oestrogen and a progestogen. Administration is oral in the form of tablets.

✚ warning: norethisterone should not be administered to patients with undiagnosed bleeding from the vagina or breast cancer, who are pregnant, or who have a history of thrombosis; it should be administered with extreme caution to those with heart, liver or kidney disease, diabetes, asthma, epilepsy, or high blood pressure (hypertension), or who are lactating.

▲ side-effects: there may be fluid and sodium retention (oedema) leading to weight gain; there may also be breast tenderness, a change in libido, irregular menstrual cycles and gastrointestinal disturbance. Headache and depression may occur; some patients take on the yellow coloration of jaundice, or suffer from skin disorders.

Related articles: BINOVUM; BREVINOR; MENOPHASE; MICRONOR; Neocon 1/35; NORIDAY; NORIMIN; NORINYL-1; ORTHO-NOVIN 1/50; Ovysmen; PRIMOLUT N; SYNPHASE; TRINOVUM; UTOVLAN.

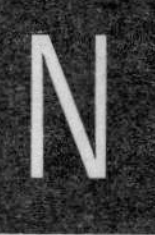

norethisterone acetate is another form of the PROGESTOGEN norethisterone, used primarily as a constituent in ORAL CONTRACEPTIVES that combine an OESTROGEN with a progestogen, but also in hormone replacement therapy to treat some menopausal symptoms.

✚/▲ warning/side-effects: *see* NORETHISTERONE.

Related articles: ANOVLAR; CONTROVLAR; GYNOVLAR; LOESTRIN; Minovlar; TRISEQUENS.

norethisterone enanthate is another form of the PROGESTOGEN norethisterone, used as a contraceptive and administered by injection to patients who prefer not to – or cannot – use ORAL CONTRACEPTIVE methods or forms of contraception that include an oestrogen.

✚/▲ warning/side-effects: *see* NORETHISTERONE.

Related article: NORISTERAT.

Norflex (*Riker*) is a proprietary SKELETAL MUSCLE RELAXANT, available only on prescription, used to relieve muscle spasm mainly in the muscles of the limbs; it works by direct action on the central nervous system. Produced in the form of sustained- release tablets and in ampoules for injection, Norflex is a preparation of orphenadrine citrate. It is not recommended for children.

✚/▲ warning/side-effects: *see* ORPHENADRINE CITRATE.

Norgesic (*Riker*) is a proprietary pain-relieving SKELETAL MUSCLE RELAXANT, available on prescription only to private patients, used to relieve muscle spasm mainly in the muscles of the limbs, and to soothe tension headache and rheumatic pains; it works by direct action on the central nervous system. Produced in the form of tablets, Norgesic is a preparation of orphenadrine citrate with the ANALGESIC paracetamol. It is not recommended for children.

✚/▲ warning/side-effects: *see* ORPHENADRINE CITRATE; PARACETAMOL.

Norgeston (*Schering*) is a proprietary progesterone-only ORAL CONTRACEPTIVE, available only on prescription, that is a preparation of the PROGESTOGEN levonorgestrel. It is produced in 35-day calendar packs that correspond to one complete menstrual cycle.

✚/▲ warning/side-effects: *see* LEVONORGESTREL.

norgestrel is a female sex hormone, a PROGESTOGEN used in ORAL CONTRACEPTIVES – in which it may or may not be combined with an oestrogen – and, also in combination with oestrogens, to treat menstrual and menopausal disorders. The hormone LEVONORGESTREL is a stronger form of norgestrel.

✚ warning: norgestrel should not be administered to patients who are pregnant, or with vascular or liver disease, cancer of the liver or of the breast, or undiagnosed bleeding the vagina. It should be administered with caution to those with heart disease or high blood pressure (hypertension), diabetes, or severe migraine.

▲ side-effects: there may be nausea and vomiting, with a headache; menstrual irregularities and breast tenderness are common, but there may also be weight gain and (occasionally) depression. Some patients experience skin disorders.

Related articles: CYCLO-PROGYNOVA; EUGYNON 50; NEOGEST; PREMPAK; PREMPAK-C.

Noriday (*Syntex*) is a proprietary progesterone-only ORAL CONTRACEPTIVE, available only on prescription, that consists of a preparation of the PROGESTOGEN norethisterone. It is produced in 28-day calendar packs that correspond to one complete menstrual cycle.

✚/▲ warning/side-effects: *see* NORETHISTERONE.

Norimin (*Syntex*) is a proprietary combined ORAL CONTRACEPTIVE,

available only on prescription, that consists of a preparation of the PROGESTOGEN norethisterone and the OESTROGEN ethinyloestradiol. It is produced in 21-day calendar packs that correspond to one complete menstrual cycle.
✚/▲ warning/side-effects: *see* ETHINYLOESTRADIOL; NORETHISTERONE.

Norinyl-1 (*Syntex*) is a proprietary combined ORAL CONTRACEPTIVE, available only on prescription, that consists of a combined preparation of the PROGESTOGEN norethisterone and the OESTROGEN mestranol. It is produced in 21-day calendar packs that correspond to one complete menstrual cycle.
✚/▲ warning/side-effects: *see* MESTRANOL; NORETHISTERONE.

Norisen (*Merck*) is a proprietary set of preparations of common allergens, including pollens, moulds, dusts, animal danders, stinging insects and house dust mites, for use in desensitizing patients who are allergic to them. Available only on prescription and administered by injection, Norisen preparations are of carefully annotated different allergenic effect, so that the process of desensitisation, as regulated by a doctor, can be progressive. Also available are preparations of 6 varieties of common grass pollen (under the name Norisen Grass) in vials of graded strength. Skin testing solutions are also available on prescription for each extract in the Norisen range.
✚ warning: injections should be administered under close medical supervision and in locations where emergency facilities for full cardio-respiratory resuscitation are immediately available.

Noristerat (*Schering*) is a proprietary CONTRACEPTIVE, available only on prescription, that consists of a preparation of the progestogen norethisterone enanthate. It is produced in ampoules for injection for short-term contraception.
✚/▲ warning/side-effects: *see* NORETHISTERONE.

Norit (*Dendron*) is a proprietary non-prescription adsorbent medium used orally to treat diarrhoea, indigestion and flatulence. Produced in the form of capsules, Norit is a preparation of activated CHARCOAL. It is not recommended for children aged under 2 years.

Normacol (*Norgine*) is a proprietary non-prescription LAXATIVE of the type known as bulking agents, which works by increasing the overall mass of faeces within the rectum, so stimulating bowel movement. It is thus used both to relieve constipation and to relieve diarrhoea, and is used also in the control of faecal consistency for patients with a colostomy. Produced in the form of granules in sachets, Normacol is a preparation of the bulk forming drug sterculia. Two compound preparations are also available, although not from the National Health Service: Normacol Standard granules with added frangula bark, and Normacol Antispasmodic with the added muscle relaxant ALVERINE CITRATE. None of these preparations is recommended for children aged under 6 years.

Normasol (*Schering*) is a proprietary non-prescription saline solution, used to clean burns and minor wounds. Produced in the form of a sterile solution, Normasol is a preparation of sodium chloride (saline). An ophthalmic form is also available (under the trade name Normasol Undine) for the washing out of harmful substances and foreign bodies from the eye.

Normax (*Bencard*) is a proprietary non-prescription LAXATIVE, used to treat constipation and to prepare patients for abdominal radiographic procedures. Produced in the form of capsules, Normax is a preparation of the stimulant danthron and the faecal softener DIOCTYL SODIUM SULPHOSUCCINATE (docusate sodium). It is not recommended for children aged under 6 years.
✚/▲ warning/side-effects: *see* DANTHRON.

Normetic (*Abbott*) is a proprietary DIURETIC, available only on prescription, used to treat congestive heart failure, high blood pressure (hypertension) and cirrhosis of the liver. Produced in the form of tablets, it is a compound of the weak but diuretic amiloride hydrochloride together with the THIAZIDE hydrochlorothiazide. It is not recommended for children.
✚/▲ warning/side-effects: *see* AMILORIDE; HYDROCHLOROTHIAZIDE.

Normison (*Wyeth*) is a proprietary HYPNOTIC drug, available on prescription only to private patients, used (in the short term) to treat insomnia especially in the elderly, and as a premedication prior to surgery. Produced in the form of capsules (in two strengths), Normison is a preparation of the benzodiazepine temazepam. It is not recommended for children.
✚/▲ warning/side-effects: *see* TEMAZEPAM.

nortriptyline is an ANTIDEPRESSANT drug that also has mild sedative properties, used primarily to treat depressive illness. Like several others of its type, however, the drug may also be used to assist in the treatment of nocturnal bedwetting by children (aged over 7 years). Administration is oral in the form of tablets, capsules, or a sugar-free dilute liquid.
✚ warning: nortriptyline should not be administered to patients with heart disese or psychosis; it should be administered with caution to those with diabetes, epilepsy, liver or thyroid disease, glaucoma or urinary retention; or who are pregnant or lactating. Withdrawal of treatment must be gradual.
▲ side-effects: common effects include a loss of concentration, movement and thought, dry mouth, and blurred vision; there may also be difficulty in urinating, sweating, and irregular heartbeat, behavioural disturbances, a rash, a state of confusion, and/or a loss of libido. Rarely, there are also blood deficiencies.
Related articles: ALLEGRON; AVENTYL.

Norval (*Bencard*) is a proprietary ANTIDEPRESSANT, available only on prescription, used to treat depressive illness especially when associated with anxiety. Produced in the form of tablets (in three strengths), Norval is a preparation of mianserin hydrochloride. It is not recommended for children.
✚/▲ warning/side-effects: *see* MIANSERIN.

noscapine is an OPIATE (although not related to morphine) used as a constituent in proprietary and non-proprietary formulations intended to relieve dry and painful coughs: such formulations are not available from the National Health Service. The drug has some effect as a cough suppressant.

✚ warning: noscapine should not be administered to patients with liver disease, asthma or chronic bronchitis.

▲ side-effects: there may be constipation

Related article: EXTIL COMPOUND.

Novantrone (*Lederle*) is a proprietary CYTOTOXIC drug, available only on prescription, used to treat certain forms of cancer including breast cancer. It works by reacting with cellular DNA and so disrupting normal cell replication. Produced in vials for intravenous infusion, Novantrone is a preparation of mitozantrone.

✚/▲ warning/side-effects: *see* MITOZANTRONE, DOXORUBICIN.

Noxyflex (*Geistlich*) is a proprietary ANTIMICROBIAL, available only on prescription, used to treat infections of the urinary tract. Produced in the form of a powder for reconstitution as a solution for instillation into the bladder, Noxyflex is a compound preparation of the ANTIBACTERIAL/ANTIFUNGAL drug noxythiolin and the local ANAESTHETIC amethocaine hydrochloride. A similar preparation but containing only noxythiolin is also available (under the name Noxyflex S).

✚/▲ warning/side-effects: *see* AMETHOCAINE HYDROCHLORIDE; NOXYTHIOLIN.

noxythiolin is an ANTIBIOTIC that has both ANTIBACTERIAL and ANTIFUNGAL properties. A derivative of urea, its primary use is in the treatment of infection in the urinary tract, and administration is most commonly in the form of a solute instillation into the bladder.

✚ warning: because there may be a stinging, burning sensation on initial instillation, the drug is sometimes administered in combination with a local anaesthetic.

Related article: NOXYFLEX.

Nozinan (*May & Baker*) is a proprietary ANTIPSYCHOTIC drug, available only on prescription, used to treat and sedate patients with schizophrenia and related psychoses, and to relieve anxiety during terminal care. Produced in ampoules for injection, Nozinan is a preparation of methotrimeprazine hydrochloride. It is not recommended for children.

✚/▲ warning/side-effects: *see* METHOTRIMEPRAZINE.

***NSAID** is an abbreviation of non-steroidal ANTI-INFLAMMATORY drug.

see ANALGESIC: ANTIRHEUMATIC.

Nubain (*Du Pont*) is a proprietary narcotic ANALGESIC, available only on prescription, used to treat moderate to severe pain, particularly during or following surgical procedures or a heart attack. Produced in ampoules for injection, Nubain is a preparation of the OPIATE nalbuphine hydrochloride. It is not recommended for children.

✚/▲ warning/side-effects: *see* NALBUPHINE.

Nuelin (*Riker*) is a proprietary non-prescription BRONCHODILATOR, used to treat asthmatic bronchospasm and chronic bronchitis. Produced in the form of tablets (not recommended for children aged under 7 years), as sustained-release tablets (in two strengths under the names Nuelin SA and Nuelin SA 250; not recommended for children aged under 6 years), and as a syrup for dilution (the potency of the liquid once diluted is retained for 14 days; not recommended for children aged under 2 years), Nuelin is a preparation of the xanthine drug theophylline.

✚/▲ warning/side-effects: *see* THEOPHYLLINE.

N

Nu-K (*Consolidated*) is a proprietary non-prescription POTASSIUM supplement, used to make up a blood deficiency of potassium (as may occur in the elderly, in patients with severe diarrhoea, or in patients being treated with diuretics). Produced in the form of sustained-release capsules, Nu-K is a preparation of POTASSIUM CHLORIDE. It is not recommended for children.

Nulacin (*Bencard*) is a proprietary non-prescription ANTACID that is not available from the National Health Service. It is used to treat peptic ulcers and inflammation of the stomach. Produced in the form of tablets, Nulacin is a compound preparation that includes calcium carbonate, magnesium carbonate, magnesium oxide ("magnesia"), magnesium trisilicate and maltose. It is not recommended for children, and should be avoided because of potential side-effects.

✚/▲ warning/side-effects: *see* CALCIUM CARBONATE; MAGNESIUM CARBONATE; MAGNESIUM TRISILICATE.

Numotac (*Riker*) is a proprietary BRONCHODILATOR, available only on prescription, used to treat bronchial asthma and chronic bronchitis. Produced in the form of sustained-release tablets, Numotac is a preparation of the BETA-RECEPTOR STIMULANT isoetharine hydrochloride. It is not recommended for children.

✚/▲ warning/side-effects: *see* ISOETHARINE.

Nupercainal (*Ciba*) is a proprietary non-prescription local ANAESTHETIC, used in topical application to treat painful skin conditions. Produced in the form of an ointment, Nupercainal is a solute preparation of cinchocaine hydrochloride.

✚/▲ warning/side-effects: *see* CINCHOCAINE.

Nurofen (*Crookes Healthcare*) is a proprietary non-prescription non-narcotic ANALGESIC containing ibuprofen.

✚/▲ warning/side-effects: *see* IBUPROFEN.

Nu-Seals Aspirin (*Lilly*) is a proprietary non-prescription non-narcotic ANALGESIC, a form of aspirin used to treat chronic pain such as that of arthritis and rheumatism. Produced in the form of tablets (in two strengths), Nu-Seals Aspirin is not recommended for children aged under 12 years.

✚/▲ warning/side-effects: *see* ASPIRIN.

Nutracel (*Travenol*) is a proprietary form of high-energy nutritional supplement, available only on prescription, intended for infusion into patients who are unable to take food via the alimentary tract such as after total gastrectomy. Produced in two strengths (under the trade names Nutracel 400 and Nutracel 800), it is a preparation of GLUCOSE with MAGNESIUM CHLORIDE and several other mineral salts.

Nutramigen (*Bristol-Myers*) is a proprietary non-prescription dietary supplement. Nutritionally complete, it is intended for patients who suffer from milk protein intolerance. Produced in the form of a powder, Nutramigen is a preparation of protein, carbohydrate, fat (corn oil), vitamins and minerals, and is lactose-, fructose- and gluten-free. It is not recommended for infants aged under 3 months.

Nutranel (*Roussel*) is a proprietary non-prescription dietary supplement. It is intended for patients who suffer from malabsorption of food (for example following gastrectomy). Produced in the form of a powder, Nutranel is a preparation of protein, fat, carbohydrate, vitamins, minerals and trace elements, and is low in lactose. It is not suitable as the sole source of nutrition for children, and is unsuitable for infants aged under 12 months.

Nutraplus (*Alcon*) is a proprietary non-prescription skin emollient (softener and soother), used to treat dry skin. Produced in the form of a cream in a water-miscible basis, Nutraplus is a preparation of the hydrating substance urea.

Nutrauxil (*KabiVitrum*) is a proprietary non-prescription dietary supplement. It is intended for patients who suffer from overall dietary insufficiency (as with anorexia nervosa) or from intractable malabsorption of food (as after the surgical removal of the stomach). Produced in the form of a liquid feed, Nutrauxil is a preparation of protein, carbohydrate, fat (sunflower oil), vitamins and minerals, and is lactose- and electrolyte-low and gluten-free. It is not suitable as the sole source of nutrition for children aged under 5 years, but nutritionally all that anyone else might need.

Nutrizym (*Merck*) is a proprietary non-prescription preparation of pancreatic enzymes, used to treat pancreatic disorders, and particularly the symptoms arising from cystic fibrosis (in which thick mucus obstructs the secretion of pancreatic juices). It is produced in the form of tablets to be taken during or after meals.

Nybadex (*Cox*) is a proprietary anti-inflammatory and ANTIFUNGAL compound, available only on prescription, used to treat skin inflammations in which infection is thought to be present. It is produced in the form of a dilute emulsifying ointment for topical application, and contains the corticosteroid hydrocortisone with the ANTIBIOTIC nystatin, the antifoaming agent DIMETHICONE and the antiseptic BENZALKONIUM CHLORIDE.

✚/▲ warning/side-effects: *see* HYDROCORTISONE; NYSTATIN.

Nydrane (*Lipha*) is a proprietary preparation of the ANTICONVULSANT drug beclamide, available only on prescription, used to treat grand mal and partial seizures in epilepsy, and associated behavioural disorders. It is produced in the form of tablets.

✚/▲ warning/side-effects: *see* BECLAMIDE.

Nyspes (*DDSA Pharmaceuticals*) is a proprietary ANTIFUNGAL preparation, available only on prescription, used to treat yeast infections of the vagina or vulva.

Produced in the form of vaginal inserts (pessaries), Nyspes is a preparation of the ANTIBIOTIC nystatin.
✚/▲ warning/side-effects: *see* NYSTATIN.

Nystadermal (*Squibb*) is a proprietary CORTICOSTEROID cream, available only on prescription, used for topical application on areas of inflamed skin, particularly in cases of eczema that have failed to respond to less powerful drugs. Nystadermal is a preparation of the steroid triamcinolone acetonide and the ANTIBIOTIC nystatin.
✚/▲ warning/side-effects: *see* NYSTATIN; TRIAMCINOLONE ACETONIDE.

Nystaform (*Bayer*) is a proprietary ANTIFUNGAL preparation, available only on prescription, used in topical application to treat fungal (particularly yeast) infections. Produced in the form of a cream and an anhydrous ointment, Nystaform is a preparation of the ANTIBIOTIC drug nystatin and one of two forms of the ANTISEPTIC chlorhexidine.
✚/▲ warning/side-effects: *see* CHLORHEXIDINE; NYSTATIN.

Nystaform-HC (*Bayer*) is a proprietary CORTICOSTEROID compound, available only on prescription, used to treat skin inflammations in which fungal and bacterial infections are suspected. Produced in the form of a water-miscible cream and an anhydrous ointment, Nystaform-HC is a preparation of the corticosteroid hydrocortisone, the ANTIFUNGAL drug nystatin, and one of two forms of the (mildly antibacterial) ANTISEPTIC chlorhexidine.
✚/▲ warning/side-effects: *see* CHLORHEXIDINE; HYDROCORTISONE; nystatin.

Nystan (*Squibb*) is the name of a proprietary group of ANTIFUNGAL preparations, available only on prescription, used to treat fungal infections (such as candidiasis, thrush). All are forms of the ANTIBIOTIC nystatin. Preparations for oral administration include tablets, a suspension, a gluten-, lactose- and sugar-free suspension, granules for reconstitution with water to form a solution, and pastilles (for treating mouth infections). For vaginal and vulval infections there is a vaginal cream, a gel, and vaginal inserts (pessaries; under the name Nystavescent). A triple pack containing tablets, gel and pessaries is available. A water-miscible cream, gel, ointment and dusting-powder are available for the topical treatment of fungal skin infections.
✚/▲ warning/side-effects: *see* NYSTATIN.

nystatin is a powerful ANTIFUNGAL ANTIBIOTIC drug, effective both in topical application and when taken orally, primarily used specifically to treat the yeast infection candidiasis (thrush). Less commonly, it is used to treat other fungal infections, particularly in and around the mouth. Administration is in many forms: tablets, a suspension, a solution, pastilles, vaginal inserts (pessaries), a cream, a gel, an ointment and a dusting-powder.
✚ warning: the full course of treatment must be completed, even if symptoms disappear earlier: recurrence of infection is common when treatment is withdrawn too hastily. Fungal infections in the urogenital

areas imply simultaneous treatment of the patient's sexual partner. Treatment with pessaries should be continued through menstruation.

▲ side-effects: treatment of the vagina may require additional medication to restore the natural acidity of the area. There may be nausea, vomiting or diarrhoea. *Related articles:* DERMOVATE-NN; GREGODERM; MULTILIND; Nystaform; NYSTAN; NYSTATIN-DOME; NYSTAVESCENT; TERRA-CORTRIL; TINADERM-M.

Nystatin-Dome (*Bayer*) is a proprietary ANTIFUNGAL preparation, available only on prescription, used to treat intestinal candidiasis (thrush) and oral infections. Produced in the form of a suspension, Nystatin-Dome is a preparation of the ANTIBIOTIC nystatin.

✚/▲ warning/side-effects: *see* NYSTATIN.

Nystavescent (*Squibb*) is a proprietary ANTIFUNGAL preparation, available only on prescription, used to treat vaginal and vulval candidiasis (thrush). Produced in the form of vaginal inserts (pessaries), Nystavescent is a preparation of the ANTIBIOTIC nystatin.

✚/▲ warning/side-effects: *see* NYSTATIN.

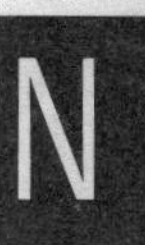

Octovit (*Smith, Kline & French*) is a proprietary non-prescription mineral-and-VITAMIN compound, used particularly as an IRON supplement (containing ferrous sulphate). Produced in the form of tablets, Octovit contains – apart from iron – calcium, magnesium and zinc, together with THIAMINE (vitamin B_1), RIBOFLAVINE (vitamin B_2), PYRIDOXINE (vitamin B_6), CYANOCOBALAMIN (vitamin B_{12}), NICOTINAMIDE (of the vitamin B complex), ASCORBIC ACID (vitamin C), CALCIFEROL (vitamin D) and TOCOPHEROL (vitamin E). Octovit should not be used simultaneously with tetracycline antibiotics.

✚/▲ warning/side-effects: *see* FERROUS SULPHATE.

octoxinol is a SPERMICIDAL drug used to assist barrier methods of contraception. In mild solution, it is produced as a jelly.

▲ side-effects: very rarely, there may be sensitivity reactions.
Related article: STAYCEPT.

Ocusert Pilo (*May & Baker*) is a proprietary form of the PARASYMPATHOMIMETIC pilocarpine hydrochloride, used to treat glaucoma. Available only on prescription (in either of two strengths), it is produced in the form of elliptical plastic inserts to be placed under the eyelid (following instructions on the pack), permitting sustained local release of the drug. Ocusert Pilo is not recommended for children.

✚/▲ warning/side-effects: *see* PILOCARPINE.

Ocusol (*Boots*) is a proprietary ANTIBACTERIAL, available only on prescription, used to treat eye infections. Produced in the form of eye-drops, Ocusol is a preparation of the sulphonamide SULPHACETAMIDE sodium together with the astringent-cleanser ZINC SULPHATE.

oestradiol is the main female sex hormone produced and secreted by the ovary. An OESTROGEN, it is used therapeutically to make up hormonal deficiencies – sometimes in combination with a PROGESTOGEN – to treat menstrual, menopausal or other gynaecological problems (such as infertility). Administration is oral in the form of tablets, or by injection.

✚ warning: oestradiol should not be administered to patients who have cancers proved to be sex-hormone-related, who have a history of thrombosis or inflammation of the womb, or who suffer from porphyria or impaired liver function. Prolonged treatment increases the risk of cancer of the endometrium (the lining of the womb). Caution should be exercised in administering oestradiol to patients who are diabetic or epileptic, who have heart or kidney disease, who are pregnant or lactating, or who have high blood pressure (hypertension) or migraine.

▲ side-effects: there may be nausea and vomiting. A common effect is weight gain, generally through fluid or sodium retention in the tissues. The breasts may become tender and enlarge slightly. There may also be headache and/or depression; sometimes a rash breaks out.
Related articles: BENZTRONE; CYCLO-PROGYNOVA; HORMONIN; PROGYNOVA; TRISEQUENS.

oestriol is a female sex hormone produced and secreted by the ovary. An OESTROGEN, it is similar in properties and uses to OESTRADIOL.
Related articles: OVESTIN; TRISEQUENS.

oestrogens are a group of STEROID hormones that promote the growth and functioning of the female sex organs and the development of female sexual characteristics. In their natural forms they are produced and secreted mainly by the ovary (and to a small extent the adrenal cortex and – in men – the testes). Natural and synthesized oestrogens are used therapeutically, sometimes in combination with PROGESTOGENS, to treat menstrual, menopausal or other gynaecological problems, and as oral contraceptives. Best known and most used are oestradiol, oestriol, ethinyloestradiol, mestranol and quinestradol.
✚/▲ warning/side-effects: *see* ETHINYLOESTRADIOL; MESTRANOL; OESTRADIOL; OESTRIOL; QUINESTRADOL; QUINESTROL.

Oilatum (*Stiefel*) is a proprietary non-prescription skin emollient (softener and soother) in the form of a water-based cream containing arachis oil and povidone. Under the same name there is a bath emulsion containing liquid paraffin and wool alcohols, for use as an emollient soaking medium.

oily cream is a general term for the kind of cream that is not water-miscible and so does not wash off so easily. Such creams are used as bases for many therapeutic preparations for topical application. Whereas an oily cream is oily, OINTMENTS are deemed to be greasy.

ointments is a general term for a group of essentially greasy preparations that are anhydrous and insoluble in water and so do not wash off. Such unguents are used as bases for many therapeutic preparations for topical application (particularly in the treatment of dry lesions or of ophthalmic complaints). Most have a form of paraffin as their base; a few contain lanolin and wool alcohols, to which a small number of patients may be sensitive.

olive oil is used therapeutically – always warmed beforehand – either to soften earwax prior to syringing the ears, or to treat the brown, flaking skin that commonly appears on the heads of very young infants (cradle cap) prior to shampooing.

Omnopon (*Roche*) is a proprietary OPIATE, a controlled drug which is a preparation of papaveretum, used primarily as premedication before surgery, but also to relieve severe pain. It is produced in the form of tablets and in ampoules for injection.
✚/▲ warning/side-effects: *see* PAPAVERETUM.

Omnopon-Scopolamine (*Roche*) is a proprietary combination of Omnopon and the powerful alkaloid SEDATIVE hyoscine (also known as scopolamine in the USA). It is a controlled drug, and is used primarily as premedication before surgery. It is produced in ampoules for injection.
✚/▲ warning/side-effects: *see* PAPAVERETUM; HYOSCINE.

Oncovin (*Lilly*) is a proprietary form of the VINCA ALKALOID vincristine sulphate, available only on prescription, used to treat acute leukaemia, lymphoma and certain sarcomas. It is produced in ampoules or as powder for reconstitution, in both cases for injection.
✚/▲ warning/side-effects: *see* VINCRISTINE SULPHATE.

One-alpha (*Leo*) is a proprietary form of the VITAMIN D analogue alfacalcidol, available only on prescription, used after renal osteodystrophy to restore and sustain calcium balance in the body due to e.g. neonatal hypocalcaemia. It is produced in the form of capsules (in two strengths) and as drops (with a diluent to adjust concentration).
✚/▲ warning/side-effects: *see* ALFACALDICOL.

Operidine (*Janssen*) is a proprietary narcotic ANALGESIC, a controlled drug used primarily as an analgesic during surgery. Produced in the form of ampoules for injection, Operidine is a preparation of phenoperidine hydrochloride.
✚/▲ warning/side-effects: *see* PHENOPERIDINE.

Ophthaine (*Squibb*) is a proprietary form of local ANAESTHETIC eye-drops, available only on prescription, commonly used during ophthalmic procedures and consisting of a preparation of proxymetacaine hydrochloride.
✚/▲ warning/side-effects: *see* PROXYMETACAINE HYDROCHLORIDE.

Ophthalmadine (*SAS Pharmaceuticals*) is a proprietary preparation, available only on prescription, used to treat Herpes simplex infections of the eye. Containing a mild solution of the antiviral agent idoxuridine, it is produced in the form of eye-drops for use during the day, and eye ointment for use overnight.
✚/▲ warning/side-effects: *see* IDOXURIDINE.

opiates are a group of drugs, derived from opium, that depress certain functions of the central nervous system. In this way, they can relieve pain (and inhibit coughing). They are also used to treat diarrhoea. Therapeutically, the most important opiate is probably morphine which, with its synthetic derivative heroin (diamorphine), is a NARCOTIC; all are potentially habituating (addictive).
✚/▲ warning/side-effects: *see* BUPRENORPHINE; CODEINE; DEXTROMORAMIDE; DIAMORPHINE; DIHYDROCODEINE; MEPTAZINOL; METHADONE; MORPHINE; PAPAVERETUM; PENTAZOCINE; PETHIDINE; PHENAZOCINE; PHENOPERIDINE.

opiate squill linctus and pastilles are a compound formulations not available from the National Health Service, combining several soothing liquids – including camphorated tincture of opium and tolu syrup – into a cough linctus (also known as Gee's linctus) and into a form of cough pastilles (also known as Gee's pastilles) made from that linctus.

Opilon (*Parke-Davis*) is a proprietary VASODILATOR, available only on prescription, used to treat neural conditions resulting from poor blood supply, particularly in the hands and feet, and in the ears (such as Regnaud's phenomenon). Produced in the form of tablets and in ampoules for injection (in two strengths), Opilon contains thymoxamine hydrochloride. It is not recommended for children.
✚/▲ warning/side-effects: *see* THYMOXAMINE.

opium alkaloids is another term for opiates.
see OPIATES.

Opobyl (*Bengué*) is a proprietary LAXATIVE available on prescription only to private patients, used to treat constipation and reduced secretion of digestive juices. Produced in the form of pills, Opobyl contains the acidic substance PODOPHYLLUM, desiccated pig's liver and bile salts. It is not recommended for children.

Opticrom (*Fisons*) is an ANTI-INFLAMMATORY preparation, available only on prescription, used to treat forms of conjunctivitis caused by allergic reactions. Produced in the form of eye-drops and eye ointment, Opticrom contains sodium cromoglycate.
✚/▲ warning/side-effects: *see* SODIUM CROMOGLUCATE.

Optimax (*Merck*) is a proprietary compound, available only on prescription, combining the ANTIDEPRESSANT drug tryptophan with PYRIDOXINE (vitamin B_6) and ASCORBIC ACID (vitamin C). By itself it is used to treat mild to moderate depressive illness; in combination with other antidepressants it is used to treat severe depressive illness. Optimax is produced in the form of tablets and as powder in sachets for reconstitution; another version of Optimax is produced without vitamins (under the name Optimax WV). It is not recommended for children.
✚/▲ warning/side-effects: *see* TRYPTOPHAN.

Optimine (*Kirby-Warrick*) is a proprietary non-prescription form of the ANTIHISTAMINE drug azatadine maleate, used to relieve the symptoms of allergic reactions such as hay fever and urticaria. Produced in the form of tablets and as a syrup for dilution, Optimine is not recommended for children aged under 12 months.
✚/▲ warning/side-effects: *see* AZATADINE MALEATE.

Opulets (*Alcon*) is the name of a proprietary brand of eye-drops which consists of a variety of different drugs. Opulets Chloramphenicol is used to treat bacterial infections in the eye and contains the ANTIBIOTIC chloramphenicol. Opulets Atropine contains the ANTICHOLINERGIC atropine sulphate and is used to dilate the pupils and paralyse the eye muscles. Opulets Cyclopentolate contains the anticholernergic cyclopentolate hydrochloride and is used to dilate the pupils and paralyse the eye muscles. Opulets Pilocarpine contains the PARASYMPATHOMIMETIC pilocarpine hydrochloride and is used to treat glaucoma. Opulets Benoxinate contains oxybuprocaine hydrochloride and has a local ANAESTHETIC effect on the eyeballs. Opulets Saline contains sodium chloride and is used as an eye-wash. Opulets Fluorescein contains fluorescein sodium and is a stain for highlighting foreign bodies on the surface of the eye. With the exception of Opulets Saline and Opulets Fluorescein, all these preparations are available only on prescription.
✚/▲ warning/side-effects: *see* ATROPINE SULPHATE; CHLORAMPHENICOL; CYCLOPENTOLATE HYDROCHLORIDE; FLOURESCEIN SODIUM; PILOCARPINE HYDROCHLORIDE; OXYBUPROCAINE HYDROCHLORIDE.

Orabase (*Squibb*) is a proprietary non-prescription ointment, used to protect sores and ulcers in and on the mouth, or in the vicinity of a stoma (an outlet on the skin surface that following the

O

surgical curtailment of the intestines). Produced in the form of paste, Orabase's active constituent is CARMELLOSE SODIUM.

Orabet (*Lagap*) is a proprietary form of the biguanide drug metformin hydrochloride, available only on prescription, used to treat adult-onset DIABETES mellitus. It works by increasing the absorption and utilization in the body of glucose, to make up for the reduction in insulin available from the pancreas, and is produced in the form of tablets (in two strengths).
✚/▲ warning/side-effects: *see* METFORMIN.

O

Orabolin (*Organon*) is a proprietary steroid preparation, available only on prescription, used to promote protein synthesis after major surgery or debilitating disease.

Oradexon (*Organon*) is a proprietary CORTICOSTEROID ANTI-INFLAMMATORY drug, available only on prescription, used to treat arthritis, joint pain, and allergies. Produced in the form of tablets (in two strengths) and in ampoules for injection, Oradexon's primary constituent is dexamethasone.
✚/▲ warning/side-effects: *see* DEXAMETHASONE.

Orahesive (*Squibb*) is a proprietary non-prescription preparation, used to protect sores and ulcers in and on the mouth, or in the vicinity of a stoma (an outlet on the skin surface that following the surgical curtailment of the intestines). Produced in the form of powder, Orahesive's active constituent is CARMELLOSE SODIUM.

oral contraceptives are prophylactic preparations taken by women to prevent conception following sexual intercourse, and commonly referred to as the "pill". Most contain both an OESTROGEN and a PROGESTOGEN – the oestrogen blocks the release of a ripened egg (ovum) from an ovary, and the progestogen blocks the remaining processes of the menstrual cycle. This type of preparation is known as the combined oral contraceptive, or combined pill, and is taken daily for 3 weeks and stopped for a week during which menstruation occurs. A second form of combined pill (the "phased formulation") is the biphasic or triphasic pill, in which the hormonal content varies according to the time of the month at which each pill is to be taken, and is reduced to the minimum still to be effective. Other types of pill contain only progestogen. A variant on this is the progestogen injection, which is renewable every 3 months. All forms may produce side-effects, and a form that is ideally suited to a patient is not always possible. Post-coital contraception is also possible in emergency by use of high-dose oestrogen preparations.
✚/▲ warning/side-effects: *see individual oestrogens and progestogens listed under* OESTROGENS *and* PROGESTOGENS.
Related articles: ANOVLAR 21; BINOVUM; BREVINOR; CONOVA 30; DEPO-PROVERA; EUGYNON 30; EUGYNON 50; FEMULEN; GYNOVLAR; Loestrin; LOGYNON; MARVELON; MICROGYNON 30; MICRONOR; MICROVAL; MINILYN; MINOVLAR; NEOCON 1/35; NEOGEST; Norgeston; NORIDAY; NORIMIN; NORINYL-1; ORTHO-NOVIN 1/50; Ovran;

OVRANETTE; OVYSMEN; PC4; SYNPHASE; TRINORDIOL; TRINOVUM.

Oral-B (*Oral B*) is a proprietary non-prescription preparation, used to relieve pain in sores and ulcers in the mouth. Produced in the form of a gel, Oral-B contains the local ANAESTHETIC lignocaine with the mouth-wash cetylpyridinium chloride and menthol.
✚/▲ warning/side-effects: CETYLPYRIDINIUM CHLORIDE; LIGNOCAINE.

Oralcer (*Vitabiotics*) is a proprietary non-prescription ANTISEPTIC preparation, used to treat infections and ulcers in the mouth. Produced in the form of lozenges, Oralcer contains clioquinol and ASCORBIC ACID (vitamin C).
✚/▲ warning/side-effects: *see* CLIOQUINOL.

Oraldene (*Warner-Lambert*) is a proprietary non-prescription ANTISEPTIC preparation, used to treat sores and ulcers in the mouth. Produced in the form of a mouth-wash, Oraldene's active constituent is HEXETIDINE.

Orap (*Janssen*) is a powerful proprietary ANTIPSYCHOTIC of complex action, available only on prescription, used with care to treat and tranquillize patients who are psychotic, particularly schizophrenic. Produced in the form of tablets (in three strengths), Orap is a preparation of pimozide.
✚/▲ warning/side-effects: *see* PIMOZIDE.

Orbenin (*Beecham*) is a proprietary ANTIBIOTIC, available only on prescription, used to treat bacterial infections, and especially staphylococcal infections that prove to be resistant to penicillin. Produced in the form of capsules (in two strengths), as a syrup for dilution, and as powder for reconstitution as injections, Orbenin's active constituent is cloxacillin.
✚/▲ warning/side-effects: *see* CLOXACILLIN.

orciprenaline is a BETA-RECEPTOR STIMULANT so acts both as a BRONCHODILATOR, commonly as an aerosol, and as a SMOOTH MUSCLE RELAXANT. Consequently it is used to treat respiratory problems associated with such conditions as asthma and emphysema, and may also be used to slow premature labour.
✚ warning: Orciprenaline should not be administered to patients who have heart disease or high blood pressure (hypertension); who have disorders of the thyroid gland or infection; who are bleeding; or who are already taking strong drugs of any kind. It should be administered with caution to those who are diabetic or pregnant. Blood pressure and pulse must be monitored constantly.
▲ side-effects: increased heart rate, reduced blood pressure, flushing and sweating are relatively common; there may also be nausea and vomiting, and/or a tremor.
Related article: ALUPENT.

Orimeten (*Ciba*) is a powerful proprietary ANTICANCER drug, available only on prescription, used to treat advanced stages of cancer of the breast in women who have reached the menopause. It is also used to treat advanced stages of cancer of the prostate gland in men. Produced in the form of tablets, Orimeten's active constituent is

aminoglutethimide.
✚/▲ warning/side-effects: *see* AMINOGLUTETHIMIDE.

Orovite (*Bencard*) is a proprietary non-prescription VITAMIN preparation that is not available from the National Health Service. It is used to treat vitamin deficiencies after illness, infection or operation. Produced in the form of tablets and as an elixir, Orovite contains THIAMINE (vitamin B_1), RIBOFLAVINE (vitamin B_2), PYRIDOXINE (vitamin B_6), NICOTINAMIDE (of the B complex) and ASCORBIC ACID (vitamin C). There is also a granular form (issued under the name Orovite 7) that includes RETINOL (vitamin A) with CALCIFEROL (vitamin D), produced in sachets for solution in water.

orphenadrine citrate is a powerful SKELETAL MUSCLE RELAXANT used to treat muscle spasm (rigidity), particularly following injury to a muscle. It works by directly affecting the central nervous system. Administration is oral in the form of tablets, or by injection. Orphenadrine citrate is not suitable for children.
✚ warning: prolonged use can reduce muscle tone in an affected muscle, leading eventually to worse disability. The drug should be administered with caution to patients with heart, kidney or liver disease, glaucoma, or urinary retention. Withdrawal of treatment must be gradual. It should not be administered to children.
▲ side-effects: there may be dry mouth and gastrointestinal disturbances; visual disturbances may also arise, with dizziness. Rarely, there is increased heart rate and/or a hypersensitive reaction, mental confusion and nervousness.
Related articles: NORFLEX; NORGESIC.

orphenadrine hydrochloride is an ANTICHOLINERGIC drug used primarily to treat the symptoms of parkinsonism (whether drug-induced or not) and drug induced extrapyramidal symptoms (*see* ANTIPARKINSONISM). It thus reduces tremor and rigidity, has a diuretic effect on the excess salivary flow, but can do little to improve slowness or awkwardness in movement. Administration of orphenadrine hydrochloride is oral in the form of tablets or as an elixir, or by injection.
✚ warning: prolonged use can reduce muscle tone in an affected muscle, leading eventually to worse disability. The drug should be administered with caution to patients with heart, kidney or liver disease, glaucoma, or urinary retention. Withdrawal of treatment must be gradual. It should not be administered to children.
▲ side-effects: there may be dry mouth and gastrointestinal disturbances; visual disturbances may also arise, with dizziness. Rarely, there is increased heart rate and/or a hypersensitive reaction, mental confusion and nervousness.
Related articles: BIORPHEN; DISIPAL.

Ortho-Creme (*Ortho-Cilag*) is a proprietary non-prescription SPERMICIDAL preparation, used as a contraceptive in conjunction with a diaphragm. Produced in the form of cream, Ortho-Creme's active constituent is an alcohol ester.

Ortho Dienoestrol (*Ortho-Cilag*)

is a proprietary OESTROGEN hormone preparation, available only on prescription, used to treat infection and irritation of the membranous surface of the vagina. Produced in the form of cream, Ortho Dienoestrol's active constituent is dienoestrol.
✚/▲ warning/side-effects: *see* DIENOESTROL.

Orthoforms (*Ortho-Cilag*) is a proprietary non-prescription SPERMICIDAL preparation, used as a contraceptive in conjunction with any of the barrier methods. Produced in the form of pessaries (vaginal inserts), Orthoforms' active constituent is an alcohol ester.

Ortho-Gynest (*Ortho-Cilag*) is a proprietary OESTROGEN preparation, available only on prescription, used to treat infection and irritation of the membranous surface of the vagina. Produced in the form of pessaries (vaginal inserts), Ortho-Gynest contains oestriol.
✚/▲ warning/side-effects: *see* OESTRIOL.

Ortho-Gyne T (*Ortho-Cilag*) is a proprietary intrauterine contraceptive device, available only on prescription. Ortho-Gyne T is a T-shaped plastic carrier with a copper wire, which has an effect on the enzyme activity on the lining of the womb necessary for implantation. The device has to be replaced after three years. Another device, Ortho-Gyne T 380 S, is available only on prescription to private patients, and needs replacement only after four years.

Ortho-Gynol (*Ortho-Cilag*) is a proprietary non-prescription spermicidal preparation, used as a contraceptive in conjunction with a diaphragm (intrauterine device). Produced in the form of jelly, Ortho-Gynol's active constituent is an alcohol ester.

Ortho Novin 1/50 (*Ortho-Cilag*) is a proprietary OESTROGEN-and-PROGESTOGEN preparation, available only on prescription, used as a combined ORAL CONTRACEPTIVE. Produced in the form of tablets in a 21 day calender pack representing one menstrual cycle, Ortho Novin 1/50 is a preparation of norethisterone and mestranol.
✚/▲ warning/side-effects: *see* MESTRANOL; NORETHISTERONE.

Orudis (*May & Baker*) is a proprietary ANTI-INFLAMMATORY non-narcotic ANALGESIC, available only on prescription, used to relieve arthritic and rheumatic pain and to treat other musculo-skeletal disorders. Produced in the form of capsules (in two strengths) and as anal suppositories, Orudis's active constituent is ketoprofen.
✚/▲ warning/side-effects: *see* KETOPROFEN.

Oruvail (*May & Baker*) is a proprietary ANTI-INFLAMMATORY non-narcotic ANALGESIC, available only on prescription, used to relieve arthritic and rheumatic pain and to treat other musculo-skeletal disorders. Produced in the form of capsules (in two strengths), Oruvail's active constituent is ketoprofen.
✚/▲ warning/side-effects: *see* KETOPROFEN.

Osmitrol (*Travenol*) is a powerful proprietary DIURETIC drug, available only on prescription, used to rid the body of accumulated fluids especially in emergency situations (such as following a drug overdose). Produced in the form of fluid for

intravenous infusion (in three strengths), Osmitrol is a preparation of mannitol.
✚/▲ warning/side-effects: *see* MANNITOL.

Osmolite (*Abbott*) is a bland, proprietary, non-prescription, gluten- and lactose-free liquid that is a complete nutritional diet for adult patients (but not for children) who are severely undernourished (such as with anorexia nervosa) or who are suffering from some problem with the absorption of food (such as following gastrectomy). Produced in cans, Osmolite contains protein, carbohydrate, fat, vitamins and minerals. It is not suitable for children aged under 12 months.

Ossopan (*Labaz*) is a proprietary non-prescription CALCIUM supplement, used to treat degenerative bone diseases. Produced in the form of tablets and powder, Ossopan is a preparation of calcium salts.

Ostobon (*Coloplast*) is a proprietary non-prescription deodorant powder, used to freshen and sanitize the appliance or bag that is attached to a stoma (an outlet on the skin surface) following ileostomy or colostomy (surgical curtailing of the intestines) or ureterostomy (surgical curtailing of the ureter between kidney and bladder).

Otosporin (*Calmic*) is a proprietary ANTIBIOTIC preparation, available only on prescription, used to treat infections and inflammation in the outer ear. Produced in the form of ear-drops, Otosporin contains the CORTICOSTEROID hydrocortisone, the ANTIBIOTIC neomycin sulphate and polymyxin B sulphate.
✚/▲ warning/side-effects: *see* HYDROCORTISONE; NEOMYCIN SULPHATE; POLYMYXIN B SULPHATE.

Ototrips (*Consolidated*) is a proprietary ANTIBIOTIC preparation, available only on prescription, used to treat inflammation and bacterial infections in the middle and outer ear. Produced in the form of ear-drops, Ototrips contains polymyxin B sulphate, the enzyme trypsin, and the secondary antibiotic bacitracin.
✚/▲ warning/side-effects: *see* POLYMYXIN B SULPHATE; TRYPSIN.

Otrivine (*Ciba*) is a proprietary SYMPATHOMIMETIC nasal DECONGESTANT, available only on prescription, and produced in the form of drops and spray. Otrivine Paediatric drops (at half the strength) are available for children. Otrivine's active constituent is xylometazoline hydrochloride.
✚/▲ warning/side-effects: *see* XYLOMETAZOLINE HYDROCHLORIDE.

Otrivine-Antistin (*Zyma*) is a proprietary non-prescription ANTIHISTAMINE drug, used to treat allergic and inflammatory ophthalmic conditions. Produced in the form of eye-drops, Otrivine-Antistin contains antazoline and xylometazoline hydrochloride. It is not recommended for children aged under 2 years. Otrivine-Antistin is produced also by Ciba in the form of nose-drops and as a nasal spray, neither of which is available from the National Health Service.
✚/▲ warning/side-effects: *see* ANTAZOLINE; XYLOMETAZOLINE HYDROCHLORIDE.

ouabain is a CARDIAC GLYCOSIDE that acts as a strong heart stimulant, and is thus used to treat heart failure and severe heartbeat irregularity. Administration is almost always by injection.
+ warning: ouabain should be administered with caution to patients who have undergone a recent heart attack, or who suffer from disorders of the thyroid gland. Dosage should be reduced for the elderly.
▲ side-effects: there may be serious effects on the heart rate. Sometimes there is nausea and vomiting.
Related article: OUABAINE ARNAUD.

Ouabaine Arnaud (*Lewis*) is a proprietary heart stimulant drug, a CARDIAC GLYCOSIDE, available only on prescription, used to treat heart attack and severe heartbeat irregularity. Produced in ampoules for injection, Ouabaine Arnaud's active constituent is ouabain.
+/▲ warning/side-effects: *see* OUABAIN.

Ovestin (*Organon*) is a proprietary OESTROGEN preparation, available only on prescription, used to treat vaginal and cervical disorders during the menopause. Produced in the form of tablets and cream, Ovestin contains oestriol.
+/▲ warning/side-effects: *see* OESTRIOL.

Ovran (*Wyeth*) is a proprietary OESTROGEN-and-PROGESTOGEN preparation, available only on prescription, used as a combined ORAL CONTRACEPTIVE and to treat menstrual problems. Produced in the form of tablets in a 21 day calender pack representing one menstrual cycle, Ovran contains levonorgestrel and ethinyloestradiol. A lower-dosage version is available under the name Ovran 30.
+/▲ warning/side-effects: *see* ETHINYLOESTRADIOL; LEVONORGESTREL.

Ovranette (*Wyeth*) is a proprietary OESTROGEN-and-PROGESTOGEN preparation (a lower dosage version of OVRAN), available only on prescription, used as a combined ORAL CONTRACEPTIVE. Produced in the form of tablets in a 21 day calender pack representing one menstrual cycle, Ovranette contains levonorgestrel and ethinyloestradiol.
+/▲ warning/side-effects: *see* ETHINYLOESTRADIOL; LEVONORGESTREL.

Ovysmen (*Ortho-Cilag*) is a proprietary OESTROGEN-and-PROGESTOGEN preparation, available only on prescription, used as an combined ORAL CONTRACEPTIVE. Produced in the form of tablets in a 21 day calender pack representing one menstrual cycle, Ovysmen contains norethisterone and ethinyloestradiol.
+/▲ warning/side-effects: *see* ETHINYLOESTRADIOL; NORETHISTERONE.

oxaminiquine is an ANTHELMINTIC drug that is effective in treating bilharziasis (schistosomiasis) caused by the intestinal fluke parasite Schistosoma mansoni, not uncommon in Africa, the West Indies, and South and Central America. Administration is oral, and toxicity is minimal.

Oxanid (*Steinhard*) is a proprietary ANXIOLYTIC or TRANQUILLIZER drug, available only on prescription to private patients, used to treat acute anxiety and attacks of phobic

panic. Produced in the form of tablets (in three strengths), Oxanid is a preparation of the BENZODIAZEPINE oxazepam.
✚/▲ warning/side-effects: *see* OXAZEPAM.

oxatomide is a relatively new ANTIHISTAMINE, used to treat hay fever, urticaria and other allergic conditions, particularly those concerned with food intake. Administration is oral in the form of tablets. It is not recommended for children aged under 5 years.
✚ warning: as with all antihistamines, oxatomide may cause drowsiness, or loss of the ability to concentrate. It should be administered with caution to patients with epilepsy, glaucoma, liver disease, or enlargement of the prostate gland. It may also enhance the effects of alcohol consumption.
▲ side-effects: there may be headache, dry mouth, gastrointestinal disturbances and/or visual disturbances. High dosage may lead to increased appetite and consequent weight gain.
Related article: TINSET.

oxazepam is a short-acting ANXIOLYTIC or TRANQUILIZER drug, one of the BENZODIAZEPINES used primarily to relieve acute anxiety or an attack of phobic panic. Administration is oral in the form of tablets or capsules.
✚ warning: oxazepam may reduce a patient's concentration and intricacy of movement or thought; it may enhance the effects of alcohol consumption. Prolonged use or abrupt withdrawal should be avoided. It should be administered with caution to patients with respiratory difficulties, glaucoma, or kidney or liver damage; who are in the last stages of pregnancy; or who are elderly or debilitated.
▲ side-effects: drowsiness usually occurs; there may also be dizziness, headache, dry mouth and shallow breathing. Hypersensitive reactions may occur. Repeated doses are, however, less cumulative in effect than with many other benzodiazepine anxiolytics.
Related article: OXANID.

oxedrine tartrate is a VASOCONSTRICTOR, a SYMPATHOMIMETIC used to treat very low blood pressure (hypotension) or cardiac arrest. Administration is oral in the form of a liquid, or by intramuscular or intravenous injection.
✚ warning: oxedrine tartrate should not be administered to patients who suffer a heart attack caused by interruption of the blood supply (myocardial infarction), or who are pregnant. An escape of the drug into the tissues at the site of the injection may cause tissue damage.
▲ side-effects: there is a risk of speeding the heart rate too much, resulting in high blood pressure (hypertension) or of reflex brachycardia (slowing of the heart rate), and associated headache and palpitations. There may be vomiting, and tingling and coolness of the skin. Prolonged treatment may result in kidney problems.
Related article: SYMPATOL.

oxerutins are mixtures of vasodilating RUTOSIDES that are thought to reduce the fragility and the permeability of the capillary blood vessels. They are used to treat disorders of the

O

veins, mostly in the legs.

oxethazaine is a minor local ANAESTHETIC used in very mild solution within other preparations to relieve incidental local pain. It is for example used in one proprietary antacid. *Related article:* MUCAINE.

oxpentifylline is a drug used to treat circulation problems in the extremities, and the attendant neural effects. Administration is oral in the form of tablets, or by injection. It is not recommended for children.
✚ warning: oxpentifylline should be administered with caution to patients with low blood pressure (hypotension).
▲ side-effects: there may be flushes, dizziness and/or nausea.
Related article: TRENTAL.

oxprenolol is a BETA-BLOCKER, a drug used to control and regulate the heart rate and and irregularities in its rhythms (arrhythmias), and to treat high blood pressure (*see* ANTI-HYPERTENSIVE) and angina. It is also used to treat the symptoms of excessive amounts of thyroid hormones in the bloodstream (including goitre). Administration is oral in the form of tablets, or by injection.
✚ warning: oxprenolol should not be administered to patients with heart disease or asthma; it should be administered with caution to those with liver or kidney disease, or who are pregnant or lactating. Withdrawal of treatment must be gradual.
▲ side-effects: there may be a slowing of the heartbeat, with coldness of the extremities. Sometimes there is respiratory depression and/or gastrointestinal disturbances.
Related articles: APSOLOX; LARACOR; SLOW-PREN; SLOW-TRASICOR; TRASICOR.

oxybenzone is a derivative of aminobenzoic acid used to protect the skin from ultraviolet radiation. It is a constituent in several suntan lotions and barrier creams for topical application.
✚/▲ warning/side-effects: *see* AMINOBENZOIC ACID.

oxybuprocaine is a widely-used local ANAESTHETIC with, particularly used in ophthalmic treatments. In the form of oxybuprocaine hydrochloride, it is administered as eye-drops.
▲ side-effects: there may be initial stinging on application.
Related articles: MINIMS BENOXINATE; OPULETS.

oxygen is an odourless, colourless gas which makes up 20% of the air at usual surface levels. Breathed into the human body through the lungs and taken up by the bloodstream, it combines chemically with glucose (or other sugars) to provide energy for metabolism. Therapeutically, oxygen is administered both to relieve respiratory problems and to maintain metabolic functions. Dosage (that is, concentration) is critical, for too much OR too little may be harmful. Too little prevents body function; too much may eventually inhibit the body's respiratory mechanism altogether. For emergency purposes (when blood gas measurements are not immediately feasible), a 35%-50% oxygen concentration is normally used, administered through a mask. Blood gas measurements should, however, be taken as soon as possible and regularly thereafter in order to achieve an optimum dosage level. Many patients who suffer from respiratory complications need an intermittent supply of oxygen daily: cylinders of oxygen, with a breathing-mask attachment, are available on prescription from the National Health Service for use at home (although counselling is normally given first about the fire risk). Also available are oxygen concentrators.

oxymetazoline is a VASOCONSTRICTOR, a potent SYMPATHOMIMETIC used primarily as a nasal decongestant. It works by constricting the blood vessels of the nose, thus in turn constricting the nasal mucous membranes. Administration is in the form of nose-drops or nasal spray.

✚ warning: prolonged use may result in tolerance, leading to even worse nasal congestion. Oxymetazoline should be administered with caution to children aged under 3 months.

▲ side-effects: there may be local irritation.
Related articles: AFRAZINE; ILIADIN-MINI.

oxymetholone is an anabolic STEROID used primarily to treat aplastic anaemia, but also to assist post-operative and convalescent recovery to full metabolic function. Administration is oral in the form of tablets.

✚ warning: the necessarily prolonged high-dosage treatment of anaemias ordinarily produces some masculinizing effects in women; such effects are, however, potentially reversible. Oxymetholone should not be administered to patients with impaired liver function or cancer of the prostate gland, or who are pregnant or lactating. It should be administered with caution to patients who are diabetic or epileptic; who have heart or kidney disease; or who suffer from migraine. Bone growth in children should be monitored for 6 months following treatment.

▲ side-effects: there may be acne, jaundice and high blood calcium levels, with fluid retention in the tissues (oedema). Prolonged treatment with high doses may in women cause menstrual problems and some degree of masculinization.
Related article: ANAPOLON 50.

Oxymycin (*DDSA Pharmaceuticals*) is a proprietary ANTIBIOTIC, available only on prescription, used to treat many serious microbial infections, such as severe acne vulgaris and exacerbations of chronic bronchitis. Produced in the form of tablets, Oxymycin's active constituent is the TETRACYCLINE oxytetracycline dihydrate.

✚/▲ warning/side-effects: *see* OXYTETRACYCLINE.

oxypertine is a powerful ANTIPSYCHOTIC drug used to treat and tranquillize psychosis (such as schizophrenia); it is suitable both for manic and hyperactive forms of behavioural disturbance, as well as for apathetic and withdrawal forms. The drug may also be used to treat severe anxiety in the short term. Administration is oral in the form of capsules or tablets.

✚ warning: oxypertine should not be administered to patients who suffer from reduction in the bone marrow's capacity for producing blood cells, or from certain types of glaucoma. It should be administered only with caution to patients with heart or vascular disease, kidney or liver disease, parkinsonism, or depression; or who are pregnant or lactating. Abrupt withdrawal should be avoided. It is not recommended for children.

▲ side-effects: patients should be warned before treatment that their judgement and powers of concentration may become defective under treatment. There may be restlessness, insomnia and nightmares; rashes and jaundice may occur; and there may be dry mouth, constipation, difficulties on urination, and blurred vision.

Related article: INTEGRIN.

oxyphenbutazone is an ANTI-INFLAMMATORY non-narcotic ANALGESIC used to relieve pain in rheumatic and arthritic joints, and in gout; in solution it is used as an eye ointment to treat local infection. Administration is oral, as eye-drops, or as anal suppositories.

✚ warning: ophthalmic treatment should not be prolonged.

▲ side-effects: oral treatment may cause nausea and dizziness, a rash and/or mouth ulcers.

Related article: TANDERIL.

oxytetracycline is a broad-spectrum ANTIBIOTIC used to treat many serious infections, particularly those of the urogenital organs and skin or membrane surfaces, of the bones, and of the respiratory passages. It may also be used to treat acne, although it is not suitable for children aged under 12 years. Administration is oral in the form of tablets or syrup.

✚ warning: oxytetracline should not be administered to patients who are pregnant, or who have kidney failure. It should be administered with caution to patients who are lactating. Some infections have now become resistant.

▲ side-effects: there may be nausea and vomiting, with diarrhoea; hypersentivity reactions may occur, as may photosensitivity (sensitivity of the skin and eyes to light), but both are rare.

Related articles: BERKMYCEN; CHEMOCYCLINE; GALENOMYCIN; Imperacin; OXYMYCIN; TERRA-CORTRIL; TERRAMYCIN; UNIMYCIN.

oxytocin is a natural HORMONE produced and secreted by the pituitary gland. Although it does not actually initiate the process, it increases the contractions of the womb during labour, and stimulates lactation in the breasts. Therapeutically, it may be administered orally or by injection to induce or assist labour (or abortion), or to stimulate lactation in women who have a hormonal insufficiency (in which case administration is by nasal spray). Sometimes it is additionally used to help stop post-natal bleeding.

✚ warning: oxytocin should not be administered to patients who suffer from muscular abnormalities of the womb or whose birth canal is obstructed in any way; or in whom the foetus is in evident distress. It should be administered with caution to those who suffer from high blood pressure (hypertension), who are about to undergo a multiple birth, or who have previously had a Caesarean section.

▲ side-effects: there may be heartbeat irregularity and cerebral pressure. High doses may lead to violent

contractions of the womb which may actually rupture the uterine wall and/or cause harm to the child.
Related articles: SYNTOCINON; SYNTOMETRINE.

O

Pabrinex (*Paines & Byrne*) is a proprietary VITAMIN preparation, available only on prescription, used to treat vitamin B and C deficiencies associated with acute feverish illnesses, with the effects of alcoholism or of certain drug treatments, or with states of confusion following severe illness or major surgery. It is produced in ampoules (in two strengths) for intramuscular injection, and in ampoules for intravenous injection.

Pacitron (*Berk*) is a proprietary ANTIDEPRESSANT, available only on prescription, used to treat mild to moderate depressive illness, although in combination with other antidepressants it may also be used to treat severe depressive illness. Produced in the form of tablets, Pacitron is a preparation of the amino acid tryptophan, and is not recommended for children.
✚/▲ warning/side-effects: *see* TRYPTOPHAN.

padimate O is a sunscreen that is capable of protecting the skin from ultraviolet radiation. For this reason, padimate O is a constituent in a number of suntan lotions. Administration is topical in the form of a solution.
✚ warning: protection is temporary, and the solution must be applied frequently. Some patients are in any case more sensitive to ultraviolet radiation than others. Padimate O is also flammable, and stains fabric.
Related article: SPECTRABAN.

Paedo-Sed (*Pharmax*) is a proprietary compound ANALGESIC, available on prescription only to private patients. Used to treat children, Paedo-Sed is a preparation of PARACETAMOL and the HYPNOTIC drug DICHLORALPHENAZONE, and is produced in the form of an elixir for dilution (the potency of the elixir once dilute is retained for 14 days).
✚/▲ warning/side-effects: *see* DICHLORALPHENAZONE; PARACETAMOL.

Palaprin Forte (*Nicholas*) is a proprietary non-prescription ANTI-INFLAMMATORY non-narcotic ANALGESIC used to relieve pain – particularly rheumatic and arthritic pain – and to treat other musculo-skeletal disorders. Produced in the form of tablets, Palaprin Forte is a preparation of the aspirin-like analgesic aloxiprin.
✚/▲ warning/side-effects: *see* ALOXIPRIN.

Paldesic (*RP Drugs*) is a proprietary non-prescription form of the non-narcotic ANALGESIC paracetamol. It is produced in the form of a syrup and is intended for hospital use only.
✚/▲ warning/side-effects: *see* PARACETAMOL.

Palfium (*MCP Pharmaceuticals*) is a proprietary narcotic ANALGESIC which, because it is a preparation of the OPIATE dextromoramide, is on the controlled drugs list. Used to relieve severe pain, especially during the final stages of terminal malignant disease, it is produced in the form of tablets (in two strengths), ampoules (in two strengths) for injection, and anal suppositories (which are not recommended for children).
✚/▲ warning/side-effects: *see* DEXTROMORAMIDE.

Paludrine (*ICI*) is a proprietary non-prescription drug used in the prevention of malaria (*see* ANTIMALARIAL). Produced in the form of tablets, Paludrine is a

preparation of proguanil hydrochloride.
✚/▲ warning/side-effects: *see* PROGUANIL.

Pamergan P100 (*Martindale*) is a proprietary narcotic ANALGESIC on the controlled drugs list, used both in the relief of pain and as a premedication prior to surgery, especially obstetrics. Produced in ampoules for injection, Pamergan P100 is a preparation of the narcotic analgesic pethidine hydrochloride and the SEDATIVE ANTIHISTAMINE promethazine hydrochloride.
✚/▲ warning/side-effects: *see* PETHIDINE; PROMETHAZINE HYDROCHLORIDE.

Pameton (*Winthrop*) is a proprietary non-prescription non-narcotic ANALGESIC, not available from the National Health Service, used to treat pain (especially for patients likely to overdose) and to reduce high body temperature. Produced in the form of tablets, Pameton is a compound preparation of PARACETAMOL and the amino acid METHIONINE (a paracetamol overdose antidote). It is not recommended for children aged under 6 years.
✚/▲ warning/side-effects: *see* METHIONINE; PARACETAMOL.

Panadeine (*Winthrop*) is a proprietary non-prescription compound ANALGESIC, not available from the National Health Service, used to treat pain and to reduce high body temperature. Produced in the form of tablets, and as effervescent tablets (under the name Panadeine Soluble), it is a preparation of paracetamol and codeine (a combination known as co-codamol), and is not recommended for children aged under 7 years. A stronger form is available only on prescription – but not from the National Health Service – (under the name Panadeine Forte), and is not recommended for children.
✚/▲ warning/side-effects: *see* CODEINE PHOSPHATE; PARACETAMOL.

Panadol (*Winthrop*) is a proprietary non-prescription non-narcotic ANALGESIC. Used to treat pain and to reduce high body temperature, it is produced in the form of tablets (of two kinds), as effervescent tablets (under the name Panadol Soluble), and as an elixir for dilution (the potency of the elixir once dilute is retained for 14 days). It is not available from the National Health Service. In all forms it is a preparation of paracetamol, and is not recommended for children aged under 3 months.
✚/▲ warning/side-effects: *see* PARACETAMOL.

Panasorb (*Winthrop*) is a proprietary non-prescription non-narcotic ANALGESIC, not available from the National Health Service, used to treat pain and high body temperature. Produced in the form of tablets in a SORBITOL base, it is a preparation of paracetamol, and is not recommended for children aged under 6 years.
✚/▲ warning/side-effects: *see* PARACETAMOL.

Pancrease (*Ortho-Cilag*) is a proprietary non-prescription form of pancreatic enzymes, used to treat enzymatic deficiency in such conditions as cystic fibrosis and chronic inflammation of the pancreas. Pancrease is produced in the form of capsules.

Pancrex (*Paines & Byrne*) is a proprietary non-prescription form of pancreatic enzymes, used to treat enzymatic deficiency in cystic fibrosis and similar diseases. Pancrex is produced in the form of granules, but (under the name Pancrex V) there are also versions available as a powder, as capsules (in two strengths, the weaker under the name Pancrex V "125"), and as tablets (in two strengths, the stronger under the name Pancrex V Forte).

pancuronium bromide is a SKELETAL MUSCLE RELAXANT used primarily under general anaesthesia for medium-duration paralysis. Administration is by injection.

✚ warning: the onset of the paralysis may be accompanied by temporarily increased heart rate: caution should be exercised in relation to patients for whom this might present difficulty. Dosage should be reduced for patients who suffer from impaired kidney function or who are obese.

▲ side-effects: paralysis is rapid in onset following injection.
Related article: PAVULON.

Panoxyl 2.5 (*Stiefel*) is a proprietary, non-prescription, topical preparation for the treatment of acne. Produced in the form of an aqueous gel, Panoxyl 2.5 is a solute preparation of the KERATOLYTIC benzoyl peroxide. A stronger version is produced also in the form of an aqueous gel and additionally as a gel in an alcohol base (under the name Panoxyl 5). And an even stronger preparation is available as an aqueous gel, as a gel in an alcohol base, and as a wash lotion in a detergent base (under the name Panoxyl 10).

✚/▲ warning/side-effects: *see* BENZOYL PEROXIDE.

Panthenol
see PANTOTHENIC ACID.

pantothenic acid, or panthenol, is an organic compound often classified as a VITAMIN of the B complex; it is a coenzyme – a catalyst in the reaction instituted by an enzyme – that assists in the metabolism of fatty acids. Dietary sources are many such as in milk, yeast, fresh vegetables and plentiful in normal life-styles; deficiency is exceptional. Pantothenic acid has no accepted therapeutic uses, although the calcium salt has been used to treat streptomycin intoxication and rheumatoid conditions.
Related articles: LIPOFLAVNOID; LIPOTRIAD; MULTIBIONTA; Solivito; VERDIVITON; VIGRANON B.

papaveretum is a compound preparation of alkaloids of opium, about half of which is made up of MORPHINE, the rest consisting proportions of CODEINE, NOSCAPINE and PAPAVERINE. It is used as a narcotic ANALGESIC primarily during or following surgery, but also as a SEDATIVE prior to an operation. Administration is oral in the form of tablets, or by injection. All proprietary preparations containing papaveretum are on the controlled drugs list: the drug is potentially addictive.

✚ warning: papaveretum should not be administered to patients who are suffering from head injury or intracranial pressure; it should be administered with caution to those with asthma, impaired kidney or liver function, hypotension (low blood pressure), or hypothyroidism (underactivity of the thyroid gland), who are pregnant or breast feeding, or who have a history of drug abuse. Dosage should be reduced for elderly or debilitated patients.

▲ side-effects: there is constipation and urinary retention, shallow breathing and cough suppression; there may also be nausea and vomiting, and drowsiness. Injections may cause pain and tissue damage at the site. Tolerance and dependence (addiction) occur readily.
Related articles: OMNOPON; OMNOPON-SCOPOLAMINE.

papaverine is an alkaloid of opium, technically an OPIATE but is unlike many others in being primarily a SMOOTH MUSCLE RELAXANT, and having little or no ANALGESIC effect. It is consequently used mostly in the treatment of the bronchospasm of asthma or to relieve other spasmodic conditions of smooth muscle, such as in indigestion or in vascular disorders of the limbs. It is present in some cough preparations. Administration is mostly (in the form of papaverine hydrochloride) as a solution for an aerosol spray or as a linctus, in combination with other anti-asthma drugs; it may sometimes be prescribed in the form of tablets.

✚ warning: papaverine should not be administered to patients with heart disease, especially if it involves heartbeat irregularities, or glaucoma.

▲ side-effects: it may cause heartbeat irregularitie, gastrointestinal disturbances, headache, sweating, vertigo and skin rash.
Related articles: ACTONORM; APP; BROVON; PAVACOL-D; Pholcomed; RYBARVIN.

paracetamol is a non-narcotic ANALGESIC used to treat all forms of mild to moderate pain; although it is also effective in reducing high body temperature it has no capacity for relieving inflammation. In many ways it is similar to ASPIRIN – except that it does not cause gastric irritation. It may (in high overdosage or prolonged use) cause liver damage. Many proprietary preparations combine the two analgesics (compound analgesics) although these are not generally recommended. Administration is oral in the form of tablets, capsules or a liquid.

✚ warning: paracetamol should be administered with caution to patients with impaired liver function or who suffer from alcoholism (which causes liver damage).

▲ side-effects: there are few side-effects if dosage is low; high overdosage or prolonged use may result in liver dysfunction.
Related articles: CAFADOL; CALPOL; CO-DYDRAMOL; DISPROL; DISTALGESIC; FEMERITAL; FORTAGESIC; LOBAK; MEDISED; MEDOCODENE; MIDRID; MIGRALEVE; MYOLGIN; NEURODYNE; NORGESIC; PAEDO-SED; PALDESIC; PAMETON; PANADEINE; PANADOL; PANASORB; PARACODOL; PARACLEAR; PARADEINE; PARAHYPON; PARAKE; PARAMAX; PARAMOL; PARDALE; PAXALGESIC; PHARMIDONE; PROPAIN; RINUREL; SAFAPRYN; SALZONE; SOLPADEINE; SYNDOL; UNIFLU; UNIGESIC; VEGANIN.

Paraclear (*Sussex Pharmaceuticals*) is a proprietary non-prescription non-narcotic ANALGESIC produced in the form of soluble tablets. It contains paracetamol.

✚/▲ warning/side-effects: *see* PARACETAMOL.

Paracodol (*Fisons*) is a pro-

prietary non-prescription compound ANALGESIC that is not available from the National Health Service. Used to treat muscular and rheumatic pain, and produced in the form of tablets for effervescent solution, it is a preparation of paracetamol and CODEINE phosphate (a combination itself known as co-codamol) and is not recommended for children aged under 6 years.
✚/▲ warning/side-effects: *see* CODEINE; PARACETAMOL.

Paradeine (*Scotia*) is a proprietary non-prescription compound ANALGESIC that is not obtainable from the National Health Service. Used to treat muscular and rheumatic pain, and produced in the form of tablets, Paradeine is a preparation of paracetamol and codeine phosphate, together with the LAXATIVE phenolphthalein.
✚/▲ warning/side-effects: *see* CODEINE PHOSPHATE; PARACETAMOL; PHENOLPHTHALEIN.

paraffin is a hydrocarbon derived from petroleum. Its main therapeutic use is as a base for ointments (in the form of yellow or white soft paraffin). As a mineral oil, liquid paraffin is used as an effective laxative (although prolonged use may have unpleasant side-effects) and as an eye ointment in cases of tear deficiency.
see LIQUID PARAFFIN.

Parahypon (*Calmic*) is a proprietary non-prescription compound ANALGESIC that is not available from the National Health Service. Used to relieve most types of pain, and produced in the form of tablets, Parahypon is a preparation of paracetamol and codeine phosphate with the stimulant caffeine. It is not recommended for children aged under 6 years.
✚/▲ warning/side-effects: *see* CAFFEINE; CODEINE PHOSPHATE; PARACETAMOL.

Parake (*Galen*) is a proprietary non-prescription compound ANALGESIC that is not available from the National Health Service. Used both to relieve pain and to reduce high body temperature, and produced in the form of tablets, Parake is a preparation of paracetamol and codeine phosphate (a combination itself known as co-codamol) and is not recommended for children.
✚/▲ warning/side-effects: *see* CODEINE PHOSPHATE; PARACETAMOL.

paraldehyde is a strong-smelling and fast-acting SEDATIVE. It is primarily used in the treatment of severe and continuous epileptic seizures (status epilepticus), and is administered generally by injection although it is sometimes instead administered via the rectum in the form of an enema.
✚ warning: paraldehyde should be administered with caution to patients with lung disease or impaired liver function. Keep away from rubber, plastics or fabric.
▲ side-effects: a rash is not uncommon. The injections may be painful.

Paramax (*Beecham*) is a proprietary non-narcotic ANALGESIC, available only on prescription, used to relieve the pain of migraine. Produced in the form of tablets and as a sugar-free powder in sachets for effervescent solution, Paramax is a preparation of paracetamol and the ANTINAUSEANT metoclopramide hydrochloride. It is not recommended for children.

✚/▲ warning/side-effects: *see* METOCLOPRAMIDE; PARACETAMOL.

Paramol (*Duncan, Flockhart*) is a proprietary compound ANALGESIC, available on prescription only to private patients, used as a painkiller and as a cough suppressant. Produced in the form of tablets, Paramol is a preparation of paracetamol and the OPIATE dihydrocodeine tartrate (a combination itself known as co-dydramol) and is not recommended for children.
✚/▲ warning/side-effects: *see* DIHYDROCODEINE TARTRATE; PARACETAMOL.

Paraplatin (*Bristol-Myers*) is a proprietary CYTOTOXIC drug, available only on prescription, used to treat certain types of solid tumour such as cancer of the ovary. Produced in the form of powder for reconstitution as a medium for injection, Paraplatin is a preparation of the CISPLATIN derivative carboplatin.
✚/▲ warning/side-effects: *see* CARBOPLATIN.

***parasympathomimetics** are drugs that have effects similar to those of the parasympathetic nervous system. They work by mimicking the actions of a natural neurotransmitter (e.g. ACETYLCHOLINE CHLORIDE) or by prolonging its duration of action (e.g. NEOSTIGMINE). Important actions include slowing of the heart, vasodilation, construction of the bronchioles, stimulation of the muscles of the intestine and bladder, dilation of the pupil and altering the focusing of the eye. ANTICHOLINERGIC drugs oppose some of these actions.

Pardale (*Martindale*) is a proprietary non-prescription compound ANALGESIC that is not available from the National Health Service. Used to relieve headaches and menstrual and rheumatic pain, and produced in the form of tablets, Pardale is a preparation of paracetamol and codeine phosphate together with the mild stimulant caffeine hydrate. It is not recommended for children.
✚/▲ warning/side-effects: *see* CAFFEINE; CODEINE PHOSPHATE; PARACETAMOL.

Parentrovite (*Bencard*) is a proprietary VITAMIN preparation, available only on prescription, used to treat vitamin B and C deficiencies associated with acute illnesses such as those that involve high body temperature, that result from alcoholism or from drug treatment, or that accompany states of confusion following severe illness or major surgery. It is produced in ampoules (in two strengths) for intramuscular injection, and in ampoules for intravenous injection.
✚/▲ warning/side-effects: *see* THIAMINE.

Parfenac (*Lederle*) is a proprietary non-steroidal ANTI-INFLAMMATORY drug, available only on prescription, used in topical application to treat mild inflammation on the skin. Produced in the form of a water-miscible cream, Parfenac is a preparation of bufexamac.
✚/▲ warning/side-effects: *see* BUFEXAMAC

Parlodel (*Sandoz*) is a proprietary preparation of the drug bromocriptine, used primarily to treat parkinsonism but not the parkinsonian symptoms caused by certain drug therapies (*see* ANTIPARKINSONISM). It may also be used to treat delayed puberty caused by hormonal insufficiency,

to relieve certain menstrual disorders, or to reduce or halt lactation. It is produced in the form of tablets (in two strengths) and capsules (in two strengths).
✚/▲ warning/side-effects: *see* BROMOCRIPTINE.

Parmid (*Lagap*) is a proprietary ANTINAUSEANT, available only on prescription, used to treat severe conditions of nausea and vomiting especially when associated with gastrointestinal disorders, during radiotherapy, or accompanying treatment with cytotoxic drugs. Produced in the form of tablets, as a syrup, and in ampoules for injection, Parmid is a preparation of metoclopramide hydrochloride. Use is restricted to patients under 20 years of age.
✚/▲ warning/side-effects: *see* METOCLOPRAMIDE.

Parnate (*Smith Kline & French*) is a proprietary ANTIDEPRESSANT drug, available only on prescription. Produced in the form of tablets, Parnate is a preparation of the MAO INHIBITOR tranylcypromine. It is not recommended for children.
✚/▲ warning/side-effects: *see* TRANYLCYPROMINE.

Paroven (*Zyma*) is a proprietary non-prescription preparation used to treat symptoms of cramps and other manifestations of poor circulation in the veins. Produced in the form of capsules, Paroven is a preparation of oxerutins and is not recommended for children.
✚/▲ warning/side-effects: *see* OXERUTINS.

Parstelin (*Smith Kline & French*) is a proprietary ANTIDEPRESSANT drug, available only on prescription, used to treat depressive illness particularly in association with anxiety. Produced in the form of tablets, Parstelin is a compound preparation of the MAO INHIBITOR tranylcypromine and the ANTI-EMETIC tranquillizer trifluoperazine. It is not recommended for children.
✚/▲ warning/side-effects: *see* TRANYLCYPROMINE; TRIFLUOPERAZINE.

Parvolex (*Duncan, Flockhart*) is a proprietary form of the amino acid acetylcysteine, available only on prescription, used in emergencies to treat paracetamol overdosage and so to try to limit liver damage. It is produced in ampoules for injection.
✚/▲ warning/side-effects: *see* ACETYLCYSTEINE.

Pavacol-D (*Boehringer Ingelheim*) is a proprietary non- prescription cough mixture. It is a sugar-free preparation of the opiates papaverine hydrochloride and pholcodine for solution with the sugar-substitute sorbitol (the potency of the mixture once dilute is retained for 14 days). It is not recommended for children aged under 12 months.
✚/▲ warning/side-effects: *see* PAPAVERINE; PHOLCODINE.

Pavulon (*Organon-Teknika*) is a proprietary SKELETAL MUSCLE RELAXANT of the type known as competitive or non-depolarizing. Available only on prescription, it is used during surgical operations, but only after the patient has been rendered unconscious. Produced in ampoules for injection, Pavulon is a preparation of pancuronium bromide.
✚/▲ warning/side-effects: *see* PANCURONIUM BROMIDE.

Paxadon (*Steinhard*) is a proprietary non-prescription VITAMIN B supplement that is not available from the National

Health Service. Used to treat vitamin deficiency and associated symptoms, Paxadon is a preparation of PYRIDOXINE hydrochloride (vitamin B_6). It is produced in the form of tablets.
✚/▲ warning/side-effects: *see* PYRIDOXINE

Paxane (*Steinhard*) is a proprietary TRANQUILLIZER and HYPNOTIC, available on prescription only to private patients, used to treat insomnia in cases where some degree of daytime sedation is acceptable, short-term use only. Produced in the form of capsules (in two strengths), Paxane is a preparation of the long-acting BENZODIAZEPINE flurazepam.
✚/▲ warning/side-effects: *see* FLURAZEPAM.

Paxofen (*Steinhard*) is a proprietary ANTI-INFLAMMATORY non-narcotic ANALGESIC, available only on prescription, used to treat the pain of rheumatic and other musculo-skeletal disorders. Produced in the form of tablets (in three strengths), Paxofen is a preparation of ibuprofen.
✚/▲ warning/side-effects: *see* IBUPROFEN.

Paynocil (*Beecham*) is a proprietary non-prescription preparation of the non-narcotic ANALGESIC aspirin that is not available from the National Health Service. Used to relieve pain and reduce high body temperature, especially in relation to rheumatic conditions. Produced in the form of tablets, Paynocil also contains the essential amino acid glycine. It is not recommended for children.
✚/▲ warning/side-effects: *see* ASPIRIN.

PC4 (*Schering*) is a proprietary form of ORAL CONTRACEPTIVE for use after sexual intercourse has already taken place. Available only on prescription as as occasional emergency measure, and produced in the form of tablets, PC4 is a preparation of the OESTROGEN ethinyloestradiol and the PROGESTOGEN norgestrel.
✚/▲ warning/side-effects: *see* ETHINYLOESTRADIOL; NORGESTREL.

Ped-El (*KabiVitrum*) is a preparation of additional electrolytes and trace elements for use in association with Vamin (proprietary) amino acid solutions for use as intravenous nutrition. Available only on prescription, Ped-El is intended primarily for paediatric use.
see VAMIN.

***pediculicidal** drugs kill lice of the genus Pediculus, which infest either the body or the scalp – or both – and cause intense itching. Scratching tends only to damage the skin surface, and may eventually cause weeping lesions or bacterial infection on top. Best known and most used pediculicides include malathion and carbaryl; the once commonly used lindane is now no longer recommended for lice on the scalp because resistant strains have emerged. Administration is topical, generally in the form of a lotion; contact between drug and skin should be as long as possible (at least two hours), which is why shampoos are less commonly used.
✚/▲ warning/side-effects: *see* BENZYL BENZOATE; CARBARYL; LINDANE; MALATHION.

pemoline is a fairly mild STIMULANT that works by direct action on the brain, and is used primarily to treat debility, lassitude, senility or fatigue. It may also be administered to prevent patients from becoming too drowsy following the administration of other drugs. Administration is oral in the form of tablets, it is not recommended and should not be used to treat depression.

✚ warning: pemoline should not be administered to patients with heart disease, glaucoma, extrapyramidal disorders, hyperexcitable states.

▲ side-effects: concentration and speed of thought and movement may be affected. There may also be sweating and slight headache. High dosage may cause heartbeat irregularities and dizziness, insomnia. agitation.

Related article: VOLITAL.

Penbritin (*Beecham*) is a proprietary form of the broad-spectrum penicillin ampicillin, available only on prescription. A powerful ANTIBIOTIC used mainly to treat infections of the respiratory passages, the middle ear and the urinary tract, it is also effective against gonorrhoea. Penbritin is produced in the form of capsules (in two strengths), as tablets for children, as a syrup (in two strengths, for dilution; the potency of the syrup once diluted is retained for 7 days), as a children's suspension for use with a pipette, and as powder for reconstitution as a solution for injections.

✚/▲ warning/side-effects: *see* AMPICILLIN.

penbutolol sulphate is a BETA-BLOCKER used as an ANTI-HYPERTENSIVE drug. Administration is in combination with the DIURETIC FRUSEMIDE, and is oral in the form of tablets.

✚ warning: propanolol should not be administered to patients withany serious form of heart disesase, or asthma. It should be administered with caution to those with impaired liver or kidney function, who are nearing the end of pregnancy, or who are lactating.

▲ side-effects: the heart rate is slowed; there may also be bronchospasm (causing asthma-like symptoms), gastrointestinal disturbances, and tingling or numbness in the fingers and toes.

Related article: LASIPRESSIN.

Pendramine (*Degussa*) is a proprietary non-steroidal ANTI-INFLAMMATORY drug, available only on prescription, used to relieve the pain and to halt the progress of severe rheumatoid arthritis. The drug may also be used as a long-term chelating agent to treat poisoning by the metals copper or lead (especially in metabolic disorders like Wilson's disease). Produced in the form of tablets (in two strengths), Pendramine is a preparation of the penicillin-derivative penicillamine.

✚/▲ warning/side-effects: *see* PENICILLAMINE.

Penetrol (*Crookes Healthcare Prooducts UK*) is a proprietary non-prescription preparation for the relief of catarrh. Produced in the form of an inhalant and as lozenges, it contains MENTHOL, eucalyptus and peppermint oils.

✚/▲ warning/side-effects: *see* PEPPERMINT OIL.

penicillamine is a breakdown product of penicillin that is an extremely effective CHELATING AGENT: it binds various metals (and mineral substances) as it passes through the body before being excreted in the normal way. It is thus used to treat various forms of metallic

P

poisoning – notably copper poisoning in Wilson's disease, lead and mercury poisoning – and can also be used to assist in the treatment of severe rheumatoid arthritis or juvenile chronic arthritis, especially when anti-inflammatory analgesics (such as aspirin) have proved unsuccessful; in the treatment of chronic hepatitis once the acute phase is over; and in the treatment of biliary cirrhosis. Administration is oral in the form of tablets.

✚ warning: penicillamine should not be administered to patients with the serious skin disorder lupus erythematosus; it should be administered with caution to those with impaired kidney function, or some forms of hypertension (high blood pressure), who are pregnant, who are taking any form of immunosuppressant drug,or who are sensitive to penicillin. Patients should be warned that treatment may take up to 12 weeks for any effect to become apparent, and up to 6 months to achieve its full therapeutic effect. Regular and frequent blood counts and urine analyses are essential.

▲ side-effects: there may be nausea, but this can be minimized by taking the drug before food or on going to bed. Between the sixth and twelfth weeks of treatment there is commonly a loss of the sense of taste. There is commonly also a rash. Some patients experience extreme weight loss, mouth ulcers, muscle weakness, fluid retention and/or blood disorders. *Related articles:* DISTAMINE; PENDRAMINE.

penicillin G is a term for the ANTIBIOTIC more commonly known as benzylpenicillin. *see* BENZYLPENICILLIN.

penicillin V is a term for the ANTIBIOTIC more commonly known as phenoxymethylpenicillin. *see* PHENOXYMETHYLPENICILLIN.

penicillin VK is a term for the potassium salt of the ANTIBIOTIC more commonly known as phenoxymethylpenicillin. *see* PHENOXYMETHYLPENICILLIN.

penicillinases are enzyme-like substances produced by some bacteria that commonly inhibit or completely neutralize the antibacterial activity of many forms of PENICILLIN. Treatment of infections caused by bacteria that produce penicillinases has generally therefore to be undertaken with other forms of antibiotic. Therapeutically, however, penicillinases can be used (in purified form) to treat sensitivity reactions to penicillin, or in tests to identify micro-organisms in blood samples taken from patients who are taking penicillin.

penicillins are effective ANTIBIOTIC drugs that work by interfering with the synthesis of bacterial cell walls. They are absorbed rapidly by most (but not all) body tissues and fluids, perfuse through the kidneys, and are excreted in the urine. One great disadvantage of penicillins is that many patients are allergic to them – allergy to one means allergy to all – and may cause reactions that range from a minor rash right up to anaphylactic shock which may be fatal. Very high dosage may rarely cause brain damage and convulsions, or may cause abnormally high body levels of sodium or potassium, with consequent symptoms. Best known and most used penicillins include benzylpenicillin

(penicillin G, the first of the penicillins), phenoxymethylpenicillin (penicillin V), cloxacillin, flucloxacillin, amoxycillin and ampicillin. Those taken orally tend to cause diarrhoea.
✚/▲ warning/side-effects: *see* AMOXYCILLIN; AMPICILLIN; AZLOCILLIN; BACAMPICILLIN HYDROCHLORIDE; BENETHAMINE PENICILLIN; BENZATHINE PENICILLIN; BENZYLPENICILLIN; CARBENICILLIN; CARFECILLIN SODIUM; CICLACILLIN; CLOXACILLIN; FLUCLOXACILLIN; MECILLINAM; METHICILLIN SODIUM; MEZLOCILLIN; PHENETHICILLIN; PHENOXYMETHYLPENICILLIN; PIPERACILLIN; PIVAMPICILLIN; PIVMECILLINAM; PROCAINE PENICILLIN; TALAMPICILLIN HYDROCHLORIDE; TICARCILLIN.

Penidural (*Wyeth*) is a proprietary ANTIBIOTIC, available only on prescription, used to treat many forms of infection (including syphilis) and to relieve the symptoms of rheumatic fever. Produced in the form of a suspension for dilution (the potency of the suspension once dilute is retained for 14 days), as drops for children, and in vials for injection (under the name Penidural-LA), Penidural is a preparation of benzathine penicillin.
✚/▲ warning/side-effects: *see* BENZATHINE PENICILLIN.

Penotrane (*Boehringer Ingelheim*) is a proprietary ANTISEPTIC that has ANTIBACTERIAL and ANTIFUNGAL properties, available only on prescription, used in topical application to treat vaginal infections. Produced in the form of vaginal inserts (pessaries), Penotrane is a preparation of the organic mercurial compound hydrargaphen.
✚/▲ warning/side-effects: *see* HYDRARGAPHEN.

pentaerythritol tetranitrate is a powerful VASODILATOR that is extremely effective in preventing and treating the symptoms of angina pectoris (heart pain). It works by dilating the veins returning blood to the heart, thus reducing the pressure within the heart and reducing its workload at the same time. Fairly short-acting, pentaerythritol tetranitrate's effect is generally extended through its preparation in sustained-release capsules to be kept under the tongue; administration is also in the form of tablets.
✚ warning: pentaerythritol tetranitrate should be administered with caution to patients with low blood pressure (hypotension) and associated conditions.
▲ side-effects: there may be headache, flushes and dizziness; some patients experience an increase in heart rate.
Related articles: CARDIACAP; MYCARDOL.

pentamidine is an ANTI-PROTOZOAL drug that is used to treat pneumonia caused by the protozoan micro-organism Pneumocystis carinii in patients whose immune system has been suppressed (either following transplant surgery or because of a condition such as AIDS). However, it is not ordinarily available in the United Kingdom.

pentazocine is a powerful narcotic ANALGESIC used to treat moderate to severe pain. Much like MORPHINE in effect and action, it is less likely to cause dependence. Administration is

P

oral in the form of capsules and tablets, topical in the form of anal suppositories, or by injection. Treatment by injection has a stronger effect than oral treatment. The proprietary form is on the controlled drugs list.

✚ warning: pentazocine should not be administered to patients who have recently had a heart attack, with high blood pressure (hypertension), heart failure, respiratory depression or head injury, who are taking any other narcotic analgesic, who are pregnant or have kidney or liver damage. Patients should be warned that hallucinations and other disturbances in thought and sensation may occur, especially following administration by injection.

▲ side-effects: there is sedation and dizziness, with nausea; injection may lead to hallucinations. There is often also constipation. Tolerance and dependence (addiction) may result from prolonged treatment.
Related article: FORTRAL

Pentostam (*Wellcome*) is a proprietary preparation of the drug sodium stibogluconate (an organic compound of antimony), available only on prescription, used to treat skin infections by protozoan micro-organisms of the genus Leishmania (leishmaniasis). It is produced in a solution for injection.

✚/▲ warning/side-effects: *see* SODIUM STIBOGLUCONATE.

Pentovis (*Parke-Davis; Warner UK*) is a proprietary female sex HORMONE preparation, available only on prescription, used to make up hormonal deficiency during and after the menopause. Produced in the form of capsules, Pentovis is a preparation of the OESTROGEN quinestradol.

✚/▲ warning/side-effects: *see* QUINESTRADOL.

peppermint oil is used to relieve the discomfort of abdominal colic and distension of severe indigestion or flatulence. It is thought to work by direct action on the smooth muscle of the intestinal walls. Administration is oral in the form of capsules.

✚ warning: peppermint oil should not be administered to patients who suffer from paralytic ileus or ulcerative colitis; a very few patients are allergic to menthol.

▲ side-effects: there may be heartburn and local irritation.
Related articles: CARBELLON; COLPERMIN; MINTEC; TERCODA.

Peptard (*Riker*) is a proprietary ANTISPASMODIC drug, available only on prescription, used to assist in the treatment of gastrointestinal disorders arising from muscular spasm of the intestinal walls. Produced in the form of sustained-release tablets, Peptard is a preparation of the HYOSCINE-like ANTICHOLINERGIC drug HYOSCYAMINE sulphate; it is not recommended for children aged under 10 years.

✚/▲ warning/side-effects: *see* ATROPINE SULPHATE

Peptisorbon (*Merck*) is a proprietary, non-prescription, sucrose-, galactose-, fructose- and gluten-free, lactose-low powder that is a complete nutritional diet for patients who have conditions involving the malabsorption of food (such as following gastrectomy). Produced in sachets for solution, Peptisorbon is a preparation of amino acids and peptides, carbohydrate, fats, and vitamins and minerals. It is not suitable for children.

Percutol (*Rorer*) is a proprietary non-prescription VASODILATOR, used to prevent recurrent attacks of angina pectoris (heart pain). Produced in the form of an ointment for use on a dressing strapped to the skin surface (on the chest, arm or thigh), Percutol is a preparation of glyceryl trinitrate. It is not recommended for children.

✚/▲ warning/side-effects: *see* GLYCERYL TRINITRATE.

Pergonal (*Serono*) is a proprietary preparation of follicle-stimulating hormone (FSH), available only on prescription, used to treat women suffering from specific hormonal deficiency to treat the resulting infertility. Produced in the form of a powder for reconstitution as a medium for injection, Pergonal is a preparation of human FSH, human luteinising hormone and lactose.

✚/▲ warning/side-effects: *see* FSH.

Periactin (*Merck, Sharp & Dohme*) is a proprietary non-prescription ANTIHISTAMINE, used both to treat the symptoms of allergic disorders like hay fever and as a tonic for stimulating appetite. Produced in the form of tablets and as a syrup for dilution (the potency of the syrup once dilute is retained for 14 days), Periactin is a preparation of cyproheptadine hydrochloride, and is not recommended for children aged under 2 years.

✚/▲ warning/side-effects: *see* CYPROHEPTADINE HYDROCHLORIDE.

pericyazine is an ANTIPSYCHOTIC drug used to tranquillize patients suffering from schizophrenia and other psychoses, particularly during behavioural disturbances. The drug may also be used in the short term to treat severe anxiety. Administration is oral in the form of tablets or a dilute elixir.

✚ warning: pericyazine should not be administered to patients with certain forms of glaucoma, whose blood-cell formation by the bone-marrow is reduced, or who are taking drugs that depress certain centres of the brain and spinal cord. It should be administered with caution to those with lung disease, cardiovascular disease, epilepsy, parkinsonism, abnormal secretion by the adrenal glands, impaired liver or kidney function, undersecretion of thyroid hormones (hypothyroidism), enlargement of the prostate gland or any form of acute infection; who are pregnant or lactating; or who are elderly. Prolonged use requires regular checks on eye function and skin pigmentation. Withdrawal of treatment should be gradual.

▲ side-effects: concentration and speed of thought and movement are affected; the effects of alcohol consumption are increased. There may be dry mouth and blocked nose, constipation and difficulty in urinating, and blurred vision; menstrual disturbances in women or impotence in men may occur, with weight gain; there may be sensitivity reactions. Some patients feel cold and depressed, and tend to suffer from poor sleep patterns. Blood pressure may be low and the heartbeat irregular. Prolonged high dosage may cause opacity in the cornea and lens of the eyes, and a purple pigmentation of the skin. Treatment by intramuscular

injection may be painful.
Related article: NEULACTIL.

Perifusin (*Merck*) is a proprietary fluid nutritional preparation, available only on prescription. Produced in the form of a solution for intravenous infusion into patients who cannot be fed via the alimentary canal because of conditions such as coma or prolonged disorders of the gastrointestinal tract. Perifusin is a preparation of amino acids with electrolytes.

Pernivit (*Duncan, Flockhart*) is a proprietary non-prescription VASODILATOR that is not available from the National Health Service. Used to treat poor circulation in the hands and feet, and produced in the form of tablets, Pernivit is a preparation of the B vitamin nicotinic acid and the synthetic vitamin K acetomenaphthone.
✚/▲ warning/side-effects: *see* NICOTINIC ACID.

Pernomol (*LAB*) is a proprietary non-prescription VASODILATOR used in topical application to treat chilblains. Produced in the form of a paint, Pernomol is a preparation of various natural oils and essences, including CHLORBUTOL and PHENOL.

per/vac is an abbreviation for pertussis vaccine (whooping cough vaccine).
see PERTUSSIS VACCINE.

perphenazine is an ANTIPSYCHOTIC drug used to tranquillize patients suffering from schizophrenia and other psychoses, particularly during behavioural disturbances. The drug may also be used in the short term to treat severe anxiety, to soothe patients who are dying, as a premedication prior to surgery, and to remedy intractable hiccups.
Alternatively, it may be used to relieve nausea and vertigo caused by disorders in the middle or inner ear. Administration is oral in the form of tablets, or by injection.
✚ warning: perphenazine should not be administered to patients with certain forms of glaucoma, whose blood-cell formation by the bone-marrow is reduced, or who are taking drugs that depress certain centres of the brain and spinal cord. It should be administered with caution to those with lung disease, cardiovascular disease, epilepsy, parkinsonism, abnormal secretion by the adrenal glands, impaired liver or kidney function, undersecretion of thyroid hormones (hypothyroidism), enlargement of the prostate gland or any form of acute infection; who are pregnant or lactating; or who are elderly. Prolonged use requires regular checks on eye function and skin pigmentation. Withdrawal of treatment should be gradual. It should not be administered to children.
▲ side-effects: concentration and speed of thought and movement are affected; the effects of alcohol consumption are increased. There may be dry mouth and blocked nose, constipation and difficulty in urinating, and blurred vision; menstrual disturbances in women or impotence in men may occur, with weight gain; there may be sensitivity reactions. Some patients feel cold and depressed, and tend to suffer from poor sleep patterns. Blood pressure may be low and the heartbeat

irregular. Prolonged high dosage may cause opacity in the cornea and lens of the eyes, and a purple pigmentation of the skin. Treatment by intramuscular injection may be painful.
Related article: FENTAZIN.

Persantin (*Boehringer Ingelheim*) is a proprietary preparation of the unusual drug dipyramidole, available only on prescription, used as an additional treatment with anticoagulants or aspirin in the prevention of thrombosis, especially during or following surgical procedures. It works by inhibiting the adhesiveness of blood platelets so that they stick neither to themselves nor to the walls of valves or tubes surgically inserted. The drug is produced in the form of tablets (in two strengths) and in ampoules for injection.
✚/▲ warning/side-effects: *see* DIPYRIDAMOLE.

Pertofran (*Geigy*) is a proprietary ANTIDEPRESSANT, available only on prescription. Produced in the form of tablets, Pertofran is a preparation of desipramine hydrochloride. It is not recommended for children.
✚/▲ warning/side-effects: *see* DESIPRAMINE HYDROCHLORIDE.

pertussis vaccine, or whooping cough VACCINE, is a suspension of dead pertussis bacteria (Bordetella pertussis) that is injected to cause the body's own defence mechanisms to form antibodies and thus provide immunity. It is available on prescription by itself, but it is most commonly administered as one element in the triple vaccination procedure involving diphtheria-pertussis-tetanus (DPT) vaccine. The vaccine remains the subject of some controversy over the number of children who may or may not have been brain-damaged by inoculation. It would in any case be extremely difficult to attribute such damage definitively to the use of the vaccine, and law suits brought to court have had to rely on solely statistical evidence of probability or possibility. However, the statistics do not make for comfortable reading by parents: in the 1980s it was estimated that permanent brain damage might be expected to occur in 1 in 300,000 vaccinations. Obviously, people would prefer to have no risk whatever, but sometimes disregard the fact that the likelihood of catching whooping cough (and possibly suffering permanent physical damage) may statistically be actually greater. Except as part of the triple vaccination, administration is by a single injection. (Available from Wellcome).
✚ warning: in general, pertussis vaccine should not be administered to children who suffer a severe local or general reaction to the initial dose, or who have a history of brain damage at birth or of cerebral irritation or seizures. It should be administered with extreme caution to children whose relatives have a history of seizures or who appear to have any form of neurological disorder.
see also DIPHTHERIA-PERTUSSIS-TETANUS (DPT) VACCINE.

Peru balsam is a mild ANTISEPTIC used in some disinfectant preparations, especially in creams or ointments for topical application for example as soothing agents or in anal suppositories.

pethidine is a narcotic ANALGESIC

used primarily for the relief of moderate to severe pain, especially in labour and childbirth. Its effect is rapid and short-lasting, so its sedative properties are made use of only as a premedication prior to surgery or to enhance the effects of other anaesthetics during or following surgery. Administration (as pethidine hydrochloride) is oral in the form of tablets, or by injection. Proprietary forms are on the controlled drugs list.

✚ warning: pethidine should not be administered to patients with head injury or intracranial pressure; it should be administered with caution to those with impaired kidney or liver function, asthma, depressed respiration, insufficient secretion of thyroid hormones (hypothyroidism) or low blood pressure (hypotension), or who are pregnant (except during labour) or breast feeding. Dosage should be reduced for the elderly or debilitated.

▲ side-effects: shallow breathing, urinary retention, constipation and nausea are all fairly common; tolerance and dependence (addiction) are possible. There may also be drowsiness and pain at the site of injection.

Related articles: PAMERGAN P100; PETHILORFAN.

Pethilorfan (*Roche*) is a proprietary narcotic ANALGESIC that is on the controlled drugs list; it is used to treat moderate to severe pain, particularly in labour and childbirth. Produced in ampoules for injection, Pethilorfan is a preparation of pethidine hydrochloride with the respiratory stimulant levallorphan tartrate.

✚/▲ warning/side-effects: *see* PETHIDINE.

Petrolagar (*Wyeth*) is a proprietary non-prescription LAXATIVE that is not available from the National Health Service. Produced in the form of a sugar-free emulsion, Petrolagar is a preparation of two forms of LIQUID PARAFFIN.

Pevaryl (*Ortho-Cilag*) is a proprietary non-prescription ANTIFUNGAL drug, used in topical application to treat fungal infections on the skin such as nail infections, and particularly in the genital areas. Produced in the form of a cream, a lotion, and a spray-powder in an aerosol unit, Pevaryl is a preparation of econazole nitrate.

✚/▲ warning/side-effects: *see* ECONAZOLE NITRATE.

Phanodorm (*Winthrop*) is a proprietary HYPNOTIC drug that is on the controlled drugs list. Used to treat severe intractable insomnia in patients already taking barbiturates, and produced in the form of tablets, Phanodorm is a preparation of the barbiturate cyclobarbitone calcium. It is not recommended for children.

✚/▲ warning/side-effects: *see* CYCLOBARBITONE CALCIUM.

Pharmalgen (*Pharmacia*) is either of two preparations – of bee venom or of wasp venom – for use in diagnosing and desensitizing patients who are allergic to them. Available only on prescription, solutions of one or the other venom are administered as injections in increasingly less dilute form so that treatment is progressive.

✚ warning: injections should be administered under close medical supervision and in locations where emergency facilities for full cardio-respiratory resuscitation are immediately available. Pharmalgen preparations should not be given to patients who are pregnant, feverish or who suffer from asthma.

Pharmidone (*Farmitalia Carlo Erba*) is a proprietary non-prescription compound ANALGESIC that is not available from the National Health Service. Used to treat headache, including migraine, and muscle or nerve pain, Pharmidone is a preparation of the analgesic paracetamol, the OPIATE codeine phosphate, the antihistamine diphenhydramine hydrochloride and the mild stimulant CAFFEINE.

✚/▲ warning/side-effects: *see* CODEINE PHOSPHATE; DIPHENHYDRAMINE HYDROCHLORIDE; PARACETAMOL.

Pharmorubicin (*Farmitalia Carlo Erba*) is a proprietary CYTOTOXIC drug that has ANTIBIOTIC properties, available only on prescription, used to treat acute leukaemia and various solid tumours. Produced in the form of a powder for reconstitution as a medium for injection (in vials of three strengths), Pharmorubicin is a preparation of epirubicin hydrochloride.

✚/▲ warning/side-effects: *see* EPIRUBICIN HYDROCHLORIDE.

Phasal (*Lagab*) is a proprietary ANTIDEPRESSANT, available only on prescription, used in the treatment and prevention of mania, in the prevention of recurrent manic-depressive bouts, and for aggressive or self-mutilating behaviour. Produced in the form of sustained-release tablets, Phasal is a preparation of the powerful drug lithium carbonate.

✚/▲ warning/side-effects: *see* LITHIUM.

Phazyme (*Stafford-Miller*) is a proprietary non-prescription ANTACID preparation, used to treat flatulence. Produced in the form of tablets, Phazyme is a preparation of the antifoaming agent DIMETHICONE.

phenazocine is a narcotic ANALGESIC used primarily for the relief of moderate to severe pain, especially pain arising from disorders of the pancreas or of the bile ducts. Administration (as phenazocine hydrobromide) is oral in the form of tablets. The proprietary form is on the controlled drugs list.

✚ warning: phenazocine should not be administered to patients with head injury or intracranial pressure; it should be administered with caution to those with impaired kidney or liver function, asthma, depressed respiration, insufficient secretion of thyroid hormones (hypothyroidism) or low blood pressure (hypotension), or who are pregnant or lactating. Dosage should be reduced for the elderly or debilitated.

▲ side-effects: shallow breathing, urinary retention, constipation and nausea are all fairly common; tolerance and dependence (addiction) are possible. There may also be drowsiness.

Related article: NARPHEN.

phenazopyridine is an ANALGESIC that relieves the pain specifically of disorders of the urinary tract such as cystitis and urethritis. It is sometimes used as a constituent in compound antibiotic preparations to treat urinary infections. Administration (as phenazopyridine hydrochloride) is oral in the form of tablets.

✚ warning: phenazopyridine hydrochloride should be administered with caution to patients with impaired liver or kidney function.

▲ side-effects: there may be gastrointestinal disturbance, with headache and dizziness. High dosage may cause blood disorders and discolour the urine. Prolonged treatment may increase the risk of urinary stones (calculi). *Related articles:* PYRIDIUM; UROMIDE.

P

phenelzine is an ANTIDEPRESSANT drug, one of the MAO INHIBITORS. It is used particularly when treatment with TRICYCLIC antidepressants (such as AMITRYPTILINE OR IMIPRAMINE) has failed, even though phenelzine is one of the safer, less stimulant MAO inhibitors. Treatment with the drug requires a strict dietary regime – in which for example a patient must avoid eating cheese, or meat or yeast extracts, or drinking alcohol – and extreme care in taking any other form of medication. Administration (as phenelzine sulphate) is oral in the form of tablets.

✚ warning: phenelzine should not be administered to patients with liver disease, epilepsy, vascular disease of the heart or brain, or abnormal secretion of hormones by the adrenal glands, or who are children. It should be administered with caution to those who are elderly or debilitated. Counselling – if not supervision – over diet and any other medication is essential. Withdrawal of treatment should be gradual.

▲ side-effects: concentration and speed of thought and movement may be affected. There may also be dizziness, particularly on standing up from lying or sitting (because of low blood pressure). Much less commonly, there may be headache, dry mouth and blurred vision, difficulty in urinating, constipation and a rash. Susceptible patients may experience agitation, tremor, or even psychotic episodes. *Related article:* NARDIL.

Phenergan (*May & Baker*) is a proprietary non-prescription ANTIHISTAMINE, used to treat the symptoms of allergies such as hay fever and for emergency treatment of reactions to drugs or injected substances. It is produced in the form of tablets (in two strengths), as an elixir for dilution (the potency of the elixir once dilute is retained for 14 days), neither of which is recommended for children aged under 6 months, and (only on prescription) in ampoules for injection, which is not recommended for children aged under 5 years. Phenergan is a preparation of promethazine hydrochloride. Under the name Phenergan Compound Expectorant, a compound linctus is also available, but not from the National Health Service, which consists of a preparation of promethazine hydrochloride and several LAXATIVE constituents; it too is not recommended for children aged under 5 years.

✚/▲ warning/side-effects: *see* PROMETHAZINE HYDROCHLORIDE.

phenethicillin is a penicillin-type ANTIBIOTIC that is used both to treat bacterial infection and to prevent it. Administration (as a potassium salt) is oral in the form of capsules or a dilute syrup.

✚ warning: phenethicillin should

not be administered to patients who are known to be allergic to penicillins; it should be administered with caution to those with impaired kidney function.

▲ side-effects: there may be sensitivity reactions ranging from a minor rash to urticaria and joint pains, diarrhoea and (occasionally) to high temperature or anaphylactic shock.

Related article: BROXIL.

phenindamine tartrate is an ANTIHISTAMINE used to treat the symptoms of allergic conditions such as hay fever and urticaria. It has only a mildly depressant action on the brain and so is less sedating than most antihistamines, and may in fact cause slight stimulation of the central nervous system. Administration is oral in the form of tablets.

✚ warning: phenindamine tartrate should not be administered to patients with glaucoma, urinary retention, intestinal obstruction, enlargement of the prostate gland, or peptic ulcer, or who are pregnant; it should be administered with caution to those with epilepsy or liver disease.

▲ side-effects: concentration and speed of thought and movement may be affected; there may be nausea, headache, and/or weight gain, dry mouth, gastrointestinal disturbances and visual problems.

Related article: THEPHORIN.

phenindione is an ANTICOAGULANT that is effective when taken orally, used in the treatment and prevention of thrombosis. However, because of the proportion of patients who are sensitive to it, its use has largely been replaced by that of WARFARIN sodium. It remains available: administration is in the form of tablets.

✚ warning: phenindione should not be administered to patients with kidney or liver disease, severe hypertension (high blood pressure), bacterial endocarditis, or a peptic ulcer; who are regularly taking anabolic steroids, aspirin, barbiturates or phytomenadione (vitamin K) supplements; who are using oral contraceptives; or who are in the first three months or last two months of pregnancy, or have had recent surgery.

▲ side-effects: there may be sensitivity reactions. Internal haemorrhaging may occur: monitoring is required.

Related article: DINDEVAN.

pheniramine maleate is an ANTIHISTAMINE used to treat the symptoms of allergic conditions such as hay fever and urticaria. Administration is oral in the form of tablets.

✚ warning: pheniramine maleate should not be administered to patients with glaucoma, urinary retention, intestinal obstruction, enlargement of the prostate gland, or peptic ulcer, or who are pregnant; it should be administered with caution to those with epilepsy or liver disease.

▲ side-effects: concentration and speed of thought and movement may be affected; there may be nausea, headache, and/or weight gain, dry mouth, gastrointestinal disturbances and visual problems.

Related article: DANERAL SA.

phenobarbitone is a powerful BARBITURATE, used as a HYPNOTIC drug to treat insomnia, as an ANXIOLYTIC to relieve anxiety, and as an ANTICONVULSANT in the prevention of recurrent epileptic seizures or the treatment of febrile convulsions. In all uses, prolonged treatment may rapidly result in tolerance and then dependence (addiction). Its use may also cause behavioural disturbances (such as hyperactivity) in children. Administration (as phenobarbitone or phenobarbitone sodium) is oral in the form of tablets and an elixir, or by injection. All proprietary preparations containing phenobarbitone are on the controlled drugs list.

✚ warning: phenobarbitone should not be administered to patients with porphyria or who are already taking drugs that depress brain function (such as alcohol) on a regular basis; it should be administered with caution to those with impaired kidney or liver function, or who have respiratory disorders, who are elderly or children, or who are lactating. Withdrawal of treatment should be gradual.

▲ side-effects: there is drowsiness and lethargy; sometimes there is also depression, muscle weakness and/or sensitivity reactions in the form of skin rashes or blood disorders. Elderly or juvenile patients may experience psychological disturbance.

Related articles: GARDENAL SODIUM; LUMINAL.

phenol, or carbolic acid, is a very early DISINFECTANT still much used for the cleaning of wounds or inflammation (such as boils and abscesses), the maintenance of hygiene in the mouth, throat or ear, and as a preservative in injections. Administration is topical in solutions, lotions, creams and ointments.

✚ warning: phenol is highly toxic if swallowed in concentrated form.

Related articles: CHLORASEPTIC; ILONIUM; SECADERM.

phenolphthalein is a LAXATIVE that works by irritating the nerve endings in the intestinal walls. Its use is now rare because of an association with blood disorders that affect the composition of the urine, with sensitivity reactions, and with a duration of effect that may continue for several days as the chemical is recycled through the liver. Proprietary preparations that contain phenolphthalein all also contain either other forms of laxative or an antacid.

Related articles: AGAROL; ALOPHEN; KEST.

phenoperidine is an narcotic ANALGESIC, a morphine-like drug used to relieve pain during surgery and particularly in combination with (to enhance) general ANAESTHETICS; its additional properties as a respiratory depressant are sometimes made use of in the treatment of patients who undergo prolonged assisted respiration. Administration (in the form of phenoperidine hydrochloride) is by injection.

✚ warning: phenoperidine should not be administered to patients who suffer from head injury or intracranial pressure; it should be administered with caution to those with impaired kidney or liver function, insufficient secretion of thyroid hormones (hypothyroidism) or low blood pressure (hypotension), or who are pregnant or lactating. Dosage should be reduced for

the elderly or debilitated.
▲ side-effects: shallow breathing, urinary retention, constipation and nausea are all fairly common; tolerance and dependence (addiction) are possible. There may also be drowsiness, and pain at the site of injection.
Related article: OPERIDINE.

phenothiazine derivatives, or phenothiazines, are a group of drugs that are chemically related but are not restricted to a single mode of activity. Many are ANTIPSYCHOTIC drugs, including some of the tranquillizers best known and most used – such as chlorpromazine, promazine, thioridazine, fluphenazine and trifluoperazine. Some of these are used also as ANTI-EMETICS. Others – such as piperazine – are ANTHELMINTICS.
✚/▲ warning/side-effects: *see* CHLORPROMAZINE; FLUPHENAZINE; METHOTRIMEPRAZINE; pericyazine; PERPHENAZINE; PIPERAZINE; PIPOTHIAZINE; PROCHLORPERAZINE; PROMAZINE; THIORIDAZINE; TRIFLUOPERAZINE.

phenoxybenzamine hydrochloride is ALPHA-BLOCKER used in conjunction with either a BETA-BLOCKER and/or a DIURETIC to reduce blood pressure and to improve conditions that result from poor circulation or from abnormal secretion of hormones by the adrenal glands. By itself it is also sometimes useful in improving urine flow in cases of benign enlargement of the prostate gland. Administration is oral in the form of capsules, or by injection.
✚ warning: phenoxybenzamine hydrochloride should be administered with caution to patients with heart disease, severe arteriosclerosis, or impaired kidney function, or who are elderly.
▲ side-effects: the heart rate increases; there may be dizziness, particularly on standing up from lying or sitting (because of low blood pressure), with lethargy. There is sometimes nasal congestion and contraction of the pupils. Rarely, there is gastrointestinal disturbance or ejaculation failure.
Related article: DIBENYLINE.

phenoxymethylpenicillin, or penicillin V, is a widely used ANTIBIOTIC particularly effective in treating tonsillitis, infection of the middle ear, and some skin infections, and to prevent the onset of rheumatic fever. Administration (as a potassium salt sometimes called phenoxymethylpenicillin VK) is oral in the form of tablets or liquids.
✚ warning: phenoxymethylpenicillin should not be administered to patients known to be allergic to penicillins; it should be administered with caution to those with impaired kidney function.
▲ side-effects: there may be sensitivity reactions ranging from a minor rash to urticaria and joint pains, and (occasionally) to high temperature or anaphylactic shock. High dosage may in any case cause convulsions.
Related articles: APSIN VK; CRYSTAPEN V; DISTAQUAINE V-K; ECONOCIL VK; STABILLIN V-K; V-CIL-K.

Phensedyl (*May & Baker*) is a proprietary non-prescription ANTITUSSIVE that is not available from the National Health Service. Produced in the form of a linctus, Phensedyl is a preparation of the ANTIHISTAMINE promethazine hydrochloride, the OPIATE codeine phosphate and the SYMPATHOMIMETIC ephedrine hydrochloride as a syrup for dilution (the potency of the syrup once dilute is retained for 14 days). It is not recommended for children aged under 2 years.

✚/▲ warning/side-effects: *see* CODEINE PHOSPHATE; EPHEDRINE HYDROCHLORIDE; PROMETHAZINE HYDROCHLORIDE.

P

Phensic (*Beecham Health Care*) is a proprietary non-prescription ANALGESIC containing aspirin and caffeine.

✚/▲ warning/side-effects: *see* ASPIRIN; CAFFEINE.

phentermine is a SYMPATHOMIMETIC drug used under medical supervision and on a short-term basis to aid weight loss in moderate to severe obesity because it acts to suppress the appetite. Administration is in the form of sustained-release capsules.

✚ warning: phentermine should not be administered to patients who suffer from glaucoma; it should be administered with caution to those with heart disease, diabetes, epilepsy, peptic ulcer, or depression.

▲ side-effects: there is commonly rapid heart rate, nervous agitation and insomnia, tremor, gastrointestinal disturbance, dry mouth, dizziness and headache.
Related articles: DUROMINE; IONAMIN.

phentolamine is an ALPHA-BLOCKER used to reduce blood pressure and to improve con-Tditions that result from poor circulation, it is particularly useful in emergency situations situations caused by abnormal secretion of hormones by the adrenal glands, by internal reactions between incompatible antidepressant drugs, or by heart failure. It is also used to test adrenal function or diagnose adrenal disorder. Administration is by injection or infusion.

▲ side-effects: there is commonly a rapid heart rate and dizziness, with low blood pressure (hypotension). High dosage may lead to nausea, nasal congestion and diarrhoea.
Related article: ROGITINE.

phenylbutazone is an ANTI-INFLAMMATORY non-narcotic ANALGESIC which, because of its sometimes severe side-effects, is used solely in the treatment of progressive fusion of the synovial joints of the spine (ankylosing spondylitis) under medical supervision in hospitals. Even for that purpose, it is used only when all other therapies have failed. Treatment then, however, may be prolonged. Administration is oral in the form of tablets.

✚ warning: phenylbutazone should not be administered to patients with cardiovascular disease, thyroid disease, or impaired liver or kidney function; who are pregnant; or who have a history of stomach or intestinal haemorrhaging. It should be administered with caution to those who are elderly or lactating. Regular and frequent blood counts are essential.

▲ side-effects: there may be gastrointestinal disturbances, nausea, vomiting, and allergic reactions such as a rash. Less often, there is inflammation of the glands of the mouth, throat and neck; pancreatitis, nephritis or hepatitis; or headache and visual

disturbances. Rarely, there is severe fluid retention (which may eventually in susceptible patients precipitate heart failure) or serious and potentially dangerous blood disorders.
Related articles: BUTACOTE; BUTAZOLIDIN; BUTAZONE.

phenylephrine is a VASOCONSTRICTOR, a SYMPATHOMIMETIC drug used in administration by injection or infusion to increase blood pressure (sometimes in emergency situations until plasma transfusion is available). It is sometimes used in the form of a spray or drops to clear nasal congestion; as eye-drops to dilate the pupil and facilitate ophthalmic examination; or as a constituent in some proprietary preparations produced to treat bronchospasm in conditions such as asthma.

✚ warning: phenylephrine should not be administered to patients with severe hypertension (high blood pressure), or from overactivity of the thyroid gland (hyperthyroidism), who are undergoing a heart attack, or who are pregnant. Leakage of the drug into the tissues following injection may cause tissue damage.

▲ side-effects: treatment by injection or infusion causes a rise in the blood pressure, which may in turn cause headache and heartbeat irregularities; there may be vomiting, and a tingling or coolness in the skin. Topical application may promote the appearance of a form of dermatitis. As nasal drops or spray, excessive use may lead to tolerance and worse congestion than previously.
Related articles: BETNOVATE; BETOPTIC; BRONCHILATOR; DIMOTANE EXPECTORANT; DIMOTAPP; DUO-AUTOHALER; HAYPHRIN; ISOPTO-FRIN; MEDIHALER-DUO; MINIMS; NEOPHRYN; NETHAPRIN DOSPAN; SOFRAMYCIN; UNIFLU; VIBROCIL; ZINCFRIN.

phenylpropanolomine is a SYMPATHOMIMETIC drug that has a strongly relaxant effect on certain muscles of the body, including especially the muscles of the bladder that contract to allow urine to escape through the urethra. The drug is therefore primarily used under medical supervision to treat urinary incontinence (of the type caused by muscular weakness). However, it is used also to relieve the symptoms of some allergic disorders, such as asthma and hay fever, often when administered with an antihistamine. Administration is oral in the form of sustained-release capsules and a dilute syrup, topical in the form of a nasal or throat spray, and by injection.

✚ warning: phenylpropanolamine should not be administered to patients with high blood pressure (hypertension), overactivity of the thyroid gland (hyperthyroidism), coronary heart disease or diabetes, or who are taking antidepressant drugs. It should be administered with caution to those who are elderly.

▲ side-effects: there may be anxiety, restlessness and insomnia, with dry mouth, sweating, and cold extremities; urinary retention may occur. Some patients experience tremor and heartbeat irregularities.
Related articles: DIMOTAPP; ESKORNADE; TRIOGESIC.

phenytoin is an ANTICONVULSANT drug that is also an ANTI-ARRHYTHMIC. It is consequently used both to treat the severer forms of epilepsy (not including petit mal), and to regularize the heartbeat (especially following the administration of a heart stimulant). The drug is also useful in assisting in the treatment of the neuropathy that sometimes accompanies diabetes. Administration (as phenytoin or phenytoin sodium) is oral in the form of tablets, chewable tablets, capsules and a suspension, or by injection.

✚ warning: phenytoin should not be administered to patients whose heart rate is excessively fast, who have heart block, liver damage or who have already been administered lignocaine hydrochloride. Monitoring of plasma concentration of the drug is essential in the initial treatment of epilepsy in order to establish an optimum administration level. Withdrawal should be gradual. Drug interactions are common.

▲ side-effects: the heart rate and blood pressure are reduced; asystole (a "missed beat") may occur. The skin and facial features may coarsen during prolonged treatment; there may also be acne, enlargement of the gums, and/or growth of excess hair. Some patients enter a state of confusion. Nausea and vomiting, headache, blurred vision, blood disorders and insomnia may occur.
Related articles: EPANUTIN; EPANUTIN READY MIXED PARENTERAL.

pHiso-Med (*Winthrop*) is a proprietary non-prescription DISINFECTANT used as a soap or shampoo substitute in acne and seborrhoeic conditions, for bathing mothers and babies in maternity units to prevent cross infection, and for pre-operative hand and skin cleansing. Produced in the form of a solution, pHiso-Med is a preparation of CHLORHEXIDINE gluconate.

✚ warning: s sensitivity may occur.

pholcodine is an OPIATE that is used as an ANTITUSSIVE constituent in cough linctuses or syrups. Although its action on the cough centre of the brain resembles that of other opiates, it has no ANALGESIC effect.

✚ warning: pholcodine should not be taken by patients with liver or kidney disease; it should be taken with caution by patients who suffer from asthma or have a history of drug abuse.

▲ side-effects: there is commonly constipation. High or prolonged dosage may lead to respiratory depression.
Related articles: COPHOLCO; DAVENOL; DIA-TUSS; EXPULIN; Galenphol; PAVACOL-D; PHOLCOMED; PHOLTEX; RUBELIX.

Pholcomed (*Medo*) is a proprietary brand of ANTITUSSIVES used to treat an irritable and unproductive cough. Produced in the form of a linctus (in two strengths, the stronger under the name Pholcomed Forte) for dilution (the potency of each linctus once dilute is retained for 14 days), as a sugar-free linctus for use by diabetics (in two strengths, under the names Pholcomed-D and Pholcomed Forte Diabetic) and as pastilles (only the last of which preparations is available from the National Health Service), Pholcomed is a compound of the ANTITUSSIVE PHOLCODINE and the

MUSCLE RELAXANT papaverine hydrochloride, both of which are OPIATES. The Forte linctuses are not recommended for children.
✚/▲ warning/side-effects: *see* PAPAVERINE; PHOLCODINE.

Pholcomed Expectorant (*Medo*) is a proprietary non-prescription ANTITUSSIVE, not available from the National Health Service, being a compound preparation of the EXPECTORANT guaiphenesin and the SYMPATHOMIMETIC methylephedrine hydrochloride.

Pholtex (*Riker*) is a proprietary ANTITUSSIVE that is not available from the National Health Service. Used to treat a dry, unproductive cough, and produced in the form of a sugar-free mixture for dilution (the potency of the mixture once dilute is retained for 14 days), Pholtex is a preparation of the OPIATE pholcodine and the ANTIHISTAMINE phenyltoloxamine.
✚/▲ warning/side-effects: *see* PHOLCODINE.

Phortinea (*Philip Harris*) is a proprietary non-prescription ANTIFUNGAL paint for topical application, used to treat fungal skin infections such as athlete's foot. Phortinea is a preparation of the drug NITROPHENOL.

phosphate infusion is administered to replace phosphates lost through disease or disorder – as may occur in diabetic emergencies. For infusion, phosphates (usually as the potassium and sodium salts) may be administered in saline or glucose solution.

phosphates may be administered orally (with CALCIFEROL) to make up for the phosphate (and vitamin D) deficiency that occurs in vitamin D-resistant rickets. Diarrhoea is a common side-effect. Rarely, phosphates may be administered in order to treat high levels of calcium in the blood, although this may lead to the deposition of calcium in kidney tissues and consequent kidney damage. Phosphates are used as enemas for bowel clearance before radiological procedues, endoscopy and surgery.

Phosphate-Sandoz (*Sandoz*) is a proprietary non-prescription phosphate supplement, which may be required in addition to vitamin D in patients with vitamin D-resistant rickets. Produced in the form of tablets, Phosphate-Sandoz is a preparation of sodium acid phosphate, SODIUM BICARBONATE and potassium bicarbonate.

Phospholine Iodide (*Ayerst*) is a proprietary form of eye-drops, available only on prescription, used to treat severe cases of glaucoma. Phospholine Iodide is a preparation of ecothiopate iodide and is produced in the form of a powder (with diluent) for reconstitution (in four strengths).
✚/▲ warning/side-effects: *see* ECOTHIOPATE IODIDE.

phosphorus is a non-metallic element whose salts are important to all forms of terrestrial life. In humans, for example, phosphates are concentrated mainly in bones and teeth, but are also essential to the conversion and storage of energy in the body, and are intimately linked with corresponding levels of CALCIUM, potassium and SODIUM in the bloodstream. Phosphates may also be administered therapeutically to treat deficiency disorders.
see PHOSPHATES.

P

phthalylsulphathiazole is a SULPHONAMIDE used primarily to treat infection of the intestines, or to act as a disinfectant before intestinal surgery. That it is effective for this purpose is due to the fact that it is poorly absorbed when taken orally – but that it is poorly absorbed means that it is now declining in use in favour of more specific drugs.

✚ warning: phthalysulphathiazole should not be administered to patients with blood disorders or impaired kidney or liver function, who are pregnant, or who are aged under 6 weeks. It should be administered with caution to those who are elderly or lactating. Regular blood counts are essential during treatment. An adequate fluid intake must be maintained.

▲ side-effects: there may be nausea and vomiting; rarely, there may be rashes, skin disorders and blood deficiencies.

Related article: THALAZOLE.

Phyllocontin Continus (*Napp*) is a proprietary non-prescription BRONCHODILATOR, used to treat asthma and chronic bronchitis. Produced in the form of sustained-release tablets (in three strengths, the weakest labelled for children, the strongest labelled Forte), Phyllocontin Continus is a preparation of aminophylline. The two stronger forms of tablets are not recommended for children; and the paediatric tablets are not recommended for children aged under 12 months.

✚/▲ warning/side-effects: *see* AMINOPHYLLINE.

Physeptone (*Calmic*) is a proprietary narcotic ANALGESIC that is on the controlled drugs list. Used to treat severe pain, and produced in the form of tablets and in ampoules for injection, Physeptone is a preparation of the OPIATE methadone hydrochloride; it is not recommended for children.

✚/▲ warning/side-effects: *see* METHADONE.

physostigmine is a vegetable alkaloid (derived from calabar beans) used in dilute solution in the form of eye-drops to treat glaucoma or to contract the pupil of the eye after it has been dilated through the use of ANTICHOLINERGICS such as ATROPINE for the purpose of ophthalmic examination. It works by improving drainage in the tiny channels of the eye processes. It is, however, potentially irritant, causing gastrointestinal disturbance and excessive salivation if absorbed, and is most commonly used in combination with other drugs, particularly pilocarpine.

Phytex (*Pharmax*) is a proprietary non-prescription ANTIFUNGAL drug, used to treat fungal infections in the skin and nails. Produced in the form of a paint for topical application, Phytex is a preparation of various natural acids, including SALICYLIC ACID, together with with METHYL SALICYLATE.

✚/▲ warning/side-effects: hypersensitivity reactions may occur.

Phytocil (*Radiol*) is a proprietary non-prescription ANTIFUNGAL drug, used in topical application to treat skin infections, especially athlete's foot. Produced in the form of a cream, and a powder in a sprinkler tin, Phytocil is a compound preparation that includes several minor antifungal constituents

including SALICYLIC ACID.
✚/▲ warning/side-effects: hypersensitivty may occur.

phytomenadione is the technical term for vitamin K, a fat-soluble vitamin essential to the production of clotting factors in the blood, and to the metabolism of the proteins necessary for the calcification of bone. Good food sources include vegetable oils, liver, pork meat and green vegetables. Deficiency causes a condition much like haemophilia, and in children may lead to irregular bone growth. Therapeutically, phytomenadione is administered to make up deficiency – especially in newborn babies whose intestines have not had to time to obtain the normal bacterial agents that synthesize the vitamin. Administration is oral in the form of tablets, or by very slow intravenous injection.
Related articles: KONAKION; VITLIPID.

PIB (*Napp*) is a proprietary compound BRONCHODILATOR, available only on prescription, used to treat bronchospasm in asthma and chronic bronchitis. Produced in a metered-dosage aerosol (in two strengths, the stronger under the name PIB Plus), it is a preparation of the SYMPATHOMIMETIC isoprenaline hydrochloride together with the BELLADONNA alkaloid atropine methonitrate. It is not recommended for children.
✚/▲ warning/side-effects: *see* ATROPINE METHONITRATE; ISOPRENALINE.

Picolax (*Nordic*) is a proprietary non-prescription LAXATIVE produced in the form of a sugar-free powder for solution. Picolax is a preparation of the stimulant laxative sodium PICOSULPHATE and the ANTACID laxative magnesium citrate.
✚/▲ warning/side-effects: *see* SODIUM PICOSULPHATE.

pilocarpine is a PARA-SYMPATHOMINETIC drug used in dilute solution in the form of eye-drops to treat glaucoma or to contract the pupil of the eye after it has been dilated for the purpose of ophthalmic examination. It works by improving drainage in the channels of the eye processes. It is, however, potentially irritant, causing eyeache and blurred vision, and even gastrointestinal disturbance and excessive salivation if absorbed especially to patients under 40 years of age. As pilocarpine hydrochloride or pilocarpine nitrate, it is commonly used in combination with other drugs, particularly PHYSOSTIGMINE.
Related articles: ISOPTO; MINIMS; OCUSERT PILO; SNO PILO.

Pimafucin (*Brocades*) is a proprietary ANTIFUNGAL drug, available only on prescription, used to treat fungal infections (such as candidiasis), particularly in the mouth, respiratory tract and vagina. Produced in the form of a sugar-free oral suspension, a suspension for inhalation, as vaginal inserts (pessaries) and as vaginal cream, and as a water-miscible cream for topical application to the skin, Pimafucin is a preparation of natamycin.
✚/▲ warning/side-effects: *see* NATAMYCIN.

pimozide is an ANTIPSYCHOTIC drug used to tranquillize patients suffering from schizophrenia and other psychoses, including paranoia and mania. It is especiaslly effective in relieving hallucinations. The drug may

also be used in the short term to treat severe anxiety.
Administration is oral in the form of tablets.

✚ warning: pimozide should not be administered to patients who suffer from certain forms of glaucoma, whose blood-cell formation by the bone-marrow is reduced, or who are taking drugs that depress certain centres of the brain and spinal cord. It should be administered with caution to those with lung disease, cardiovascular disease, epilepsy, parkinsonism, abnormal secretion by the adrenal glands, impaired liver or kidney function, undersecretion of thyroid hormones (hypothyroidism), enlargement of the prostate gland or any form of acute infection; who are pregnant or lactating; or who are elderly. Prolonged use requires regular checks on eye function and skin pigmentation. Withdrawal of treatment should be gradual.

▲ side-effects: concentration and speed of thought and movement are affected; the effects of alcohol consumption are enhanced. There may be dry mouth and blocked nose, constipation and difficulty in urinating, and blurred vision; menstrual disturbances in women or impotence in men may occur, with weight gain; there may be sensitivity reactions. Some patients feel cold and depressed, and tend to suffer from poor sleep patterns. Blood pressure may be low and the heartbeat irregular.
Related article: ORAP.

pindolol is a BETA-BLOCKER, a drug used to control and regulate the heart rate and to treat hypertension (high blood pressure). It is also used to treat the symptoms of angina pectoris (heart pain) and to assist in relieving the symptoms of the neuropathy that sometimes accompanies diabetes.
Administration is oral in the form of tablets.

✚ warning: pindolol should not be administered to patients who have heart disease or asthma; it should be administered with caution to those with liver or especially kidney disease, or who are pregnant or lactating. Withdrawal of treatment must be gradual.

▲ side-effects: there may be a slowing of the heartbeat, with coldness of the extremities. Sometimes there is respiratory depression and/or gastrointestinal disturbances.
Related articles: VISKALDIX; VISKEN.

pipenzolate bromide is an ANTICHOLINERGIC drug used to assist in the treatment of gastrointestinal disorders that involve muscle spasm of the intestinal wall. Administration is oral in the form of tablets, or a suspension.

✚/▲ warning/side-effects: *see under* ATROPINE
Related articles: PIPTAL; PIPTALIN.

piperacillin is a broad-spectrum penicillin-type ANTIBIOTIC closely related to AMPICILLIN, used to treat many serious or compound forms of bacterial infection, and to prevent infection during or following surgery.
Administration is by injection or infusion.

✚ warning: piperacillin should not be administered to patients known to be allergic to penicillins; it should be administered with caution to those with impaired kidney function.

▲ side-effects: there may be sensitivity reactions ranging from a minor rash to urticaria and joint pains, and (occasionally) to high temperature or anaphylactic shock. High dosage may in any case cause convulsions.
Related article: PIPRIL.

piperazine is an ANTHELMINTIC drug, one of the PHENOTHIAZINE derivatives, used to treat infestation by roundworms or threadworms. Treatment should take no longer than seven days: in the treatment of some species a single dose is sufficient. Administration (as piperazine citrate, piperazine hydrate or piperazine phosphate) is oral in the form of tablets, a syrup or a dilute elixir.

✚ warning: piperazine should not be administered to patients with liver disease or epilepsy; it should be administered with caution to those with impaired kidney function, neurological disease or psychiatric disorders.

▲ side-effects: there may be nausea and vomiting, with diarrhoea; there may also be urticaria. Rarely, there is dizziness and lack of muscular co-ordination.
Related articles: ANTEPAR; ASCALIX; PRIPSEN.

piperazine oestron sulphate is a female sex hormone, an OESTROGEN used to make up hormonal deficiency during or following the menopause. Administration is oral in the form of tablets.

✚ warning: piperazine oestron sulphate should not be administered to patients who have cancers proved to be sex-hormone-linked, who have a history of thrombosis or inflammation of the womb, or with porphyria or impaired liver function. It should be administered with caution to those who are diabetic or epileptic, who have heart or kidney disease, or who have hypertension (high blood pressure) or recurrent severe migraine. Prolonged treatment increases the risk of cancer of the endometrium (the lining of the womb).

▲ side-effects: there may be nausea and vomiting. A common effect is weight gain, generally through fluid or sodium retention in the tissues. The breasts may become tender and enlarge slightly. There may also be headache and/or depression; rash, liver function disorders, jaundice.
Related article: HARMOGEN.

piperidolate hydrochloride is an ANTICHOLINERGIC drug used to assist in the treatment of gastrointestinal disorders that involve muscle spasm of the intestinal wall. Administration is oral in the form of tablets.

✚ warning: piperidolate hydrochloride should not be administered to patients with glaucoma; it should be administered with caution to those with heart problems and rapid heart rate (tachycardia), ulcerative colitis, urinary retention or enlargement of the prostate gland; who are elderly; or who are lactating.

▲ side-effects: there is commonly dry mouth and thirst; there may also be visual disturbances, flushing, irregular heartbeat and difficulty in urination and constipation. Rarely, there may be high temperature

accompanied by delirium.
Related article: DACTIL.

Piportil Depot (*May & Baker*) is a proprietary ANTIPSYCHOTIC drug, available only on prescription, used in maintenance therapy for patients who suffer from psychotic disorders such as chronic schizophrenia and related psychoses. Produced in ampoules for long-acting depot injections, Piportil Depot is a preparation of the PHENOTHIAZINE DERIVATIVE pipothiazine palmitate; it is not recommended for children.
✚/▲ warning/side-effects: *see* CHLORPROMAZINE.

P

pipothiazine palmitate is an ANTIPSYCHOTIC drug, one of the PHENOTHIAZINE derivatives used in maintenance therapy for patients who suffer from schizophrenia and other related psychoses. Administration is by injection.
✚/▲ warning/side-effects: *see* CHLORPROMAZINE.
Related article: PIPORTIL DEPOT.

Pipril (*Lederle*) is a proprietary broad-spectrum penicillin-type ANTIBIOTIC, available only on prescription, used to treat many serious or compound forms of bacterial infection, and to prevent infection during or following surgery. Produced in the form of a powder in vials (in two strengths) and in an infusion bottle, Pipril is a preparation of piperacillin.
✚/▲ warning/side-effects: *see* PIPERACILLIN.

Piptal (*MCP Pharmaceuticals*) is a proprietary ANTISPASMODIC drug, available only on prescription, used to assist in the treatment of gastrointestinal disorders arising from muscular spasm of the intestinal walls. Produced in the form of tablets, Piptal is a preparation of the ANTICHOLINERGIC drug pipenzolate bromide; it is not recommended for children.
✚/▲ warning/side-effects: *see* PIPENZOLATE BROMIDE.

Piptalin (*MCP Pharmaceuticals*) is a proprietary ANTISPASMODIC drug, available only on prescription, used to assist in the treatment of gastrointestinal disorders arising from muscular spasm of the intestinal walls. Produced in the form of a sugar-free suspension for dilution (the potency of the suspension once dilute is retained for 14 days), Piptalin is a preparation of the ANTICHOLINERGIC pipenzolate bromide together with the antifoaming agent DIMETHICONE.
✚/▲ warning/side-effects: *see* PIPENZOLATE BROMIDE.

pirbuterol is a BRONCHODILATOR, of the type known as a selective BETA-RECEPTOR STIMULANT, used to treat asthmatic bronchospasm, emphysema and chronic bronchitis. It has fewer cardiac side-effects than some others of its type, and is administered orally in the form of capsules, as a syrup or by aerosol inhalation.
✚ warning: pirbuterol should be administered with caution to patients with disorders of the thyroid gland, from heart disease or hypertension (high blood pressure), who are elderly, or who are pregnant. It is important not to exceed the recommended dose.
▲ side-effects: there may be headache and nervous tension, associated with tingling of the fingertips and a fine tremor of the muscles of the hands. Administration other than by inhalation may cause an

increase in the heart rate.
Related article: EXIREL.

pirenzepine is a relatively new drug used in the treatment of gastric and duodenal ulcers. It it is an ANTICHOLINERGIC drug, but with properties different from many others in this class, and works by inhibiting the receptors in the stomach lining that ordinarily evoke the production of gastric acids and digestive juices from the stomach, so reducing the overall acidity around the ulcerated area. Administration is oral in the form of tablets to be taken before meals.

✚ warning: in resistant cases it may be used simultaneously with drugs like CIMETIDINE, which are thought to form a protective layer over the healing ulcer.

▲ side-effects: side-effects are uncommon, but there may be dry mouth and slight visual disturbance. Blood disorders have been reported.
Related article: GASTROZEPIN.

piretanide is a DIURETIC used primarily to treat mild to moderate high blood pressure (*see* ANTIHYPERTENSIVE). Administration is oral in the form of sustained-release capsules.

✚ warning: piretanide should not be administered to patients who have any form of electrolyte imbalance; this is because the drug itself tends to cause a reduction in blood potassium. Regular checks on liver and kidney function during treatment are therefore essential.

▲ side-effects: side-effects are rare, but there may be nausea and vomiting, with diarrhoea and gastrointestinal disturbances; some patients experience sensitivity reactions such as rashes. High dosage in the elderly may lead to excessive diuresis and consequent circulatory disorders.
Related article: ARELIX.

Piriton (*Allen & Hanburys*) is a proprietary non-prescription preparation of the ANTIHISTAMINE chlorpheniramine maleate, used to treat allergic conditions such as hay fever and urticaria. It is produced in the form of tablets, as sustained-release tablets ("spandets", not recommended for children), and as a syrup for dilution (the potency of the syrup once dilute is retained for 14 days); it is also produced in ampoules for injection, but in that form is available only on prescription, and is not recommended for children.

✚/▲ warning/side-effects: *see* CHLORPHENIRAMINE.

piroxicam is a non-steroidal ANTI-INFLAMMATORY ANALGESIC used to treat pain and inflammation in rheumatic disease and other musculo-skeletal disorders (such as acute gout). Administration is oral in the form of capsules and soluble (dispersible) tablets, and topical in the form of anal suppositories.

✚ warning: piroxicam should be administered with caution to patients with allergies, gastric ulceration or impaired liver or kidney function, or who are pregnant. Prolonged high dosage increases the risk of gastrointestinal disturbances.

▲ side-effects: there may be nausea and gastrointestinal disturbance, either or both of which may be reduced by taking the drug with milk or food. Some patients experience sensitivity reactions (such as headache, ringing in the ears

P

– tinnitus – and vertigo), fluid retention, and/or blood disorders.
Related articles: FELDENE; LARAPAM.

Pitressin (*Parke-Davis Medical*) is a proprietary preparation of the HORMONE argipressin, which is a synthetic version of vasopressin. Available only on prescription, it is administered primarily to diagnose or to treat pituitary-originated diabetes insipidus, and to treat the haemorrhaging of varicose veins in the oesophagus (the tubular channel for food between throat and stomach). Produced in ampoules for injection (generally in hospitals only).
✚/▲ warning/side-effects: *see* VASOPRESSIN.

pivampicillin is a more active form of the ANTIBIOTIC ampicillin that is converted in the body to ampicillin after absorption. It has similar actions and uses.
✚/▲ warning/side-effects: *see* AMPICILLIN.
Related articles: MIRAXID; PONDOCILLIN.

pivmecillinam hydrochloride is a form of the ANTIBIOTIC mecillinam that can be taken orally. It has similar actions and uses.
✚/▲ warning/side-effects: *see* MECILLINAM.
Related articles: MIRAXID; SELEXID.

Piz Buin (*Ciba*) is a proprietary non-prescription brand of barrier creams for topical application, containing constituents able to protect the skin from ultraviolet radiation (such as with radiotherapy or as a sunscreen). A lipstick having similar constituents is also available.

pizotifen is an ANTIHISTAMINE structurally related to TRICYCLIC antidepressant drugs. It is used to treat and prevent headaches, particularly those in which blood pressure inside the blood vessels plays a part – such as migraine. Administration is oral in the form of tablets and an elixir.
✚ warning: pizotifen should not be administered to patients with closed-angle glaucoma or urinary retention. The effects of alcohol may be enhanced.
▲ side-effects: concentration and speed of thought and movement may be affected. There may be drowsiness, dry mouth and blurred vision, with constipation and difficulty in urinating; sometimes there is muscle pain and/or nausea. Patients may put on weight.
Related article: SANOMIGRAN.

PK Aid 1 (*Scientific Hospital Supplies*) is a proprietary non-prescription nutritional supplement for patient who suffer from amino acid abnormalities (such as phenylketonuria). It contains essential and non-essential amino acids – except phenylalanine.

Plaquenil (*Sterling Research*) is a proprietary ANTI-INFLAMMATORY drug, available only on prescription, used primarily to treat rheumatoid arthritis and forms of the skin disease lupus erythematosus. Treatment of rheumatoid arthritis may take up to 6 months to achieve full effect. The drug is also used in the prevention and treatment of malaria. Produced in the form of tablets, Plaquenil is a preparation of hydroxychloroquine sulphate.
✚/▲ warning/side-effects: *see* HYDROXYCHLOROQUINE.

Plasma-Lyte (*Travenol*) is the name of a selection of proprietary infusion fluids for the intravenous nutrition of a patient in whom feeding via the alimentary tract is not possible. All contain glucose in the form of dextrose, and water.

Platosin (*Nordic*) is a proprietary CYTOTOXIC drug, available only on prescription, used to treat certain solid tumours (such as cancer of the ovary or of the testes). It works by damaging the DNA of newly forming cells and is especially used to treat cancers that are metastatic and have failed to respond to other forms of therapy. Produced in the form of a powder in vials (in three strengths) for injection, and as a powder for reconstitution as a medium for injection, Platosin is a preparation of the drug cisplatin.
✚/▲ warning/side-effects: *see* CISPLATIN.

Plesmet (*Napp*) is a proprietary non-prescription preparation of ferrous glycine sulphate, used as an IRON supplement in the treatment of iron-deficiency anaemia, and produced in the form of a syrup for dilution (the potency of the syrup once dilute is retained for 14 days).
✚/▲ warning/side-effects: *see* FERROUS GLYCINE SULPHATE.

Plex-Hormone (*Consolidated*) is a proprietary androgenic sex HORMONE preparation, available only on prescription, used primarily to make up a hormonal deficiency in underdeveloped adolescent boys. Produced in the form of tablets, Plex-Hormone is a preparation of hormones and other steroids, together with tocopheryl acetate (vitamin E).
✚/▲ warning/side-effects: *see* ETHINYLOESTRADIOL; METHYLTESTOSTERONE; TOCOPHERYL ACETATE.

plicamycin, formerly called mithramycin, is a CYTOTOXIC drug that has ANTIBIOTIC properties. It is no longer used as a cytotoxic drug but now is used solely in the emergency treatment of excessive levels of calcium in the blood caused by malignant disease. Administration is by injection.
✚ warning: the drug is toxic: dosage should be the least that is effective. Regular blood counts are essential during treatment.
▲ side-effects: there may be nausea and vomiting, with hair loss. The blood-cell producing capacity of the bone-marrow is reduced.
Related article: MITHRACIN.

pneumococcal vaccine is a VACCINE against pneumonia, consisting a suspension of polysaccharides from a number of capsular types of pneumococci, administered by subcutaneous or intramuscular injection. Like the influenza vaccine, it is intended really only for those people at risk from infection in a community – and at risk from an identified pneumococcal strain prevalent within that community. Immunity is reckoned to last for about 5 years.
✚ warning: vaccination should not be given to patients who are aged under 2 years, who have any form of infection, or who are pregnant. It should be administered with caution to those with cardiovascular or respiratory disease. Some patients experience sensitivity reactions, which may be serious. Although protection may last for only 5 years, revaccination should be

avoided because of the risk of adverse reactions.

Pneumovax (*Morson*) is a proprietary form of the pneumococcal vaccine, available only on prescription for the immunization of personnel for whom the risk of contracting pneumococcal pneumonia is unusually high.
✚ warning: see PNEUMOCOCCAL VACCINE.

podophyllin is a non-proprietary compound paint for the topical treatment of verrucas (plantar warts) and warts in the ano-genital region. It is a solute preparation of podophyllum resin, a highly acidic substance.
✚ warning: the paint should not be used on the face, or on warts on the genitals during pregnancy. The maximum duration for paint to remain on the skin is 6 hours: it should then be washed off. Avoid areas of normal skin. Do not attempt to treat a large number or a whole area of warts at any one time: the highly acidic drug may be absorbed. Pregnant patients are advised NOT to use the paint.
▲ side-effects: application may cause pain (because of the acidity).
Related article: POSALFILIN.

podophyllum resin is the highly acidic substance from which podophyllin compound paint is derived. The resin is also a constituent of a proprietary laxative.
✚/▲ warning/side-effects: *see* PODOPHYLLIN.
see also OPOBYL.

Point-Two (*Hoyt*) is a proprietary non-prescription form of fluoride supplement for administration in areas where the water supply is not fluoridated, especially to growing children. Produced in the form of a mouth-wash, Point-Two is a preparation of SODIUM FLUORIDE.

poldine methylsulphate is an ANTICHOLINERGIC and ANTISPASMODIC drug used to assist in the treatment of gastrointestinal disorders that involve muscle spasm of the intestinal wall. Administration is oral in the form of tablets.
✚ warning: poldine methylsulphate should not be administered to patients with glaucoma; it should be administered with caution to those with heart problems and rapid heart rate, ulcerative colitis, urinary retention or enlargement of the prostate gland; who are elderly; or who are breast feeding.
▲ side-effects: there is commonly dry mouth and thirst; there may also be visual disturbances, flushing, irregular heartbeat and constipation. Rarely, there may be high temperature accompanied by delirium.
Related article: NACTON.

poliomyelitis vaccine is a VACCINE available in two types. Poliomyelitis vaccine, inactivated, is a suspension of dead viruses injected into the body for the body to generate antibodies and so become immune. Poliomyelitis vaccine, live, is a suspension of live but attenuated polio viruses (of polio virus types 1, 2 and 3) for oral administration. In the United Kingdom, the live vaccine is the medium of choice, and the administration is generally simultaneous with the administration of the diphtheria-pertussis-tetanus (DPT) vaccine

– three times during the first year of life, and a booster at school entry age. The inactivated vaccine remains available for those patients for whom there are contra-indications.

✚ warning: poliomyelitis vaccine should not be administered to patients known to have immunodeficiency disorders, who have diarrhoea or cancer, where there is infection, or who are pregnant. Parents of a recently inoculated baby must take extra hygienic precautions when changing its nappies.

Pollinex (*Bencard*) is a proprietary set of 12 grass pollen preparations for use in desensitizing patients who are allergic to one or more of such substances (and so suffer from hay fever or similar symptoms). Available only on prescription, and administered by injection, Pollinex preparations are of carefully annotated different allergenic strength, so that the process of desensitization, as regulated by a doctor, can be progressive.

✚ warning: injections should be administered under close medical supervision and in locations where emergency facilities for full cardio respiratory resuscitation are immediately available.

pol/vac (inact) is an abbreviation for poliomyelitis vaccine, inactivated.
see POLIOMYELITIS VACCINE.

pol/vac (oral) is an abbreviation for poliomyelitis vaccine, live (oral).
see POLIOMYELITIS VACCINE.

Polyalk Revised Formula (*Galen*) is a proprietary non-prescription compound ANTACID used to treat severe indigestion, heartburn, and to relieve the symptoms of gastric or duodenal ulcers. Produced in the form of a suspension, Polyalk Revised Formula is a preparation of ALUMINIUM HYDROXIDE and magnesium oxide ("magnesia") – both fair antacids in their own right – and is not recommended for children.

Polybactrin (*Calmic*) is a proprietary ANTIBIOTIC, available only on prescription, used either as a powder for reconstitution as a solution for bladder irrigation to prevent bladder and urethral infections, or in the form of a powder spray as a topical treatment for minor burns and wounds. In each case, active constituents are POLYMYXIN B sulphate, NEOMYCIN sulphate and bacitracin.

Polycal (*Cow & Gate*) is a proprietary non-prescription nutritional supplement for patients with renal failure, liver cirrhosis, disorders of amino acid metabolism and protein intolerance, and who require a high-energy, low-fluid diet. Produced in the form of a powder for solution, Polycal contains glucose, maltose and polysaccharides.

Polycose (*Abbott*) is a proprietary non-prescription nutritional supplement for patients with renal failure, liver cirrhosis, disorders of amino acid metabolism and protein intolerance, and who require a high-energy, low-fluid diet. Produced in the form of a powder for solution, Polycose contains GLUCOSE polymers.

Polycrol (*Nicholas*) is a proprietary non-prescription ANTACID. Used to treat severe indigestion, heartburn, stomach acidity and flatulence, and produced in the form of tablets (in two strengths, the stronger under the name Polycrol Forte) and a sugar-free gel (in two strengths, the stronger under the name Polycrol Forte Gel), Polycrol is a preparation that contains aluminium hydroxide, MAGNESIUM HYDROXIDE, and the antifoaming agent DIMETHICONE. Most of these preparations are not recommended for children aged under 12 months.

P

polyestradiol phosphate is a compound OESTROGEN used to treat cancer of the prostate gland. Because this type of cancer is linked to the presence of androgens (male sex hormones), administration of this female sex hormone – although it produces some symptoms of feminization – is an effective counter-measure. Administration is by injection.
- ✚ warning: caution should be exercised in administering polyestradiol to patients who are diabetic or epileptic, who have heart or kidney disease, or who have high blood pressure (hypertension) or recurrent severe migraine.
- ▲ side-effects: there may be nausea and vomiting. A common effect is weight gain, generally through fluid or sodium retention in the tissues. There may also be headache and/or depression; sometimes a rash breaks out.
- ✚/▲ warning/side-effects: *see ethinyloestradiol*

Polyfax (*Calmic*) is a proprietary ANTIBACTERIAL drug, available only on prescription, used in topical application to treat infections in the skin and the eye. Produced in the form of an ointment in a paraffin base, and as an eye ointment, Polyfax is a preparation of polymyxin B sulphate and bacitracin zinc.
- ✚/▲ warning/side-effects: *see* POLYMIXIN B.

polygeline is a special refined, partly degraded, form of the hydrolized animal protein gelatin, used in infusion with saline (sodium chloride) as a means of expanding overall blood volume in patients whose blood volume is dangerously low through shock, particularly in cases of severe burns or septicaemia.
- ✚ warning: polygeline should not be administered to patients with congestive heart failure, severely impaired kidney function, or certain blood disorders; ideally, blood samples for cross-matching should be taken before administration.
- ▲ side-effects: rarely, there are hypersensitive reactions.

Related article: HAEMACCEL.

polymyxin B is an ANTIBIOTIC used to treat several forms of bacterial infection. Its use would be more popular were it not so toxic. Because of its toxicity, administrationn (as polymyxin B sulphate) virtually always to be topical in the form of solutions (as in eye-drops and ear-drops) or ointments, or by injection.
- ✚ warning: polymyxin B should not be administered to patients with the neuromuscular disease myasthenia gravis; it should be administered with caution to those with impaired kidney function.
- ▲ side-effects: there may be numbness and tingling in the limbs, blood and protein in the urine, dizziness, breathlessness and overall weakness.

Related articles: AEROSPORIN;

GREGODERM; MAXITROL; NEOSPORIN; OTOSPORIN; OTOTRIPS; POLYBACTRIN; POLYFAX; POLYTRIM; TERRA-CORTRIL; TRIBIOTIC; UNIROID.

polynoxylin is an ANTISEPTIC ANTIFUNGAL agent that also has some ANTIBACTERIAL properties. It is used primarily to treat fungal infections of the mouth and throat (such as thrush). Administration is oral in the form of lozenges.
Related articles: ANAFLEX; PONOXYLAN.

polysaccharide-iron complex is an IRON-rich compound used to restore iron to the blood (in the form of haemoglobin) in cases of iron-deficiency anaemia. Once a patient's blood haemoglobin level has reached normal, treatment should nevertheless continue for at least three months to replenish fully the reserves of iron in the body.
✚ warning: polysaccharide-iron complex should not be administered to patients already taking tetracycline antibiotics.
▲ side-effects: large doses may cause gastrointestinal upset and diarrhoea; there may be vomiting. Prolonged treatment may result in constipation.
Related article: NIFEREX.

polystyrene sulphonate resins are used to treat excessively high levels of potassium in the blood such as dialysis patients. Administration is oral in the form of a solution, or topical in the form of a retention enema (to be retained for as long as 9 hours, if possible). Adequate fluid intake during oral treatment is essential, to prevent impaction of the resins.
✚ warning: resins that contain calcium should be avoided in patients with metastatic cancer or abnormal secretion by the parathyroid glands. Resins that contain sodium should be avoided by patients with congestive heart failure or impaired kidney function.
▲ side-effects: some patients treated by enema experience rectal ulcers.
Related articles: CALCIUM RESONIUM; RESONIUM A.

Polytar Emollient (*Stiefel*) is a proprietary non-prescription brand of preparations used to treat non-infective skin inflammations, including psoriasis and eczema. The standard form is produced in the form of a bath additive, and is a preparation of ANTISEPTICS and natural oils including COAL TAR and ARACHIS OIL. An alcohol-based shampoo is also available (under the name Polytar Liquid), as is a gelatin-based shampoo (under the name Polytar Plus Liquid).

polythiazide is a DIURETIC, one of the THIAZIDES, used to treat fluid retention in the tissues (oedema), hypertension (high blood pressure) and mild to moderate heart failure. Because all thiazides tend to deplete body reserves of potassium, polythiazide may be administered in combination either with potassium supplements or with diuretics that are complementarily potassium-sparing. Administration is oral in the form of tablets.
✚ warning: polythiazide should not be administered to patients with kidney failure or urinary retention, or who are lactating. It should be administered with caution to those who are pregnant. It may aggravate conditions of diabetes or gout.
▲ side-effects: there may be

tiredness and a rash. In men, temporary impotence may occur.
Related article: NEPHRIL.

Polytrim (*Wellcome*) is a proprietary ANTIBIOTIC, available only on prescription, used in the form of eye-drops to treat bacterial infections in the eye. Polytrim is a preparation of the powerful drugs trimethoprim and polymyxin B sulphate.
✚/▲ warning/side-effects: *see* POLYMYXIN B; TRIMETHOPRIM.

polyvinyl alcohol is used as a surfactant tear-distributor, administered in the form of eye-drops to patients whose lachrymal apparatus is dysfunctioning. It works by helping the aqueous layer provided by the lachrymal apparatus (tear fluid) to spread across an eyeball on which the normal mucous surface is patchy or missing.
Related articles: HYPOTEARS; LIQUIFILM TEARS; SNO TEARS.

Polyvite (*Medo*) is a proprietary multivitamin supplement, available on prescription only to private patients. Produced in the form of capsules, Polyvite is a preparation of RETINOL (vitamin A), THIAMINE (vitamine B_1), RIBOFLAVINE (vitamin B_2), PYRIDOXINE (vitamin B_6), NICOTINAMIDE (of the B complex), calcium pantothenate (of the vitamin B complex), ASCORBIC ACID (vitamin C), and ERGOCALCIFEROL (vitamin D).

Ponderax (*Servier*) is a proprietary APPETITE SUPPRESSANT, available only on prescription, used as a short-term additional treatment in medical therapy for obesity. Produced in the form of sustained-release capsules ("Pacaps"), Ponderax is a preparation of the potentially addictive drug fenfluramine hydrochloride. It is not recommended for children.
✚/▲ warning/side-effects: *see* FENFLURAMINE HYDROCHLORIDE.

Pondocillin (*Burgess*) is a proprietary ANTIBIOTIC, available only on prescription, used to treat systemic bacterial infections and infections of the upper respiratory tract, of the ear, nose and throat, and of the urogenital tracts. Produced in the form of tablets, as a sugar-free suspension, and as granules in sachets, Pondocillin is a preparation of the broad-spectrum PENICILLIN pivampicillin.
✚/▲ warning/side-effects: *see* PIVAMPICILLIN.

Ponoxylan (*Berk*) is a proprietary non-prescription ANTIFUNGAL and ANTIBACTERIAL drug, used in topical application to treat skin infections. Produced in the form of a gel, Ponoxylan is a preparation of polynoxylin.
✚/▲ warning/side-effects: *see* POLYNOXYLIN.

Ponstan (*Parke-Davis*) is a proprietary ANTI-INFLAMMATORY non-narcotic ANALGESIC, available only on prescription, used to treat pain in rheumatoid arthritis, osteoarthritis and other musculo-skeletal disorders. Produced in the form of capsules, as tablets, as soluble (dispersible) tablets (under the name Ponstan Dispersible), and as a children's suspension for dilution (the potency of the suspension once dilute is retained for 14 days), Ponstan is a preparation of mefenamic acid. None of these products is recommended for children aged under 6 months.

✚/▲ warning/side-effects: *see* MEFENAMIC ACID.

Portagen (*Bristol-Myers*) is a proprietary non-prescription powdered nutritionally complete diet, used to treat patients whose metabolisms have difficulty in absorbing fats and are unable to tolerate lactose, such as in liver cirrhosis and after surgery of the intestine. Portagen is a preparation of proteins, glycerides, sucrose, vitamins and minerals, and is glucose- and lactose-free.

Posalfilin (*Norgine*) is a proprietary non-prescription compound ointment for topical application, intended to treat and remove anogenital warts and verrucas (plantar warts). Posalfilin is a preparation of the KERATOLYTIC salicylic acid and the highly acidic substance PODOPHYLLUM RESIN. It should not be used for facial warts.
✚/▲ warning/side-effects: *see* SALICYLIC ACID.

Potaba (*Glenwood*) is a proprietary preparation of potassium aminobenzoate, available only on prescription, used to treat scleroderma (hardening and contraction of connective tissue anywhere in the body). Produced in the form of capsules, as tablets and as a powder in sachets ("envules"), Potaba is not recommended for children. Its therapeutic value is debatable.
✚/▲ warning/side-effects: *see* POTASSIUM AMINOBENZOATE.

potassium is a metallic element that occurs naturally only in compounds. In the body, a highly sensitive balance is maintained between potassium within the cells and sodium in the fluids outside the cells (although chemically the two elements are very similar). Nerve impulses are transmitted by means of an almost instantaneous transference of potassium and sodium across cell membranes that sets up a momentary electric current. Deficiency or excess of potassium thus interferes with the actions of most nerves, and particularly those of the heart. Fluid loss from the body results in potassium loss – and therapeutically most potassium is administered to make up such losses, especially following the use of some potassium-depleting drugs (such as the THIAZIDE DIURETICS or CORTICOSTEROIDS). Compounds most used as potassium supplements are potassium bicarbonate and potassium chloride (the latter being a good substitute for natural salt – sodium chloride).

potassium aminobenzoate is a drug most commonly used in the treatment of conditions in which body tissues anywhere in the body become fibrous or hardened (scleroderma) , and contract. How it works – and even whether it works – remains the subject of some debate. Administration is oral in the form of capsules, tablets or in solution.
✚ warning: potassium aminobenzoate should not be administered to patients who are already taking sulphonamide antibiotics; it should be administered with caution to those with impaired kidney function.
▲ side-effects: there may be nausea. Treatment should be withdrawn if serious weight loss occurs.
Related article: POTABA.

potassium canrenoate is a diuretic used to treat the fluid retention associated with heart or liver disease or disorder. Administration is by injection.

✚ warning: potassium canrenoate should not be administered to patients with high levels of potassium in the blood or impaired kidney function. It should be administered with caution to those who are pregnant.

▲ side-effects: there may be nausea and vomiting, especially following high doses. Injection may cause pain.

Related article: SPIROCTAN-M.

P

potassium chloride is used primarily as a POTASSIUM supplement to treat conditions of potassium deficiency, especially during or following severe loss of body fluids or treatment with drugs that deplete body reserves. It may also be used as a substitute for natural salt (sodium chloride) in cases where sodium is for one reason or another inadvisable. Administration is oral, or by injection or infusion.

Related articles: BRINALDIX-K; BURINEX-K; CENTYL-K; Dextrolyte; DIARREST; DIORALYTE; DIUMIDE-K CONTINUS; ELECTROSOL; ESIDREX-K; GLANDOSANE; HYGROTON-K; KEY-CEE-L; K-CONTIN CONTINUS; KLOREF; LASIKAL; LASIX; LEO-K; MICRO-K; NAVIDREX-K; NEO-NACLEX-K; NU-K; RAUTRAX; REHIDRAT; RUTHINOL; SANDO-K; SELORA; SLOW-K.

potassium citrate administered orally has the effect of making the urine alkaline instead of acid. This is of use in relieving pain in some infections of the urinary tract or the bladder. Administration is in the form of tablets or a non-proprietary liquid mixture.

✚ warning: potassium citrate should be administered with caution to patients with heart disease or impaired kidney function.

▲ side-effects: there may be mild diuresis. Prolonged high dosage may lead to excessively high levels of potassium in the blood.

Related article: EFFERCITRATE.

potassium hydroxyquinoline sulphate is a drug that has both ANTIBACTERIAL and ANTIFUNGAL properties – and is pleasant-smelling with it. It is used mostly as a constituent in anti-inflammatory and antibiotic creams and ointments that also contain corticosteroids, such as preparations used to treat acne. Rarely, it causes sensitivity reactions.

Related articles: QUINOCORT; QUINODERM; QUINOPED.

potassium perchlorate was formerly used to treat overactivity of the thyroid gland (hyperthyroidism) and the consequent symptoms (thyrotoxicosis). It works by blocking the uptake of iodine by the thyroid gland, so preventing the production and secretion of thyroid hormones. However, treatment was then proved to be associated with the risk of anaemia, and there are now no proprietary forms available in the United Kingdom.

potassium permanganate is a general DISINFECTANT used in solution for cleaning burns and abrasions and maintaining asepsis in wounds that are suppurating or weeping.

✚ warning: avoid splashing mucous membranes, to which it is an irritant. It also stains skin and fabric.

povidone-iodine is a complex of iodine on an organic carrier, used as an ANTISEPTIC in topical application to the skin, especially in sensitive areas (such as the vulva), and as a mouth wash. Produced in the form of a gel, a solution, or vaginal inserts (pessaries), it works by slowly releasing the iodine it contains.

✚ warning: povidone-iodine should not be used during pregnancy or while lactating.

▲ side-effects: rarely, there may be sensitivity reactions.
Related articles: BETADINE; DISADINE DP; VIDENE.

practolol is a BETA-BLOCKER used as an ANTIARRHYTHMIC drug used to treat tachycardia (fast heart rate), especially following a heart attack. It works by inhibiting the contractile capacity of the heart muscle. Administration is by slow intravenous injection.

✚ warning: practolol should not be administered to patients who have already been given the anti-arrhythmic CALCIUM ANTAGONIST verapamil; it should be administered with caution to those who have had long-term respiratory depression.

▲ side-effects: the heart rate and blood pressure are reduced; there may rarely be heart failure and/or bronchospasm (producing asthma- like symptoms).
Related article: ERALDIN.

Pragmatar (*Bioglan*) is a proprietary non-prescription ointment used in topical application to treat chronic eczema and psoriasis. It is a preparation of various mildly KERATOLYTIC and antibiotic agents including SALICYLIC ACID in a water-miscible base.

pralidoxime mesylate is an unusual drug that is used virtually solely in combination with the belladonna alkaloid ATROPINE in the treatment of severe poisoning by organophosphoric compounds (such as those used as insecticides). The drug is particularly effective in reversing the dangerous muscular paralysis that may affect the entire body. Diagnosis is critical, in that the use of atropine and pralidoxime mesylate to treat poisoning by other compounds used as insecticides may have no effect whatever and can be dangerous. Administration is by injection; repeated doses may be required.

✚ warning: pralidoxime mesylate should be administered with caution to patients with the neuromuscular disease myasthenia gravis, or impaired kidney function.

▲ side-effects: there is drowsiness, dizziness and visual disturbances, muscular weakness, nausea and headache, and rapid heart and breathing rate.

Praxilene (*Lipha*) is a proprietary VASODILATOR that affects principally the blood vessels of the feet and hands, but also affects the blood supply to the brain. It is therefore used to relieve the symptoms of both cerebral and peripheral vascular disease. Produced in the form of capsules, and in ampoules for injection (under the name Praxilene Forte), it is a preparation of naftidrofuryl oxalate, and is not recommended for children.

✚/▲ warning/side-effects: *see* NAFTIDROFURYL OXALATE.

prazepam is an ANXIOLYTIC drug, one of the BENZODIAZEPINES, used primarily in the short-term to treat anxiety and states of nervous tension. Administration is oral in the form of tablets.

✚ warning: prazepam should be administered with caution to patients with severe respiratory difficulties, muscle weakness, glaucoma, or kidney or liver damage; who are in the last stages of pregnancy or are lactating; who are elderly or debilitated; or who have a history of drug abuse. Prolonged use or abrupt withdrawal of the drug should be avoided.

▲ side-effects: concentration and speed of reaction are affected. Drowsiness, dizziness, headache, dry mouth and shallow breathing are all fairly common. Elderly patients may enter a state of confusion. Sensitivity reactions may occur.
Related article: CENTRAX.

P

praziquantel is a synthetic ANTHELMINTIC drug used to rid the body of an infestation of tapeworms. Administration is by a single oral dose, but the drug is not available in the United Kingdom.

prazosin is a VASODILATOR, an ANTIHYPERTENSIVE drug of the alpha-blocker class used to treat both high blood pressure (hypertension) and congestive heart failure. It works as a MUSCLE RELAXANT that is so specific in action that it affects mainly the muscles that surround the smaller arteries. Administration is oral in the form of tablets.

✚ warning: the initial reduction in blood pressure may be precipitous and cause collapse due to hypotension (low blood pressure) (for which reason, extreme caution should be observed in the treatment of patients with impaired kidney function). Later dosage may lead to rapid heart rate.

▲ side-effects: blood pressure may be reduced, causing dizziness on standing up from lying or sitting. There may be weakness.
Related article: HYPOVASE.

Precortisyl (*Roussel*) is a proprietary CORTICOSTEROID preparation, available only on prescription, used to treat inflammation especially in allergic and rheumatic conditions (particularly those affecting the joints) and collagen disorders. It may also be used for systemic corticosteroid therapy. Produced in the form of tablets (in three strengths, the strongest under the name Precortisyl Forte), its active ingredient is the glucocorticoid steroid prednisolone. It is not recommended for children aged under 12 months.

✚/▲ warning/side-effects: *see* PREDNISOLONE.

Predenema (*Pharmax*) is a proprietary CORTICOSTEROID preparation, available only on prescription, used to treat inflammation of the rectum and anus, and associated with haemorrhoids and ulcerative colitis. Produced in the form of a retention enema, Predenema is a preparation of the glucocorticoid steroid prednisolone metasulphobenzoate sodium. It is not recommended for children.

✚/▲ warning/side-effects: *see* PREDNISOLONE.

Prednesol (*Glaxo*) is a proprietary CORTICOSTEROID preparation, available only on prescription, used to treat inflammation especially in allergic and rheumatic conditions (particularly those affecting the joints) and collagen disorders. It may also be used for systemic corticosteroid therapy. Produced

in the form of tablets, its active ingredient is the glucocorticoid steroid prednisolone disodium phosphate. It is not recommended for children aged under 12 months.
✚/▲ warning/side-effects: *see* PREDNISOLONE.

prednisolone is a synthetic CORTICOSTEROID, a glucocorticoid used to treat inflammation especially in rheumatic and allergic conditions (particularly those affecting the joints or the bronchial passages) and collagen disorders, but also effective in the treatment of ulcerative colitis, or rectal or anal inflammation. It may also be used for systemic corticosteroid therapy. Administration (as prednisolone, prednisolone acetate, prednisolone sodium phosphate or prednisolone steaglate) is oral in the form of tablets, or topical in the form of creams, lotions and ointments, as anal suppositories and a retention enema, or by injection.
✚ warning: prednisolone should not be administered to patients with psoriasis; it should be administered with caution to the elderly (in whom overdosage can cause osteoporosis, "brittle bones"). In children, administration of prednisolone may lead to stunting of growth. The effects of potentially serious infections may be masked by the drug during treatment. Withdrawal of treatment must be gradual. In children, administration may result in suppression of growth.
▲ side-effects: treatment of susceptible patients may engender a euphoria, or a state of confusion or depression. Rarely, there is peptic ulcer.
Related articles: ANACAL; CODELSOL; DELTACORTRIL; DELTALONE; DELTA-PHORICOL; DELTASTAB; MINIMS; PRECORTISYL; PREDENEMA; PREDNESOL; PREDSOL; SCHERIPROCT; SINTISONE.

prednisone is a synthetic CORTICOSTEROID that is converted in the body to the glucocorticoid PREDNISOLONE, and is used to treat inflammation especially in rheumatic and allergic conditions (particularly those affecting the joints or the bronchial passages). Administration is oral in the form of tablets.
✚/▲ warning/side-effects: *see* PREDNISOLONE.
Related articles: DECORTISYL; ECONOSONE.

Predsol (*Glaxo*) is a proprietary CORTICOSTEROID preparation, available only on prescription, used either to treat ulcerative colitis and inflammations of the rectum and anus especially in Crohn's disease, or to treat non-infected inflammatory ear and eye conditions. Produced in the form of a retention enema and anal suppositories, and as ear- or eye-drops, Predsol is a preparation of the glucocorticoid prednisolone sodium phosphate. Ear- and eye-drops that additionally contain the antibiotic neomycin sulphate are also available (under the name Predsol-N).
✚/▲ warning/side-effects: *see* NEOMYCIN; PREDNISOLONE.

Prefil (*Norgine*) is a proprietary non-prescription bulking agent, used orally in the medical treatment of obesity. It is intended to work by causing a patient to feel full. Produced in the form of granules for solution, Prefil is a preparation of sterculia.
✚/▲ warning/side-effects: *see* STERCULIA.

Pregaday (*Duncan, Flockhart*) is a proprietary non-prescription VITAMIN-and-mineral supplement, used to prevent iron and folic acid deficiencies in pregnancy. Produced in the form of tablets, Pregaday is a preparation of FERROUS FUMARATE and FOLIC ACID.

Pregestimil (*Bristol-Myers*) is a proprietary non-prescription nutritionally complete dietary preparation, used by patients whose metabolisms are unable to tolerate sucrose, lactose or protein, and who in addition have difficulty in absorbing fats following surgery of the intestine. Produced in the form of a powder, Pregestimil is a preparation of glucose, the milk fat casein, corn oil, modified starch, vitamins and minerals, and is gluten-, sucrose- and lactose-free.

Pregnavite Forte F (*Bencard*) is a proprietary compound IRON and VITAMIN preparation that is not usually available from the National Health Service. It is used mainly by patients during pregnancy to avoid iron and folic acid deficiency. Produced in the form of tablets, Pregnavite Forte F is a preparation of FERROUS SULPHATE, RETINOL (vitamin A), THIAMINE (vitamin B_1), RIBOFLAVINE (vitamin B_2), PYRIDOXINE (vitamin B_6), NICOTINAMIDE (of the B complex), FOLIC ACID, ASCORBIC ACID (vitamin C), CALCIFEROL (vitamin D) and calcium phosphate.

Premarin (*Ayerst*) is a proprietary preparation of female sex HORMONES, available only on prescription, used to treat vaginal and cervical disorders during the menopause. Produced in the form of tablets (in three strengths) and as a vaginal cream for topical application, Premarin is a preparation of conjugated oestrogens.

Premence-28 (*Viabiotics*) is a proprietary non-prescription formulation of nutrients for the days preceeding menstruation. It contains, VITAMIN B, magnesium and IRON.

✚/▲ warning/side-effects: *see* MAGNESIUM.

Prempak (*Wyeth*) is a proprietary HORMONE preparation, available only on prescription, used for the replacement of female sex hormones in women during and following the menopause and to treat atrophic vaginitis or urethritis. Produced in the form of tablets (in three strengths, the two stronger ones under the name Prempak-C), Prempak is a preparation of conjugated OESTROGENS together with the PROGESTOGEN norgestrel.

✚/▲ warning/side-effects: *see* NORGESTREL.

prenylamine is a VASODILATOR used primarily to prevent recurrent attacks of angina pectoris (heart pain). It works as a CALCIUM ANTAGONIST by inhibiting the contractile capacity of the heart muscle. Administration is oral in the form of tablets.

✚ warning: prenylamine should not be administered to patients with severely impaired liver or kidney function or severe heart disease. Blood counts to check on blood potassium levels are advisable during treatment.

▲ side-effects: there may be nausea and vomiting, with diarrhoea. Some patients faint through a condition corresponding to rapid heartbeat combined with low potassium levels. It should therefore not be considered as a first-line drug. Withdrawal should be gradual.

Related article: SYNADRIN.

Pressimmune (*Hoechst*) is a powerful proprietary immunosuppressant, available only on prescription (but generally only in hospitals). Synthesized as an antilymphocyte immunoglobulin from plasma taken from immunized horses, and produced in ampoules for injection, Pressimmune is used to prevent tissue rejection following transplant surgery.
✚/▲ warning/side-effects: *see* IMMUNOGLOBULINS.

Prestim (*Leo*) is a proprietary ANTIHYPERTENSIVE compound, available only on prescription, used to treat mild to moderate high blood pressure (hypertension). Produced in the form of tablets (in two strengths, the stronger under the name Prestim Forte), it is a preparation of the BETA-BLOCKER timolol maleate and the diuretic THIAZIDE bendrofluazide. It is not recommended for children.
✚/▲ warning/side-effects: *see* BENDROFLUAZIDE; TIMOLOL.

Priadel (*Delandale*) is a proprietary drug, available only on prescription, used to treat mania and to prevent some of the more violent outward manifestations of manic-depressive illnesses such as aggressive and self-mutilating behaviour. Produced in the form of sustained-release tablets, Priadel is a preparation of the powerful drug lithium carbonate. It is not recommended for children.
✚/▲ warning/side-effects: *see* LITHIUM.

prilocaine is primarily a local ANAESTHETIC, the drug of choice for very many topical or minor surgical procedures, especially in dentistry (because it is absorbed directly through mucous membranes). Administration is (in the form of a solution of prilocaine hydrochloride) by injection or topically as a cream.
✚ warning: prilocaine should not be administered to patients with the neural disease myasthenia gravis; it should be administered with caution to those with heart or liver failure (in order not to cause depression of the central nervous system and convulsions), or from epilepsy. Dosage should be reduced for the elderly and the debilitated. Full facilities for emergency cardio-respiratory resuscitation should be on hand during anaesthetic treatment.
▲ side-effects: there is generally a slowing of the heart rate and a fall in blood pressure. Some patients under anaesthetic become agitated, others enter a state of euphoria. Sometimes there is respiratory depression and convulsions.
Related articles: CITANEST; CITANEST WITH OCTAPRESSIN; EMLA.

Primalan (*May & Baker*) is a proprietary ANTIHISTAMINE, available only on prescription, used to treat allergic symptoms in such conditions as hay fever. Produced in the form of tablets, Primalan is a preparation of the phenothiazine-type antihistamine mequitazine; it is not recommended for children.
✚/▲ warning/side-effects: *see* MEQUITAZINE.

primaquine is an ANTIMALARIAL drug used to administer the coup de grace to benign tertian forms of malaria following initial treatment with the powerful drugs CHLOROQUINE and/or AMODIAQUINE.

Administration is oral in the form of tablets.
✚ warning: a blood count is essential before administration to check that a patient has sufficient blood levels of a specific enzyme, without which the presence of the drug may cause blood disorders. Primaquine should be administered with caution to patients who are pregnant.
▲ side-effects: there may be nausea and vomiting, anorexia and jaundice. Rarely, there are blood disorders or depression of the bone- marrow's capacity for forming new blood cells.

P

primidone is an ANTICONVULSANT drug used in the treatment of all forms of epilepsy (except absence seizures) and of tremors due to old age or infirmity. It is converted in the body to the BARBITURATE phenobarbitone, and its actions and effects are thus identical to those of that drug.
✚/▲ warning/side-effects: *see* PHENOBARBITONE.
Related article: MYSOLINE.

Primolut N (*Schering*) is a proprietary HORMONAL preparation, available only on prescription, used primarily to treat dysmenorrhoea and pre-menstrual syndrome, although it can additionally be used to make up a hormonal deficiency during or following the menopause. Produced in the form of tablets, Primolut N is a preparation of the PROGESTOGEN norethisterone.
✚/▲ warning/side-effects: *see* NORETHISTERONE.

Primoteston Depot (*Schering*) is a proprietary preparation of the ANDROGEN (male sex hormone) testosterone enanthate , available only on prescription, used to treat hormonal deficiency in men and inoperable breast cancer in women. It is produced in ampoules for long-acting (depot) injection.
✚/▲ warning/side-effects: *see* TESTOSTERONE.

Primperan (*Berk*) is a proprietary ANTINAUSEANT, available only on prescription, used to treat nausea and vomiting especially in gastrointestinal disorders, during treatment for cancer with cytotoxic drugs or radiotherapy, or in association with migraine. Produced in the form of tablets, as a sugar-free syrup for dilution (the potency of the syrup once dilute is retained for 14 days) and in ampoules for injection, Primperan is a preparation of metoclopramide hydrochloride. It is not recommended for children aged under 5 years.
✚/▲ warning/side-effects: *see* METOCLOPRAMIDE.

Prioderm (*Napp*) is a proprietary non-prescription drug used to treat infestations of the scalp and pubic hair by lice (pediculosis), or of the skin by the itch-mite (scabies). Produced in the form of a lotion in an alcohol base, and as a cream shampoo, Prioderm is a preparation of the insecticide malathion.
✚/▲ warning/side-effects: *see* MALATHION.

Pripsen (*Reckitt & Colman*) is a proprietary non-prescription ANTHELMINTIC, used to treat infections by threadworm and roundworm. Produced in the form of an oral powder, Pripsen is a preparation of the phenothiazine derivative piperazine phosphate with various stimulant LAXATIVES, and is not recommended for children aged under 3 months.
✚/▲ warning/side-effects: *see* PIPERAZINE.

Pro-Actidil (*Wellcome*) is a proprietary non-prescription ANTIHISTAMINE drug used to treat the symptoms of various allergic conditions, particularly hay fever and urticaria. Produced in the form of sustained-release tablets, Pro-Actidil is a preparation of the antihistamine triprolidine hydrochloride; it is not recommended for children.
✚/▲ warning/side-effects: *see* TRIPROLIDINE.

Pro-Banthine (*Gold Cross*) is a proprietary ANTICHOLINERGIC ANTISPASMODIC drug, available only on prescription, used to assist in the treatment of gastrointestinal disorders arising from muscular spasm of the intestinal walls. As a SMOOTH MUSCLE RELAXANT, it is also sometimes used to treat children for nocturnal bedwetting (because the bladder sphincter muscles have to contract to let urine through) or with retention enemas. Produced in the form of tablets, Pro-Banthine is a preparation of propantheline bromide.
✚/▲ warning/side-effects: *see* PROPANTHELINE BROMIDE.

probenecid is a drug that promotes the excretion of uric acid in the urine; it is therefore used in the treatment of gout, and other conditions that also result from an excess of uric acid in the bloodstream. The drug can also be used to inhibit the excretion through the kidneys of penicillin and cephalosporin antibiotics, thus prolonging the antibiotics' effects. Administration is oral in the form of tablets.
✚ warning: probenecid should not be administered to patients with blood disorders or kidney stones, who are undergoing an acute attack of gout, or who are already taking salicylate drugs (such as aspirin). It should be administered with caution to patients with peptic ulcer. The drug is ineffective in a patient with impaired kidney function. Initial administration should be accompanied by the administration of colchicine to ward off acute gout attacks. Adequate fluid intake is essential.
▲ side-effects: side-effects are uncommon, but there may be nausea and vomiting, headache and flushing, dizziness and a rash, and frequent urination. Some patients experience blood disorders.
Related article: BENEMID.

probucol is a drug used to treat high levels of cholesterol or other lipids (fats) within the bloodstream. It works by inhibiting the uptake of fats by the liver. Administration is oral in the form of tablets.
✚ warning: probucol should not be administered to patients who are lactating. Pregnancy should be avoided during treatment and for 6 months afterwards.
▲ side-effects: there may be nausea, vomiting, flatulence, abdominal pain and diarrhoea. Rarely there are sensitivity reactions – which may be serious.
Related article: LURSELLE.

procainamide is a BETA-BLOCKER, used as an ANTIARRHYTHMIC drug to treat heartbeat irregularities especially after a heart attack. Administration (as procainamide hydrochloride) is oral in the form of tablets and sustained-release tablets, or by injection.
✚ warning: procainamide should not be administered to patients

P

with heart failure, heart block, or low blood pressure; it should be administered with caution to those with asthma, the neuromuscular disease myasthenia gravis or impaired kidney function, or who have already received treatment with lignocaine.

▲ side-effects: there may be nausea, diarrhoea, high temperature, slow heart rate and rashes. In susceptible patients there may be heart failure and/or skin or blood disorders, especially after prolonged treatment.
Related articles: PROCAINAMIDE DURULES; PRONESTYL.

P

Procainamide Durules (*Astra*) is a proprietary ANTIARRHYTHMIC drug, available only on prescription, used to treat heartbeat irregularities especially after a heart attack. Produced in the form of sustained-release tablets, Procainamide Durules is a preparation of the BETA-BLOCKER procainamide hydrochloride; it is not recommended for children.

✚/▲ warning/side-effects: *see* PROCAINAMIDE.

procaine is a local ANAESTHETIC that is now seldom used. Once popular, it has been overtaken by anaesthetics that are longer-lasting and better absorbed through mucous membranes. Because of this poor absorption it cannot be used as a surface anaesthetic. It remains available, however, and may be used for regional anaesthesia or by infiltration, usually in combination with adrenaline. Administration (as procaine hydrochloride) is by injection.

✚ warning: the metabolite of procaine inhibits the action on the body of sulphonamide drugs.

▲ side-effects: rarely, there are sensitivity reactions – which may be serious.

procaine penicillin is a penicillin-type ANTIBIOTIC that is a derivative of benzylpenicillin. It is primarily used in long- lasting (depot) injections to treat conditions such as syphilis and gonorrhoea, but may also be used to treat the equally serious condition gas gangrene following amputation. Administration is by intramuscular injection.

✚/▲ warning/side-effects: *see* BENZYLPENICILLIN.
Related articles: BICILLIN; DEPOCILLIN.

procarbazine is a CYTOTOXIC drug used to treat the lymphatic cancer Hodgkin's disease, other lymphatic growths, and some small solid tumours, such as of the bronchus. Administration is oral in the form of capsules.

✚ warning: dietary counselling is essential before treatment with procarbazine. Alcohol consumption must be avoided during treatment. Regular blood counts are advisable. A reduced dose should be used in patients with kidney damage.

▲ side-effects: there is a reduction in the capacity of the bone-marrow for producing new blood cells. There may also be nausea, vomiting and hair loss. Treatment should be withdrawn if a rash denoting hypersensitivity appears.
Related article: NATULAN.

prochlorperazine is a phenothiazine derivative used as an ANTIPSYCHOTIC drug in the treatment of psychosis (such as schizophrenia); as an ANXIOLYTIC in the short-term treatment of anxiety; and as an ANTI-EMETIC in the prevention of nausea caused by gastrointestinal disorder, by chemotherapy and radiotherapy in the treatment of cancer, by motion within a vehicle, or by the vertigo that results from infection of the middle or inner ear. Administration (as prochlorpromazine maleate or prochlorpromazine mesylate) is oral in the form of tablets, sustained-release capsules and syrups, topical in the form of anal suppositories, or by injection.

✚ warning: prochlorpromazine should not be administered to patients with certain forms of glaucoma, whose blood-cell formation by the bone-marrow is reduced, or who are taking drugs that depress certain centres of the brain and spinal cord. It should be administered with caution to those with lung disease, cardiovascular disease, epilepsy, parkinsonism, abnormal secretion by the adrenal glands, impaired liver or kidney function, undersecretion of thyroid hormones (hypothyroidism), enlargement of the prostate gland, or any form of acute infection; who are pregnant or lactating; or who are elderly. Prolonged treatment requires checks on eye function and skin pigmentation. Withdrawal of treatment should be gradual.

▲ side-effects: concentration and speed of thought and movement may be affected. High doses may cause neuromuscular disorders, especially in children, the elderly or the debilitated. *Related articles:* STEMETIL; VERTIGON.

Proctofibe (*Roussel*) is a proprietary non-prescription LAXATIVE that is not available from the National Health Service. A bulking agent – which works by increasing the overall mass of faeces within the rectum, so stimulating bowel movement – Proctofibe is a preparation of grain fibre and citrus fibre. Produced in the form of tablets, it is not recommended for children aged under 3 years, and counselling is advised before use.

Proctofoam HC (*Stafford-Miller*) is a proprietary CORTICOSTEROID compound with ANALGESIC properties, available only on prescription, used to treat, dress and soothe various painful conditions of the anus and rectum. Produced in the form of a foam in an aerosol, Proctofoam HC is a preparation of the corticosteroid hydrocortisone acetate and the ANAESTHETIC pramoxine hydrochloride. It is not recommended for children.

✚/▲ warning/side-effects: *see* HYDROCORTISONE ACETATE.

Proctosedyl (*Roussel*) is a proprietary CORTICOSTEROID compound with ANALGESIC properties, available only on prescription, used to treat, dress and soothe various painful conditions of the anus and rectum. Produced in the form of suppositories and as an ointment, Proctosedyl is a preparation that includes the corticosteroid hydrocortisone, the ANAESTHETIC cinchocaine hydrochloride, and the antibiotic framycetin sulphate.

✚/▲ warning/side-effects: *see* CINCHOCAINE; FRAMYCETIN; HYDROCORTISONE.

procyclidine is a powerful ANTICHOLINERGIC drug used to relieve some of the symptoms of parkinsonism, specifically the tremor of the hands, the overall rigidity of the posture, and the tendency to produce an excess of saliva. (The drug also has the capacity to treat these conditions in some cases where they are produced by drugs.) It is thought to work by compensating for the lack of dopamine in the brain that is the major cause of such parkinsonian symptoms. Administration – which may be in parallel with the administration of levodopa – is oral in the form of tablets or a syrup or by injection.

✚ warning: procyclidine should not be administered to patients who suffer not merely from tremor but from distinct involuntary movements; it should be administered with caution to those with impaired kidney or liver function, cardiovascular disease, glaucoma, or urinary retention. Withdrawal of treatment must be gradual.

▲ side-effects: there may be dry mouth, dizziness and blurred vision, and/or gastrointestinal disturbances. Some patients experience sensitivity reactions and anxiety. Rarely, and in susceptible patients, there may be confusion, agitation and psychological disturbance (at which point treatment MUST be withdrawn). *Related articles:* ARPICOLIN; KEMADRIN.

P

Prodexin (*Bencard*) is a proprietary non-prescription ANTACID compound that is not available from the National Health Service. It is used to treat acid stomach and indigestion and to soothe pain from peptic ulcer. Produced in the form of tablets, Prodexin is a preparation of ALUMINIUM GLYCINATE and MAGNESIUM CARBONATE and is not recommended for children.

✚ warning: should not be given at the same time as other drugs as they will reduce absorption. May cause constipation.

Profasi (*Serono*) is a proprietary preparation of human chorionic gonadotrophin (HCG), available only on prescription, used to treat undescended testicles in boys, and to treat women suffering from specific hormonal deficiency for infertility. It is produced in the form of a powder for reconstitution as a medium for injection.

✚/▲ warning/side-effects: *see* HCG.

proflavine cream is a non-proprietary formulation that includes beeswax, wool fat, liquid paraffin and some mild antibacterial agents; it is used in topical application as a dressing for minor skin infections, burns and abrasions.

✚ warning: wool fat causes sensitivity reactions in some patients.

Progesic (*Lilly*) is a proprietary non-steroidal ANTI-INFLAMMATORY non-narcotic ANALGESIC used to relieve pain – particularly arthritic and rheumatic pain – and to treat other musculo-skeletal disorders. Available only on prescription, and produced in the form of tablets, Progesic is a preparation of fenoprofen (as a calcium salt). It is not recommended for children.

✚/▲ warning/side-effects: *see* FENOPROFEN.

progesterone is a sex HORMONE, a PROGESTOGEN found predominantly in women, but that has a role in the sexual make-up also of men. In women it is produced and secreted mainly by the corpus luteum of the ovary, and is responsible for the preparation of the lining of the womb (the endometrium) once every menstrual cycle to receive a fertilized ovum. Most cycles come and go without fertilization (conception), but if a fertilized ovum does implant in the endometrium, the resultant formation of a placenta ensures the continuation of the supply of progesterone and so prevents further menstrual cycles while the pregnancy lasts. In men, small quantities of progesterone are secreted by the testes and by the adrenal glands. Therapeutically, progesterone is administered to women chiefly to treat premenstrual syndrome, but may also be used to prevent recurrent miscarriage or abnormal bleeding from the vagina. Administration is by anal or vaginal suppositories (pessaries), or by injection.

✚ warning: progesterone should not be administered to patients who suffer from undiagnosed vaginal bleeding or from sex-hormone- linked cancer, or who have a history of thrombosis. It should be administered with caution to those with high blood pressure (hypertension), diabetes, impaired liver or kidney function, or heart disease.

▲ side-effects: there may be acne, urticaria, fluid retention and consequent weight gain, and gastrointestainal disturbances; there may also be breast tenderness, irregular menstruation and a change in libido. Injection may cause pain.

Related articles: CYCLOGEST; GESTONE.

progestogens are sex hormones that oppose or modify the action of some OESTROGENS. There are two main groups of progestogens: the natural progestogen PROGESTERONE and those like it (allyloestrenol, dydrogesterone, hydroxyprogesterone and medroxyprogesterone) and the analogues of TESTOSTERONE (such as norethisterone). All are synthesized for therapeutic use – and can therefore be taken orally – to prevent recurrent miscarriage, to relieve the symptoms of premenstrual syndrome or menstrual difficulty, or to treat lack of menstruation (amenorrhoea) or abnormal bleeding from the womb through the vagina. But perhaps the most widely used mode of application is as constituents (with or without accompanying oestrogens) in ORAL CONTRACEPTIVES, because progestogens prevent ovulation.

✚/▲ warning/side-effects: *see* PROGESTERONE.

Related articles: ALLYLOESTRENOL; DYDROGESTERONE; HYDROXYPROGESTERONE HEXANOATE; LEVONORGESTREL; LYNOESTRENOL; MEDROXYPROGESTERONE ACETATE; NORETHISTERONE; NORETHISTERONE ACETATE; NORGESTREL.

proguanil is an ANTIMALARIAL drug used to try to prevent the contraction of malaria by travellers in tropical countries. Its effectiveness is not guaranteed, and the traveller is advised to take measures as far as possible to avoid being bitten by mosquitoes. Administration (as proguanil hydrochloride) is oral in the form of tablets.

✚ warning: proguanil should be administered with caution to patients who suffer from impaired kidney function.

▲ side-effects: there may be mild gastric disorder.

Related article: PALUDRINE.

Progynova (*Schering*) is a proprietary OESTROGEN

preparation available only on prescription, used to treat vaginal and cervical disorders during the menopause. Produced in the form of tablets (in two strengths), Progynova is a preparation of oestradiol valerate.

✚/▲ warning/side-effects: *see* OESTRADIOL.

prolintane is a weak STIMULANT used as a constituent in some proprietary vitamin preparations, and intended to assist in the treatment of fatigue or lethargy. Prolonged or high dosage, however, may lead to a state of arousal and/or anxiety.
Related article: VILLESCON.

Proluton Depot (*Schering*) is a proprietary form of the PROGESTOGEN (sex hormone) hydroxyprogesterone hexanoate, available only on prescription, used to treat recurrent miscarriage. It is produced in ampoules (in two strengths) for long-lasting (depot) injection.

✚/▲ warning/side-effects: *see* HYDROXYPROGESTERONE HEXANOATE.

promazine hydrochloride is an ANTIPSYCHOTIC drug used to tranquillize agitated patients, especially patients who are elderly. The drug is also used in the short term to treat severe anxiety, or to soothe patients who are dying. Administration is oral in the form of a suspension, or by injection.

✚ warning: promazine hydrochloride should not be administered to patients with certain forms of glaucoma (closed-angle), whose blood-cell formation by the bone-marrow is reduced, or who are taking drugs that depress certain centres of the brain and spinal cord. It should be administered with caution to those with lung disease, cardiovascular disease, epilepsy, parkinsonism, abnormal secretion by the adrenal glands, impaired liver or kidney function, undersecretion of thyroid hormones (hypothyroidism), enlargement of the prostate gland or any form of acute infection; who are pregnant or lactating; or children. Prolonged use requires regular checks on eye function and skin pigmentation. Withdrawal of treatment should be gradual.

▲ side-effects: concentration and speed of thought and movement are affected; the effects of alcohol consumption are enhanced. There may be dry mouth and blocked nose, constipation and difficulty in urinating, rash, jaundice and blurred vision; menstrual disturbances in women or impotence in men may occur, with weight gain; there may be sensitivity reactions. Some patients feel cold and depressed, and tend to suffer from poor sleep patterns. Blood pressure may be low and the heartbeat irregular. Treatment by intramuscular injection may be painful.
Related article: SPARINE.

promethazine hydrochloride is a powerful ANTIHISTAMINE that also has HYPNOTIC and ANTITUSSIVE properties. Consequently, although it is used to treat the symptoms of allergic conditions (such as hay fever and urticaria, but additionally including the emergency treatment of anaphylactic shock), it is used also to induce sleep in the treatment of insomnia (especially in children) or as a premedication prior to surgery, and as a cough suppressant in cough linctuses. It may also be used in the treatment of parkinsonism, and as an ANTI-EMETIC in the prevention of nausea due to motion sickness or to ear infection. Its effect is comparatively long-lasting. Administration is oral in the form of tablets and a dilute elixir, or by injection.

✚ warning: promethazine should be administered with caution to patients with epilepsy, glaucoma, liver disease or enlargement of the prostate gland. During treatment, alcohol consumption must be avoided.

▲ side-effects: concentration and speed of thought and movement may be affected. There may be headache, drowsiness and dry mouth, with gastrointestinal disturbances. Some patients experience blurred vision and/or sensitivity reactions on the skin.

Related articles: MEDISED; PAMERGAN P100; PHENERGAN; Phensedyl; SOMINEX.

promethazine theoclate is a salt of the powerful ANTIHISTAMINE promethazine, used primarily to prevent nausea and vomiting caused by motion sickness or infection of the ear. It is slightly longer-acting than the hydrochloride, but otherwise is similar in every respect.

✚/▲ warning/side-effects: *see* PROMETHAZINE HYDROCHLORIDE.

Related article: AVOMINE.

Prominal (*Winthrop*) is a proprietary form of the BARBITURATE methylphenobarbitone, and is on the controlled drugs list. Produced in the form of tablets (in three strengths), Prominal is used to treat tonic-clonic and partial seizure epilepsy. It is not recommended for children.

✚/▲ warning/side-effects: *see* METHYLPHENOBARBITONE.

Prondol (*Wyeth*) is a proprietary ANTIDEPRESSANT drug, available only on prescription, used to treat depressive illness and associated symptoms. Produced in the form of tablets (in two strengths), Prondol is a preparation of the TRICYCLIC drug iprindole hydrochloride; it is not recommended for children.

✚/▲ warning/side-effects: *see* IPRINDOLE.

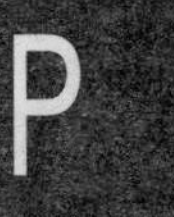

Pronestyl (*Squibb*) is a proprietary ANTIARRHYTHMIC drug, available only on prescription, used to treat irregularities in the heartbeat, especially after a heart attack. Produced in the form of tablets and in vials for injection, Pronestyl is a preparation of the PROCAINE derivative procainamide hydrochloride. It is not recommended for children.

✚/▲ warning/side-effects: *see* PROCAINAMIDE.

Propaderm (*Allen & Hanburys*) is a proprietary brand of CORTICOSTEROID preparations, available only on prescription, used in topical application to treat severe non-infective skin inflammation such as eczema, especially in patients whose conditions have not responded to less powerful corticosteroids. Produced in its standard form of a cream and ointment, Propaderm is a preparation of the steroid beclomethasone dipropionate. An ointment additionally containing the ANTIBACTERIAL drug chlortetracycline hydrochloride (under the name Propaderm-A) is available for infective skin

inflammation, and a cream and an ointment additionally containing the iodine-rich ANTISEPTIC clioquinol (under the name Propaderm-C) are also available.
✚/▲ warning/side-effects: *see* BECLOMETHASONE DIPROPIONATE; CHLORTETRACYCLINE; CLIOQUINOL.

Propain (*Panpharma*) is a proprietary non-prescription compound ANALGESIC that is not available from the National Health Service. It is used to treat many forms of pain, including headache, migraine, muscular pain and menstrual problems. Produced in the form of tablets, Propain is a compound that includes the OPIATE codeine phosphate, the ANTIHISTAMINE diphenhydramine hydrochloride, the ANALGESIC paracetamol and the STIMULANT caffeine. It is not recommended for children.
✚/▲ warning/side-effects: *see* CAFFEINE; CODEINE PHOSPHATE; DIPHENHYDRAMINE HYDROCHLORIDE; PARACETAMOL.

propamidine isethionate is an ANTIBIOTIC drug used specifically in the form of eye-drops to treat bacterial infections of the eyelids (blepharitis) or conjunctiva (conjunctivitis).
Related article: BROLENE.

propantheline bromide is an ANTICHOLINERGIC drug used to assist in the treatment of gastrointestinal disorders that involve muscle spasm of the intestinal wall (and by the same token to increase the duration of enema retention in patients who suffer from diarrhoea). It is also used to treat urinary incontinence and nocturnal bedwetting in children. Administration is oral in the form of tablets.
✚ warning: propantheline bromide should not be administered to patients with glaucoma; it should be administered with caution to those with heart problems and rapid heart rate, ulcerative colitis and other gastro-intestinal disorders, urinary retention or enlargement of the prostate gland; who are elderly; or who are breast feeding.
▲ side-effects: there is commonly dry mouth and thirst; there may also be visual disturbances, flushing, irregular heartbeat, urinary retention and constipation. Rarely, there may be high temperature accompanied by delirium.
Related article: PRO-BANTHINE.

Propine (*Allergan*) is a proprietary SYMPATHOMIMETIC, available only on prescription, used in the form of eye-drops to treat glaucoma by relieving intra-ocular pressure. Propine is a preparation of the ADRENALINE derivative dipivefrine hydrochloride which passes more readily through the cornea and is then converted to adrenaline. It is not recommended for children.
✚/▲ warning/side-effects: *see* DIPIVEFRINE.

Pro-Plus (*Ashe Consumer Products*) is a proprietary non-prescription preparation of caffeine for use in reducing fatigue.
✚/▲ warning/side-effects: *see* CAFFEINE.

propofol is a general ANAESTHETIC used specifically for the initial induction of anaesthesia. Recovery after treatment is rapid and without any hangover effect. Administration is by injection.

- ✚ warning: intravenous injection must be carried out with caution in order to avoid thrombophlebitis.
- ▲ side-effects: there may sometimes be pain on injection, which can be overcome by prior administration of suitable premedication (such as a narcotic analgesic). Urine may turn green.

Related article: DIPRIVAN.

propranolol is a BETA-BLOCKER, used primarily to regularize the heartbeat and to treat and prevent angina pectoris (heart pain) and hypertension (*see* ANTIHYPERTENSIVE). It may additionally be used to relieve the symptoms of excess thyroid hormones in the bloodstream (thyrotoxicosis), or of migraine, and it is also often used to relieve anxiety (particularly if there is tremor or palpitations). Administration (as propranolol hydrochloride) is oral in the form of tablets and sustained-release capsules, or by injection.

- ✚ warning: propranolol should not be administered to patients with any serious form of heart disease, or asthma. It should be administered with caution to those with impaired liver or kidney function, who are nearing the end of pregnancy, or who are lactating.
- ▲ side-effects: the heart rate is slowed; there may also be bronchospasm (causing asthma-like symptoms), gastrointestinal disturbances, and tingling or numbness in the fingers and toes.

Related articles: ANGILOL; APSOLOL; BEDRANOL; BERKOLOL; HALF-INDERAL LA; INDERAL; INDERAL-LA; INDERETIC; INDEREX; SLOPROLOL; SPIROPROP.

propylthiouracil is a drug that prevents the production or secretion of the HORMONE thyroxine by the thyroid gland, so treating an excess in the blood of thyroid hormones and the symptoms that it causes (thyrotoxicosis). Treatment may be on a maintenance basis over a long period (dosage adjusted to optimum effect), or may be merely preliminary to surgical removal of the thyroid gland. Administration is oral in the form of tablets.

- ✚ warning: propylthiouracil should not be administered to patients with obstruction of the upper respiratory tract, and should be administered with extreme caution to patients who are pregnant or lactating.
- ▲ side-effects: an itching rash may indicate a need for alternative treatment. There may also be nausea and headache; occasionally there is jaundice or hair loss. Rarely, there may be a tendency to haemorrhage.

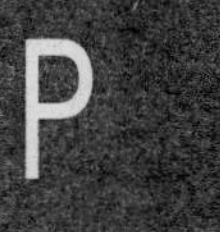

Prosigmin (*Roche*) is a proprietary preparation of neostigmine, available only on prescription. The drug prolongs the action of the natural neurotransmitter acetylcholine, and can thus be used both in the diagnosis of disorders of the neurotransmission process caused by disease such as myesthesia gravis or by drug treatments (through a comparison of its effect with the effect of its absence), and as an antidote to muscle relaxants and anaesthetics which block the action of the neurotransmitter (in which case, atropine should be administered simultaneously). It

is produced in ampoules (in two strengths) for injection (in the form of neostigmine methylsulphate) and as tablets (as neostigmine bromide).
✚/▲ warning/side-effects: *see* NEOSTIGMINE.

Prosobee (*Bristol-Myers*) is a proprietary food product that is nutritionally a complete diet, for use by patients whose metabolic processes are unable to tolerate milk or lactose. Produced in the form of a liquid concentrate, it is a preparation of protein (soya protein), carbohydrate (corn syrup solids), fat (soya oil, coconut oil), VITAMINS, minerals and trace elements, and is gluten-, sucrose-, fructose- and lactose-free. Prosobee is also produced as a powder containing protein (soya protein), carbohydrate (corn syrup solids), fat (coconut oil, corn oil) and vitamins and minerals that is also gluten-, sucrose-, fructose- and lactose-free.

Prosparol (*Duncan, Flockhart*) is a proprietary nutritional preparation for patients requiring a high energy, low fluid and low electrolyte diet. Produced in the form of an emulsion, Prosparol is a preparation of ARACHIS OIL in water.

prostacyclin is a technical term for the drug and naturally occuring compound more commonly known as epoprostenol.
see EPOPROSTENOL.

Prostin E2 (*Upjohn*) is a proprietary drug of the HORMONE-like PROSTAGLANDIN E1, available only on prescription, used because of its property of causing uterine contractions mainly to induce and augment labour and therapeutic abortion. Produced in the form of tablets, as vaginal tablets (pessaries), as a vaginal gel (in two strengths), in ampoules (in two strengths) for intravenous injection, and in ampoules for extra-amniotic injection for hospital use only, Prostin E2 is a preparation of dinoprostone.
✚/▲ warning/side-effects: *see* DINOPROSTONE.

Prostin F2 alpha (*Upjohn*) is a proprietary form of the naturally occuring HORMONE-like PROSTAGLANDIN F2 alpha, available only on prescription, used because of its property of causing uterine contractions mainly to induce and augment labour and therapeutic abortion. Produced in ampoules for intravenous injection, and in ampoules for intra-amniotic injection for hospital use only, Prostin F2 alpha is a preparation of dinoprost.
✚/▲ warning/side-effects: *see* DINOPROST.

Prostin VR (*Upjohn*) is a proprietary hormonal drug, available only on prescription, used to maintain newborn babies born with heart defects while preparations are rapidly made for corrective surgery in intensive care. Produced in ampoules for injection or infusion, Prostin VR is a preparation of the PROSTAGLANDIN alprostadil (prostaglandin E1).
✚/▲ warning/side-effects: *see* ALPROSTADIL.

protamine sulphate is essentially a coagulant, in that its primary use is as an antidote to an overdose of the ANTI-COAGULANT heparin. However, it too – in overdosage – has an anticoagulant effect. Administration is by slow

intravenous injection.
✚ warning: dosage is critical: administration must be of enough to neutralize the heparin, but not so much as to contribute to further anticoagulation.
▲ side-effects: there is a reduction in heart rate and blood pressure; there is often also flushing.

Protaphane, Human
see HUMAN PROTAPHANE.

Prothiaden (*Boots*) is a proprietary ANTIDEPRESSANT drug, available only on prescription, used to treat depressive illness especially in cases where some degree of sedation is deemed necessary. Produced in the form of tablets and capsules, Prothiaden is a preparation of dothiepin hydrochloride. It is not recommended for children.
✚/▲ warning/side-effects: *see* DOTHIEPIN HYDROCHLORIDE.

prothionamide is an ANTITUBERCULAR drug also used to treat leprosy. It is no longer available in the United Kingdom.

protirelin, or thyrotrophin-releasing hormone (TRH), is a natural HORMONE produced and secreted by the thalamus; it acts on the pituitary gland in turn to produce and secrete thyrotrophin, a hormone that then causes the production and secretion of yet other hormones in the body. Therapeutically it is used primarily to assess thyroid function in patients who suffer from underactivity of the pituitary gland (hypopituitarism) or from overactivity of the thyroid gland (hyperthyroidism). Administration is oral in the form of tablets, or it can be given by injection.
✚ warning: protirelin should be administered with caution to patients with severe underactivity of the pituitary gland or heart failure, or who are in early pregnancy; oral administration is advised for patients with breathing difficulties.
▲ side-effects: there is commonly nausea. Treatment by injection may cause flushing, dizziness, faintness, a strange taste in the mouth, and a desire to urinate. Occasionally there may be bronchospasm.
Related article: TRH.

protriptyline is an ANTIDEPRESSANT drug used because it has a stimulant effect particularly to treat depressive illness that disposes towards apathy and withdrawal. Administration (as protriptyline hydrochloride) is oral in the form of tablets.
✚ warning: protriptyline should not be administered to patients with heart disease or psychosis, as it may aggravate tension and cause insomnia; it should be administered with caution to patients with diabetes, epilepsy, liver or thyroid disease, glaucoma or urinary retention; or who are pregnant or lactating; or who are elderly. Withdrawal of treatment must be gradual.
▲ side-effects: common effects include loss of intricacy in movement or thought, dry mouth and blurred vision, an increased heart rate, irregular heartbeat, and a raised body temperature; there may also be difficulty in urinating, a rash, behavioural disturbances, insomnia, anxiety, state of confusion, and/or a loss of libido. Rarely, there are also blood deficiencies.
Related article: CONCORDIN.

Pro-Vent (*Wellcome*) is a proprietary non-prescription BRONCHODILATOR, used to treat the bronchospasm of asthma, emphysema and chronic bronchitis. Produced in the form of sustained-release capsules, Pro-Vent is a preparation of the xanthine drug theophylline. It is not recommended for children.
✚/▲ warning/side-effects: *see* THEOPHYLLINE.

Provera (*Upjohn*) is a proprietary preparation of the PROGESTOGEN medroxyprogesterone acetate, available only on prescription, used as a hormonal supplement in women whose progestogen level requires boosting, as at menopause, and (in higher doses) to treat sex-hormone-linked cancer, such as cancer of the breast or of the womb-lining. It is produced in tablets (in four strengths).
✚/▲ warning/side-effects: *see* MEDROXYPROGESTERONE.

Pro-Viron (*Schering*) is a proprietary ANDROGEN (male sex hormone), available only on prescription, used primarily to make up hormonal deficiency and thus treat male infertility. Produced in the form of tablets, Pro-Viron is a preparation of mesterolone.
✚/▲ warning/side-effects: *see* MESTEROLONE.

proxymetacaine is a widely-used local ANAESTHETIC with particular application to ophthalmic treatments. Administered in the form of eye-drops (and as proxymetacaine hydrochloride) it generally causes little initial stinging and is therefore useful for treating children.
▲ side-effects: there may be slight stinging on initial application.
Related article: OPHTHAINE.

pseudoephedrine is a VASOCONSTRICTOR, a SYMPATHOMIMETIC drug that is also a BRONCHODILATOR, used mainly in the treatment of asthma, chronic bronchitis and similar conditions (especially allergy-based ones). In all respects its actions and effects are identical to those of the closely-related drug ephedrine hydrochloride.
✚/▲ warning/side-effects: *see* EPHEDRINE HYDROCHLORIDE.
Related articles: BENYLIN DECONGESTANT; DIMOTANE PLUS; DIMOTANE WITH CODEINE; GALPSEUD; SUDAFED.

pseudomonic acid is a term for the drug more commonly known as mupirocin.
see MUPIROCIN.

Psoradrate (*Norwich Eaton*) is a proprietary non-prescription preparation, used in topical application to treat chronic and mild forms of psoriasis. Produced in a powder-in-cream base containing the natural DIURETIC urea (in three strengths), Psoradrate is a preparation of dithranol.
✚/▲ warning/side-effects: *see* DITHRANOL.

Psoriderm (*Dermal*) is a proprietary ANTISEPTIC used to treat non-infective skin conditions such as psoriasis. Produced in the form of a cream, a scalp lotion (used as a shampoo), and a bath emulsion, Psoriderm's active constituent is COAL TAR.

PsoriGel (*Alcon*) is a proprietary ANTISEPTIC used to treat non-infective skin conditions such as psoriasis and chronic eczema. Produced in the form of a gel, PsoriGel is a preparation of a

COAL TAR solution in an emollient alcohol base.

Psorin (*Thames*) is a proprietary, non-prescription compound preparation used in topical application to treat chronic and mild forms of the troublesome skin disorder psoriasis. Produced in the form of an ointment in an emollient base, Psorin is a combination of dithranol, salicylic acid and COAL TAR.
✚/▲ warning/side-effects: *see* DITHRANOL; SALICYLIC ACID.

Pulmadil (*Riker*) is a proprietary BRONCHODILATOR, available only on prescription, used to treat bronchospasm in asthma and chronic bronchitis. Produced in a metered-dosage aerosol, and in metered-dosage cartridges (under the name Pulmadil Puto), Pulmadil is a preparation of the SYMPATHOMIMETIC rimiterol hydrobromide.
✚/▲ warning/side-effects: *see* RIMITEROL.

Pulmicort (*Astra*) is a proprietary CORTICOSTEROID preparation, available only on prescription, used to treat the inflammatory symptoms of bronchial asthma. Produced in a metered-dosage aerosol (in two strengths, the weaker labelled for children and named Pulmicort LS), Pulmicort is a preparation of budesonide.
✚/▲ warning/side-effects: *see* BUDESONIDE.

Pump-Hep (*Burgess*) is a proprietary preparation of the natural ANTICOAGULANT heparin sodium, available only on prescription, used to treat and prevent various forms of thrombosis. It is produced in ampoules for intravenous infusion.
✚/▲ warning/side-effects: *see* HEPARIN.

Puri-Nethol (*Wellcome*) is a proprietary CYTOTOXIC drug, available only on prescription, used to treat acute leukaemia, especially in children. It works by combining with new-forming cells in a way that prevents normal cell replication. Produced in the form of tablets, Puri-Nethol is a preparation of mercaptopurine.
✚/▲ warning/side-effects: *see* MERCAPTOPURINE.

Pyopen (*Beecham*) is a proprietary ANTIBIOTIC, available only on prescription, used mainly to treat infections of the urinary tract and upper respiratory tract, and septicaemia. Produced in the form of a powder for reconstitution as a medium for injection, Pyopen is a preparation of the PENICILLIN carbenicillin.
✚/▲ warning/side-effects: *see* CARBENICILLIN.

Pyralvex (*Norgine*) is a proprietary non-prescription ANTI-INFLAMMATORY preparation, used in topical application to treat inflammation in and around the mouth. Produced in the form of a paint, Pyralvex is a preparation of various glycosides with the anti-inflammatory salicylic acid.
✚/▲ warning/side-effects: *see* SALICYLIC ACID.

pyrantel is a broad-spectrum ANTHELMINTIC drug used in the treatment of infections by roundworm, threadworm, hookworm and whipworm. Administration is oral in the form of tablets.
✚ warning: pyrantel should not be administered to patients with liver disease, or to children aged under 6 months.
▲ side-effects: pyrantel rarely has side-effects, but it may

P

occasionally produce mild nausea.
Related article: COMBANTRIN.

pyrazinamide is an ANTIBACTERIAL that is one of the major forms of treatment for tuberculosis, and particularly tuberculous meningitis. It is used generally in combination (to cover resistance and for maximum effect) with other powerful drugs such as ISONIAZID or RIFAMPICIN. Treatment lasts for between 6 and 18 months, depending on the severity of the condition and on the specific drug combination. Administration is oral in the form of tablets.

✚ warning: pyrazinamide should not be administered to patients with liver disease; it should be administered with caution to patients with impaired liver function, diabetes or gout. Regular checks on liver function are essential.

▲ side-effects: there may be symptoms of liver malfunction, including high temperature, severe weight loss and jaundice. There may be nausea and vomiting, sensitivity reactions such as urticaria, and/or blood disorders.
Related article: ZINAMIDE.

Pyridium (*Parke-Davis*) is a proprietary non-prescription preparation, used to relieve pain stemming from disorder in the urinary tract. Produced in the form of tablets, Pyridium is a preparation of phenazopyridine hydrochloride; it is not recommended for children.

✚/▲ warning/side-effects: *see* PHENAZOPYRIDINE.

pyridostigmine is a drug that has the effect of increasing the activity of the neurotransmitters which transmit the neural instructions of the brain to the muscles. It works by inhibiting the "switching-off" of the neural impulses as they pass from one nerve cell to another, therefore increasing transmission. Its main use is in the treatment of the neuromuscular disease myasthenia gravis (which causes extreme muscle weakness amounting even to paralysis); it is also used to reverse the effects of muscle relaxants administered during surgical operations. Occasionally the drug is used to stimulate intestinal motility and so promote defecation. Administration is oral in the form of tablets, or by injection.

✚ warning: pyridostigmine bromide should not be administered to patients with intestinal or urinary blockage; it should be administered with caution to those with epilepsy, asthma, parkinsonism, hypotension (low blood pressure) or a slow heart rate, who have recently had a heart attack, or who are pregnant.

▲ side-effects: there may be nausea and vomiting, diarrhoea and abdominal cramps, and an excess of saliva in the mouth. Overdosage may cause gastrointestinal disturbance, an excess of bronchial mucus, sweating, faecal and urinary incontinence, vision disorders, excessive dreaming, nervous agitation and muscular weakness.
Related article: MESTINON.

pyridoxine is the chemical name for vitamin B_6, a VITAMIN that is essential in the diet for the metabolism of amino acids and the maintenance of body cells. Good food sources include fish, liver, peas and beans, yeast and whole grains. A deficiency – rare in the Western world but which

P

may occur due to certain drug treatments, such as with isoniazid – may dispose a patient towards nerve or blood disorders, and in children might eventually cause convulsions. Therapeutically, it is administered to make up a vitamin deficiency (and especially if that deficiency has resulted in neuritis or anaemia); to treat premenstrual syndrome. An increased dietary intake may be required during pregnancy or breast-feeding, or during childhood growth.

✚ warning: pyridoxine should not be administered to patients who are taking the anti-parkinsonism drug levodopa.

Related articles: ABIDEC; ALLBEE WITH C; BC 500; BECOSYM; BENADON; BRAVIT; COMPLOMENT CONTINUS; CONCAVIT; DALIVIT; HEPACON-PLEX; JUVEL; KETOVITE; LIPOFLAVONOID; LIPOTRIAD; OCTOVIT; OROVITE 7; PABRINEX; PARENTROVITE; PAXADON; POLYVITE; SURBEX T; TONIVITAN B; VERDIVITON; VI-DAYLIN.

pyrimethamine is an ANTIMALARIAL drug used primarily to prevent contraction of malaria by travellers in tropical countries. However, if the disease is contracted, the drug is effective in treating forms of malaria that are resistant to treatment with the more commonly-prescribed drug chloroquine, and additionally prevents most relapses of benign tertiary forms. Pyrimethamine can also be used to treat the rotozoan infection toxoplasmosis. Administration is oral in the form of tablets.

✚ warning: pyrimethamine should be administered with caution to patients with impaired liver or kidney function, or who are taking folic acid supplements (for example, during pregnancy). High doses require regular blood counts.

▲ side-effects: suppression of the bone-marrow's capacity for forming new blood cells occurs with prolonged treatment. There may be rashes.

Related articles: DARAPRIM; FANSIDAR; MALOPRIM.

pyrithione zinc shampoos are ANTIMICROBIAL scalp preparations used to treat dandruff.

Pyrogastrone (*Winthrop*) is a proprietary preparation, available only on prescription, used to treat gastric ulcers in young and middle-aged people. Thought to work by creating a protective coating over the mucous lining of the stomach, Pyrogastrone is produced in the form of tablets and as a liquid mixture. It is a preparation of carbenoxolone sodium and various ANTACIDS (including ALUMINIUM HYDROXIDE, MAGNESIUM TRISILICATE and SODIUM BICARBONATE). It is not recommended for children.

✚/▲ warning/side-effects: *see* CARBENOXOLONE SODIUM.

P

Quellada (*Stafford-Miller*) is a proprietary non-prescription preparation of the antiparasitic lindane, used to treat infestation of the skin of the trunk and limbs by itch-mites (scabies) or by lice (pediculosis). It is also used to treat hair lice infestations. Produced in the form of a lotion, it is also available as a shampoo (under the name Quellada Application PC). Neither is recommended for children aged under 1 month. Children under 6 months should be treated only under medical supervision. Both are for external use only.
✚/▲ warning/side-effects: LINDANE.

Q

Questran (*Bristol-Myers*) is a proprietary ANTIDIARRHOEAL RESIN, available only on prescription, used to treat diarrhoea associated with inflammation of the small intestines, or resulting from a reduction in gastric secretions following gastrointestinal surgery, or diarrhoea following radiation treatment. It is also used alternatively to relieve itching in liver disease, and to lower blood cholesterol concentrations. Produced in the form of powder in sachets, Questran is a preparation of cholestyramine. Use with other drugs should be avoided. It is not recommended for children aged under 6 years.
✚/▲ warning/side-effects: *see* CHOLESTYRAMINE.

Quiksol (*Boots*) is a proprietary non-prescription preparation of very pure beef neutral insulin, used to treat and maintain diabetic patients. It may be used in emergency cases when blood sugar levels are dangerously high (hyperglycaemia). It is produced in vials for injection.
✚/▲ warning/side-effects: *see* INSULIN.

Quinaband (*Seton*) is a proprietary non-prescription form of bandaging impregnated with ZINC OXIDE, CALAMINE and CLIOQUINOL, used to treat and dress ulcers, burns and scalds. (Further bandaging is required to keep it in place.)

quinalbarbitone sodium is a BARBITURATE with a rapid onset of action, used as a HYPNOTIC to promote sleep in conditions of severe intractable insomnia. It is a dangerous and potentially addictive drug, administered orally in the form of capsules. It is also used in the compound barbiturate Tuinal.
✚ warning: quinalbarbitone sodium should not be administered to patients who have insomnia caused by pain, or porphyria, who are pregnant or lactating, or to the elderly or debilitated, or to children. In fact, usage should be avoided altogether where possible. It should be administered with caution to patients with respiratory difficulties, or liver or kidney disease. Tolerance, followed by dependence, occurs readily. Repeated doses have cumulative effect; abrupt withdrawal of treatment may precipitate serious withdrawal symptoms (including fits and delirium). It should not be used in patients with a history of alcohol abuse.
▲ side-effects: drowsiness, dizziness, lack of power to co-ordinate body movements, shallow breathing and headache are all fairly common, especially in elderly patients. There may be allergic/sensitivity reactions.
Related article: SECONAL SODIUM; TUINAL.

quinestradol is an OESTROGEN, a

female sex HORMONE, used in replacement therapy to relieve symptoms in women during and after the menopause (such as inflammation or erosion of the vagina, and urinary incontinence due to oestrogen deficiency). Administration is oral in the form of capsules.

✚ warning: quinestradol should not be administered to patients with inflammation of the womb lining, impaired liver function, porphyria, undiagnosed bleeding from the vagina, thrombosis, or oestrogen-dependent cancer of the breast. It should be administered with caution to those with epilepsy, diabetes, heart or kidney disease, from high blood pressure (hypertension), or migraine, or who are pregnant or lactating. Many doctors will not prescribe quinestradol for patients who wear contact lenses. Treatment may cause misleading results in thyroid-function tests.

▲ side-effects: there may be nausea and vomiting, breast tenderness, fluid and sodium retention leading to weight gain, a rash and/or headache. Some patients experience impaired liver function or depression. Withdrawal of treatment may cause haemorrhage. Prolonged treatment of women after the menopause may give rise to a predisposition towards cancer of the womb lining.

Related article: PENTOVIS.

quinestrol is an OESTROGEN, a female sex HORMONE that is a derivative of oestradiol, formerly used to suppress lactation in women following childbirth. (Such use was discontinued when an association was made between the oestrogens and some forms of thrombosis.) Administration is oral in the form of tablets.

✚ warning: quinestrol should not be administered to patients with inflammation of the womb lining, impaired liver function, porphyria, undiagnosed bleeding from the vagina, thrombosis, or oestrogen-dependent cancer of the breast. It should be administered with caution to those with epilepsy, diabetes, heart or kidney disease, high blood pressure (hypertension), or migraine, or who are pregnant or lactating. Many doctors will not prescribe quinestrol for patients who wear contact lenses. Treatment may cause misleading results in thyroid-function tests.

▲ side-effects: there may be nausea and vomiting, breast tenderness, fluid and sodium retention leading to weight gain, a rash and/or headache. Some patients experience impaired liver function or depression. Withdrawal of treatment may cause haemorrhage.

Related article: ESTROVIS.

Quinicardine (*Lewis*) is a proprietary ANTIARRHYTHMIC drug, available only on prescription, used to treat heartbeat irregularities and to prevent an increase in the heart rate. Produced in the form of tablets – the interval between doses being the regulating factor to suit each individual patient – Quinicardine is a preparation of quinidine sulphate.

✚/▲ warning/side-effects: *see* QUINIDINE.

quinidine is an alkaloid of cinchona much like QUININE, but is used specifically in treatments that take advantage of its effect

Q

on the heart. It is used (in the form of quinidine sulphate) as an ANTIARRHYTHMIC drug, to treat heartbeat irregularities and regularize the heart rate. However, the drug may itself precipitate some disorders of the heart rhythm and should accordingly be administered only on specialist advice and under strict medical supervision. Rarely, the drug is also used as an equivalent of quinine in the emergency treatment of severe malaria. Administration is oral in the form of tablets, sustained-release tablets and sustained-release capsules.

✚ warning: quinidine should not be administered to patients with heart block. An initial test dose is usually administered to detect any sensitivity reactions and check tolerance.

▲ side-effects: there may be high temperature, nausea, diarrhoea, a rash, ringing in the ears (tinnitus), visual disturbances and vertigo; there may also be impaired heart activity, more serious skin disorders and confusion. In some patients the white blood cell count is diminished, and it may cause types of anaemia.

Related articles: KIDITARD; KINIDIN DURULES; QUINICARDINE.

quinine is an alkaloid of cinchona which was for years used as the main treatment for malaria. Now synthetic and less toxic drugs – like chloroquine and proguanil – have replaced it almost entirely, although it is still used (in the form of quinine sulphate or quinine hydrochloride) in cases that prove to be resistant to the newer drugs or for emergency cases in which large doses are necessary. Administration is oral in the form of tablets, or by injection.

✚ warning: quinine should not be administered to patients who suffer from inflammation of the optic nerves or any condition that produces blood in the urine; it should be administered with caution to those who suffer from heart block or atrial fibrillation ("palpitations"), or who are pregnant.

▲ side-effects: toxic effects – corporately called cinchonism – include nausea, headache and abdominal pain, visual disturbances, ringing in the ears (tinnitus), a rash and confusion. Some patients may experience visual disturbances and temporary blindness, others may undergo further sensitivity reactions.

Quinocort (*Quinoderm*) is a proprietary ANTIFUNGAL and ANTIBACTERIAL STEROID preparation, available only on prescription, used to treat inflammation, particularly when associated with fungal infections. Produced in the form of vanishing cream for topical application, Quinocort is a combination of the steroid hydrocortisone and the antifungal, antibacterial and deodorant potassium hydroxyquinoline sulphate.

✚/▲ warning/side-effects: *see* HYDROCORTISONE; POTASSIUM HYDROXYQUINOLINE SULPHATE.

Quinoderm (*Quinoderm*) is a proprietary, non-prescription, topical preparation for the treatment of acne. Produced in the form of a cream (in two strengths in an astringent vanishing cream basis) and a lotio-gel (in two strengths in an astringent creamy basis),

Quinoderm is a combination of the keratolytic benzoyl peroxide and the antifungal, antibacterial and deodorant potassium hydroxyquinoline sulphate. Another form is available, only on prescription, to treat severe and inflamed acne (under the name Quinoderm with Hydrocortisone). As its name suggests, this additionally contains the CORTICOSTEROID hydrocortisone; it too is produced in an astringent vanishing cream basis.
✚/▲ warning/side-effects: *see* BENZOYL PEROXIDE; HYDROCORTISONE; POTASSIUM HYDROXYQUINOLINE SULPHATE.

Quinoped (*Quinoderm*) is a proprietary, non-prescription, topical ANTIFUNGAL preparation for the treatment of skin infections such as athlete's foot. Produced in the form of a cream in an astringent basis, Quinoped is a compound of the KERATOLYTIC benzoyl peroxide and the antifungal, ANTIBACTERIAL and deodorant potassium hydroxyquinoline sulphate.
✚/▲ warning/side-effects: *see* BENZOYL PEROXIDE; POTASSIUM HYDROXY-QUINOLONE SULPHATE.

Q

rabies vaccine is specifically a VACCINE and not a treatment for rabies, administered to medical workers and relatives who may come into contact with hydrophobic patients or to patients who have been bitten by an animal that might or might not be rabid. It should be routinely administered to people who work with animals (e.g. vets) to prevent rabies. The vaccine is of a type known as a human diploid cell vaccine and has no known contra-indications. It is freeze-dried and produced in vials with a diluent for injection. The timing of injections within courses of injections depends on whether treatment is simply preventive (in which case the regime is usually two doses over 1 month a third dose after 6-12 months, and possibly a booster every 3 years, depending on the risk of infection), or if rabies in a patient is suspected or confirmed (in which case medical workers and their relatives are injected on days 0, 3, 7, 14, 30 and 90 after exposure).

Rabro (*Sinclair*) is a proprietary non-prescription compound drug containing ANTACIDS and a constituent of liquorice. It is used to soothe the symptoms of peptic ulcers. Produced in the form of tablets, the antacid constituents are CALCIUM CARBONATE, MAGNESIUM OXIDE (magnesia). It is not recommended for children.

Ramodar (*Wyeth*) is a proprietary non-narcotic ANALGESIC, available only on prescription, used to treat both acute and chronic rheumatoid arthritis. Produced in the form of tablets, Ramodar is a preparation of the non-steroidal ANTI-INFLAMMATORY drug etodolac. It is not recommended for children.

✚/▲ warning/side-effects: *see* ETODOLAC.

ranitidine is a powerful drug used to assist in the treatment of peptic ulcers and to relieve heartburn in cases of oesophagitis caused by peptic disturbance. It works by reducing the secretion of gastric acids (by blocking histamine H_2 receptors – *see* ANTIHISTAMINE), so reducing bleeding from gastric or duodenal ulcers and giving them a chance to heal. However, treatment with ranitidine should not be given before full diagnosis of gastric bleeding, because its action in restricting gastric secretions may possibly mask the presence of stomach cancer. Administration is oral in the form of tablets and soluble (dispersible) tablets, or by injection.

✚ warning: ranitidine should be administered with caution to patients with impaired liver or kidney function. A course of treatments lasts usually from 4 to 8 weeks, but may be repeated if necessary.

▲ side-effects: side-effects are rare. But there may be nausea, constipation and headache; a very few patients experience a temporary state of mild confusion. Even more rarely there are allergic/sensitivity reactions.

Related article: ZANTAC.

Rapifen (*Janssen*) is a proprietary ANALGESIC which, because it is also a NARCOTIC, is on the controlled drugs list. It is used especially in outpatient surgery, short operational prodeedures, and for the enhancement of anaesthesia. Produced in the form of ampoules for injection, Rapifen is a preparation of alfentanil. A weaker paediatric injection is also available.

✚/▲ warning/side-effects: *see* ALFENTANIL.

Rapitard MC (*Novo*) is a

proprietary non-prescription preparation of highly purified beef-with-pork insulin, used to treat and maintain diabetic patients. Rapitard MC is produced in the form of vials for regular injection.

✚/▲ warning/side-effects: *see* INSULIN.

Rastinon (*Hoechst*) is a proprietary form of the SULPHONYLUREA tolbutamide, available only on prescription, used to treat adult-onset diabetes mellitus. It works by augmenting what remains of insulin production in the pancreas, and is produced in the form of tablets.

✚/▲ warning/side-effects: *see* TOLBUTAMIDE.

Rautrax (*Squibb*) is a proprietary compound ANTIHYPERTENSIVE drug, available only on prescription, used to treat high blood pressure (hypertension) and to slow the heart rate. It also has a sedative effect. Produced in the form of tablets, Rautrax is a preparation of Rauwolfia serpentina, the THIAZIDE DIURETIC hydroflumethiazide, and the potassium supplement potassium chloride. It is not recommended for children.

✚/▲ warning/side-effects: *see* HYDROFLUMETHIAZIDE; POTASSIUM CHLORIDE; RAUWOLFIA ALKALOIDS.

Rauwiloid (*Riker*) is a proprietary ANTIHYPERTENSIVE drug, available only on prescription, used to treat high blood pressure (hypertension) and to slow the heart rate. Produced in the form of tablets, Rauwiloid is a preparation of alseroxylon, a derivative of Rauwolfia serpentina. It is not recommended for children.

✚/▲ warning/side-effects: *see* RAUWOLFIA ALKALOIDS.

Rauwolfia alkaloids are medications derived from the root of the plant Rauwolfia serpentina. In all, the main active constituent is the substance reserpine, which is used increasingly less often as an ANTIHYPERTENSIVE drug to treat high blood pressure (hypertension) and to slow the heart rate; it works by direct action upon the nervous system. These drugs are also used as major TRANQUILLIZERS, though rarely these days. Many proprietary preparations contain two or more Rauwolfia alkaloids. Administration is oral in the form of tablets.

✚ warning: Rauwolfia alkaloids should not be administered to patients with peptic ulcers, parkinsonism or depression; they should be administered with caution to those who are pregnant or lactating.

▲ side-effects: there may be dry mouth and blocked nose, sedation with low blood pressure (hypotension), and fluid retention leading to weight gain.

Related articles: ABICOL; DECASERPYL; HYPERCAL; RAUTRAX; Rauwiloid; SERPASIL; SERPASIL-ESIDREX.

razoxane is a synthetic CYTOTOXIC drug used (infrequently) in combination with radiotherapy to treat some forms of cancer, including leukaemia. Administration is oral in the form of tablets.

✚ warning: an anti-emetic should be administered simultaneously to lessen the risk of nausea and vomiting. Monitoring of kidney function, blood counts and the sense of hearing is advisable. It should not be used in patients with psoriasis. Protective gloves should be worn when handling tablets, and they should not be handled at all by pregnant women.

▲ side-effects: there may be nausea and vomiting, progressive deafness and symptoms of kidney dysfunction. The blood-forming capacity of the bone marrow may be suppressed and there may be blood disorders (and treatment should not be repeated within 4 weeks).
Related article: RAZOXIN.

Razoxin (*ICI*) is a proprietary preparation of the CYTOTOXIC drug razoxane, available only on prescription, used (infrequently) in combination with radiotherapy to treat some cancers and acute leukaemia. It is produced in the form of tablets.
✚/▲ warning/side-effects: *see* RAZOXANE.

R.B.C. (*Rybar*) is a proprietary non-prescription ANTIHISTAMINE, used to treat skin irritation (itching and nettlerash), stings and bites, and sunburn. Produced in the form of a cream, R.B.C. contains the antihistamine ANTAZOLINE hydrochloride, the antiseptic CETRIMIDE, CALAMINE and camphor.

Redeptin (*Smith Kline & French*) is a proprietary preparation of the powerful ANTIPSYCHOTIC drug fluspirilene. Available only on prescription, it is used to treat and tranquillize psychoses. Produced in ampoules for injection, Redeptin is not recommended for children.
✚/▲ warning/side-effects: *see* FLUSPIRILENE.

Redoxon (*Roche*) is a proprietary non-prescription VITAMIN C preparation that is not available from the National Health Service. It is used to treat the symptoms of vitamin C deficiency (such as scurvy). Produced in the form of tablets (in four strengths) and as tablets for effervescent solutions. Redoxon contains ASCORBIC ACID.

Refolinon (*Farmitalia Carlo Erba*) is a proprietary preparation of the vitamin B FOLINIC ACID, available only on prescription, used to treat body deficiency of the vitamin (as occurs in certain types of anaemia). It is produced in the form of tablets and in ampoules for injection.

Regulan (*Gold Cross*) is a proprietary LAXATIVE of the type known as a bulking agent, which works by increasing the overall mass of faeces within the rectum, so stimulating bowel movement. It is used both to relieve constipation and to relieve diarrhoea, and also in the control of faecal consistency for patients with a colostomy. Produced in the form of gluten-free powder in sachets for effervescent solution in water, Regulan is a preparation of ispaghula husk. It is not recommended for children aged under 6 years, except on medical advice.
✚/▲ warning/side-effects: *see* ISPAGHULA HUSK.

Regulettes (*Cupal*) is a proprietary non-prescription LAXATIVE produced in the form of tablets and as chocolate. Both preparations contain phenylpathaline.

Rehibin (*Thames*) is a proprietary preparation of the drug cyclofenil (an anti-oestrogen), available only on prescription, used under strict medical supervision to treat certain conditions of infertility in which the presence of OESTROGENS may be preventing hormonal

activity necessary for ovulation. It is produced in the form of tablets.
✚/▲ warning/side-effects: *see* CYCLOFENIL.

Rehidrat (*Searle*) is a proprietary non-prescription fluid-replacement supplement, used to treat patients suffering from dehydration and sodium depletion caused by acute diarrhoea, gastro-enteritis and conditions that lead to salt deficiency. Produced in the form of a (lemon-, lime- or orange-flavoured) powder in sachets for reconstitution with water for drinking, Rehidrat contains SODIUM CHLORIDE, POTASSIUM CHLORIDE, SODIUM BICARBONATE, citric acid, GLUCOSE, sucrose and FRUCTOSE.

Relaxit (*Pharmacia*) is a proprietary non-prescription form of micro-enema administered rectally to soften the faeces and promote bowel movement. Produced in the form of single-dose disposable packs with a nozzle, Relaxit is a compound preparation that includes SODIUM CITRATE. For children aged under 3 years there are special instruction for the use of this enema.

Relefact LH-RH (*Hoechst*) is a proprietary preparation of gonadotrophin-releasing hormone, available only on prescription, used as a diagnostic aid in assessing the functioning of the pituitary gland and its secretions. Produced in ampoules for intravenous injection, Relefact LH-RH contains the hormonal substance gonadorelin. Another form, which additionally contains the thryotrophin-releasing hormone protirelin, is also produced (under the name Relefact LH-RH/TRH).
✚/▲ warning/side-effects: *see* GONADORELIN; PROTIRELIN.

Remnos (*DDSA Pharmaceuticals*) is a proprietary TRANQUILLIZER and hypnotic available on prescription only to private patients, used to treat insomnia in cases where some degree of daytime sedation is acceptable. Produced in the form of tablets (in two strengths), Remnos is a preparation of the long-acting benzodiazepine nitrazepam.
✚/▲ warning/side-effects: *see* NITRAZEPAM.

Rendells (*Rendell*) is a proprietary non-prescription SPERMICIDAL preparation, for use only in combination with barrier methods of contraception (such as a condom or diaphragm). Produced in the form of vaginal inserts (pessaries), Rendells is a preparation of alcohol esters in palm kernel oil.

Rennie (*Nicholas Kiwi*) is a proprietary non-prescription ANTACID produced in the form of tablets. It contains calcium carbonate and magnesium carbonate.
✚/▲ warning/side-effects: *see* CALCIUM CARBONATE; MAGNESIUM CARBONATE.

reproterol hydrochloride is a BRONCHODILATOR, a SYMPATHOMIMETIC that is useful in treating all forms and stages of asthma and other conditions that involve obstruction of the air passages. It is also used to treat spasm of the airways. Administration is oral in the form of tablets; as a dilute elixir, which must be diluted (and is then potent for 14 days); topical in the form of an inhalant spray; or as a respirator solution.
✚ warning: reproterol hydrochloride should be

R

administered with caution to patients with heart disease or high blood pressure (hypertension), bleeding or infection, an excess of thyroid hormones in the blood (thyrotoxicosis), who are already taking antihypertensive drugs or beta-blockers, with diabetes, who are undergoing treatment with corticosteroids or diuretics, or who are elderly. Regular blood counts and blood pressure monitoring are essential, as is monitoring of blood glucose in diabetics.

▲ side-effects: there may be nausea and vomiting, flushing and sweating, restlessness, and a tremor. High dosage may cause an increase in the heart rate, with high blood pressure.

Related article: BRONCHODIL.

R

Rescufolin (*Nordic*) is a proprietary preparation of the vitamin B-like compound folinic acid, available only on prescription, used primarily as a supplement to treat body deficiency of the vitamin (as occurs in certain types of anaemia). It is produced in the form of tablets and as a powder for reconstitution as a medium for injection.

✚ warning: *see* FOLINIC ACID.

reserpine is the principal constituent of the Rauwolfia alkaloids, a drug used mainly to treat high blood pressure or, more rarely, to treat anxiety (although it may take some time to achieve full effect). It is now administered less frequently, however, because it may cause depression in some patients, and because there is a wider choice of drugs available to treat high blood pressure. Administration is oral in the form of tablets, or by injection.

✚/▲ warning/side-effects: *see* RAUWOLFIA ALKALOIDS.

Resolve (*Beecham Health Care*) is a proprietary, non-prescription formulation for the relief of "morning after" hangover symptoms. Produced in the form of a powder, it contains citric acid, vitamin C, glucose, paracetamol and the ANTACIDS sodium carbonate, sodium bicarbonate and potassium bicarbonate.

✚/▲ warning/side-effects: *see* GLUCOSE, ASCORBIC ACID, PARACETAMOL, SODIUM CARBONATE.

Resonium-A (*Winthrop*) is a proprietary non-prescription sodium supplement used to treat high blood levels of POTASSIUM, particularly in patients who suffer from fluid retention or who undergo kidney dialysis. It is produced in the form of a powdered resin, consisting of a preparation of sodium polystyrene sulphonate.

resorcinol is an astringent drug that in topical application causes skin to peel (it is a KERATOLYTIC) and relieves itching (it is antipruritic); it is most used in ointments and lotions to treat acne or remove dandruff.

✚ warning: prolonged usage, leading to absorption, may cause underactivity of the thyroid gland (hypothyroidism) with resultant symptoms (myxoedema) and eventual convulsions.

Related articles: DOME-ACNE; ESKAMEL.

Restandol (*Organon*) is a proprietary preparation of the male sex hormone testosterone undecanoate, available only on

prescription, used to treat sexually undeveloped men, and conditions of osteoporosis ("brittle bones") caused by lack of ANDROGENS. It is produced in the form of capsules.
✚/▲ warning/side-effects: *see* TESTOSTERONE.

Retcin (*DDSA Pharmaceuticals*) is a proprietary ANTIBIOTIC, available only on prescription, used to treat many infections (including serious infections such as legionnaires' disease and inflammation of the prostate gland) and to prevent others (such as diphtheria or whooping cough), especially in patients who are allergic to penicillin-type antibiotics. Produced in the form of tablets, Retcin is a preparation of the erythromycin.
✚/▲ warning/side-effects: *see* ERYTHROMYCIN.

Retin-A (*Ortho-Cilag*) is a proprietary preparation of the VITAMIN A-type compound tretinoin, available only on prescription, used to treat severe acne and to prevent excessive scarring by it. Produced in the form of a cream (for dry or fair skin), a gel (for more severe acne or dark and oily skin) or a lotion (for treating large areas such as the back), it is not recommended for children.
✚/▲ warning/side-effects: *see* TRETINOIN.

retinol is the chemical term for VITAMIN A, a fat-soluble vitamin that is found in meats and milk products, and is also synthesized in the body from constituents in green vegetables and carrots. Essential for growth and the maintenance of mucous surfaces, retinol is particularly useful in supporting the part of the eye's retina that allows vision in the dark; a deficiency may thus cause night blindness, dry eyes and stunted growth. Conversely, however, an excess may cause hair loss, peeling of the skin, joint pain and liver damage. It is administered therapeutically to make up vitamin deficiency – which is rare in Western countries – mostly orally in the form of capsules or as an emulsion, but also by injection. Some people absorb vitamin A poorly and thus show deficiency signs. Vitamin A may be used topically to treat acne.
Related articles: HALIBUT-LIVER OIL; HALYCITROL; RO-A-VIT.

Rheomacrodex (*Pharmacia*) is a proprietary form of the plasma substitute dextran, available only on prescription, used in infusion with either saline (sodium chloride) or glucose to make up a deficiency in the overall volume of blood in a patient, to improve blood flow or to prevent thrombosis (blood clots) following surgery. It is produced in flasks (bottles) for infusion.
✚/▲ warning/side-effects: *see* DEXTRAN.

Rheumacin LA (*CP Pharmaceuticals*) is a proprietary non-steroidal ANTI-INFLAMMATORY non-narcotic ANALGESIC, available only on prescription, used to relieve pain – particularly rheumatic and arthritic pain – and to treat other musculo-skeletal disorders (including gout, and inflammation of joints and tendons). Produced in the form of sustained-release capsules, Rheumacin LA is a preparation of indomethacin.
✚/▲ warning/side-effects: *see* INDOMETHACIN.

Rheumox (*Robins*) is a proprietary non-steroidal ANTI-INFLAMMATORY non-narcotic ANALGESIC, available only on

prescription, used to relieve pain – particularly rheumatic and arthritic pain – and to treat other musculo-skeletal disorders (including the prevention and treatment of gout). It is a preparation of azapropazone and is produced in the form of capsules and tablets.
✚/▲ warning/side-effects: *see* AZAPROPAZONE.

Rhinocort (*Astra*) is a proprietary nasal spray, available only on prescription, used to treat nasal congestion caused by allergy. Consisting of a preparation of the CORTICOSTEROID budesonide, it is produced in an aerosol with a nasal adaptor for metered inhalation, and is not recommended for children.
✚/▲ warning/side-effects: *see* BUDESONIDE.

rhubarb in powdered form is sometimes used as a constituent in non-proprietary formulations (with sodium bicarbonate and other constituents); it has a mildly LAXATIVE effect. Rarely, it is also used in small quantity as an astringent bitter.

riboflavine is a chemical name for VITAMIN B_2, a water-soluble vitamin that is important for carbohydrate and protein metabolism, and for maintaining the mucous membranes. Deficiency is rare, but may cause skin rashes, cracked lips, and some types of anaemia. Good dietary sources include eggs, liver, milk products and cereals. Administered therapeutically, riboflavine is a constituent of very many vitamin and mineral-and-vitamin supplements.
Related articles: ABIDEC; ALLBEE WITH C; ALUZYME; BC 500; BECOSYM; BRAVIT; CALCIMAX; CONCAVIT; DALIVIT; HEPACON-PLEX; JUVEL; LIPOFLAVONOID; LIPOTRIAD; TONIVITAN B; VIGRANON B; WALLACHOL; KETOVITE; MINAMINO; MULTIVITAMINS; OCTOVIT; OROVITE; PABRINEX; PARENTROVITE; POLYVITE; SURBEX T; VERDIVITON; VI-DAYLIN; VITAVEL.

Rifadin (*Merrell*) is a proprietary ANTITUBERCULAR drug, available only on prescription, generally used in combination with other antitubercular drugs. It may also be used to treat leprosy in dapsone-resistant cases. Produced in the form of capsules (in two strengths), as a syrup, and in the form of a powder for reconstitution as a medium for intravenous infusion, Rifadin is a preparation of the ANTIBIOTIC rifampicin.
✚/▲ warning/side-effects: *see* RIFAMPICIN.

rifampicin is an ANTIBIOTIC that is one of the major forms of treatment for tuberculosis. Even so, it is used generally in combination (to cover resistance and for maximum effect) with other antitubercular drugs such as ISONIAZID or STREPTOMYCIN. Treatment lasts for between 6 and 18 months depending on severity and on the specific drug combination, but the use of rifampicin tends to imply the shorter duration. The drug is also effective in the treatment of leprosy in cases where the usual antileprotic drug DAPSONE has failed. Administration is oral in the form of capsules, tablets or a syrup, or by injection or infusion.
✚ warning: rifampicin should not be administered to patients with jaundice; it should be administered with caution to those with impaired liver function, who are alcoholic, or who are pregnant or lactating. One other effect of the drug is

that soft contact lenses may become discoloured.
▲ side-effects: there are often gastrointestinal problems involving nausea, vomiting, diarrhoea and weight loss; many patients also undergo the symptoms of flu, which may also lead to breathlessness. Rarely, there is kidney failure, liver dysfunction, jaundice, alteration in the composition of the blood and/or discoloration of the urine, saliva and other body secretions. Sensitivity reactions, such as a rash or urticaria, can occur.
Related articles: RIFADIN; RIFATER; RIFINAH; RIMACTANE; RIMACTAZID.

Rifater (*Merrell*) is a proprietary ANTITUBERBULAR drug, available only on prescription, used to treat pulmonary tuberculosis in the initial intensive phase. Produced in the form of tablets, Rifater is a combined preparation of rifampicin, isoniazid and pyrazinamide. It is not recommended for children.
✚/▲ warning/side-effects: *see* ISONIAZID; PYRAZINAMIDE; RIFAMPICIN.

Rifinah (*Merrell*) is a proprietary ANTITUBERCULAR drug, available only on prescription, used to treat tuberculosis. Produced in the form of tablets (in two strengths, under the trade names Rifinah 150 and Rifinah 300), Rifinah is a combined preparation of rifampicin and isoniazid.
✚/▲ warning/side-effects: *see* ISONIAZID; RIFAMPICIN.

Rikospray Balsam (*Riker*) is a proprietary non-prescription barrier skin protectant, used to treat skin infections, cracked nipples and bedsores, or to protect and sanitize a stoma (an outlet on the skin surface following the surgical curtailment of the intestines). Produced in the form of a pressurized aerosol pack for spray application, Rikospray Balsam is a preparation of two natural resinous substances, one of which is BENZOIN.

Rikospray Silicone (*Riker*) is a proprietary non-prescription barrier skin protectant, used to treat bedsores and nappy rash, or to protect and sanitize a stoma (an outlet on the skin surface following the surgical curtailment of the intestines). Produced in a pressurized aerosol pack for spray application, Rikospray Silicone is a preparation of the ANTIBIOTIC CETYLPYRIDINIUM CHLORIDE together with the astringent ANTIPERSPIRANT aluminium dihydroxyallantoinate in a water-repellent basis containing the antifoaming agent DIMETHICONE.

Rimactane (*Ciba*) is a proprietary ANTITUBERCULAR drug, available only on prescription, used in combination with other antitubercular drugs. Produced in the form of capsules (in two strengths), as a syrup and in the form of a powder for reconstitution as a medium for intravenous infusion, Rimactane is a preparation of the ANTIBIOTIC rifampicin.
✚/▲ warning/side-effects: *see* RIFAMPICIN.

Rimactazid (*Ciba*) is a proprietary ANTITUBERCULAR drug, available only on prescription, used singly or in combination with other antitubercular drugs. It may also be used to treat certain other bacterial infections. Produced in the form of tablets (in two strengths, under the

R

names Rimactazid 150 and Rimactazid 300), Rimactazid is a combined preparation of the ANTIBIOTICS rifampicin and isoniazid.
✚/▲ warning/side-effects: *see* ISONIAZID; RIFAMPICIN.

Rimevax (*Smith, Kline & French*) is a proprietary VACCINE against measles (rubeola), available only on prescription. It is a powdered preparation of live but attenuated measles viruses for administration with a diluent by injection to provide active immunization. Rimevax is not recommended for children aged under 12 months.
✚ warning: Rimevax should not be administered to patients with any infection, particularly tuberculosis and other infections of the airways; who are allergic to eggs (the viruses are cultured in chick-embryo tissue); who have known immune-system abnormalities, including leukemia; who are known to be allergic to neomycin; who are pregnant; or who are already taking corticosteroid drugs, cytotoxic drugs or undergoing radiation treatment. It should be administered with caution to those with epilepsy (especially children) or any other condition potentially involving convulsive fits, and those who have recently had a blood transfusion.
▲ side-effects: there may be inflammation at the site of injection. Rarely, there may be high temperature, headache, a rash, swelling of the lymph glands, pain in the joints and/or a cough. Very rarely, there are allergic reactions, and in a few patients convulsions have followed the high fever.

Rimifon (*Roche*) is a proprietary ANTITUBERCULAR drug, available only on prescription, used in combination with other antitubercular drugs. Produced in ampoules for injection, Rimifon is a preparation of the ANTIBIOTIC isoniazid.
✚/▲ warning/side-effects: *see* ISONIAZID.

rimiterol is a BRONCHODILATOR, a SYMPATHOMIMETIC that is useful in treating all forms and stages of asthma and other conditions that involve obstruction in the air passages, and to prevent spasm of the airways. Administration (in the form of rimiterol hydrobromide) is topical in the form of an inhalant spray.
✚ warning: rimiterol should not be administered to patients with heart disease or high blood pressure (hypertension), bleeding or infection, an excess of thyroid hormones in the blood (thyrotoxicosis), or who are already taking antihypertensive drugs or beta-blockers. It should be administered with caution to those with diabetes, who are undergoing treatment with corticosteroids or diuretics, or who are elderly.
▲ side-effects: there may be nausea and vomiting, flushing and sweating, and a tremor. Overdosage may cause an increase in the heart rate, with high blood pressure.
Related article: PULMADIL.

Rimso-50 (*Britannia*) is a proprietary organic solution that is intended for bladder washouts. Available only on prescription, such bladder irrigation is used to relieve the symptoms of cystitis (inflammation of the bladder) or of bladder ulcers. Its active constituent is dimethyl sulphoxide.

Ringer's solution is a non-proprietary solution for injection that is intended as a SODIUM CHLORIDE (saline) supplement in patients with sodium depletion. It contains the chlorides of sodium, potassium and calcium.

Rite-Diet (*Welfare Foods*) is a brand of special foods for special diets. For patients who require a gluten-free diet there are sweet biscuits and crackers, digestive biscuits, savoury biscuits, bread, bread with soya bran, high-fibre bread, a bread mix, and a flour mix. For patients on a low-protein diet there is macaroni, spaghetti (in two sizes), a flour mix, a bread mix, bread, bread with soya bran, bread without salt, white bread with added fibre, sweet biscuits, crackers, cream-filled biscuits and cream wafers. Most of these are also available specially prepared for patients on a combined gluten-free low-protein diet. Finally, for patients on a low-sodium diet, there is another form of bread.

ritodrine hydrochloride is a BETA-RECEPTOR STIMULANT that affects principally the muscles of the womb: it is therefore used mainly to prevent or stall the uterine contractions of premature labour, although it is also used in cases where a foetus may be in danger of asphyxiation through excessive contractility of the womb muscles. Administration is oral in the form of tablets, or by injection.

✚ warning: ritodrine hydrochloride should not be administered to patients with heart disease, high blood pressure (hypertension), pre-eclampsia, excess thyroid hormones in the bloodstream (thyrotoxicosis), or infection of any kind; who are bleeding; or who are already taking antidepressants, beta-blockers or drugs against high blood pressure. It should be administered with caution to those with diabetes, or who are undergoing treatment with corticosteroids, diuretics or anaesthetics. Blood pressure and pulse should be monitored during treatment.

▲ side-effects: there may be nausea and vomiting, flushing and sweating, and a tremor; high doses may increase the heart rate and lower the blood pressure.

Related article: YUTOPAR.

Rivotril (*Roche*) is a proprietary ANTICONVULSANT, available only on prescription, used to treat all forms of epilepsy. It is produced in the form of tablets (in two strengths) and in ampoules (with diluent) for injection, and is a preparation of the BENZODIAZEPINE clonazepam.

✚/▲ warning/side-effects: *see* CLONAZEPAM.

Roaccutane (*Roche*) is a proprietary preparation of the vitamin A derivative isotretinoin, available only on prescription (and generally only in hospitals), used to treat severe acne that proves to be unresponsive to the more common antibiotic therapy. It is produced in the form of capsules (in two strengths), and is not recommended for children.

✚/▲ warning/side-effects: *see* ISOTRETINOIN.

Ro-A-Vit (*Roche*) is a proprietary preparation of RETINOL (vitamin A), available only on prescription, used to treat and prevent vitamin A deficiency. It is produced in the form of tablets and as an oily solution in ampoules for injection. Injections are used when absoption of oral Ro-A-Vit is poor.

Robaxin 750 (*Robins*) is a proprietary MUSCLE RELAXANT, available only on prescription, used to relieve muscle spasm mainly in the muscles of the limbs; it works by direct action on the central nervous system. Produced in the form of tablets and in ampoules for injection, Robaxin 750 is a preparation of methocarbamol. It is not recommended for children; lower doses are recommended for the elderly.
✚/▲ warning/side-effects: *see* METHOCARBAMOL.

Robaxisal Forte (*Robins*) is a proprietary compound ANALGESIC, available on prescription only to private patients, used to relieve muscle spasm and pain, mainly in the muscles of the limbs; it works by direct action on the central nervous system. Produced in the form of tablets, Robaxisal Forte is a preparation of methocarbamol and aspirin. It is not recommended for children. Lower doses are recommended for the elderly.
✚/▲ warning/side-effects: *see* ASPIRIN; METHOCARBAMOL.

Robinul (*Robins*) is a proprietary ANTICHOLINERGIC drug, available only on prescription, used to treat rigidity (spasm) or hyperactivity of the muscles of the colon. Produced in the form of tablets and in ampoules for injection, Robinul is a preparation of the MUSCLE RELAXANT glycopyrronium bromide. It is not recommended for children.
✚/▲ warning/side-effects: *see* GLYCOPYRRONIUM BROMIDE.

RoC Total Sunblock (*RoC*) is a proprietary non-prescription cream containing constituents that protect the skin from ultraviolet radiation and radiotherapy. Patients whose skin condition is such as to require this sort of protection may be prescribed RoC Total Sunblock at the discretion of their doctors. Its major active constituent is ZINC OXIDE.

Rocaltrol (*Roche*) is a proprietary form of the vitamin D analogue calcitriol, available only on prescription, used to restore and sustain calcium balance in the body. It is produced in the form of capsules (in two strengths) and the appropriate dose for children has not been established.
✚ warning: *see* CALCITRIOL.

Roccal (*Winthrop*) is a proprietary non-prescription DISINFECTANT, used to cleanse the skin before operations, to cleanse wounds, to sterilize dressings, to cleanse breast and nipple shields, and also as a vaginal douche. Produced in the form of a solution, Roccal is a preparation of BENZALKONIUM CHLORIDE. A concentrated form is available (under the name Roccal Concentrate 10X) for the preparation of the same solution, using purified water. Roccal should not be used with soap.

Roferon-A (*Roche*) is a proprietary preparation of the viral inhibitor and cellular disrupter interferon (in the form of alfa interferon), available only on prescription, and used mainly to treat some kinds of leukaemia and AIDS-related Kaposi's sarcoma (a type of skin cancer). Administration is by injection. As with virtually all anticancer drugs, some side-effects are inevitable.
✚/▲ warning/side-effects: *see* INTERFERON.

Rogitine (*Ciba*) is a proprietary ANTIHYPERTENSIVE drug, available only on prescription, used to treat both high blood pressure (hypertension) and heart failure. Produced in ampoules for injection, Rogitine is a preparation of the ALPHA-BLOCKER phentolamine mesylate.

✚/▲ warning/side-effects: *see* PHENTOLAMINE.

Rohypnol (*Roche*) is a proprietary TRANQUILLIZER, available on prescription only to private patients, used for the short-term treatment of insomnia and sleep disturbance in cases where some degree of daytime sedation is acceptable. Produced in the form of tablets, Rohypnol is a preparation of the BENZODIAZEPINE flunitrazepam. It is not recommended for children.

✚/▲ warning/side-effects: *see* FLUNITRAZEPAM.

Ronicol (*Roche*) is a proprietary non-prescription VASODILATOR, used to relieve circulatory disorders (e.g. of the fingers and toes) and to treat the condition of excess fats (lipids) in the blood, and to treat Raynaud's disease, spasm of blood vessels, chilblains, Ménière's syndrome and eye conditions caused by poor circulation. Produced in the form of tablets, and as sustained-release tablets (under the name Ronicol Timespan), Ronicol is a preparation of the nicotinic acid derivative nicotinyl alcohol tartrate. It is not recommended for children.

✚/▲ warning/side-effects: *see* NICOTINYL ALCOHOL.

rosaxacin is another name for the antibacterial agent acrosoxacin. *see* ACROSOXACIN.

rose bengal is a form of dye which (in solution), when placed in contact with the cornea of the eye, makes obvious any lesion or foreign body (particularly on the conjunctiva and the cornea). Administration is thus ordinarily in the form of eye-drops.
Related article: MINIMS.

Roter (*Roterpharma*) is a proprietary non-prescription ANTACID, not available from the National Health Service, used to treat peptic ulcers and gastritis. Produced in the form of tablets, Roter is a compound in which the major active constituents are magnesium carbonate, SODIUM BICARBONATE and BISMUTH SUBNITRATE. It is not recommended for children.

Rotersept (*Roterpharma*) is a proprietary non-prescription DISINFECTANT, used to treat sore and cracked nipples before and after breast-feeding. Produced in the form of spray in an aerosol, Rotersept is a preparation of chlorhexidine gluconate.

✚/▲ warning/side-effects: *see* CHLORHEXIDINE.

Rowachol (*Tillotts*) is a proprietary non-prescription preparation of essential oils, used to treat gallstones and bile and liver disorders, especially when surgery is not possible or available. It is produced in the form of a liquid (in a dropper bottle). Another form is available only on prescription, produced in the form of capsules, and used as an additional therapy for dispersing stones in the bile duct. Neither of these products is recommended for children.

✚ warning: Rowachol should be used with caution by pregnant women, and by patients on anticoagulants.

Rowatinex (*Tillotts*) is a proprietary non-prescription preparation of volatile oils, used to treat renal and urinary disorders and in the prevention of urinary stone formation. It is produced in the form of a liquid (in a dropper bottle) and as capsules. Neither form is recommended for children.

rubefacient is another term for a COUNTER-IRRITANT.

Rubelix (*Pharmax*) is a proprietary non-prescription compound ANTITUSSIVE that is not available from the National Health Service. Produced in the form of a syrup for dilution (the potency of the mixture once dilute is retained for 14 days), Rubelix is a compound of the cough suppressant pholcodine and the sympathomimetic ephedrine hydrochloride. It is not recommended for children aged under 12 months.

✚/▲ warning/side-effects: *see* EPHEDRINE HYDROCHLORIDE; PHOLCODINE.

rubella vaccine is a VACCINE against German measles (rubella) that is medically recommended for pre-pubertal girls between the ages of 10 and 14, and for medical staff who as potential carriers might put pregnant women at risk from infection, and also for women of child-bearing age, because German measles during pregnancy constitutes a serious risk to the foetus. Vaccination should not take place if the patient is pregnant or likely to become pregnant within the following 3 months, because initially the vaccine can have similar effects to German measles. The vaccine is prepared as a freeze-dried suspension of live but attenuated viruses grown in cell cultures; administration is by injection.

rub/vac is an abbreviation for rubella vaccine.
see RUBELLA VACCINE.

Ruthmol (*Cantassium*) is a proprietary non-prescription substitute for common salt (sodium chloride) for patients who are on a low-sodium diet. Looking remarkably like salt, and used in similarly in and on food, Ruthmol is the similar compound POTASSIUM CHLORIDE.

rutosides are derivatives of rutin, a vegetable substance. They work by reducing the fragility and permeability of certain blood vessels and may thus be effective in preventing small haemorrhages and swellings. In mixtures called OXERUTINS, they are used especially to treat disorders of the veins of the legs, such as cramps, swollen ankles, and varicose veins.

Rybarvin (*Rybar*) is a proprietary non-prescription compound BRONCHODILATOR, used to treat asthma. Produced in the form of an inhalant solution (for its own special "inhalor"), Rybarvin is a preparation of several drugs: the ANTICHOLINERGIC atropine methonitrate, the SYMPATHOMIMETIC adrenaline, the MUSCLE RELAXANT papaverine hydrochloride, and the local ANAESTHETIC benzocaine in a saline (sodium chloride) base. An identical preparation but without the papaverine is also available (under the trade name Rybarvin Inhalant).

✚/▲ warning/side-effects: *see* ADRENALINE; ATROPINE METHONITRATE; BENZOCAINE.

Rynacrom (*Fisons*) is a proprietary non-prescription preparation used to treat allergic nasal congestion. Produced in the form of a nasal spray (with a metered-dose pump), as nasal drops, and in cartridges for nasal insufflation, Rynacrom is a preparation of sodium

cromoglycate. A similar nasal spray additionally containing the ANTIHISTAMINE xylometazoline hydrochloride is also available (under the name Rynacrom Compound).
✚/▲ warning/side-effects: *see* SODIUM CROMOGLYCATE; XYLOMETAZOLINE HYDROCHLORIDE.

Rythmodan (*Roussel*) is a proprietary ANTIARRHYTHMIC drug, available only on prescription, used to treat heartbeat irregularities and to prevent speeding up of the heart rate (tachycardia). Produced in the form of capsules (in two strengths), as sustained-release tablets (under the name Rythmodan Retard), and in ampoules for injection, Rythmodan is a preparation of disopyramide. It is not recommended for children.
✚/▲ warning/side-effects: *see* DISOPYRAMIDE.

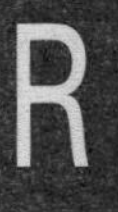

Sabidal SR 270 (*Zyma*) is a proprietary non-prescription BRONCHODILATOR, used to treat asthmatic bronchospasm, emphysema and chronic bronchitis. Produced in the form of sustained-release tablets, Sabidal SR 270 is a preparation of the xanthine drug choline theophyllinate. It is not recommended for children.
✚/▲ warning/side-effects: *see* CHOLINE THEOPHYLLINATE.

Salactol (*Dermal*) is a proprietary non-prescription compound preparation in the form of a paint for topical application, intended to remove warts (particularly verrucas) and hardened skin. With its own special applicator, Salactol's major active constituent is the ANTIBACTERIAL KERATOLYTIC salicylic acid.
✚/▲ warning/side-effects: *see* SALICYLIC ACID.

Salazopyrin (*Pharmacia*) is a proprietary preparation, available only on prescription, used primarily to induce a remission in the symptoms of ulceration of the intestinal wall (generally in the colon) and, having induced it, to maintain it. Because the drug also has ANTI-INFLAMMATORY properties, it is additionally used to treat rheumatoid arthritis (although there are some haematological side-effects). Produced as tablets (in two forms, one enteric-coated under the name Salazopyrin EN-tablets), as suppositories, and as a retention enema in a disposable pack, Salazopyrin is a preparation of the SULPHONAMIDE sulphasalazine.
✚/▲ warning/side-effects: *see* SULPHASALAZINE.

salbutamol is a BRONCHODILATOR, of the type known as a selective BETA-RECEPTOR STIMULANT, used to treat asthmatic bronchospasm, emphysema and chronic bronchitis. It is sometimes also used to prevent or stall premature labour. It has fewer cardiac side-effects than some others of its type, and is administered orally in the form of tablets, as sustained-release tablets, as a sugar-free liquid, and as an inhalant from aerosol, nebulizer, inhalation cartridge or ventilator; it is also administered by injection or infusion.
✚ warning: salbutamol should be administered with caution to patients with disorders of the thyroid gland, heart disease or hypertension (high blood pressure), who are elderly, or who are pregnant.
▲ side-effects: there may be headache and nervous tension, associated with tingling of the fingertips and a fine tremor of the hands. Administration other than by inhalation may cause an increase in the heart rate; infusion may lower blood potassium levels. There may be headache, peripheral vasidilation and pain in the injection site.
Related articles: ASMAVEN; COBUTOLIN; SALBULIN; VENTIDE; VENTOLIN.

salcatonin is a synthesized form of the thyroid hormone calcitonin that is particularly suited to long-term therapy of certain bone disorders.
see CALCITONIN.

salicylic acid is an ANTIBACTERIAL and ANTIFUNGAL drug that is used to treat minor skin infections such as athlete's foot, and may also assist in the treatment of major skin disorders such as psoriasis. It also has useful KERATOLYTIC properties in removing dry, hard or scaly skin, dandruff, or warts (especially verrucas). Administration is topical, in the form of a solution, a collodion (paint or gel), as an ointment – or, in combination with precipitated sulphur, as an ointment or a cream – as a shampoo, and even in an impregnated adhesive plaster.

✚ warning: in applying salicylic acid topically, areas of healthy skin and the anogenital region should be avoided. Application to large areas is also inadvisable (absorption through the skin may lead to gastrointestinal disturbance and ringing in the ears).

▲ side-effects: side-effects are rare, confined largely to the effects of too widescale an application (see above) and to sensitivity reactions.

Related articles: ANTHRANOL; CUPLEX; DITHROLAN; DUOFILM; IONIL T; KERALYT; PHYTEX; PHYTOCIL; PRAGMATAR; PSORIN; PYRALVEX; SALACTOL; VERRUGON.

Salonair (*Salonpas*) is a proprietary non-prescription COUNTER-IRRITANT which, in the form of a spray (from an aerosol) applied to the skin, produces an irritation of the sensory nerve endings that offsets the pain of underlying muscle or joint ailments. Active constituents include two salts of SALICYLIC ACID, menthol, and camphor.

salsalate is a long-acting non-narcotic ANALGESIC much like aspirin but without so many gastric side-effects, used primarily to treat inflammation and pain in rheumatic and other musculo-skeletal disorders. Administration is oral in the form of capsules.

✚ warning: salsalate should not be administered to patients who suffer from peptic ulcers, or who are aged under 12 years. It should be administered with caution to those with severely impaired function of the kidneys or the liver, or who are dehydrated; who are elderly; who have known allergies; who are pregnant or breast feeding; or who are already taking oral anticoagulant drugs.

▲ side-effects: side-effects are not as common as they are with aspirin, but may include gastrointestinal disturbance or bleeding, hearing difficulties and ringing in the ears (tinnitus), and/or vertigo. There may also be sensitivity reactions, resulting in asthma-like symptoms and a rash.

Related article: DISALCID.

***salt substitutes** may be used instead of true salt (sodium chloride) by patients who are on a medically-supervised low-sodium diet. In general, they consist of potassium chloride with or without additives (such as calcium silicate).

Related articles: RUTHMOL; SELORA.

Saltair (*Salt*) is the name of a series of proprietary non-prescription products for the care, freshening and sanitization of a stoma (an outlet in the skin surface following the surgical curtailment of the intestines). There is a dusting powder, a lotion (for sore or excoriated skin), a cleansing soap, and an antiseptic spray (under the name Saltair "Protect" Friar's Balsam Spray).

Saluric (*Merck, Sharp & Dohme*) is a proprietary DIURETIC, available only on prescription, used to treat hypertension (*see* ANTIHYPERTENSIVE) and the accumulation of fluid within the tissues (oedema). Produced in the

S

form of tablets, it is a preparation of the THIAZIDE chlorothiazide.
✚/▲ warning/side-effects: *see* CHLOROTHIAZIDE.

Salzone (*Wallace*) is a proprietary non-prescription preparation of the non-narcotic ANALGESIC paracetamol, used to treat pain anywhere in the body. It is produced in the form of an elixir for dilution (the potency of the elixir once dilute is retained for 14 days).
✚/▲ warning/side-effects: *see* PARACETAMOL.

Sandimmun (*Sandoz*) is a proprietary preparation of the powerful immunosuppressant cyclosporin, available only on prescription, used to prevent tissue rejection following donor grafting or transplant surgery, specifically in bone-marrow, liver, kidney, pancreas, heart, or heart-and-lung transplant operations. It is administered as an oral solution.
✚/▲ warning/side-effects: *see* CYCLOSPORIN.

Sandocal (*Sandoz*) is a proprietary non-prescription calcium supplement, used to make up depleted calcium levels following certain surgical operations (such as gastrectomy) and to treat calcium-deficient conditions such as osteomalacia, osteoporosis, rickets; it may also be helpful when taken during pregnancy or when breast-feeding. Produced in the form of tablets, Sandocal's active constituents include CALCIUM (in the form of calcium lactate gluconate), POTASSIUM bicarbonate and SODIUM BICARBONATE. It should be avoided in patients with renal impairment.

Sandoglobulin (*Sandoz*) is a proprietary preparation of human normal immunoglobulin (HNIG), available only on prescription, used in infusion to make up globulin deficiencies in newborn infants or to correct blood levels of thrombocytes in patients who are unable to tolerate intramuscular injections. Treatment may take place over several consecutive days.
✚ warning: *see* HNIG.

Sando-K (*Sandoz*) is a proprietary non-prescription POTASSIUM supplement, used to make up deficient blood levels of potassium. Produced in the form of tablets for effervescent solution in water, it contains POTASSIUM CHLORIDE and potassium bicarbonate, and is not recommended for children.

Sanomigran (*Sandoz*) is a proprietary preparation of the ANTIHISTAMINE pizotifen, a drug related to some of the antidepressants. It is used to treat headaches, particularly those in which blood pressure inside the blood vessels plays a part – such as migraine. Available only on prescription, and produced in the form of tablets (in two strengths) and as a sugar-free elixir, Sanomigran is not recommended for children aged under 5 years.
✚/▲ warning/side-effects: *see* PIZOTIFEN.

Saventrine (*Pharmax*) is a proprietary heart stimulant, available only on prescription, used to treat a dangerously low heart rate, or heart block. A preparation of the SYMPATHOMIMETIC isoprenaline, it works by increasing both the heart rate and the force of contractility of the heart muscle. Saventrine is produced in the form of sustained-release tablets and (under the name Saventrine

I.V.) in ampoules for infusion following dilution.
✚/▲ warning/side-effects: *see* ISOPRENALINE.

Savloclens (*ICI*) is a proprietary non-prescription ANTISEPTIC used to prevent infection of wounds and burns. Produced in the form of sachets of sterile solution, Savloclens is a compound preparation of the disinfectants chlorhexidine gluconate and cetrimide. It is generally available only in hospitals.
✚/▲ warning/side-effects: *see* CETRIMIDE; CHLORHEXIDINE GLUCONATE.

Savlodil (*ICI*) is a proprietary non-prescription ANTISEPTIC used to prevent infection of wounds and burns. Produced in the form of sachets of sterile solution, Savlodil is a compound preparation of the disinfectants chlorhexidine gluconate and cetrimide. (It is a weaker preparation than the similar Savloclens.)
✚/▲ warning/side-effects: *see* CETRIMIDE; CHLORHEXIDINE GLUCONATE.

Savlon Hospital Concentrate (*ICI*) is a proprietary non-prescription ANTISEPTIC used to prevent infection of wounds and burns, and to prepare skin prior to surgery. Produced in the form of sachets of sterile solution, Savlon Hospital Concentrate is a compound preparation of the disinfectants chlorhexidine gluconate and cetrimide, and may be used in dilute form.
✚/▲ warning/side-effects: *see* CETRIMIDE; CHLORHEXIDINE GLUCONATE.

***scabicidal** drugs are used to treat infestations by itch-mites (Sarcoptes scabiei). The female mite tunnels into the top surface of the skin in order to lay eggs, causing severe irritation as she does so. Newly hatched mites, also causing irritation with their secretions, then pass easily from person to person on direct contact. Treatment is (almost always) with local applications of HEXACHLOROPHANE or BENZYL BENZOATE in the form of a cream: these kill the mites. Every member of an infected household should be treated, and clothing and bedding should also be disinfested.

Schering PC4 (*Schering*) is a proprietary ORAL CONTRACEPTIVE, available only on prescription, used – unusually – after sexual intercourse has taken place. (It is a post-coital or "morning-after" pill.) Produced in the form of tablets (two to be taken not later than 72 hours after intercourse, and two more after another 12 hours), Schering PC4 is particularly useful in treating patients who have been subjected to rape. Like certain other oral contraceptives it combines an OESTROGEN (ethinyloestradiol) and a PROGESTOGEN (levonorgestrel).
✚/▲ warning/side-effects: *see* ETHINYLOESTRADIOL; LEVONORGESTREL.

Scheriproct (*Schering*) is a proprietary CORTICOSTEROID-ANTIHISTAMINE compound with ANAESTHETIC properties, available only on prescription, and made up of the steroid prednisolone hexanoate, with the antihistamine clemizole undecenoate and the local anaesthetic cinchocaine. Produced in the form of ointment and as anal suppositories, Scheriproct is used to treat piles (haemorrhoids), anal fissure and infection of the anal region.
✚/▲ warning/side-effects: *see* PREDNISOLONE.

Scoline (*Duncan Flockhart*) is a proprietary SKELETAL MUSCLE RELAXANT, available only on prescription, that has an effect for only 5 minutes, and is thus used – following the initial injection of an intravenous BARBITURATE in order to control pain – for short, complete and predictable paralysis (mostly during diagnostic or surgical procedures). Produced in ampoules for injection, Scoline is a preparation of suxamethonium chloride.
✚/▲ warning/side-effects: *see* SUXAMETHONIUM CHLORIDE.

scopolamine is another name for the powerful alkaloid drug hyoscine.
see HYOSCINE.

SDV (*Bencard*) is a proprietary series of VACCINES containing specific allergens; they may be injected into patients who are allergic in order – over time and a course of treatment – to reduce their sensitivity. There is a choice of more than 200 specific allergens, produced in vials for injection (and available only on prescription) at a maximum of 8 allergens in any one vial.

Sea-Legs (*Bioceuticals*) is a proprietary non-prescription anti-motion sickness preparation. It contains the ANTIHISTAMINE meclozine.
✚/▲ warning/side-effects: *see* MECLOZINE.

Secaderm (*Radiol*) is a proprietary non-prescription ANTISEPTIC used in topical application to treat boils and abscesses. But it also has the property of improving underlying blood circulation, and is therefore also used to treat such disorders as chilblains, varicose veins or whitlows. Produced in the form of an ointment (salve), Secaderm's active constituents include phenol and turpentine oil.

Secadrex (*May & Baker*) is a proprietary compound ANTIHYPERTENSIVE, available only on prescription, used to treat mild to moderate hypertension (high blood pressure). Produced in the form of tablets (in two strengths), Secadrex is a preparation of the BETA-BLOCKER acebutolol hydrochloride together with the THIAZIDE DIURETIC hydrochlorothiazide.
✚/▲ warning/side-effects: acebutolol; HYDROCHLOROTHIAZIDE.

Seclodin (*Whitehall Laboratories*) is a proprietary non-prescription ANALGESIC preparation that contains ibuprofen.
✚/▲ warning/side-effects: *see* IBUPROFEN.

Seconal Sodium (*Lilly*) is a proprietary BARBITURATE, and on the controlled drugs list, used as a HYPNOTIC to treat persistent and intractable insomnia. A dangerous and potentially addictive drug, it is produced in the form of capsules (in two strengths) and is a preparation of quinalbarbitone sodium. It is not recommended for children.
✚/▲ warning/side-effects: *see* QUINALBARBITONE SODIUM.

Sectral (*May & Baker*) is a proprietary ANTIHYPERTENSIVE drug, available only on prescription, used to treat hypertension (high blood pressure), heartbeat irregularities, and angina pectoris (heart pain). Produced in the form of capsules (in two strengths) and tablets, and in ampoules for injection, Sectral is a preparation of the BETA-BLOCKER acebutolol hydrochloride. It is not

recommended for children.
✚/▲ warning/side-effects: *see* ACEBUTOLOL.

Securon (*Knoll*) is a proprietary ANTIARRHYTHMIC drug, available only on prescription, used to treat hypertension (high blood pressure), heartbeat irregularities, and angina pectoris (heart pain). It works primarily by decreasing oxygen demand. Produced in the form of tablets (in five strengths, the strongest under the name Securon SR), Securon is a preparation of the calcium antagonist verapamil hydrochloride.
✚/▲ warning/side-effects: *see* VERAPAMIL HYDROCHLORIDE.

Securopen (*Bayer*) is a proprietary ANTIBIOTIC of the penicillin type, available only on prescription, used primarily to treat infections of the urinary tract, upper respiratory tract, and septicaemia. Produced in the form of powder in vials for reconstitution as a medium for infusion, Securopen is a preparation of azlocillin.
✚/▲ warning/side-effects: *see* AZLOCILLIN.

***sedatives** are drugs that calm and soothe, relieving anxiety and nervous tension, and disposing towards drowsiness. They are used particularly for premedication prior to surgery. Many are hypnotic drugs (such as BARBITURATES) used in doses lower than those administered to induce sleep. The term TRANQUILLIZER is more commonly used of the sedatives (such as BENZODIAZEPINES) that do not tend to cause dependence (addiction).

Select-A-Jet Dopamine (*International Medication Systems*) is a potent proprietary preparation of the SYMPATHOMIMETIC drug dopamine hydrochloride, used to treat cardiogenic shock following a heart attack or during heart surgery. Dosage is critical – too much OR too little may have harmful effects. It is produced as a liquid in vials for dilution and infusion.
✚/▲ warning/side-effects: *see* DOPAMINE.

Select-A-Jet Multiple Vitamin Solution (*International Medication Systems*) is a proprietary MULTIVITAMIN solution for addition to infusion solutions in patients who require additional nutrition but cannot be fed via the alimentary canal. In vials for injection, it contains several forms of vitamin B (THIAMINE, RIBOFLAVINE, PYRIDOXINE, NICOTINAMIDE and DEXPANTHENOL), ASCORBIC ACID (vitamin C), CALCIFEROL (vitamin D) and TOCOPHEROL (vitamin E). It is available only on prescription.

selegiline is a drug that has the effect of inhibiting the enzyme that breaks down the neurotransmitter dopamine in the brain, and is accordingly used in combination with LEVODOPA (which is converted to dopamine in the brain) to treat the symptoms of parkinsonism (*see* ANTIPARKINSONISM). In this way it supplements and extends the action of levodopa, also (in many patients) succesfully reducing some side-effects.
✚ warning: in some patients the side-effects are in fact aggravated by the combination of drugs, and the dosage of levodopa may have to be reduced.
▲ side-effects: there may be nausea and vomiting, with agitation and hypotension (low

S

blood pressure); some patients experience a state of confusion.
Related article: ELDEPRYL.

selenium sulphide is a substance thought to act as an antidandruff agent, and used accordingly as the active constituent in some shampoos.
✚ warning: selenium sulphide, or preparations containing it, should not be used within 48 hours of a hair colorant or a permanent wave.

Selexid (*Leo*) is a proprietary ANTIBIOTIC of the penicillin type, available only on prescription, used to treat many forms of infection, but particularly salmonellosis and infections of the urinary tract. Produced in the form of tablets and as a suspension (in sachets), Selexid is a preparation of the drug pivmecillinam hydrochloride.
✚/▲ warning/side-effects: *see* PIVMECILLINAM HYDROCHLORIDE.

Selexidin (*Leo*) is a proprietary ANTIBIOTIC of the penicillin type, available only on prescription, used to treat many forms of infection, but particularly those of the intestines and the urinary tract. Produced in the form of a powder for reconstitution as a medium for injections, Selexidin is a preparation of the drug mecillinam.
✚/▲ warning/side-effects: *see* MECILLINAM.

Selora (*Winthrop*) is a proprietary non-prescription substitute for common salt (sodium chloride) for patients who are on a low-sodium diet. Looking very much like salt, and used in the same way in and on food, Selora is the very similar compound potassium chloride.

Selsun (*Abbott*) is a proprietary non-prescription shampoo containing SELENIUM SULPHIDE, a substance thought to act as an antidandruff agent. Selsun should not be used within 48 hours of a hair colorant or a permanent wave.

Semi-Daonil (*Hoechst*) is a proprietary form of the SULPHONYLUREA glibenclamide, available only on prescription, used to treat adult-onset diabetes mellitus. It works by augmenting what remains of insulin production in the pancreas, and is produced in the form of tablets (at half the strength of DAONIL tablets).
✚/▲ warning/side-effects: *see* GLIBENCLAMIDE.

Semitard MC (*Novo*) is a proprietary non-prescription preparation of highly purified pork insulin zinc suspension, used to treat and maintain diabetic patients. It is produced in vials for injection.
✚/▲ warning/side-effects: *see* INSULIN.

senna is a powerful stimulant LAXATIVE which acts by increasing the muscular activity of the intestinal walls. It is still in fairly common use, but may take between 8 and 12 hours to have any relieving effect on constipation. Senna preparations also may be administered to evacuate the bowels before an abdominal X-ray or prior to endoscopy or surgery.
✚ warning: senna preparations should not be administered to patients who suffer from intestinal blockage or who are pregnant; they should be administered with caution to children.
▲ side-effects: the urine may be coloured red. Senna may cause

abdominal cramp and prolonged use of such a stimulant can eventually wear out the muscles on which it works, thus causing severe intestinal problems in terms of motility and absorption.
Related articles: AGIOLAX; SENOKOT; X-PREP.

Senokot (*Reckitt & Colman*) is a proprietary LAXATIVE containing preparations of senna derivatives (sennosides), used to treat constipation or administered to prepare patients for X-ray, endoscopy or surgery. Non-prescription preparations are produced in the form of granules or as a syrup for dilution (the potency of the syrup once dilute is retained for 14 days). Senokot in tablet form is available only on prescription. It is not recommended in any form for children aged under 2 years.
✚/▲ warning/side-effects: *see* SENNA.

Sential (*Pharmacia*) is a proprietary CORTICOSTEROID cream for topical application, used mostly to treat mild inflammation of the skin and to assist in the treatment of eczema. Available only on prescription, Sential is a compound preparation of the steroid hydrocortisone, together with the DIURETIC urea and sodium chloride, in a water-miscible base.
✚/▲ warning/side-effects: *see* HYDROCORTISONE.

Septex No.2 (*Norton*) is a proprietary ANTIBACTERIAL cream, available only on prescription, used for topical application on minor skin infections and as an antiseptic on abrasions and burns. Active constituents include ZINC OXIDE and the SULPHONAMIDE sulphathiazole.

Septrin (*Wellcome*) is a proprietary SULPHONAMIDE, available only on prescription, used to treat bacterial infections, especially of the urinary tract, infections such as sinusitis and bronchitis, and infections of bones and joints. Produced in the form of tablets (in three strengths), as soluble (dispersible) tablets, as a suspension (in two strengths) for dilution (the potency of either suspension once dilute is retained for 14 days), and in ampoules for injection or (following dilution) infusion, Septrin is a preparation of the compound drug co-trimoxazole, made up of the sulphonamide sulphamethoxazole with the ANTIBACTERIAL agent trimethoprim.
✚/▲ warning/side-effects: *see* CO-TRIMOXAZOLE.

Serc (*Duphar*) is a proprietary ANTI-EMETIC, available only on prescription, used to relieve symptoms of nausea caused by the vertigo and loss of balance experienced in infections of the middle and inner ears. Produced in the form of tablets, Serc is a preparation of the VASODILATOR betahistine hydrochloride. It is not recommended for children.
✚/▲ warning/side-effects: *see* BETAHISTINE.

Serenace (*Searle*) is a proprietary series of preparations of the ANTIPSYCHOTIC drug haloperidol, all available only on prescription, and used to treat most forms of mental disturbance from short-term anxiety to long-term psychosis (including schizophrenia and mania, in emergency and maintenance modes of treatment). Serenace is produced as tablets (in four strengths), as capsules, as a liquid for swallowing, and in ampoules for injection (in two strengths). In all forms except that of the liquid, Serenace is not recommended for children.

✚/▲ warning/side-effects: *see* HALOPERIDOL.

Serophene (*Serono*) is a proprietary hormonal preparation used to treat the kind of infertility in women caused by a deficiency in the hormonal contact between the hypothalamus and the pituitary gland (which produces the GONADOTROPHINS) such that ovulation does not occur. Available only on prescription, Serophene is produced in the form of tablets containing a preparation of clomiphene citrate.

✚/▲ warning/side-effects: *see* CLOMIPHENE CITRATE.

Serpasil (*Ciba*) is a proprietary ANTIHYPERTENSIVE drug, available only on prescription, used to treat all forms of hypertension (high blood pressure). Produced in the form of tablets, Serpasil is a preparation of the RAUWOLFIA ALKALOID reserpine – a powerful drug that causes its antihypertensive effects by acting on the brain and thus may have psychological effects. It is not recommended for children.

✚/▲ warning/side-effects: *see* RESERPINE.

Serpasil-Esidrex (*Ciba*) is a proprietary ANTIHYPERTENSIVE drug, available only on prescription, used to treat all forms of hypertension (high blood pressure). Produced in the form of tablets, Serpasil is a compound preparation of the RAUWOLFIA ALKALOID reserpine together with the THIAZIDE DIURETIC hydrochlorothiazide. It is not recommended for children.

✚/▲ warning/side-effects: *see* HYDROCHLOROTHIAZIDE; RESERPINE.

Setlers (*Beecham Health Care*) is a proprietary non-prescription ANTACID containing calcium carbonate and magnesium carbonate.

✚/▲ warning/side-effects: *see* CALCIUM CARBONATE; MAGNESIUM CARBONATE.

SH 420 (*Schering*) is a proprietary PROGESTOGEN, available only on prescription, used to assist in the treatment of breast cancer (and especially in cases that are inoperable). Produced in the form of tablets, SH 420 is a preparation of norethisterone acetate.

✚/▲ warning/side-effects: *see* NORETHISTERONE ACETATE.

Siloxyl (*Martindale*) is a proprietary non-prescription ANTACID compound that is not available from the National Health Service. It is used to treat acid stomach, indigestion and flatulence, and to soothe a peptic ulcer. Produced in the form of tablets and as a suspension, Siloxyl is a preparation of ALUMINIUM HYDROXIDE together with the antifoaming agent DIMETHICONE.

silver nitrate is a salt that has astringent and ANTISEPTIC properties useful in topical application to wounds and burns, and is also used as a styptic (to stop bleeding or suppuration) or as a caustic (to cauterize warts). Administration is thus topical, mostly in creams and ointments, or in solution, but also in the form of sticks. In other countries silver nitrate is sometimes used in mild solution in eye-drops.

✚ warning: silver nitrate is toxic if ingested; prolonged

application discolours the skin (and fabrics). Solutions should be protected from light.

silver protein is a minor constituent of some nose-drops and a nasal spray, used to treat nasal infections. It has some astringent and ANTISEPTIC properties, but prolonged treatment may lead to silver poisoning (argyria).

silver sulphadiazine is a compound preparation of silver with the SULPHONAMIDE sulphadiazine. In the form of a cream for topical application, it thus has broad-spectrum ANTIBACTERIAL capability as well as the atringent and ANTISEPTIC qualities of the silver, and is used primarily to treat skin infections and to protect wounds, burns and bedsores.

✚ warning: silver sulphadiazine should not be administered to patients who are allergic to sulphonamides; it should be administered with caution to those with impaired function of the liver or kidneys.

▲ side-effects: side-effects are rare, but there may be sensitivity reactions including rashes.

Related article: FLAMAZINE.

Simeco (*Wyeth*) is a proprietary non-prescription ANTACID compound that is not available from the National Health Service. It is used to treat acid stomach, indigestion and flatulence, and to soothe a peptic ulcer. Produced in the form of tablets and as a suspension, Simeco is a preparation of magnesium carbonate, magnesium hydroxide and ALUMINIUM HYDROXIDE with the antifoaming agent DIMETHICONE.

✚/▲ warning/side-effects: *see* MAGNESIUM CARBONATE; MAGNESIUM HYDROXIDE.

Simpla Sassco (*Simpla*) is a proprietary non-prescription gel used to protect and sanitize a stoma (an outlet in the skin surface after the surgical curtailment of the intestines).

simple eye ointment is a bland, sterile formulation of liquid paraffin and wool fat, used both as a night-time eye lubricant (in conditions that cause dry eyes) and to soften the crusts of infections of the eyelids (blepharitis).

✚ warning: wool fat may cause sensitivity reactions in some patients.

simple linctus is a non-proprietary formulation of fairly standard constituents that together make an ANTITUSSIVE as good as many proprietary ones. The constituents include citric acid, anise water, amaranth solution and chloroform spirit.

simple ointment is a bland, sterile formulation of liquid paraffin, wool fat and stearyl alcohol, used as a household ointment for topical application on minor wounds and burns, and areas of dry or cracked skin.

✚ warning: wool fat may cause sensitivity reactions in some patients.

Simplene (*Smith & Nephew*) is a proprietary preparation of the SYMPATHOMIMETIC hormone adrenaline, in very mild solution, in the form of eye-drops within a viscous vehicle. Available only on prescription, it is used to treat all forms of glaucoma except closed-angle glaucoma.

✚/▲ warning/side-effects: *see* ADRENALINE.

Sinemet (*Merck, Sharp & Dohme*) is a proprietary preparation of the powerful drug levodopa in combination with the enyzyme inhibitor CARBIDOPA; it is available only on prescription. Sinemet is used to treat parkinsonism, but not the parkinsonian symptoms induced by drugs (*see* ANTIPARKINSONISM): the carbidopa prevents too rapid a breakdown of the levodopa (into dopamine) in the periphery, thus allowing more levodopa to reach the brain to make up the deficiency (of dopamine) that is the major cause of parkinsonian symptoms. Sinemet is produced in the form of tablets with a levodopa/carbidopa ratio of 10:1 (in two strengths) or (under the name Sinemet-Plus) of 4:1.
✚/▲ warning/side-effects: *see* LEVODOPA.

Sinequan (*Pfizer*) is a proprietary ANTIDEPRESSANT drug, available only on prescription. Used especially in cases where sedation is deemed necessary. Produced in the form of capsules (in four strengths), Sinequan is a preparation of doxepin. It is not recommended for children.
✚/▲ warning/side-effects: *see* DOXEPIN.

Sinthrome (*Geigy*) is a proprietary oral ANTICOAGULANT, available only on prescription, used to prevent or treat conditions of thrombosis and to improve blood circulation through the brain and the heart. Produced in the form of tablets (in two strengths), Sinthrome is a preparation of the synthesized anticoagulant nicoumalone. It is not recommended for children.
✚/▲ warning/side-effects: *see* NICOUMALONE.

Sintisone (*Farmitalia Carlo Erba*) is a proprietary CORTICOSTEROID preparation, available only on prescription, used to treat inflammation (particularly rheumatoid arthritis and inflammatory skin diseases) and to suppress the symptoms of allergy (particularly those of asthma). Produced in the form of tablets, Sintisone is a preparation of the cortisone-derivative prednisolone.
✚/▲ warning/side-effects: *see* PREDNISOLONE.

Siopel (*Care*) is a proprietary non-prescription barrier cream used to treat and dress itching skin and skin infections, nappy rash and bedsores, or to protect and sanitize a stoma (an outlet on the skin surface following the surgical curtailment of the intestines). It contains the antiseptic CETRIMIDE and the antifoaming agent DIMETHICONE.

***skeletal muscle relaxants** act on voluntary (skeletal) muscles of the body. Some are used during operations to aid surgery (e.g. tubocurarine) and act by interfering with the actions of the neurotransmitter acetylcholine at sites between nerve and muscle. Others used in the treatment of painful muscle spasms act within the central nervous system (e.g. DIAZEPAM). Drugs of this class are quite distinct from SMOOTH MUSCLE RELAXANTS.

Slo-Indo (*Generics*) is a proprietary ANTI-INFLAMATORY non-narcotic ANALGESIC, available only on prescription, used to relieve the pain of rheumatic disease, gout, and other inflammatory musculo-skeletal disorders. Produced in the form of sustained-release capsules, Slo-Indo is a preparation of indomethacin.
✚/▲ warning/side-effects: *see* INDOMETHACIN.

Slo-Phyllin (*Lipha*) is a proprietary non-prescription BRONCHODILATOR, used to treat asthmatic bronchospasm, emphysema and chronic bronchitis. Produced in the form of sustained-release capsules (in three strengths), Slo-Phyllin is a preparation of the xanthine drug theophylline. It is not recommended for children aged under 2 years.
✚/▲ warning/side-effects: *see* THEOPHYLLINE.

Sloprolol (*CP Pharmaceuitcals*) is a proprietary ANTIHYPERTENSIVE drug, available only on prescription, used to treat hypertension (high blood pressure) and angina pectoris (heart pain), heartbeat irregularities and the effects of an excess of thyroid hormones in the bloodstream (thyrotoxicosis), and to assist in the prevention of migraine and secondary heart attacks. Produced in the form of sustained-release capsules, Sloprolol is a preparation of the BETA-BLOCKER propranolol hydrochloride.
✚/▲ warning/side-effects: *see* PROPRANOLOL.

Slow-Fe (*Ciba*) is a proprietary non-prescription IRON supplement, used to treat iron deficiency in the bloodstream. Produced in the form of sustained-release tablets, Slow-Fe is a preparation of ferrous sulphate. It is not recommended for children aged under 12 months.
✚/▲ warning/side-effects: *see* FERROUS SULPHATE.

Slow-Fe Folic (*Ciba*) is a proprietary IRON-and-VITAMIN supplement, used to prevent a deficiency of iron and vitamin B, particularly during pregnancy. Produced in the form of sustained-release tablets, Slow-Fe is a combination of ferrous sulphate and folic acid. It should not be taken by patients already taking tetracycline antibiotics.
✚/▲ warning/side-effects: *see* FERROUS SULPHATE.

Slow-K (*Ciba*) is a proprietary non-prescription POTASSIUM supplement, used to make up a blood deficiency of potassium (as may occur in the elderly, in patients with severe diarrhoea, or in patients being treated with diuretics). Produced in the form of sustained-release tablets, Slow-K is a preparation of potassium chloride.

Slow-Pren (*Norton*) is a proprietary ANTIHYPERTENSIVE drug, available only on prescription, used to treat hypertension (high blood pressure), angina pectoris and heartbeat irregularities, and to assist in the treatment of excess levels of thyroid hormones (thyrotoxicosis). Produced in the form of sustained- release tablets, Slow-Pren is a preparation of the BETA-BLOCKER oxprenolol hydrochloride.
✚/▲ warning/side-effects: *see* OXPRENOLOL.

Slow Sodium (*Ciba*) is a proprietary non-prescription preparation of SODIUM CHLORIDE (saline, or salt) used to treat patients suffering from a salt deficiency, or to prevent salt deficiency in hot climates. It is produced in the form of sustained-release capsules.

Slow-Trasicor (*Ciba*) is a proprietary ANTIHYPERTENSIVE drug, available only on prescription, used to treat hypertension (high blood pressure), angina pectoris and heartbeat irregularities, and to

relieve anxiety. Produced in the form of sustained-release tablets, Slow-Trasicor is a preparation of the BETA-BLOCKER oxprenolol hydrochloride.
✚/▲ warning/side-effects: *see* OXPRENOLOL.

smallpox vaccine is now retained only in specialist centres for researchers working with dangerous viruses (and in a possible emergency on doctors who may be called to treat suspected cases of smallpox) – for smallpox has officially been eradicated. Technically, however, smallpox vaccine is still available on prescription, and consists of a suspension of live (but attenuated) viruses, freeze-dried and supplied with a diluent for reconstitution. Administration is through a short linear scratch, or by "multiple pressure inoculation".
✚ warning: smallpox vaccine should not be administered to patients who are pregnant or aged under 12 months, or with any infection or immune system deficiency.

***smooth muscle relaxants** act on the involuntary muscles throughout the body to reduce spasm (an ANTISPASMODIC) or induce relaxation. Thus they may be used to dilate blood vessels and improve circulation in the extremities, lower blood pressure (antihypertensive), or relieve the strain on the heart of angina pectoris. They can induce brochodilation in the treatment of asthma, and may help spasm of the intestine or uterus. Drugs of this class are quite distinct from SKELETAL MUSCLE RELAXANTS.

Sno Phenicol (*Smith & Nephew*) is a proprietary ANTIBIOTIC used to treat bacterial infections. It is a preparation of the potentially toxic drug chloramphenicol.
✚/▲ warning/side-effects: *see* CHLORAMPHENICOL.

Sno-Pilo (*Smith & Nephew*) is a proprietary form of eye-drops, available only on prescription, used to treat most types of glaucoma. It is a dilute solution of the PARASYMPATHOMIMETIC pilocarpine hydrochloride in a viscous fluid.
✚/▲ warning/side-effects: *see* PILOCARPINE.

Sno Tears (*Smith & Nephew*) is a proprietary non-prescription form of synthetic tears administered in drops to lubricate the surface of the eye in patients whose lachrymal glands or ducts are dysfunctioning. It is a preparation of POLYVINYL ALCOHOL.

sodium acid phosphate is an acid DIURETIC, although its main use is in combination either with other phosphorus salts as a phosphorus supplement, or with HEXAMINE to treat infections of the urinary tract.

Sodium Amytal (*Lilly*) is a proprietary preparation of the BARBITURATE amylobarbitone sodium, a drug on the controlled drugs list, used to relieve intractable insomnia in cases other than where pain is the cause. Side-effects may be severe – it is not recommended for children – and dependence (addiction) occurs readily. It is produced in the form of capsules (in two strengths) or tablets (in two strengths), or as a powder for reconstitution as a medium for injection.
see AMYLOBARBITONE SODIUM.

sodium aurothiomalate is the form in which the metallic element gold may be prescribed to treat severe conditions of active rheumatoid arthritis. Unlike ANTI-INFLAMMATORY non-narcotic ANALGESICS, however, gold works slowly so that full effects are achieved only after four or five months. Improvement then is significant, not only in the reduction of joint inflammation but also in associated inflammations. Administration is by intramuscular injection.

✚ warning: sodium aurothiomalate should not be administered to patients who suffer from blood disorders; regular blood counts during treatment are essential. It should be administered with caution to those with impaired function of the liver or kidneys, eczema or colitis; who are elderly; or who are pregnant or lactating. Weekly test doses should be administered to establish changing levels of tolerance within the body; treatment under such monitoring – unless relapse occurs – may then continue for life.

▲ side-effects: about one in every twenty patients experiences severe reactions, especially blood disorders; in all patients there may be skin reactions, mouth ulcers, the accumulation of fluid in the tissues (oedema) and/or neural effects in the extremities.
Related article: MYOCRISIN.

sodium bicarbonate is an ANTACID used for the rapid relief of indigestion and acid stomach. For this purpose it is readily available in the form of powder (for solution), as tablets or as a mixture (liquid). Sodium bicarbonate is also sometimes used in infusion (together with sodium chloride) to relieve conditions of severe metabolic acidosis – when the acidity of body fluids is badly out of balance with the alkalinity as may occur in renal failure or diabetic coma.

✚ warning: sodium bicarbonate should not be taken by patients with impaired kidney function, or who are on a low-sodium diet. Prolonged use is to be avoided, or the cramps and muscular weakness of alkalosis may occur.

▲ side-effects: following the intake of sodium bicarbonate as an antacid, belching is virtually inevitable through the liberation of carbon dioxide.

sodium calciumedetate is a CHELATING AGENT, an antidote to poisoning by heavy metals, especially by lead. It works by forming chemical complexes, binding (and so neutralizing) metal ions to the drug which can then be excreted safely in the usual fashion. Administration is by injection or by topical application in the form of a cream (on areas of skin that have become broken or sensitive through contact with the metal).

✚ warning: sodium calciumedetate should be administered with caution to patients with impaired kidney function.

▲ side-effects: there may be nausea and/or cramp. Overdosage causes kidney damage.
Related article: LEDCLAIR.

sodium carboxymethyl cellulose is another name for carmellose sodium.
see CARMELLOSE SODIUM.

sodium cellulose phosphate is a drug used to help reduce high levels of calcium in the blood. It effects this by inhibiting calcium absorption from food, although a low-calcium diet is also essential. Administration is in the form of a powder (marketed in sachets) to be sprinkled on food.

✚ warning: sodium cellulose phosphate should not be administered to patients with impaired function of the kidneys, or congestive heart failure. Reduction in blood calcium may result in an imbalance in the blood of phosphates, with associated detrimental effects.

▲ side-effects: there may be diarrhoea.
Related article: CALCISORB.

S

sodium chloride is a vital constituent of the human body, in both blood and tissues, and is the major form in which the mineral element sodium appears. (Sodium is involved in the balance of extracellular fluids, maintains electrical potentials in the nervous system, and is essential for the functioning of the muscles). Sodium chloride, or salt, is contained in many foods; too much salt in the diet may lead to the accumulation of fluids in the tissues (oedema), dehydration, and/or high blood pressure (hypertension). Therapeutically, sodium chloride is widely used as saline solution (0.9%) or as dextrose saline (to treat dehydration and shock), as a medium with which to effect bladder irrigation (specifically to dissolve blood clots), as a sodium supplement in patients with low sodium levels, as an eye-wash, as nose-drops, and as a mouth-wash, to topical application in solution as a cleansing lotion.

✚ warning: sodium chloride should be administered with caution to patients with heart failure, high blood pressure (hypertension), fluid retention, or impaired kidney function.

▲ side-effects: overdosage may lead to high blood pressure (hypertension), dehydration, and the accumulation of fluid within the tissues (oedema).

sodium citrate is an alkaline compound, used to treat infections of the urinary tract (especially cystitis) in which the urine is acid. It is also used in the treatment of gout to promote the excretion of uric acid, and may additionally be used to assist in the dissolution of blood clots within the bladder. Administration is oral, in the form of granules (marketed in sachets) for solution in water.

✚ warning: sodium citrate should be administered with caution to patients with impaired kidney function or heart disease, or who are pregnant.

▲ side-effects: there may be dry mouth and mild diuresis.
Related articles: BENILYN DECONGESTANT; BENILYN EXPECTORANT; Dextrolyte; URISAL.

sodium cromoglycate is a drug used to prevent recurrent asthma attacks. How it works is not fully understood though it seems to prevent release of inflammatory mediators, but its BRONCHODILATOR and ANTISPASMODIC effect is particularly marked in allergic conditions. It is used solely prophylactically: the drug has no remedial value in acute attacks. Advice to this effect – that administration must be regular whether symptoms are present or not – is generally given by the prescribing doctor. Administration is usually in the form of inhalation, either from an aerosol or nebulizer, or from an applicator that squirts dry powder.

✚ warning: dosage is adjusted to

the requirements of individual patients (but administration is generally 4 times a day).

▲ side-effects: there may be coughing accompanied by temporary bronchospasm. Inhalation of the dry powder preparation may cause irritation of the throat.
Related article: INTAL.

sodium fluoride is the normal form of fluoride in toothpastes and added to many water supplies to assist in the prevention of tooth decay. Because many water authorities now add fluoride to their region's drinking-water, sodium fluoride should be administered therapeutically only in relation to levels each patient would naturally be receiving anyway. Administration is oral in the form of tablets, as drops, as a gel, or as a mouth-wash.

✚ warning: in general, sodium fluoride is normally prescribed only in areas where the water is not fluoridated at source.

▲ side-effects: some patients eventually notice white flecks on their teeth; overdosage may cause yellow-brown discoloration.
Related articles: EN-DE-KAY; FLUOR-A-DAY LAC; FLUORIGARD; POINT-TWO; ZYMAFLUOR.

sodium fusidate is a narrow-spectrum ANTIBIOTIC used most commonly in combination with other antibiotics to treat staphylococcal infections – especially skin infections, abscesses and infections of bone – that prove to be resistant to penicillin. Administration is oral in the form of tablets and as a suspension, or by infusion.

✚ warning: regular monitoring of liver function is essential during treatment.

▲ side-effects: there may be nausea with vomiting; a rash may occur. Some patients experience temporary kidney dysfunction.
Related article: FUCIDIN.

sodium hypochlorite solutions are used as DISINFECTANTS for cleansing abrasions, burns and ulcers. They differ only in concentration. Non-proprietary solutions are available in 8% and 1% (chlorine) concentrations; both must be diluted before use, for normal skin can tolerate no more than 0.5% available chlorine in topical application.

sodium ironedetate is a form in which IRON can be made available to the body, an iron supplement used to treat iron deficiency and associated anaemia. Administration is oral in the form of a sugar-free elixir.

✚ warning: sodium ironedetate should not be administered to patients already taking tetracycline antibiotics.

▲ side-effects: large doses may cause gastrointestinal upset and diarrhoea; there may be vomiting. Prolonged treatment may result in constipation.
Related article: SYTRON.

sodium lactate was formerly used to treat diabetic coma and the acidosis (the high ratio of acid to alkali in the body and the loss of sodium, potassium and ketones in the urine) associated with the diabetic condition. Containing sodium lactate as the active constituent, a preparation suitable for intravenous infusion was known as Hartmann's or M/6 solution. Now, however, a solution of sodium bicarbonate is preferred. Instead, sodium lactate presently is a minor constituent of one or two sodium supplements.

▲ side-effects: administration of sodium lactate may produce another form of acidosis in patients with poor circulation or impaired function of the liver.
Related article: DEXTROLYTE.

sodium nitrite is a VASODILATOR used in an emergency, often in combination with sodium thiosulphate, to treat cyanide poisoning. It was formerly also used to treat angina pectoris (heart pain). Administration is by injection of a mild aqueous solution.
▲ side-effects: there may be flushing and headache, caused by the vasodilating effect of the drug. Some patients experience gastrointestinal disturbance, dizziness and a loss of sensation in the extremities.

S

sodium nitroprusside is a VASODILATOR used in an emergency to treat apoplexy (a hypertensive crisis); but it may be used more ordinarily to treat heart failure, and during surgery to effect a controlled low blood pressure. Administration is by infusion.
✚ warning: sodium nitroprusside should not be administered to patients with impaired liver function or body deficiency in cyanocobalamin (vitamin B_{12}); it should be administered with caution to those with impaired kidney function, impaired blood circulation through the brain, or the effects of an insufficient supply of thyroid hormones (hypothyroidism), or who are elderly. Strict observation of patients is essential throughout treatment, and should include blood counts.
▲ side-effects: headache, dizziness, sweating, nausea and heartbeat irregularities are all fairly common; there may also be abdominal pain and, in some patients, anxiety.
Related article: NIPRIDE.

sodium perborate is an ANTISEPTIC (and deodorant) powder that is soluble in water. As a mouth-wash the solution has a cleansing effect because it tends to froth on contact with plaque and other oral debris.
✚ warning: sodium perborate should not be used continuously for more than about 4 weeks or borate poisoning may occur.
Related article: BOCASAN.

sodium picosulphate is a stimulant LAXATIVE which works by direct action on the nerve endings within the intestinal walls of the colon. Prescribed not only to relieve constipation and to prepare patients for X-ray, endoscopy or surgery, the drug is administered orally in the form of an elixir or a solution.
✚ warning: sodium picosulphate should not be administered to patients who suffer from intestinal blockage or who are pregnant; it should be administered with caution to children.
▲ side-effects: prolonged use may eventually precipitate the onset of atonic non-functioning colon.
Related articles: LAXOBERAL; PICOLAX.

sodium salicylate is a soluble non-narcotic ANALGESIC and ANTI-INFLAMMATORY agent used in both capacities to treat rheumatic and other musculo-skeletal disorders. Administration is oral in the form of a non-proprietary mixture (liquid).
✚ warning: sodium salicylate should not be administered to

patients with peptic ulcers or who are aged under 12 years; it should be administered with caution to those with severely impaired function of the kidneys or the liver, allergies or dehydration, who are pregnant or lactating, who are elderly, or who are already taking anticoagulant drugs.

▲ side-effects: gastrointestinal upset is common; there may also be nausea, hearing disturbances and vertigo; some patients experience ulceration and bleeding. Rarely, there is a state of confusion, sensitivity reactions (such as asthma-like attacks or a rash), inflammation of the heart, or blood disorders.

sodium stibogluconate is a powerful compound drug used to treat forms of the tropical disease leishmaniasis or kala-azar (caused by parasitic protozoans transmitted in sandfly bites) that leave extensive or unsightly lesions on the skin surface, or that have a similar effect internally. Administration is by slow intravenous injection (which must immediately be halted if there is an attack of coughing or the onset of chest pain).

✚ warning: sodium stibogluconate should not be administered to patients with hepatitis, pneumonia, kidney disease or inflammation of the heart.

▲ side-effects: there may be vomiting, coughing and chest pain; continued treatment may lead to severe weight loss (anorexia).

Related article: PENTOSTAM.

sodium tetradecyl sulphate is a drug used in sclerotherapy – a technique to treat varicose veins by the injection of an irritant solution. The resultant inflammation of the vein promotes the obliteration of the vein by thrombosis.

✚ warning: sodium tetradecyl sulphate should not be injected into patients whose varicose veins are already inflamed or so painful as to prevent walking, who are obese, or who are taking oral contraceptives.

▲ side-effects: some patients experience sensitivity reactions.

Related article: STD.

sodium thiosulphate is a compound used in an emergency, often in combination with sodium nitrite, to treat cyanide poisoning. Administration is by injection of a mild aqueous solution.

▲ side-effects: there may be flushing and headache, caused by the vasodilating effect of the drug. Some patients experience gastrointestinal disturbance, dizziness and a loss of sensation in the extremities.

sodium valproate is an ANTICONVULSANT drug used to treat epilepsy. It is particularly effective in controlling grand mal (tonic-clonic) seizures in primary generalized epilepsy, although it is used to treat all forms of the disorder. The drug is also occasionally used to treat the rare cases of recurrent febrile convulsions in children, to whom it may be administered prophylactically. Administration is oral in the form of tablets and as a liquid (or dilute syrup).

✚ warning: sodium valproate should not be administered to patients with liver disease: liver function should be monitored for at least the first 6 months of treatment. The drug may cause some blood count readings to be misleading in relation to diabetic patients.

▲ side-effects: there may be nausea and gastrointestinal disturbance, increased appetite and consequent weight gain, temporary hair loss, and impaired liver function. If severe vomiting and weight loss occur, treatment should be withdrawn at once.
Related article: EPILIM.

Sofradex (*Roussel*)is a proprietary compound ANTIBIOTIC, available only on prescription, used to treat inflammation and infection in the eye or outer ear. Produced in the form of drops and as an ointment, Sofradex is a combination of the CORTICOSTEROID dexamethasone and the broad-spectrum antibiotic framycetin.

✚/▲ warning/side-effects: *see* DEXAMETHASONE; FRAMYCETIN.

Soframycin (*Roussel*) is a proprietary ANTIBIOTIC, available only on prescription, used to treat many forms of infection. Major uses include disinfection of the intestines (especially prior to intestinal surgery), topical application on the skin, injection into the membranes that surround the spinal cord, as eye-drops and eye ointment, and as a cream for use in the outer ear. Produced in the form of tablets, as a powder for reconstitution as a medium for injection or for topical application, as drops, as an ointment and as a water-miscible cream, Soframycin in all forms is a preparation of the broad-spectrum antibiotic framycetin sulphate.

✚/▲ warning/side-effects: *see* FRAMYCETIN.

Solarcaine (*Plough*) is a proprietary non-prescription local ANAESTHETIC used in topical application to treat local pain and skin irritation. Produced in the form of a cream, as a lotion, and as a spray, Solarcaine is a combination of benzocaine with the DISINFECTANT TRICLOSAN.

✚ warning: see BENZOCAINE.

Solis (*Galen*) is a proprietary ANXIOLYTIC drug, available on prescription only to private patients, used to treat anxiety and insomnia, and to assist in the treatment of acute alcohol withdrawal symptoms. Also a MUSCLE RELAXANT, Solis is sometimes also used to relieve muscle spasm. Produced in the form of capsules (in two strengths), it is a preparation of the BENZODIAZEPINE diazepam.

✚/▲ warning/side-effects: *see* DIAZEPAM.

Solivito (*KabiVitrum*) is a proprietary VITAMIN supplement, available only on prescription, used in injection or infusion. It contains almost all forms of VITAMIN B together with ASCORBIC ACID (vitamin C), and is produced in the form of a powder for reconstitution either with water or with glucose (or an equivalent medium).

Soliwax (*Martindale*) is a proprietary non-prescription form of ear-drops designed to soften and dissolve ear-wax (cerumen), and commonly prescribed for use at home two nights consecutively before syringing of the ears in a doctor's surgery. Its solvent constituent is DIOCTYL SODIUM SULPHOSUCCINATE (also called docusate sodium).

✚ warning: soliwax should not be used if there is inflammation in the ear, or where there is any chance that the eardrum has been perforated.

Solpadeine (*Sterling Research*) is a proprietary non-prescription compound ANALGESIC that is not available from the National Health Service. It is used to relieve the pain of headaches, and of rheumatism and other musculo-skeletal disorders. Produced in the form of tablets for effervescent solution (in two strengths, the stronger under the trade name Solpadeine Forte and available on prescription only to private patients), Solpadeine is a combination of paracetamol, codeine phosphate and caffeine.
✚/▲ warning/side-effects: *see* CAFFEINE; CODEINE PHOSPHATE; PARACETAMOL.

Solprin (*Reckitt & Colman*) is a proprietary non-prescription preparation of the non-narcotic ANALGESIC aspirin that is not available from the National Health Service. It is used to relieve mild to moderate pain, and is produced in the form of soluble (dispersible) tablets.
✚/▲ warning/side-effects: *see* ASPIRIN.

Solu-Cortef (*Upjohn*) is a proprietary CORTICOSTEROID preparation, available only on prescription, used to make up natural steroid deficiency, to suppress inflammation or allergic symptoms, or to treat shock. Produced in the form of powder for reconstitution as a medium for injection, Solu-Cortef is a form of hydrocortisone.
✚/▲ warning/side-effects: *see* HYDROCORTISONE.

Solu-Medrone (*Upjohn*) is a proprietary CORTICOSTEROID preparation, available only on prescription, used to suppress inflammation or allergic symptoms, to relieve fluid retention around the brain, or to treat shock. Produced in the form of powder for reconstitution as a medium for injection, Solu-Medrone is a form of methylprednisolone.
✚/▲ warning/side-effects: *see* METHYLPREDNISOLONE.

Solvazinc (*Thames*) is a proprietary non-prescription ZINC supplement used to make up a body deficiency of that mineral. Produced in the form of tablets for effervescent solution, Solvazinc is a preparation of zinc sulphate.
✚/▲ warning/side-effects: *see* ZINC SULPHATE.

Somatonorm 4IU (*KabiVitrum*) is a proprietary preparation of human growth HORMONE (HGH, or somatotrophin) in its synthetic form, somatrem, available only on prescription, used to treat hormonal deficiency and associated symptoms (in particular short stature). It is produced in the form of a powder for reconstitution as a medium for injection.
✚/▲ warning/side-effects: *see* SOMATREM.

somatotrophin is a chemical name for human growth HORMONE (HGH). Not viable for therapeutic use, it is synthesized in the form of SOMATREM.
see HGH.

somatrem is a synthesized form of human growth HORMONE (HGH, or somatotrophin), prepared by genetic engineering for therapeutic use because the natural hormone secreted by the pituitary gland is not viable in treatment. It is produced using sequences of DNA to create what is known as a growth hormone of human sequence, and is used to treat dwarfism and other problems of short stature caused by hormone deficiency.

Administration is by injection.

✚ warning: somatrem should not be administered to patients who suffer from diabetes mellitus. Treatment is possible only for younger patients whose long bones have not fully fused and are thus capable of growth in the normal fashion – the ends lengthening independently of the shaft.

▲ side-effects: there is a risk of the formation of antibodies. *Related article:* SOMATONORM 4IU.

Sominex (*Beecham*) is a proprietary non-prescription TRANQUILLIZER used to relieve occasional insomnia. Produced in the form of tablets, it is a preparation of the ANTIHISTAMINE promethazine hydrochloride; it is not recommended for children aged under 16 years.

✚/▲ warning/side-effects: *see* PROMETHAZINE HYDROCHLORIDE.

Somnite (*Norgine*) is a proprietary HYPNOTIC, available on prescription only to private patients, used in the short term to treat insomnia in patients for whom daytime sedation is not appropriate. Produced in the form of a suspension (for swallowing), Somnite is a preparation of the BENZODIAZEPINE nitrazepam. It is not recommended for children.

✚/▲ warning/side-effects: *see* NITRAZEPAM.

Soneryl (*May & Baker*) is a proprietary sedative, a BARBITURATE on the controlled drugs list, used as a HYPNOTIC to treat intractable insomnia. Produced in the form of tablets, it is a preparation of butobarbitone. It is not recommended for children or the elderly.

✚/▲ warning/side-effects: *see* BUTOBARBITONE.

Soni-Slo (*Lipha*) is a proprietary non-prescription VASODILATOR, used to prevent or to treat recurrent attacks of angina pectoris (heart pain). Produced in the form of sustained-release capsules (in two strengths), Soni-Slo is a preparation of isosorbide dinitrate. It is not recommended for children.

✚/▲ warning/side-effects: *see* ISOSORBIDE DINITRATE.

Sorbichew (*Stuart*) is a proprietary non-prescription VASODILATOR, used to treat attacks of angina pectoris (heart pain). Produced in the form of tablets, Sorbichew is a preparation of isosorbide dinitrate. Sorbichew is not recommended for administration to children.

✚/▲ warning/side-effects: *see* ISOSORBIDE DINITRATE.

Sorbid SA (*Stuart*) is a proprietary non-prescription VASODILATOR, used to prevent attacks of angina pectoris (heart pain). Produced in the form of sustained-release tablets, Sorbid SA is a preparation of isosorbide dinitrate. Sorbid SA is not recommended for administration to children.

✚/▲ warning/side-effects: *see* ISOSORBIDE DINITRATE.

sorbitol is a sweet-tasting carbohydrate that is used as a sugar-substitute (particularly by diabetics) and as the carbohydrate in some nutritional supplements administered by injection or infusion.

✚ warning: large oral doses may cause gastrointestinal disturbance.

Sorbitrate (*Stuart*) is a proprietary non-prescription VASODILATOR, used to prevent attacks of angina pectoris (heart pain). Produced in the form of tablets (in two strengths), Sorbitrate is a preparation of isosorbide dinitrate. It is not recommended for children.

✚/▲ warning/side-effects: *see* ISOSORBIDE DINITRATE.

Sotacor (*Bristol-Myers*) is a proprietary BETA-BLOCKER, an ANTIHYPERTENSIVE drug, available only on prescription, used to treat high blood pressure (hypertension), heartbeat irregularities and angina pectoris (heart pain), and to prevent secondary heart attacks. Produced in the form of tablets (in two strengths), Sotacor is a preparation of the beta-blocker sotalol hydrochloride.

✚/▲ warning/side-effects: *see* SOTALOL HYDROCHLORIDE.

sotalol hydrochloride is a BETA-BLOCKER, an ANTIHYPERTENSIVE drug used to treat high blood pressure (hypertension), heartbeat irregularities and angina pectoris (heart pain), and to prevent secondary heart attacks. It is also useful in relieving the symptoms of excess thyroid hormones in the bloodstream (thyrotoxicosis). Administration is oral in the form of tablets, or by injection.

✚ warning: sotalol hydrochloride should not be administered to patients with asthma, heart failure or heart block; it should be administered with caution to those with impaired liver or kidney function, who are diabetic, or who are pregnant or lactating. Withdrawal of treatment should be gradual.

▲ side-effects: there may be gastrointestinal disturbances, slow heart rate and cold fingertips and toes, and symptoms much like asthma.

Related articles: BETA-CARDONE; SOTACOR.

Sotazide (*Bristol-Myers*) is a proprietary ANTIHYPERTENSIVE drug, available only on prescription, used to treat mild to moderate high blood pressure (hypertension). Produced in the form of tablets, Sotazide is a preparation of the BETA-BLOCKER sotalol hydrochloride together with the THIAZIDE DIURETIC hydrochlorothiazide.

✚/▲ warning/side-effects: *see* HYDROCHLOROTHIAZIDE; SOTALOL HYDROCHLORIDE.

Sparine (*Wyeth*) is a proprietary ANTIPSYCHOTIC drug, available only on prescription, used to soothe agitation (particularly in the elderly or the dying) and for the short-term relief of acute, severe anxiety. It is also sometimes used to calm children prior to cardiac investigation or electro-encephalography. Produced in the form of tablets (in three strengths), as a suspension for dilution (the potency of the suspension once dilute is retained for 14 days) and in ampoules for injection, Sparine is a preparation of promazine hydrochloride. It is not recommended for children other than for the purpose outlined above.

✚/▲ warning/side-effects: *see* PROMAZINE HYDROCHLORIDE.

Spasmonal (*Norgine*) is a proprietary non-prescription ANTISPASMODIC drug used to treat muscle spasm in both the gastrointestinal tract (leading to abdominal pain and constipation) and the uterus or vagina (leading to menstrual problems). Produced in the form of capsules, Spasmonal is a preparation of alverine citrate. It is not recommended for children and its

use should be avoided in patients with paralytic ileus.
✚ warning: *see* ALVERINE CITRATE.

spectinomycin is an ANTIBIOTIC used almost solely to treat gonorrhoea caused by organisms resistant to penicillin, or in patients who are allergic to penicillin. Administration is by injection.
✚ warning: it is essential that both sexual partners undergo treatment even if only one shows symptoms. (Dosage for women is twice that for men.)
▲ side-effects: there may be nausea with vomiting, high temperature and dizziness; some patients experience urticaria or itching skin.
Related article: TROBICIN.

Spectraban (*Stiefel*) is the name of two proprietary non-prescription lotions containing constituents that are able to protect the skin from ultraviolet radiation. Patients whose skin condition is such as to require this sort of protection may be prescribed Spectraban at the discretion of their doctors. The two lotions differ: Spectraban 4 is a preparation of the substance padimate O in an alcohol base; Spectraban 15 is a compound preparation of padimate O and aminobenzoic acid in an alcohol base.
✚ warning: *see* AMINOBENZOIC ACID; PADIMATE O.

Spectralgen (*Pharmacia*) is a proprietary set of 4 grass pollen preparations and 3 tree dust preparations for use in desensitising patients who are allergic to one or more of such substances (and so suffer from hay fever or similar symptoms). Available only on prescription, and administered by injection, Spectralgen preparations are of carefully annotated different allergenic strength, so that the process of desensitization, as regulated by a doctor, can be progressive.
✚ warning: injections should be administered under close medical supervision and in locations where emergency facilities for full cardio-respiratory resuscitation are immediately available.

***spermicidal** drugs kill sperm and are used to assist contraception, but should never be regarded themselves as a means of contraception. They are intended to accompany barrier methods, such as the condom (sheath), or diaphragm (Dutch cap). Most spermicidal preparations consist of a spermicide – generally an alcohol ester – within an inhibitory liquid or cream base. Administration is in the form of vaginal inserts (pessaries), creams, gels, pastes, foams in aerosols, and soluble films.
Related articles: C-FILM; DELFEN; DOUBLE CHECK; DURACREME; DURAGEL; EMKO; GENEXOL; GYNOL II; ORTHO-CREME; ORTHOFORMS; ORTHO-GYNOL; RENDELLS; STAYCEPT; TWO'S COMPANY.

Spiretic (*DDSA Pharmaceuticals*) is a proprietary DIURETIC of the type that retains (rather than depletes) potassium in the body. Available only on prescription, it is used to treat fluid retention caused by cirrhosis of the liver, congestive heart failure, high blood pressure (*see* ANTIHYPERTENSIVE) or kidney disease. It is produced in the form of tablets (in two strengths), and is a preparation of the comparatively weak diuretic spironolactone.
✚/▲ warning/side-effects: *see* SPIRONOLACTONE.

Spiroctan (*MCP Pharmaceuticals*) is a proprietary DIURETIC of the type that retains (rather than depletes) potassium in the body. Available only on prescription, it is used to treat fluid retention caused by cirrhosis of the liver, congestive heart failure, high blood pressure (*see* ANTIHYPERTENSIVE) or kidney disease. It is produced in the form of tablets (in two strengths) and as capsules, and is a preparation of the comparatively weak diuretic spironolactone.
✚/▲ warning/side-effects: *see* SPIRONOLACTONE.

Spiroctan-M (*MCP Pharmaceuticals*) is a proprietary DIURETIC of the type that retains (rather than depletes) potassium in the body. Available only on prescription, it is used to treat fluid retention caused by cirrhosis of the liver, congestive heart failure, high blood pressure (*see* ANTIHYPERTENSIVE) or kidney disease. It is produced in the form of ampoules for injection, and is transformed to a metabolite of spironolactone.
✚/▲ warning/side-effects: *see* SPIRONOLACTONE.

Spirolone (*Berk*) is a proprietary DIURETIC of the type that retains (rather than depletes) potassium in the body. Available only on prescription, it is used to treat fluid retention caused by cirrhosis of the liver, congestive heart failure, high blood pressure (*see* ANTIHYPERTENSIVE) or kidney disease. It is produced in the form of tablets (in three strengths), and is a preparation of the comparatively weak diuretic spironolactone.
✚/▲ warning/side-effects: *see* SPIRONOLACTONE.

spironolactone is a DIURETIC of the type that retains (rather than depletes) potassium in the body, used primarily to treat fluid retention caused by cirrhosis of the liver, congestive heart failure, high blood pressure (*see* ANTIHYPERTENSIVE) or kidney disease. It is also used to treat the symptoms of an excess of the hormone aldosterone in the blood acting by antagonizing this hormone. Administration is oral in the form of tablets or capsules, or by injection. Comparatively weak by itself, spironolactone is often used in combination with other diuretics that are potassium-depleting (such as any of the THIAZIDES) and potentiates their effect.
✚ warning: spironolactone should not be administered to patients with kidney failure or an excess of potassium in the body; it should be administered with caution to those who are pregnant or lactating.
▲ side-effects: many patients experience gastrointestinal disturbances. In male patients the breasts may enlarge (gynaecomastia); female patients may have irregular periods.
Related articles: ALDACTIDE 50; ALDACTONE; DIATENSEC; LARACTONE; LASILACTONE; SPIRETIC; SPIROCTAN; SPIROCTAN-M; SPIROLONE; SPIROPROP.

Spiroprop (*Searle*) is a proprietary compound ANTIHYPERTENSIVE drug, available only on prescription, used to treat mild to moderate high blood pressure (hypertension). Produced in the form of tablets, it is a combination of the BETA-BLOCKER propranolol hydrochloride and the potassium-sparing DIURETIC spironolactone.
✚/▲ warning/side-effects: *see* PROPRANOLOL; SPIRONOLACTONE.

Sprilon (*Pharmacia*) is a proprietary non-prescription barrier spray for topical application to leg ulcers, bedsores, fissures in the skin or eczema, or to skin areas potentially requiring protection from urine or faeces (as in nappy rash or around a stoma – an outlet on the skin suface following the surgical curtailment of the intestines). Produced in the form of an aerosol, Sprilon is a compound of ZINC OXIDE, the antifoaming agent DIMETHICONE, wool fat, wood alcohols and paraffins.
✚ warning: some patients may be sensitive to the wool fat constituent.

S

Stabillin V-K (*Boots*) is a proprietary preparation of the penicillin-type ANTIBIOTIC phenoxymethylpenicillin, used primarily to treat infections of the head and throat, and some skin conditions; it may also be used to prevent a patient's temperature from rising too high and to prevent infections following rheumatic fever. Available only on prescription, it is produced in the form of tablets and as an elixir (in three strengths) for dilution (the potency of the elixir once dilute is retained for 7 days).
✚/▲ warning/side-effects: *see* PHENOXYMETHYLPENICILLIN.

Stafoxil (*Brocades*) is a proprietary ANTIBIOTIC, available only on prescription, used to treat bacterial infections of the skin and of the ear, nose and throat, and especially staphylococcal infections that prove to be resistant to penicillin. Produced in the form of capsules (in two strengths), Stafoxil is a preparation of flucloxacillin. It is not recommended for children aged under 2 years.
✚/▲ warning/side-effects: *see* FLUCLOXACILLIN.

stanozolol is an anabolic STEROID that also has ANTICOAGULANT properties, used to assist the metabolic synthesis of protein in the body following major surgery or long-term debilitating disease, to treat osteoporosis, or to treat various circulatory disorders. It is also used in the treatment of certain forms of anaemia although how it works in this respect – and even whether it works – remains the subject of some debate: variations in patient response are wide. Administration is oral in the form of tablets, or by injection.
✚ warning: stanozolol should not be administered to patients with impaired liver function or cancer of the prostate gland, or who are pregnant or lactating; it should be administered with caution to those with heart or kidney disease, diabetes, epilepsy, high blood pressure (hypertension) or circulatory problems, or migraine. In the treatment of children, monitoring of bone growth is essential every half-year.
▲ side-effects: there may be fluid retention in the tissues (oedema), high levels of calcium in the blood, and acne; prolonged treatment in female patients may cause menstrual irregularites and eventual slight signs of masculinization.
Related article: STROMBA.

Staphcil (*Lederle*) is a proprietary ANTIBIOTIC, available only on prescription, used to treat bacterial infections and especially staphylococcal infections that prove to be resistant to penicillin. Produced in the form of capsules (in two strengths) and in vials for injection, Staphcil is a

preparation of flucloxacillin.
✚/▲ warning/side-effects: *see* FLUCLOXACILLIN.

Staycept (*Syntex*) is a proprietary non-prescription SPERMICIDAL preparation for use in combination with one of the barrier methods of contraception (such as a condom or diaphragm). Produced in the form of vaginal inserts (pessaries) and as a jelly, Staycept's active constituent is an alcohol ester.

STD (*STD Pharmaceutical*) is a proprietary form of the drug sodium tetradecyl sulphate, available only on prescription, used in scleropathy – a technique to treat varicose veins by the injection of an irritant solution. The resultant inflammation of the vein promotes the obliteration of the vein by thrombosis. STD is produced in ampoules for injection.
✚/▲ warning/side-effects: *see* SODIUM TETRADECYL SULPHATE.

Stelazine (*Smith, Kline & French*) is a proprietary form of the powerful ANTIPSYCHOTIC drug trifluoperazine. Available only on prescription, it is used to treat and tranquillize psychoses (such as schizophrenia) including the control of behavioural disturbances. It may be used alternatively to treat anxiety in the short term. Stelazine is produced in the form of tablets (in two strengths), as sustained-release capsules (spansules, in three strengths), as a sugar-free syrup for dilution (the potency of the syrup once dilute is retained for 14 days), as a liquid concentrate for dilution (the potency of the syrup once dilute is retained for a period dependent on the diluent), and in ampoules for injection.
✚/▲ warning/side-effects: *see* TRIFLUOPERAZINE.

Stemetil (*May & Baker*) is a proprietary ANTI-EMETIC, available only on prescription, used to relieve symptoms of nausea caused by the vertigo and loss of balance experienced in infections of the inner and middle ears, or by cytotoxic drugs in the treatment of cancer. Produced in the form of tablets (in two strengths), as a syrup for dilution (the potency of the syrup once dilute is retained for 14 days), as anal suppositories (in two strengths), and in ampoules for injection, Stemetil is a preparation of the major TRANQUILLIZER prochlorperazine.
✚/▲ warning/side-effects: *see* PROCHLORPERAZINE.

sterculia is a vegetable gum capable of absorbing up to 60 times its own volume of water, useful in patients who cannot tolerate bran. Used as a LAXATIVE, it has the effect of increasing the overall mass and compaction of faeces, so promoting bowel movement; exactly the same effect is beneficial in treating diarrhoea and diverticular disease, and in maintaining faecal consistency for patients who have undergone colostomy or ileostomy. But more controversially sterculia may also be medically prescribed to treat serious obesity, in the intention that small amounts of food ingested may be bulked up internally, making the patient feel full. Administration is in the form of granules to be taken with water.
✚ warning: sterculia should not be administered to patients who suffer from intestinal blockage or a disorder of the

muscles of the intestinal walls; it should be administered with caution to those who suffer from ulcerative colitis. Adequate fluid intake must be maintained.
▲ side-effects: there may be flatulence, even to the point of abdominal distension.
Related articles: NORMACOL; PREFIL.

Steribath (*Stuart*) is a proprietary, non-prescription, concentrated solution for use in the bath as a DISINFECTANT and cleansing agent. Its active constituent is a form of IODINE.

Sterogyl-15 (*Roussel*) is a proprietary non-prescription form of the plant-derived vitamin D, ERGOCALCIFEROL, that is not available from the National Health Service. Produced in the form of a solution (for swallowing), it is used to make up CALCIFEROL (vitamin D) deficiency.

***steroids** are a class of naturally occuring and synthetic agents whose structure is based on the chemical sterone. In the body they include HORMONES of the adrenal cortex and sex glands (such as OESTROGENS and PROGESTOGENS), bile acids and VITAMINS of the D group. Many types of drug are available based on the steroids, and they are used to treat many types of disorder (including sex-hormone linked disorders, rheumatic pain and certain skin disorders).

Ster-Zac (*Hough*) is the name of three proprietary DISINFECTANT cleansing products. Ster-Zac Powder is a non-prescription dusting powder used to prevent infection in minor wounds and bedsores; it contains the antiseptic hexachlorophane, the mild astringent zinc oxide, and starch. Ster-Zac Bath Concentrate is a mild solution of the antiseptic TRICLOSAN, available without prescription, used to treat staphylococcal skin infections. And Ster-Zac DC Skin Cleanser, available only on prescription, is intended for use instead of soap either for surgeons to scrub up with before undertaking surgical operations, or for patients who suffer from acne and skin infections; it is the antiseptic hexachlorophane in the form of a cream.
✚/▲ warning/side-effects: *see* HEXACHLOROPHANE.

Stesolid (*CP Pharmaceuticals*) is a proprietary ANXIOLYTIC drug, available only on prescription, used to treat anxiety and insomnia, to act as a premedication before surgery, and to assist in the treatment of acute alcohol withdrawal symptoms. Also a muscle relaxant and an ANTICONVULSANT, Stesolid is used to treat muscle spasm and – more seriously – convulsions due to poisoning and to epileptic seizures. Produced in the form of tubes (for rectal insertion) and in ampoules for injection, Stesolid is a preparation of the BENZODIAZEPINE diazepam. It is not recommended for children aged under 12 months.
✚/▲ warning/side-effects: *see* DIAZEPAM.

Stiedex (*Stiefel*) is a proprietary CORTICOSTEROID cream, available only on prescription, used for topical application to skin inflammations and allergic skin disorders. It consists of the steroid desoxymethasone (in two strengths, the weaker under the trade name Stiedex LP) in an oily cream base. A third version, additionally containing the

antiseptic NEOMYCIN, is also produced (under the name Stiedex LPN).
✚/▲ warning/side-effects: *see* DESOXYMETHASONE.

stilboestrol is a synthesized OESTROGEN that is useful in hormone replacement therapy in women following the menopause, and is now used less commonly to treat breast cancer. It was formerly in popular use also for the suppression of lactation. In men it is widely used in low dosage to treat cancer of the prostate gland. Administration is oral in the form of tablets, as vaginal inserts (pessaries), or by injection.
✚ warning: stilboestrol should not be administered to patients with oestrogen-dependent cancers, porphyria, impaired liver function or thrombosis. It should be administered with caution to those with epilepsy, diabetes, high blood pressure (hypertension), heart or kidney disease, or migraine; who are pregnant or lactating; or who wear contact lenses.
▲ side-effects: there may be nausea and vomiting, breast enlargement and tenderness in women, weight gain through sodium retention, and a rash; some women patients experience headache and depression. There is a risk of thrombosis. Rarely, treatment encourages the development of cancer of the womb lining. Treatment of breast cancer may cause high blood levels of calcium, and bone pain. In men, treatment causes impotence and the appearance of some feminine characteristics, particularly in the development of the breasts (gynaecomastia).
Related article: TAMPOVAGAN STILBOESTROL AND LACTIC ACID.

***stimulants** are agents that activate body systems or functions. In general, the term is applied to drugs that stimulate the central nervous system. The result may be increased energy, increased enthusiasm, and euphoria, but the effects are only temporary and the return to ordinary actuality may eventually lead to a psychotic state. Yet patients who suffer from narcolepsy, and hyperactive children, may well derive some therapeutic benefit from the administration of certain types of stimulant, although in children they may also retard growth. Central nervous system stimulants include the amphetamines (such as DEXAMPHETAMINE SULPHATE) and the drug found in tea and coffee, CAFFEINE.

Stomahesive (*Squibb*) is a proprietary non-prescription paste intended for the filling and sealing of skin creases round a stoma (an outlet on the skin surface following the surgical curtailment of the intestines).

Stomabar (*Raymed*) is a proprietary non-prescription barrier cream intended for the protection and sanitization of a stoma (an outlet on the skin surface following the surgical curtailment of the intestines).

Stomogel (*Raymed*) is a proprietary non-prescription deodorant gel intended for the freshening and sanitization of a stoma (an outlet on the skin surface following the surgical curtailment of the intestines).

Stomosol (*Raymed*) is a proprietary non-prescription ANTISEPTIC liquid intended for the disinfection and sanitization of a stoma (an outlet on the skin surface following the surgical curtailment of the intestines).

Strepsils (*Crookes Healthcare*) are proprietary non-prescription throat lozenges that contain the ANTISEPTICS 2,4-dichlorobenzyl alcohol and amylmetacresol.

Streptase (*Hoechst*) is a proprietary FIBRINOLYTIC, available only on prescription, used primarily to treat thrombosis and embolism. Produced in the form of powder for reconstitution as a medium for injection, Streptase is a preparation of the enzyme streptokinase.

✚/▲ warning/side-effects: *see* STREPTOKINASE.

S

streptokinase is an enzyme that is used therapeutically as an FIBRINOLYTIC drug because it has the property of breaking up blood clots (by actuating plasmin formation which then degrades the clot component fibrin). It is very useful in treating thrombosis and embolisms. Administration is by injection or infusion.

✚ warning: streptokinase should not be administered to patients with blood disorders involving defective coagulation, or with streptococcal infections; who are liable to bleed (either by menstruation or because of recent trauma or surgery); or who are pregnant. It should be administered with caution to those who suffer from heart disease.

▲ side-effects: there may be allergic reaction, incorporating a rash and a high temperature.

Related articles: KABIKINASE; STREPTASE.

streptokinase-streptodornase is a combination of FIBRINOLYTIC enzymes that together have the property of breaking up blood clots and other exudates liable otherwise to congeal (such as pus). It is used primarily to clean wounds, ulcers and sores, and to slough off surrounding lesioned skin. Administration is by topical application in the form of a dampened powder (or in solution via a catheter).

✚/▲ warning/side-effects: *see* STREPTOKINASE.

streptomycin is an aminoglycoside ANTIBIOTIC now used almost solely for the treatment of tuberculosis, for which it is administered in combination with other antibiotics. Treatment of tuberculosis takes between 6 and 18 months. Administration of streptomycin is by injection. In the rare treatment of urinary and intestinal infections (with or without penicillin) it is administered orally.

✚ warning: streptomycin should not be administered to patients who are pregnant, and should be administered with extreme caution to patients with impaired kidney function. Regular blood counts are essential to check dosage and for signs of toxicity.

▲ side-effects: there may be hearing difficulties and dysfunction of the kidneys, particularly in elderly patients. Prolonged treatment may cause an excess of magnesium in the body.

Streptotriad (*May & Baker*) is a proprietary compound ANTIBACTERIAL, available only on prescription, used to treat any of several serious infections including meningococcal meningitis and bacillary dysentery; it is also used

prophylactically, on medical staff and relatives at high risk of infection, and on convalescing patients who may or may not become carriers of dangerous bacterial infections. Produced in the form of tablets, Streptotriad combines the aminoglycoside streptomycin with the three SULPHONAMIDES sulphadiazine, sulphathiazole and sulphadimidine.
✚/▲ warning/side-effects: *see* STREPTOMYCIN; SULPHADIAZINE; SULPHADIMIDINE.

Stromba (*Sterling Research*) is a proprietary form of the anabolic STEROID stanozolol, available only on prescription, used to assist the metabolic synthesis of protein in the body following major surgery or long-term debilitating disease, to treat osteoporosis ("brittle bones"), or to treat various circulatory disorders. It is also used in the treatment of certain forms of anaemia although how it works in this respect – and even whether it works – remains the subject of some debate: variations in patient response are wide. It is produced in the form of tablets and (in suspension) in ampoules for injection.
✚/▲ warning/side-effects: *see* STANOZOLOL.

Stugeron (*Janssen*) is a proprietary non-prescription preparation of the ANTIHISTAMINE cinnarizine, used to treat nausea caused by the vertigo and loss of balance experienced in infections of the middle and inner ears. It is produced in the form of tablets. A stronger version of cinnarizine (produced under the trade name Stugeron Forte) is also used to treat circulatory problems of the extremities.
✚/▲ warning/side-effects: *see* CINNARIZINE.

Sublimaze (*Janssen*) is a narcotic ANALGESIC on the controlled drugs list, primarily used to enhance the effect of a BARBITURATE general ANAESTHETIC, allowing the barbiturate dose to be smaller. Produced in ampoules for injection, Sublimaze is a preparation of the morphine-like fentanyl.
✚/▲ warning/side-effects: *see* FENTANYL.

sucralfate is a drug used to treat gastric and duodenal ulcers (its name derives from aluminium sucrose sulphate). Unlike antacids, it is thought to work by forming a protective barrier over an ulcer, so allowing healing underneath. Treatment lasts for more than 4 weeks. Administration is oral in the form of tablets.
✚ warning: sucralfate should be administered with caution to patients with kidney disease.
▲ side-effects: constipation is not uncommon.
Related article: ANTEPSIN.

Sudafed (*Calmic*) is a proprietary non-prescription nasal DECONGESTANT; unlike most decongestants, however, it is produced in the form of tablets (for swallowing) and an elixir for dilution (the potency of the elixir once dilute is retained for 14 days). Both forms are preparations of the ephedrine derivative pseudoephedrine hydrochloride.
✚/▲ warning/side-effects: *see* EPHEDRINE HYDROCHLORIDE.

Sudocrem (*Tosara*) is a proprietary non-prescription skin emollient (softener and soother) used to treat nappy rash, bedsores and eczema, and sometimes to dress burns. Produced in the form of a cream, its active constituents include

ZINC oxide, benzyl benzoate and wool fat.
✚ warning: wool fat may cause sensitivity reactions in some patients.

sulconazole nitrate is an ANTIFUNGAL drug, one of the IMIDAZOLES, used to treat skin infections. Administration is by topical application in the form of a water-miscible cream.
✚ warning: keep well away from the eyes.
▲ side-effects: some patients experience sensitivity reactions, especially skin irritation.
Related article: EXELDERM.

S

Suleo-C (*International Labs*) is a proprietary non-prescription drug used to treat infestations of the scalp and pubic hair by lice. Produced in the form of a lotion and a shampoo, Suleo-C is a preparation of the pediculicide carbaryl.
✚ warning: *see* CARBARYL.

Suleo-M (*International Labs*) is a proprietary non-prescription drug used to treat infestations of the scalp and pubic hair by lice (pediculosis), or of the skin by the itch-mite (scabies). Produced in the form of a lotion, Suleo-M is a preparation of the insecticide malathion in an alcohol solution.
✚ warning: *see* MALATHION.

sulfadoxine is an ANTIBACTERIAL, a long-acting SULPHONAMIDE, used solely in combination with PYRIMETHAMINE to prevent or treat malaria.

sulfametopyrazine is an ANTIBACTERIAL, a long-acting SULPHONAMIDE, used primarily in the treatment of chronic bronchitis and infections of the urinary tract. Administration is oral in the form of tablets.
✚ warning: sulfametopyrazine should not be administered to patients with liver or kidney failure, or blood disorders, who are pregnant, or who are aged under 6 weeks; it should be administered with caution to those who are elderly, or who are lactating. Adequate fluid intake must be maintained; regular blood counts are essential during prolonged treatment.
▲ side-effects: there may be nausea with vomiting, skin disorders and changes in the composition of the blood.
Related article: KELFIZINE W.

Sulfamylon (*Winthrop*) is a proprietary ANTIBACTERIAL, available only on prescription, used in topical application to treat infectious burns. Produced in the form of a water-miscible cream, Sulfamylon is a preparation of the SULPHONAMIDE mafenide.
✚/▲ warning/side-effects: *see* MAFENIDE.

Sulfomyl (*Winthrop*) is a proprietary non-prescription form of ANTIBACTERIAL eye-drops used to treat local infections. It is a preparation of the SULPHONAMIDE mafenide.
✚/▲ warning/side-effects: *see* MAFENIDE.

sulindac is a non-steroidal ANTI-INFLAMMATORY non-narcotic ANALGESIC drug used to treat pain and inflammation in rheumatic disease and other musculo-skeletal disorders.
Administration is by injection.
✚ warning: sulindac should be administered with caution to patients with impaired liver or kidney function, gastric ulcers or allergic conditions, or who are pregnant.
▲ side-effects: there may be

nausea and gastrointestinal disturbance; internal haemorrhage may occur. Some patients experience sensitivity reactions such as a rash, headache, asthma-like symptoms, and even vertigo or ringing in the ears (tinnitus). Rarely, there is fluid retention leading to weight gain, or a minor change in the composition of the blood.
Related article: CLINORIL.

sulphacetamide is an ANTIBACTERIAL, one of the SULPHONAMIDES, used (in solution) primarily in the form of eye-drops and eye ointment to treat local bacterial infections. It is also used in combination with other sulphonamides to treat infections of the vagina and cervix. Ophthalmic administration is most commonly in the form of drops during the daytime, and as ointment for overnight treatment; treatment for vaginal infections is in the form either of vaginal tablets (pessaries) or as a cream.

sulphadiazine is an ANTIBACTERIAL, one of the SULPHONAMIDES, used to treat serious bacterial infections – particularly meningococcal meningitis or resistant infections of the eye. Administration is oral in the form of tablets, or by infusion.

✚ warning: sulphadiazine should not be administered to patients with liver or kidney failure, or disorders of the blood, who are pregnant, or who are aged under 6 weeks; it should be administered with caution to those with impaired kidney function or sensitivity to light, who are elderly, or who are lactating. Adequate fluid intake is essential, as are regular blood counts during prolonged courses of treatment.

▲ side-effects: there may be nausea and vomiting, with skin disorders; changes in the composition of the blood may occur.
Related articles: STREPTOTRIAD; SULPHATRIAD.

sulphadimethoxine is a long-acting ANTIBACTERIAL, one of the SULPHONAMIDES, used to treat many serious bacterial infections – particularly infections of the urinary tract, or the eye disorder trachoma. Administration is oral in the form of tablets.

✚ warning: sulphadimethoxine should not be administered to patients with liver or kidney failure, or disorders of the blood, who are pregnant, or who are aged under 6 weeks; it should be administered with caution to those with impaired kidney function or sensitivity to light, who are elderly, or who are lactating. Adequate fluid intake is essential, as are regular blood counts during prolonged courses of treatment.

▲ side-effects: there may be nausea and vomiting, with skin disorders; changes in the composition of the blood may occur.
Related article: MADRIBON.

sulphadimidine is an ANTIBACTERIAL, one of the SULPHONAMIDES, used to treat serious bacterial infections – particularly infections of the urinary tract – and to prevent meningococcal meningitis in patients at high risk from infection. Among the least toxic of the sulphonamides, sulphadimidine is especially useful in the treatment of children. Administration is oral in the form of tablets, or by injection.

✚ warning: sulphadimidine should not be administered to patients who suffer from liver or kidney failure, or disorders of the blood, who are pregnant, or who are aged under 6 weeks; it should be administered with caution to those with impaired kidney function or sensitivity to light, who are elderly, or who are lactating. Adequate fluid intake is essential, as are regular blood counts during prolonged courses of treatment.

▲ side-effects: there may be nausea and vomiting, with skin disorders; changes in the composition of the blood may occur.

Related articles: STREPTOTRIAD; SULPHAMEZATHINE.

S

sulphafurazole is an ANTIBACTERIAL, one of the SULPHONAMIDES, used to treat serious bacterial infections – particularly infections of the urinary tract. Administration is oral in the form of tablets or as a syrup.

✚ warning: sulphafurazole should not be administered to patients with liver or kidney failure, or from disorders of the blood, who are pregnant, or who are aged under 6 weeks; it should be administered with caution to those with impaired kidney function or sensitivity to light, who are elderly, or who are lactating. Adequate fluid intake is essential, as are regular blood counts during prolonged courses of treatment.

▲ side-effects: there may be nausea and vomiting, with skin disorders; changes in the composition of the blood may occur.

Related article: GANTRISIN.

sulphaguanidine is an ANTIBACTERIAL, one of the SULPHONAMIDES, formerly in widespread use to treat intestinal infections or to prepare patients for intestinal surgery (because absorption into the body is poor, and does not occur early in the digestive processes). Administration is oral in the form of (non-proprietary) tablets.

✚ warning: sulphaguanidine should not be administered to patients with liver or kidney failure, or disorders of the blood, who are pregnant, or who are aged under 6 weeks; it should be administered with caution to those with impaired kidney function or sensitivity to light, who are elderly, or who are lactating. Adequate fluid intake is essential, as are regular blood counts during prolonged courses of treatment.

▲ side-effects: there may be nausea and vomiting, with frequent skin rashes; changes in the composition of the blood may occur.

sulphamethoxazole is an ANTIACTERIAL, one of the SULPHONAMIDES, that in combination with the antibacterial agent TRIMETHOPRIM – forming a compound drug called co-trimoxazole – is in widespread use to treat many serious infections, especially infections of the bones and joints, of the urinary tract and of the upper respiratory tract, and such infections as gonorrhoea and typhoid fever. Rarely, sulphamethoxazole is used by itself in the treatment of urinary infections; administration is oral in the form of tablets, and patients should be advised to increase fluid intake during treatment.

see CO-TRIMOXAZOLE.

Sulphamezathine (*ICI*) is a proprietary ANTIBACTERIAL, available only on prescription, used to treat serious bacterial infections – particularly bacillary dysentery and infections of the urinary tract – and to prevent meningococcal meningitis in patients at high risk from infection. Produced in ampoules for injection, Sulphamezathine is a preparation of the SULPHONAMIDE sulphadimidine.
✚/▲ warning/side-effects: *see* SULPHADIMIDINE.

sulphasalazine is an ANTIBACTERIAL, one of the SULPHONAMIDES, used primarily to induce a remission of the symptoms of ulceration of the intestinal wall (generally in the colon) and, having induced it, to maintain it. Because the drug also has anti-inflammatory properties, it is additionally used to treat rheumatoid arthritis (although there are some haematological side-effects). Administration is oral in the form of (enteric-coated or plain) tablets, or in suppositories, or as a retention enema.
✚ warning: sulphasalazine should not be administered to patients known to be sensitive to salicylates (aspirin-type drugs) or to sulphonamides; it should be administered with caution to those with liver or kidney disease, or who are pregnant or lactating. Adequate fluid intake must be maintained.
▲ side-effects: side-effects are common with higher doses. There may be nausea with vomiting and other gastrointestinal disturbance; headache, vertigo, ringing in the ears (tinnitus) and high temperature; and a rash. A change in the composition of the blood may cause a form of anaemia and a discoloration of the urine and of the tear-fluid lubricating the eyes. Even more seriously, there may be inflammation of the pancreas or of the heart.
Related article: SALAZOPYRIN.

Sulphatriad (*May & Baker*) is a proprietary compound ANTIBACTERIAL, available only on prescription, used to treat any of several serious infections including meningococcal meningitis. Produced in the form of tablets, Sulphatriad is a combination of the three SULPHONAMIDES sulphadiazine, sulphamerazine and sulphathiazole.
✚/▲ warning/side-effects: *see* SULPHADIAZINE.

sulphaurea is an ANTIBACTERIAL, one of the SULPHONAMIDES, used primarily to treat infections of the urinary tract. Administration is oral in the form of tablets (generally also containing the ANALGESIC PHENAZOPYRIDINE).
✚ warning: sulphaurea should not be administered to patients with liver or kidney failure, or disorders of the blood, who are pregnant, or who are aged under 6 weeks; it should be administered with caution to those with impaired kidney function or sensitivity to light, who are elderly, or who are lactating. Adequate fluid intake is essential, as are regular blood counts during prolonged courses of treatment.
▲ side-effects: there may be nausea and vomiting, with skin disorders; changes in the composition of the blood may occur.
Related article: UROMIDE.

sulphinpyrazone is a drug used

to treat and prevent excesses of uric acid in the bloodstream and the gout that results from it. It works by promoting the excretion of uric acid in the urine. Once treatment has started, it is continued indefinitely (so potentially preventing acute attacks of gout). Administration is oral in the form of tablets.

✚ warning: sulphinpyrazone should not be administered to patients with kidney stones or blood disorders, who are in the middle of an acute attack of gout, or who are already taking aspirin-type drugs. Initial administration may be painful (and require simultaneous administration of an analgesic). Adequate fluid intake must be maintained. Regular blood counts are advisable.

▲ side-effects: there may be gastrointestinal disturbance; a few patients experience sensitivity reactions.

Related article: ANTURAN.

S

sulphonamides, or sulpha drugs, are derivatives of a red dye called sulphanilamide that have the property of preventing the growth of bacteria. Most are administered orally and are rapidly absorbed in the stomach and small intestine, are short-acting, and thus may have to be taken several times a day. Their quick progress through the body and excretion in the urine makes them particularly suited to the treatment of urinary infections. One or two sulphonamides are long-acting (and may be used to treat diseases such as malaria or leprosy), and another one or two are poorly absorbed (for which reason they were until recently used to treat intestinal infections). Best known and most used sulphonamides include sulphadiazine, sulphadimidine and sulphafurazole. Sulphonamides tend to cause side-effects – particularly nausea, vomiting, diarrhoea and headache – some of which (especially sensitivity reactions) may become serious; bone-marrow damage may result from prolonged treatment. As a general rule, patients being treated with sulphonamides should try to avoid exposure to sunlight. As antibacterial agents they are distinct from ANTIBIOTICS, and in some cases the one class of drug may be substituted for the other when there are adverse side-effects.

see MAFENIDE; SULFADOXINE; SULFAMETOPYRAZINE; SULPHACETAMIDE; SULPHADIAZINE; SULPHADIMETHOXINE; SULPHADIMIDINE; SULPHAFURAZOLE; SULPHAGUANIDINE; SULPHAMETHOXAZOLE; SULPHASALAZINE; SULPHAUREA.

sulphones are closely related to the SULPHONAMIDES, have much the same therapeutic action, and are thus used for much the same purposes. They are particularly successful in preventing the growth of the bacteria responsible for leprosy, malaria and tuberculosis. Best known and (possibly) most used is dapsone.

see DAPSONE.

sulphonylureas are drugs derived from a SULPHONAMIDE that have the effect of reducing blood levels of glucose. They work by promoting the secretion of INSULIN from the pancreas, and are thus useful in treating the form of hyperglycaemia that occurs in adult-onset diabetes mellitus where there is still some insulin production. Best known and most used sulphonylureas include chlorpropamide, glibenclamide, glipizide, tolazamide and tolbutamide. Side-effects are not

common, although sensitivity reactions occur. But the list of drugs with which sulphonylureas must not be taken simultaneously is long, and includes relatively commonly prescribed drug-types such as corticosteroids, diuretics, anticoagulants, sulphonamides and aspirin-type antibiotics.
see ACETOHEXAMIDE; CHLORPROPAMIDE; GLIBENCLAMIDE; GLIBORNURIDE; GLICLAZIDE; GLIPIZIDE; GLIQUIDONE; GLYMIDINE; TOLAZAMIDE; TOLBUTAMIDE.

sulphur is a non-metallic element thought to be active against external parasites and fungal infections of the skin. Its common use in creams, ointments or lotions for treating skin disorders such as acne, dermatitis and psoriasis would appear to have little scientific basis.

sulpiride is an ANTIPSYCHOTIC drug used to treat the symptoms of schizophrenia. In low doses, it increases an apathetic, withdrawn patient's awareness and tends to generate a true consciousness of events. In high doses it is used also to treat other conditions that may cause tremor, tics, involuntary movements or involuntary utterances (such as the relatively uncommon Gilles de la Tourette syndrome). Administration is oral in the form of tablets.

✚ warning: sulpiride should not be administered to patients with reduction in the bone marrow's capacity to produce blood cells, or suffering from certain types of glaucoma. It should be administered only with caution to those with heart or vascular disease, kidney or liver disease, epilepsy, parkinsonism, or depression; or who are pregnant or lactating. It is not recommended for children.

▲ side-effects: patients should be warned before treatment that their judgement and powers of concentration may become defective under treatment. There may be restlessness, insomnia and nightmares; rashes and jaundice may appear; and there may be dry mouth, gastrointestinal disturbance, difficulties in urinating, and blurred vision. Muscles in the neck and back, and sometimes the arms, may undergo spasms. Some patients experience impaired kidney function.
Related article: DOLMATIL; SULPITIL.

Sulpitil (*Tillotts*) is a proprietary ANTIPSYCHOTIC drug used to treat the symptoms of schizophrenia. In low doses, it increases an apathetic, withdrawn patient's awareness and tends to generate a true consciousness of events. In high doses it is used also to treat other conditions that may cause tremor, tics, involuntary movements or involuntary utterances (such as the relatively uncommon Gilles de la Tourette syndrome). Produced in the form of tablets, Sulpitil is a preparation of sulpiride. It is not recommended for children.

✚/▲ warning/side-effects: *see* SULPIRIDE.

Sultrin (*Ortho-Cilag*) is a proprietary ANTIBACTERIAL, available only on prescription, used to treat bacterial infections of the vagina or the cervix, or to prevent infection following gynaecological surgery. Produced in the form of vaginal tablets (pessaries) and as a cream (with its own applicator), Sultrin is a compound of three SULPHONAMIDE antibacterial agents, sulphacetamide,

S

sulphabenzamide and sulphathiazole.

Suprefact (*Hoechst*) is a proprietary form of gonadotrophin-releasing HORMONE, available only on prescription, used to treat later stages of cancer of the prostate gland. It works by effectively suppressing the production and secretion of the male sex hormone testosterone which contributes to the growth and metastasis of the cancer. Produced in the form of a nasal spray and in vials for injection, Suprefact is a preparation of buserelin.
✚/▲ warning/side-effects: *see* BUSERELIN.

S

suramin is a powerful drug used in the treatment of infestations by filaria (threadlike nematode worms that parasitize the connective and lymphatic tissues of the body following transmission through the bite of a bloodsucking insect). It is also used to treat the early stages of trypanosomiasis (a tropical protozoan infection such as sleeping sickness, transmitted through bites of the tsetse fly). Administration is initially by infusion, and then by injection.
✚ warning: suramin is toxic to the kidneys; a course of treatment lasts a maximum of 5 weeks, and regular urine analysis is essential.

Surbex T (*Abbott*) is a proprietary non-prescription MULTIVITAMIN supplement that is not available from the National Health Service. Produced in the form of tablets it contains THIAMINE (vitamin B_1), RIBOFLAVINE (vitamin B_2), PYRIDOXINE (vitamin B_6), NICOTINAMIDE (of the B complex), and ASCORBIC ACID; (vitamin C).

Surem (*Galen*) is a proprietary HYPNOTIC, available on prescription only to private patients, used in the short term to treat insomnia in patients for whom daytime sedation is not appropriate. Produced in the form of capsules, Surem is a preparation of the BENZODIAZEPINE nitrazepam. It is not recommended for children.
✚/▲ warning/side-effects: *see* NITRAZEPAM.

Surgam (*Roussel*) is a proprietary non-narcotic ANALGESIC, available only on prescription, used to treat the pain of rheumatic disease and other musculo-skeletal disorders. Produced in the form of tablets (in two strengths, under the names Surgam 200 and Surgam 300), it is a preparation of the non-steroidal ANTI-INFLAMMATORY agent tiaprofenic acid.
✚/▲ warning/side-effects: *see* TIAPROFENIC ACID.

Surmontil (*May & Baker*) is a proprietary ANTIDEPRESSANT, available only on prescription, used to treat depressive illness (especially in cases where there is a need for sedation), and severe insomnia. Produced in the form of tablets (in two strengths) and as capsules, Surmontil is a preparation of the TRICYCLIC drug trimipramine maleate. It is not recommended for children.
✚/▲ warning/side-effects: *see* TRIMIPRAMINE.

Suscard Buccal (*Pharmax*) is a proprietary non-prescription VASODILATOR, used to treat congestive heart failure and angina pectoris (heart pain). It is produced in the form of sustained- release tablets (in four strengths) to be held between the upper lip and the gum until they dissolve, consisting of a preparation of glyceryl trinitrate.

It is not recommended for children.
✚/▲ warning/side-effects: *see* GLYCERYL TRINITRATE.

Sustac (*Pharmax*) is a proprietary non-prescription VASODILATOR, used to treat angina pectoris (heart pain). It is produced in the form of sustained-release tablets (in three strengths), consisting of a preparation of glyceryl trinitrate. It is not recommended for children.
✚/▲ warning/side-effects: *see* GLYCERYL TRINITRATE.

Sustamycin (*MCP Pharmaceuticals*) is a proprietary broad-spectrum ANTIBIOTIC, available only on prescription, used to treat many forms of infection. Produced in the form of sustained-release capsules, Sustamycin is a preparation of tetracycline hydrochloride. It is not recommended for children.
✚/▲ warning/side-effects: *see* TETRACYCLINE.

Sustanon (*Organon*) is a proprietary preparation of the male sex HORMONE testosterone, available only on prescription, used to treat hormonal deficiency in men, inoperable breast cancer in women (rarely now because of its masculinizing effects), and conditions of osteoporosis ("brittle bones") caused by lack of androgens. Produced in ampoules (in two strengths, under the names Sustanon 100 and Sustanon 250) for injection, administration is from fortnightly to monthly.
✚/▲ warning/side-effects: *see* TESTOSTERONE.

suxamethonium chloride is a SKELETAL MUSCLE RELAXANT that has an effect for only 5 minutes, and is thus used – following the initial injection of an intravenous BARBITURATE – for short, complete and predictable paralysis (mostly during diagnostic or surgical procedures). Recovery is spontaneous. Administration is by injection or infusion.
✚ warning: suxamethonium chloride should not be administered to patients with severe liver disease or severe burns. Premedication is usually with atropine. During treatment, the paralysis is irreversible.
▲ side-effects: blood levels of potassium rise temporarily under treatment. There may be muscle pain afterwards. Repeated doses may cause prolonged muscle paralysis.
Related articles: ANECTINE; SCOLINE.

Sween (*Francol*) is a proprietary non-prescription deodorant spray used to freshen and sanitize the appliance or bag attached to a stoma (an outlet on the skin surface following the surgical curtailment of the intestines).

Symmetrel (*Geigy*) is a proprietary preparation of the powerful drug amantadine hydrochloride, available only on prescription, used to treat parkinsonism, but not the parkinsonian symptoms induced by drugs (*see* ANTIPARKINSONSISM). Effective on some patients, but not on others, Symmetrel is produced in the form of capsules and as a syrup for dilution (the potency of the syrup once dilute is retained for 4 weeks).
✚/▲ warning/side-effects: *see* AMANTADINE HYDROCHLORIDE.

***sympathomimetics** are drugs that have effects mimicking those of the sympathetic nervous system. There are two main types, although several

sympathomimetics belong to both types. Alpha-adrenergic sympathomimetics (such as phenylephrine) are VASOCONSTRICTORS and are particularly used in nasal decongestants. Beta-adrenergic sympathomimetics (such as salbutamol, see BETA-RECEPTOR STIMULANTS) are frequently SMOOTH MUSCLE RELAXANTS, particularly on bronchial smooth muscle, and are used especially as BRONCHODILATORS.
see ADRENALINE; DOBUTAMINE HYDROCHLORIDE; DOPAMINE; EPHEDRINE HYDROCHLORIDE; FENOTEROL; ISOETHARINE HYDROCHLORIDE; ISOPRENALINE; METARAMINOL; METHOXAMINE HYDROCHLORIDE; NORADRENALINE; ORCIPRENALINE SULPHATE; OXEDRINE TARTRATE; PHENYLEPHRINE; PIRBUTEROL; REPROTEROL; RIMITEROL; SALBUTAMOL; TERBUTALINE.

Sympatol (*Lewis*) is a proprietary VASOCONSTRICTOR, available only on prescription, used to treat low blood pressure (hypotension). Produced in the form of a liquid (for swallowing) and in ampoules for injection, Sympatol is a preparation of the SYMPATHOMIMETIC drug oxedrine tartrate.
✚/▲ warning/side-effects: *see* OXEDRINE TARTRATE.

Synacthen (*Ciba*) is a proprietary form of a HORMONE that stimulates the adrenal gland into functioning to produce corticosteroid hormones (corticotrophin). This may be useful therapeutically in cases of anaphylactic shock or to stimulate the adrenal gland which may be suppressed by chronic corticosteroid administration, but in fact Synacthen is primarily used merely to test adrenal gland function. Consisting of a preparation of tetracosactrin, and produced in ampoules for injection, it is not recommended for children.
✚/▲ warning/side-effects: *see* TETRACOSACTRIN.

Synacthen Depot (*Ciba*) is a proprietary form of a HORMONE that stimulates the adrenal gland into functioning to produce either adrenaline and noradrenaline, or corticosteroid hormones (corticotrophin). Administered on a regular basis, the dosage monitored and adjusted for effect, the hormone has been used to treat several disorders that depend on hormonal factors. Such disorders include rheumatic disease, gout, ulcerative colitis and chronic skin disorders, as well as allergic conditions although now it is used more commonly as a DIAGNOSTIC AGENT of adrenal function. It is a preparation of tetracosactrin acetate and a zinc complex, produced in ampoules for injection.
✚/▲ warning/side-effects: *see* TETRACOSACTRIN.

Synadrin (*Hoechst*) is a proprietary VASODILATOR, available only on prescription, used to prevent recurrent attacks of angina pectoris (heart pain). Produced in the form of tablets, Synadrin is a preparation of prenylamine lactate. It is not recommended for children.
✚/▲ warning/side-effects: *see* PRENYLAMINE.

Synalar (*ICI*) is a series of proprietary CORTICOSTEROID ointments and creams, available only on prescription, for topical application on skin infections or inflammation. All contain the steroid fluocinolone acetonide. The standard form is a 0.025%

solution, in both ointment and cream. Synalar Cream 1:10 is a cream (only) consisting of a 0.0025% solution; Synalar Cream 1:4 is a cream (only) consisting of a 0.00625% solution. Synalar C is both ointment and cream as the standard version, but with the addition of the ANTIFUNGAL agent CLIOQUINOL. Synalar N is both ointment and cream as the standard version, but with the addition of the ANTIBIOTIC agent NEOMYCIN. There is also a similar gel with which to massage the scalp; its content is the same as the standard ointment and cream.
✚/▲ warning/side-effects: *see* FLUOCINOLONE ACETONIDE.

Synandone (*ICI*) is a proprietary CORTICOSTEROID ointment and cream, available only on prescription, for topical application on skin infections and inflammations (especially between courses of more powerful corticosteroid drugs). It is a preparation of the steroid fluocinolone acetonide in a 0.01% solution.
✚/▲ warning/side-effects: *see* FLUOCINOLONE ACETONIDE.

Syndol (*Merrell*) is a proprietary non-prescription compound analgesic that is not available from the National Health Service. It is used particularly to treat headache and toothache, and pain following surgery. Produced in the form of tablets, Syndol is a compound that includes paracetamol, codeine phosphate and caffeine. It is not recommended for children.
✚/▲ warning/side-effects: *see* CAFFEINE; CODEINE PHOSPHATE; PARACETAMOL.

Synergel (*Servier*) is a proprietary non-prescription ANTACID that is not available from the National Health Service. It is produced in the form of a gel and is based on an aluminium salt.

Synflex (*Syntex*) is a proprietary non-narcotic ANALGESIC, available only on prescription, used to treat migraine and menstrual and inflammatory pain, and pain following surgery. Produced in the form of tablets, it is a preparation of the non- steroidal ANTI-INFLAMMATORY drug naproxen sodium.
✚/▲ warning/side-effects: *see* NAPROXEN.

Synkavit (*Roche*) is a proprietary non-prescription form of the water-soluble VITAMIN K substitute menadiol sodium phosphate. It is as good as the real vitamin (phytomenadione) in making up vitamin deficiency and thus ensuring properly effective blood clotting. It is produced in the form of tablets and in ampoules for injection.
✚ warning: *see* MENADIOL SODIUM PHOSPHATE.

Synogist (*Townendale*) is a proprietary non-prescription medicated shampoo containing an ANTIBIOTIC, used to treat conditions of the scalp associated with bacterial or fungal infection (particularly of the sebaceous glands).
✚ warning: keep the shampoo away from the eyes.

Synphase (*Syntex*) is a proprietary supply of ORAL CONTRACEPTIVE tablets for one month that follows a carefully phased scheme. It is presented as a calendar pack: each of 21 tablets is numbered, and the first tablet is to be taken on the fifth day of the mestrual cycle. The contents of the pills varies according to the stage of the cycle reached, but is a combinat on of

the OESTROGEN ethinyloestradiol and the PROGESTOGEN norethisterone. Synphase is available only on prescription.
✚/▲ warning/side-effects: *see* ETHINYLOESTRADIOL; NORETHISTERONE.

Syntaris (*Syntex*) is a proprietary nasal spray, available only on prescription, used to treat the symptoms of nasal allergy (such as hay fever). Consisting of a preparation of the CORTICOSTEROID flunisolide, it is produced in a bottle with a pump and applicator. It is not recommended for children aged under 5 years.
✚/▲ warning/side-effects: *see* FLUNISOLIDE.

S

Synthamin (*Travenol*) is a proprietary series of nutritional supplements for infusion into patients unable to take food via the alimentary canal. They are all a preparation of amino acids; most also contain electrolytes. Available only on prescription, each should be administered only by qualified personnel.

Syntocinon (*Sandoz*) is a proprietary preparation of the natural HORMONE oxytocin, which causes increased contraction of the womb during labour and stimulates lactation in the breasts. Available only on prescription, it may be administered therapeutically to induce or assist labour, to control postnatal bleeding, and (in the form of a nasal spray) to promote lactation. Medical supervision is essential during treatment. It is produced in ampoules for injection (in three strengths) and as a nasal spray.
✚/▲ warning/side-effects: *see* OXYTOCIN.

Syntometrine (*Sandoz*) is a proprietary preparation of the vegetable alkaloid ergometrine maleate together with the natural HORMONE oxytocin. Available only on prescription, it may be administered to assist the second and final stages of labour (birth and the delivery of the afterbirth), and to control postnatal bleeding. Medical supervision is essential during treatment. It is produced in ampoules for injection.
✚/▲ warning/side-effects: *see* ERGOMETRINE MALEATE; OXYTOCIN.

Syntopressin (*Sandoz*) is a proprietary preparation of lypressin, one of the derivatives of the antidiuretic HORMONE vasopressin. Available only on prescription, it is used to treat pituitary-originated diabetes insipidus, and is produced in the form of a nasal spray.
✚/▲ warning/side-effects: *see* VASOPRESSIN.

Synuretic (*DDSA Pharmaceuticals*) is a proprietary compound DIURETIC, available only on prescription, used for general diuresis. Produced in the form of tablets, it is a combination of the THIAZIDE diuretic hydrochlorothiazide with a complementary potassium-sparing diuretic amiloride hydrochloride.
✚/▲ warning/side-effects: *see* AMILORIDE; HYDROCHLOROTHIAZIDE.

Syraprim (*Wellcome*) is a proprietary ANTIBACTERIAL drug, available only on prescription, used to treat serious bacterial infections, particularly those of the upper respiratory tract and of the urinary tract. Produced in the form of tablets (in two strengths) and in ampoules for injection, Syraprim is a

preparation of the antibacterial agent trimethoprim.
✚/▲ warning/side-effects: *see* TRIMETHOPRIM.

Sytron (*Parke-Davis*) is a proprietary non-prescription iron supplement, used to make up IRON deficiency (and so treat anaemia). Produced in the form of a sugar-free elixir for dilution (the potency of the elixir once dilute is retained for 14 days), it consits of sodium ironedetate.
✚/▲ warning/side-effects: *see* SODIUM IRONEDETATE.

Tachostyptan (*Consolidated*) is a proprietary preparation of the blood factor thromboplastin which, in the presence of a wound, converts the otherwise inert blood constituent prothrombin into the enzyme thrombin, so initiating the blood clotting process. It is used therapeutically to control bleeding, or to prevent excessive bleeding during or following surgery. Available only on prescription, Tachostyptan is produced in ampoules for injection.

Tachyrol (*Duphar*) is a proprietary non-prescription preparation of CALCIFEROL (vitamin D) in the form of its analogue dihydrotachysterol. Used to restore and sustain the calcium balance mechanism in the body, Tachyrol is produced in the form of tablets.
✚ warning: *see* DIHYDROTACHYSTEROL.

Tagamet (*Smith, Kline & French*) is a proprietary preparation of the drug cimetidine, available only on prescription, used to treat peptic ulcers (in the stomach or duodenum, or on a stoma) and persistent acid stomach. It works by reducing the secretion of gastric acids. It is produced in the form of tablets (in three strengths), as a syrup for dilution (the potency of the syrup once dilute is retained for 28 days), in ampoules for injection, and in bags for infusion. It is not recommended for children aged under 12 months.
✚/▲ warning/side-effects: *see* CIMETIDINE.

talampicillin is a broad-spectrum penicillin-type ANTIBIOTIC, a derivative of AMPICILLIN, used to treat severe bacterial infections (such as chronic bronchitis, gonorrhoea, infection of the middle ear, and infections of the urinary tract). Administration is oral in the form of tablets and as a dilute syrup.
✚ warning: talampicillin should not be administered to patients known to be sensitive to penicillins; it should be administered with caution to those with any allergy at all, or to those with impaired kidney function.
▲ side-effects: there may be sensitivity reactions. Some patients experience diarrhoea.
Related article: TALPEN.

Talpen (*Beecham*) is a proprietary ANTIBIOTIC of the penicillin type, available only on prescription, used to treat severe bacterial infections (such as chronic bronchitis, gonorrhoea, infection of the middle ear, and infections of the urinary tract). Produced in the form of tablets, and as a syrup for dilution (the potency of the syrup once dilute is retained for 7 days), Talpen is a preparation of the ampicillin-derivative talampicillin.
✚/▲ warning/side-effects: *see* TALAMPICILLIN.

Tambocor (*Riker*) is a proprietary ANTIARRHYTHMIC drug, available only on prescription, used to treat all forms of heartbeat irregularities. Produced in the form of tablets, and in ampoules for injection, Tambocor is a preparation of the local ANAESTHETIC LIGNOCAINE analogue flecainide acetate.
✚/▲ warning/side-effects: *see* FLECAINIDE ACETATE.

Tamofen (*Tillotts*) is a proprietary preparation of the powerful drug tamoxifen, available only on prescription, which because it inhibits or blocks the effect of OESTROGENS, is used primarily to treat cancers that depend on the presence of oestrogen in women, particularly breast cancer. But it may also be used (under strict medical supervision) to treat certain conditions of infertility in which the presence of oestrogens may be preventing other hormonal activity. It is produced in the form of tablets (in three strengths, under the names Tamofen, Tamofen-20 and Tamofen-40).

✚/▲ warning/side-effects: *see* TAMOXIFEN.

tamoxifen is a drug that inhibits or blocks the effect of OESTROGENS, and is thus used primarily to treat cancers that depend on the presence of oestrogen in women, particularly breast cancer. But it may also be used (under strict medical supervision) to treat certain conditions of infertility in which the presence of oestrogens may be preventing other hormonal activity. Administration is oral in the form of tablets.

✚ warning: tamoxifen should not be administered to patients who are pregnant.

▲ side-effects: the effect of treatment is much the same as that of surgical removal of the ovaries: menstruation ceases in pre-menopausal women. Other effects are comparatively rare, but the blood level of calcium may rise (and so cause pain in patients who suffer from the calcareous type of metastatic tumour). *Related articles:* NOLTAM; NOLVADEX; TAMOFEN.

Tampovagan Stilboestrol and Lactic Acid (*Norgine*) is a proprietary preparation of the OESTROGEN stilboestrol, available only on prescription, used to treat conditions of eroded or irritant skin in the vulva caused by hormonal deficiency (generally because of the menopause). It is produced in the form of vaginal inserts (pessaries), but dosage should be reduced as much, and as soon, as possible.

✚/▲ warning/side-effects: *see* STILBOESTROL.

Tancolin (*Ashe*) is a proprietary non-prescription ANTITUSSIVE that is not available from the National Health Service. Orange-flavoured, its active constituents include the BRONCHODILATOR theophylline, the NARCOTIC cough suppressant dextromethorphan, the ANTACID sodium citrate, and ASCORBIC ACID (vitamin C).

✚/▲ warning/side-effects: *see* DEXTROMETHORPHAN; SODIUM CITRATE; THEOPHYLLINE.

Tanderil (*Zyma*) is a proprietary eye ointment, available only on prescription, used to treat inflammation in and around the eye. It is a preparation of the non-steroid oxyphenbutazone (in solution). Another version is produced (under the name Tanderil Chloramphenicol) that additionally contains the ANTIBIOTIC chloramphenicol (in solution) to treat inflammation in which bacterial infection is also present.

✚/▲ warning/side-effects: *see* CHLORAMPHENICOL; OXYPHENBUTAZONE.

Taractan (*Roche*) is a proprietary ANTIPSYCHOTIC drug, available only on prescription, used to treat psychoses such as schizophrenia, to tranquillize patients undergoing behavioural disturbance, and in the short term to soothe severe anxiety. Produced in the form of tablets (in two strengths) Taractan is a preparation of the chlorpromazine-related drug chlorprothixene.

✚/▲ warning/side-effects: *see* CHLORPROTHIXENE.

Tarband (*Seton*) is a proprietary non-prescription form of impregnated bandaging incorporating ZINC PASTE and COAL TAR, used to dress conditions of chronic eczema and psoriasis. Further bandaging is required to hold it in place.
✚ warning: it should not be used to cover broken or inflamed skin.
▲ side-effects: there may be skin sensitivity. The dressing may stain skin and hair (and fabric).

Tarcortin (*Stafford-Miller*) is a proprietary cream, available only on prescription, for topical application to conditions of chronic eczema and psoriasis and other dermatoses. It is a compound of the CORTICOSTEROID hydrocortisone with the cleansing agent COAL TAR.
✚/▲ warning/side-effects: *see* HYDROCORTISONE.

Tavegil (*Sandoz*) is a proprietary non-prescription ANTIHISTAMINE used to treat allergic conditions such as hay fever, dermatitis and urticaria, or sensitivity reactions to drugs. Produced in the form of tablets, and as a sugar-free elixir for dilution (the potency of the elixir once dilute is retained for 14 days), Tavegil is a preparation of clemastine fumarate.
✚/▲ warning/side-effects: *see* CLEMASTINE.

Tears Naturale (*Alcon*) is a proprietary non-prescription form of synthetic tear-fluid, produced in the form of drops, used to make up for a deficiency in the lachrymal apparatus of the eye. It is a compound of the plasma substitute DEXTRAN with the artificial tears liquid HYPROMELLOSE.

Tedral (*Warner*) is a proprietary compound BRONCHODILATOR, available only on prescription, used to treat conditions such as chronic bronchitis and asthma. Produced in the form of tablets, and as a sugar-free elixir for dilution (the potency of the elixir once dilute is retained for 28 days), it is a preparation that includes the bronchodilator theophylline and the SYMPATHOMIMETIC SMOOTH MUSCLE RELAXANT ephedrine hydrochloride.
✚/▲ warning/side-effects: *see* EPHEDRINE HYDROCHLORIDE; THEOPHYLLINE.

Teejel (*Napp*) is a proprietary non-prescription gel containing both an ANTISEPTIC and an ANALGESIC, used to treat mouth ulcers, sore gums or inflammation of the tongue. The gel is intended to be massaged in gently. It consists of a compound of the analgesic CHOLINE SALICYLATE with the antiseptic cetalkonium chloride (both in solution). It is not recommended for children aged under 4 months.

Tegretol (*Geigy*) is a proprietary preparation of the ANTICONVULSANT drug carbamazapine, available only on prescription, used to treat almost all forms of epilepsy, and to relieve trigeminal neuralgia (pain in the side of the face). It is produced in the form of tablets (in three strengths) and as a sugar-free liquid for dilution (the potency of the liquid once dilute is retained for 14 days).
✚/▲ warning/side-effects: *see* CARBAMAZEPINE.

temazepam is a relatively short-acting HYPNOTIC drug, one of the BENZODIAZEPINES, used as a TRANQUILLIZER to treat insomnia (particularly in the elderly) and as an ANXIOLYTIC premedication prior to surgery. Administration is oral in the form of capsules or as a dilute elixir.

✚ warning: temazepam should be administered with caution to patients with lung disease or shallow breathing, or impaired liver or kidney function, who are pregnant or lactating, or who are elderly and debilitated.

▲ side-effects: concentration and speed of reaction are affected. There may also be drowsiness and dizziness. Some patients experience sensitivity reactions. Prolonged use may eventually result in tolerance, and finally dependence.
Related article: NORMISON.

Temetex (*Roche*) is a proprietary CORTICOSTEROID ointment and cream, available only on prescription, used for topical application on eczema and psoriasis, and on various other serious skin disorders responsive to corticosteroids. In all forms, Temetex is a preparation of the steroid diflucortolone valerate; the cream is water-miscible, the ointment is either anhydrous-based or water-based with a paraffin diluent.
✚/▲ warning/side-effects: *see* DIFLUCORTOLONE VALERATE.

Temgesic (*Reckitt & Colman*) is a proprietary narcotic ANALGESIC, available only on prescription, used to treat all forms of pain. Produced in the form of tablets to be retained under the tongue, and in ampoules for injection, it is a preparation of the OPIATE buprenorphine hydrochloride.
✚/▲ warning/side-effects: *see* BUPRENORPHINE.

Tempulin (*Boots*) is a proprietary non-prescription form of long-acting insulin, used to treat and maintain diabetic patients. It is a preparation of beef insulin zinc suspension, and is produced in vials for injection.
✚/▲ warning/side-effects: *see* INSULIN.

Tenavoid (*Burgess*) is a proprietary form of the powerful ANXIOLYTIC drug meprobamate with the THIAZIDE DIURETIC bendrofluazide – a combination which is potentially addictive – it is on the controlled drugs list. It is used to treat anxiety, and especially that associated with premenstrual tension, and is produced in the form of tablets. It is not recommended for children.
✚/▲ warning/side-effects: *see* BENDROFLUAZIDE; MEPROBAMATE.

Tenoret 50 (*Stuart*) is a proprietary ANTIHYPERTENSIVE compound drug, available only on prescription, used primarily to treat high blood pressure (hypertension), especially in the elderly, but also to treat angina pectoris (heart pain) and heartbeat irregularities. Produced in the form of tablets, it is a combination of the BETA-BLOCKER atenolol with the THIAZIDE DIURETIC chlorthalidone. It is not recommended for children.
✚/▲ warning/side-effects: *see* ATENOLOL; CHLORTHALIDONE.

Tenoretic (*Stuart*) is a proprietary ANTIHYPERTENSIVE compound drug, available only on prescription, used primarily to treat high blood pressure (hypertension). Produced in the form of tablets, it is a combination of the BETA-BLOCKER atenolol together with the THIAZIDE DIURETIC chlorthalidone (in twice the proportions contained in the same manufacturer's Tenoret 50). It is not recommended for presciption to children.

✚/▲ warning/side-effects: *see* ATENOLOL; CHLORTHALIDONE.

Tenormin (*Stuart*) is a proprietary ANTIHYPERTENSIVE drug, available only on prescription, used primarily to treat high blood pressure (hypertension). Produced in the form of tablets (in two strengths, the weaker under the name Tenormin LS), as a sugar-free lemon-and-lime-flavoured syrup, and in ampoules for injection, it is a preparation of the BETA-BLOCKER atenolol. It is not recommended for children.
✚/▲ warning/side-effects: *see* ATENOLOL.

Tensilon (*Roche*) is a proprietary preparation of the anticholinesterase drug edrophonium chloride, available only on prescription. The drug prolongs the action of the natural neurotransmitter acetylcholine, and can thus be used both in the diagnosis of disorders of the neurotransmission process caused by disease or by drug treatments (through a comparison of its effect with the effect of its absence), and as an antidote to muscle relaxants which block the action of the neurotransmitter at the end of operations (in which case, atropine should be administered simultaneously). It is produced in ampoules for injection.
✚/▲ warning/side-effects: *see* EDROPHONIUM CHLORIDE.

Tensium (*DDSA Pharmaceuticals*) is a proprietary ANXIOLYTIC drug, available on prescription only to private patients. It is used to treat insomnia and anxiety, and to relieve the effects of acute alcohol withdrawal symptoms. Produced in the form of tablets (in three strengths), Tensium is a preparation of the powerful and long-acting BENZODIAZEPINE diazepam.
✚/▲ warning/side-effects: *see* DIAZEPAM.

Tenuate Dospan (*Merrell*) is a proprietary preparation of the amphetamine-related drug diethylpropion hydrochloride, used as an appetite-suppressant in the medical treatment of obesity. On the controlled drugs list, it is produced in the form of sustained-release tablets. Treatment must be in the short term and under strict medical supervision.
✚/▲ warning/side-effects: *see* DIETHYLPROPION HYDROCHLORIDE.

Teoptic (*Dispersa*) is a proprietary form of eye-drops, available only on prescription, used to treat glaucoma. It is a preparation of the BETA-BLOCKER carteolol hydrochloride (in two strengths), and is not recommended for children.
✚/▲ warning/side-effects: *see* CARTEOLOL HYDROCHLORIDE.

terbutaline is a BETA-RECEPTOR STIMULANT and BRONCHODILATOR that is especially useful in treating all forms and stages of asthma. As a SYMPATHOMIMETIC drug and a SMOOTH MUSCLE RELAXANT, however, terbutaline (in the form of terbutaline sulphate) is also used to prevent – or at least delay – the onset of premature labour by inhibiting uterine contractions. Administration is oral in the form of tablets, sustained-release tablets and a dilute syrup, as an inhalant via an aerosol or nebuliser, or by injection or infusion.
✚ warning: terbutaline should not be administered to patients with heart disease or high blood pressure

(hypertension), bleeding or infection, an excess of thyroid hormones in the blood (thyrotoxicosis), or who are already taking antihypertensive drugs or beta-blockers. It should be administered with caution to those with diabetes, who are undergoing treatment with corticosteroids or diuretics, or who are elderly. Regular blood counts and blood pressure monitoring are essential.

▲ side-effects: there may be nausea and vomiting, flushing and sweating, and a tremor. High dosage may cause an increase in the heart rate, with high blood pressure. *Related articles:* BRICANYL; MONOVENT.

Tercoda (*Sinclair*) is a proprietary non-prescription cough elixir that is not available from the National Health Service. Active constituents include codeine phosphate and the EXPECTORANT terpin hydrate.

✚/▲ warning/side-effects: *see* CODEINE PHOSPHATE.

Tercolix (*Vestric*) is a proprietary non-prescription cough elixir that is not available from the National Health Service. Active constituents include codeine phosphate and menthol and the EXPECTORANT terpin hydrate.

✚/▲ warning/side-effects: *see* CODEINE PHOSPHATE.

terfenadine is a relatively new ANTIHISTAMINE used to treat the symptoms of allergic disorders. Unlike most, it has little sedative effect. Administration is oral in the form of tablets or as a dilute suspension.

✚ warning: terfenadine should be administered with caution to patients with epilepsy, glaucoma, liver disease or enlargement of the prostate gland.

▲ side-effects: side-effects are comparatively uncommon, but there may be headache. *Related article:* TRILUDAN.

terlipressin is a derivative of the antidiuretic HORMONE VASOPRESSIN, and is similarly a VASOCONSTRICTOR. It is used primarily to halt bleeding from varicose veins in the oesophagus - the part of the alimentary tract between the throat and the stomach. Administration is by intravenous injection.

✚ warning: terlipressin should not be administered to patients with chronic kidney disease or vascular disease; it should be administered with caution to those with epilepsy, asthma, migraine or heart failure.

▲ side-effects: There may be nausea, cramp, and an urge to defecate; some patients experience sensitivity reactions. If the vasoconstriction affects the coronary arteries, there may be heartbeat irregularities. *Related article:* GLYPRESSIN.

terodiline hydrochloride is an ANTICHOLINERGIC drug used to treat excessive frequency of urination, and urinary incontinence. It works mainly by reducing the effect of the parasympathetic nervous system on the bladder, although it also has CALCIUM ANTAGONIST properties. Administration is oral in the form of tablets.

✚ warning: terodiline hydrochloride should not be administered to patients with urinary obstruction or any kind of liver disease; it should be administered with caution to those with excess thyroid hormones in the bloodstream

T

(thyrotoxicosis), fast heart rate (tachycardia), gastrointestinal blockage, high temperature or retention of food within the stomach.

▲ side-effects: there may be dry mouth and difficulty in swallowing, pressure within the eyeballs and sensitivity to light, flushing and dry skin, heartbeat irregularities and constipation.

Related article: TEROLIN.

Terolin (*KabiVitrum*) is a proprietary preparation of the ANTICHOLINERGIC drug terodiline hydrochloride, available only on prescription, used to treat excessive frequency of urination and urinary incontinence. It works mainly by reducing the effect of the parasympathetic nervous system on the bladder, although it also has CALCIUM ANTAGONIST properties. Produced in the form of tablets, it is not recommended for children.

✚/▲ warning/side-effects: *see* TERODILINE HYDROCHLORIDE.

Teronac (*Sandoz*) is a proprietary preparation of the stimulant drug mazindol, used as an APPETITE-SUPPRESSANT in the medical treatment of obesity. On the controlled drugs list (because it is potentially addictive and anorective), it is produced in the form of tablets. Treatment must be in the short term and under strict medical supervision.

✚/▲ warning/side-effects: *see* MAZINDOL.

Terpoin (*Hough*) is a proprietary cough elixir, available on prescription only to private patients. Active constituents include codeine phosphate, the EXPECTORANT guaiphenesin, and menthol.

✚/▲ warning/side-effects: *see* CODEINE PHOSPHATE.

Terra-Cortril (*Pfizer*) is the name of several CORTICOSTEROID preparations that are also ANTIBIOTIC, available only on prescription, used for local or topical application to treat skin disorders in which bacterial or other infection is also implicated. The standard form, produced as an ointment and as a spray in an aerosol, combines the steroid hydrocortisone and the TETRACYCLINE antibiotic oxytetracycline. Terra-Cortril Ear Suspension also contains the antibiotic polymyxin B sulphate. Terra-Cortril Nystatin is a cream that is a combination of hydrocortisone and oxytetracycline with the ANTIFUNGAL agent nystatin.

✚/▲ warning/side-effects: *see* HYDROCORTISONE; NYSTATIN; OXYTETRACYCLINE; POLYMYXIN B.

Terramycin (*Pfizer*) is a proprietary ANTIBIOTIC, available only on prescription, used to treat bacterial and other infections. Produced in the form of capsules and tablets, it is a preparation of the TETRACYCLINE oxytetracycline hydrochloride.

✚/▲ warning/side-effects: *see* OXYTETRACYCLINE.

Tertroxin (*Glaxo*) is a proprietary preparation of the thyroid HORMONE triiodothyronine (in the form of liothyronine sodium), available only on prescription, used to make up hormonal deficiency (hypothyroidism) and thus to treat the associated symptoms (myxoedema). It is produced in the form of tablets.

✚/▲ warning/side-effects: *see* LIOTHYRONINE SODIUM.

testosterone is an ANDROGEN, the principal male sex HORMONE, produced mainly in the testes and, with other androgens, promoting the development of and maintenance of the male sex organs and the development of the secondary male sexual characteristics. Therapeutically it may be administered to treat hormonal deficiency (but only following careful investigation and under strict medical supervision), particularly in cases of delayed puberty in boys; it is no longer in general use to treat cancer of the breast in women because of its masculinizing effects. Administration is oral in the form of capsules, or by injection, depot injection, or as surgical implants.

✚ warning: testosterone should not be administered to male patients who suffer from kidney disease, cancer of the prostate gland or cancer of the breast, or to female patients who are pregnant or lactating; it should be administered with caution to those with impaired function of the heart, liver or kidney, circulatory disorders and/or high blood pressure (hypertension), epilepsy or diabetes, thyroid disorders, or migraine.

▲ side-effects: there may be fluid retention in the tissues (oedema) leading to weight gain. Increased levels of calcium in the body may cause bone growth (and in younger patients may fuse bones before fully grown) and the symptoms of hypercalcaemia. In elderly patients there may be (increased) enlargement of the prostate gland. High doses halt the production of sperm in men and cause the visible masculinization of women.
Related articles: PRIMOTESTON DEPOT; RESTANDOL; SUSTANON; VIRORMONE.

tetanus vaccine stimulates the formation in the body of the appropriate antitoxin – that is, an antibody produced in response to the presence of the toxin of the tetanus bacterium, rather than to the presence of the bacterium itself. Its effectiveness is improved by being adsorbed on to a mineral carrier (such as aluminium hydroxide or calcium phosphate). Its most common form of administration is as one constituent of the triple vaccine against diphtheria, whooping cough (pertussis) and tetanus (the DIPHTHERIA-PERTUSSIS-TETANUS, or DPT, vaccine) administered during early life, although it is administered by itself at any age for those at special risk, or administered as a double vaccine with the DIPHTHERIA VACCINE for those who wish not to be given the whooping cough vaccine. Administration is by injection. Tetanus vaccinations should not be renewed within 5 years.

Tetavax (*Merieux*) is a proprietary preparation of adsorbed TETANUS VACCINE, produced in syringes and vials for injection.

tet/vac/ads is an abbreviation for the kind of tetanus vaccine that is adsorbed on to a mineral carrier for injection.
see TETANUS VACCINE.

tet/vac/ft is an abbreviation for tetanus vaccine formol toxoid, the plain vaccine (that is not adsorbed on to a carrier).
see TETANUS VACCINE.

tetrabenazine is a powerful drug used to assist a patient to regain voluntary control of movement – or at least to lessen the extent of involuntary movements – in Huntington's chorea and related disorders. It is thought to work by reducing the amount of DOPAMINE in the nerve endings in the brain. Administration is oral

T

in the form of tablets.
✚ warning: tetrabenazine should not be administered to patients who are lactating or who are already taking drugs that contain levodopa or reserpine.
▲ side-effects: there may be drowsiness and postural hypotension. Some patients experience depression.
Related article: NITOMAN.

Tetrabid-Organon (*Organon*) is a proprietary broad-spectrum ANTIBIOTIC, available only on prescription, used to treat many forms of infection but particularly those of the urinary tract, of the genital organs, pustular acne or chronic bronchitis. Produced in the form of sustained-release capsules, it is a preparation of the TETRACYCLINE tetracycline hydrochloride. It is not suitable for children aged under 12 years.
✚/▲ warning/side-effects: *see* TETRACYCLINE.

Tetrachel (*Berk*) is a proprietary broad-spectrum ANTIBIOTIC, available only on prescription, used to treat many forms of infection but particularly those of the urinary tract, of the genital organs, pustular acne or chronic bronchitis. Produced in the form of capsules and tablets, it is a preparation of the TETRACYCLINE tetracycline hydrochloride. It is not suitable for children aged under 12 years.
✚/▲ warning/side-effects: *see* TETRACYCLINE.

tetrachloroethylene is an ANTHELMINTIC drug, used to treat infestations by hookworms (parasitical worms that attach to the inner wall of the small intestine, feeding not only on the passing food-mass but also on blood from the intestine wall).
✚ warning: tetrachloroethylene should not be administered to the elderly or the debilitated, or to children. Absorption of tetrachloroethylene may cause toxic side-effects; however, absorption is unlikely if patients avoid alcohol and fatty foods following treatment.
▲ side-effects: there may be nausea and headache, with drowsiness.

tetracosactrin is a synthetic HORMONE that acts on the adrenal glands to release CORTICOSTEROIDS, especially HYDROCORTISONE. Like its natural equivalent corticotrophin, tetracosactrin is useful in the treatment of allergic disorders, inflammation and especially asthma (particularly in patients who for one reason or another cannot tolerate the natural substance). It may also be used to test adrenal function. In the treatment of rheumatic disease in patients who are still growing, tetracosactrin has an advantage over corticosteroids in that it does not cause as much stunting of growth.
▲ side-effects: there is high blood pressure (hypertension), sodium and water retention (oedema) leading to weight gain, loss of blood potassium and muscle weakness.

tetracycline is a broad-spectrum ANTIBIOTIC that gave its name to a group of similar antibiotics. It is used to treat many forms of infection caused by several types of micro-organism; conditions it is used particularly to treat include infections of the urinary tract, of the respiratory tract, and of the genital organs, and acne. Administration is oral in the form of capsules, tablets and liquids, or by injection.

✚ warning: tetracycline should not be administered to patients who are aged under 12 years, who are pregnant, or who have impaired kidney function; it should be administered with caution to those who are lactating.

▲ side-effects: there may be nausea and vomiting, with diarrhoea. Occasionally there is sensitivity to light or other sensitivity reaction. These side-effects may still occur even if the causative organism of the disorder being treated proves to be resistant to the drug.

Related articles: ACHROMYCIN; ACHROMYCIN V; AUREOCORT; CHYMOCYCLAR; DETECLO; ECONOMYCIN; MYSTECLIN; SUSTAMYCIN; TETRABID-ORGANON; TETRACHEL; TETREX; TOPICYCLINE.

tetracyclines are broad-spectrum ANTIBIOTICS used to treat infection by many organisms, but especially bacteria. They are particularly used in the treatment of serious infections of the urinary tract, of the genital organs, of the respiratory tract (and especially chronic bronchitis). One or two are effective against meningitis. However, perhaps through over-use of the drugs, bacterial resistance has grown considerably and the tetracyclines are no longer as efficacious as they once were. Moreover, most tetracyclines are more difficult to absorb in a stomach that contains milk, antacids, calcium salts or magnesium salts; they tend to make kidney disease worse; and they may be deposited on growing bone and teeth (causing staining and potential deformity), so they should not be administered to children aged under 12 years. Best known and most used tetracyclines include tetracycline (which they were all named after), doxycycline and oxytetracycline. Administration is oral in the form of capsules, tablets or liquids.
see CHLORTETRACYCLINE HYDROCHLORIDE; CLOMOCYCLINE SODIUM; DEMECLOCYCLINE HYDROCHLORIDE; DOXYCYCLINE; LYMECYCLINE; MINOCYCLINE; OXYTETRACYCLINE; TETRACYCLINE.

Tetralysal (*Farmitalia Carlo Erba*) is a proprietary broad-spectrum ANTIBIOTIC, available only on prescription, used to treat many forms of infection but particularly those of the skin and soft tissues, the ear, nose or throat, or conditions such as pustular acne. Produced in the form of capsules (in two strengths, the stronger under the name Tetralysal 300), it represents a preparation of the soluble TETRACYCLINE complex lymecycline. It is not recommended for children aged under 12 years.

✚/▲ warning/side-effects: *see* LYMECYCLINE.

Tetrex (*Bristol-Myers*) is a proprietary broad-spectrum ANTIBIOTIC, available only on prescription, used to treat many forms of infection but particularly those of the urinary tract or genital organs, pustular acne or chronic bronchitis. Produced in the form of capsules and tablets, it is a preparation of the TETRACYCLINE tetracycline hydrochloride. It is not recommended for children aged under 12 years.

✚/▲ warning/side-effects: *see* TETRACYCLINE.

T/Gel (*Neutrogena*) is a proprietary non-prescription medicated shampoo designed to treat scaling skin on the scalp, as occurs with dandruff or with psoriasis. Its principal constituent is COAL TAR.

Thalamonal (*Janssen*) is a proprietary preparation of the TRANQUILLIZER droperidol and the narcotic ANALGESIC fentanyl, and is accordingly on the controlled drugs list. It is used on patients about to undergo diagnostic or minor surgical procedures that may be difficult or painful. It is produced in ampoules for injection.
✚/▲ warning/side-effects: *see* DROPERIDOL; FENTANYL.

Thalazole (*May & Baker*) is a proprietary ANTIBACTERIAL, available only on prescription, used (formerly much more commonly) in the treatment of intestinal infections and to disinfect the colon prior to examination or surgery. Produced in the form of tablets, Thalazole is a preparation of the poorly-absorbed SULPHONAMIDE phthalylsulphathiazole.
✚/▲ warning/side-effects: *see* PHTHALYLSULPHATHIAZOLE.

Thavoline (*Ilon*) is a proprietary non-prescription skin emollient (softener and soother) that also relieves itching. It may be used to provide a protective covering over burns, bedsores or nappy rash. Produced in the form of an ointment and as an aerosol spray for topical application, Thavoline contains WOOL FAT, ZINC OXIDE and KAOLIN.

Theodrox (*Riker*) is a proprietary non-prescription BRONCHODILATOR used to treat conditions such as asthma and bronchitis and to relieve the symptoms of partial heart failure. Produced in the form of tablets containing the antacid ALUMINIUM HYDROXIDE in order to prolong the effect, Theodrox has as its principal constituent the short-acting xanthine, aminophylline. It is not recommended for children.
✚/▲ warning/side-effects: *see* AMINOPHYLLINE.

Theo-Dur (*Astra*) is a proprietary non-prescription BRONCHODILATOR used to treat conditions such as asthma and chronic bronchitis. Produced in the form of sustained-release tablets (in two strengths) for prolonged effect, Theo-Dur has as its principal constituent the short-acting xanthine, theophylline.
✚/▲ warning/side-effects: *see* THEOPHYLLINE.

Theograd (*Abbott*) is a proprietary non-prescription BRONCHODILATOR used to treat conditions such as asthma and chronic bronchitis. Produced in the form of sustained-release tablets for prolonged effect, Theograd has as its principal constituent the short-acting xanthine, theophylline.
✚/▲ warning/side-effects: *see* THEOPHYLLINE.

theophylline is a BRONCHODILATOR used mostly in sustained-release forms of administration, generally to treat conditions such as asthma and bronchitis over periods of around 12 hours at a time. Administration is oral in the form of tablets, capsules, or a liquid. Many proprietary preparations are not recommended for children.
✚ warning: treatment should initially be gradually progressive in the quantity administered. Theophylline should be administered with caution to patients who suffer from heart or liver disease, or peptic ulcer; or who are

pregnant or lactating.
▲ side-effects: there may be nausea and gastrointestinal disturbances, an increase or irregularity in the heartbeat, and/or insomnia.
Related articles: BIOPHYLLINE; FRANOL; FRANOL EXPECT; FRANOL PLUS; LASMA; NUELIN; PRO-VENT; SABIDAL SR 270; SLO-PHYLLIN; TEDRAL; THEO-DUR; THEOGRAD; UNIPHYLLIN CONTINUS.

Thephorin (*Sinclair*) is a proprietary non-prescription ANTIHISTAMINE used in oral administration to treat allergic conditions such as hay fever and urticaria. Produced in the form of tablets, it is a preparation of the very mildly stimulant phenindamine tartrate. It is not recommended for children.
✚/▲ warning/side-effects: *see* PHENINDAMINE TARTRATE.

Theraderm (*Westwood*) is a proprietary non-prescription preparation for the treatment of acne. Produced in the form of a gel for topical application (in two strengths), its active constituent is the KERATOLYTIC agent benzoyl peroxide.
✚/▲ warning/side-effects: *see* BENZOYL PEROXIDE.

thiabendazole is a drug used in the treatment of infestations by worm-parasites, particularly those of the Strongyloides and Ancylostoma species that reside in the intestines but may migrate into the tissues. The usual course of treatment is intensive and lasts for 3 days; side-effects are inevitable.
✚ warning: thiabendazole should be administered with caution to patients with impaired kidney or liver function. Treatment should be withdrawn if hypersensitivity reactions occur.
▲ side-effects: there may be nausea, vomiting, diarrhoea and weight loss; dizziness and drowsiness are not uncommon; there may also be headache and itching (pruritus). Possible hypersensitivity reactions include fever with chills, rashes and other skin disorders, and occasionally ringing in the ears (tinnitus) or liver damage.
Related article: MINTEZOL.

thiamine, or aneurin, is the technical name for VITAMIN B_1. Essential in the diet, the vitamin assists in the normal functioning of nerve cells and the heart muscle; it also maintains aspects of the metabolism of carbohydrates. Deficiency leads to the unpleasant disorder beriberi (in which there is either emaciation or bloating, with widescale nerve damage). Good food sources include yeast, grains, nuts, peas and beans, potatoes and pork. Thiamine is a common constituent in many proprietary vitamin B supplements, and may be administered therapeutically to thin children, to pregnant women or to lactating mothers. Administration (often in the form of thiamine hydrochloride) is oral or by injection.
Related articles: ALUZYME; BECOSYM; BENERVA; HEPACON-PLEX; LIPOFLAVONOID; LIPOTRIAD; TONIVITAN B; VIGRANON B; WALLACHOL.

thiazides are effective DIURETICS used mainly to treat the symptoms of heart disease, such as fluid retention in the tissues and high blood pressure (hypertension) or to assist a failing kidney. They work by inhibiting the reabsorption of sodium and chloride ions within

one specific part of the kidney. The result is a moderate diuresis that includes the excretion also of potassium. Potassium supplements are often administered simultaneously, or the thiazide may be combined with another type of diuretic that actively promotes the retention of potassium. Best known and most used thiazides include hydrochlorothiazide and bendrofluazide. Unlike some types of diuretics, the thiazides can be used for prolonged courses of treatment with no residual effects.
see BENDROFLUAZIDE; CHLOROTHIAZIDE; CYCLOPENTHIAZIDE; HYDROCHLOROTHIAZIDE; HYDROFLUMETHIAZIDE; METHYCLOTHIAZIDE; POLYTHIAZIDE.

T

thiethylperazine is an ANTI-EMETIC drug used to relieve nausea and vomiting that may be caused by the vertigo associated with infections of the inner or middle ear, or by therapy with cytotoxic drugs in the treatment of cancer. Administration is oral in the form of tablets, topical as anal suppositories, or by injection.
✚ warning: thiethylperazine should not be administered to patients who are in a coma, or have glaucoma or impaired capacity of the bone-marrow to produce blood cells. It should be administered with caution to those with heart or lung disease, dysfunction of the adrenal glands in the secretion of hormones, epilepsy, parkinsonism, impaired kidney or liver function, undersecretion of thyroid hormones, or enlargement of the prostate gland. Regular ophthalmic checks and monitoring of skin pigmentation are required. Treatment should be withdrawn gradually.
▲ side-effects: there is commonly drowsiness; there may also be dry mouth and dizziness on rising from sitting or lying down (caused by low blood pressure). Some patients, particularly young women, experience muscle spasms.
Related article: TORECAN.

thioguanine is a CYTOTOXIC drug used to assist in the treatment of leukaemia, in which it is often effective in achieving a remission. Administration is oral in the form of tablets.
✚ warning: as with all cytotoxic drugs, thioguanine interferes with the bone-marrow's capacity to provide red blood cells: this may be an added complication to the leukaemia, and certainly tends to cause some loss of immunity to infection. Regular blood counts are essential.
▲ side-effects: gastric upsets with nausea and vomiting are common; there may also be hair loss (even to temporary total baldness).
Related article: LANVIS.

thiopentone sodium is a widely used general ANAESTHETIC used for general anaesthesia during operations. It has no analgesic properties. Because the drug is exceptionally powerful, however, inadvertent overdosage does occur from time to time, causing respiratory depression and depression of the heart rate. Both initial induction of anaesthesia and awakening afterwards are smooth and rapid, although some sedative effects may endure for up to 24 hours. Administration is by injection.
✚ warning: thiopentone sodium should not be given to patients whose respiratory tract is

obstructed, those in severe shock, or those with porphyria (poor porphyrin metabolism). Caution should be taken when administering the drug to patients with severe liver or kidney disease, with metabolic disorders, or who are elderly.

▲ side-effects.there may be respiratory depression, and means for treating respiratory failure should be available. During induction with thiopentone sodium, sneezing, coughing and bronchial spasm may occur.

Related article: INTRAVAL SODIUM.

thioridazine is a powerful ANTIPSYCHOTIC drug used to treat and tranquillize psychosis (such as schizophrenia), in which it is particularly suitable for treating manic forms of behavioural disturbance, especially in order to effect emergency control. The drug may also be used to treat anxiety in the short term and to calm agitated elderly patients. Administration is oral in the form of tablets or a liquid.

✚ warning: thioridazine should not be administered to patients who suffer from a reduction in the bone-marrow's capacity to produce blood cells, or from certain types of glaucoma. It should be administered only with caution to those with heart or vascular disease, kidney or liver disease, parkinsonism, or depression; or who are pregnant or lactating. It is not recommended for children.

▲ side-effects: concentration and speed of thought and movement are affected. Rashes and jaundice may occur; and there may be dry mouth, gastrointestinal disturbance, difficulties in urinating, a reduction in blood pressure, and blurred or discoloured vision.

Related article: MELLERIL.

thiotepa is a CYTOTOXIC drug used mainly to treat tumours in the bladder or malignant effusions in other body cavities. It works by interfering with the DNA of new-forming cells, so preventing normal cell replication. Administration is in the form of instillation in the body cavity, for retention for as long as possible.

✚ warning: prolonged use may cause sterility in men and an early menopause in women; in both sexes it may lead to permanent bone-marrow damage. Prolonged treatment has also been associated with the incidence of leukaemia following simultaneous irradiation treatment. Blood count monitoring is essential. Dosage should be the minimum still to be effective.

▲ side-effects: there is commonly nausea and vomiting; there may also be (temporary) hair loss. The blood-cell-producing capacity of the bone-marrow is impaired.

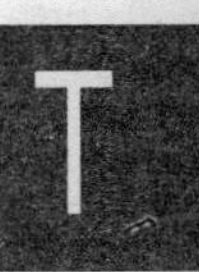

thymol is an aromatic crystalline form of the essential oil of the plant thyme (sometimes in combination with oils of other plants). It is used chiefly as an ANTISEPTIC, and particularly in preparations for oral or dental hygiene.

thymoxamine is a VASODILATOR that principally affects the blood vessels of the limbs, and especially the hands. It is accordingly used to treat circulatory disorders of these areas. In the form of thymoxamine hydrochloride, however, the drug, which is an ALPHA-BLOCKER, is administered in order to restore the pupil of the eye to its normal size following the prior administration of the mydriatic phenylephrine (which is used to dilate the pupil in order to carry out an ophthalmic examination). Administration is thus both systemic in the form of tablets and by injection, and topical in the form of eye-drops.

✚ warning: thymoxamine should be administered with caution to patients with coronary heart disease or diabetes mellitus.

▲ side-effects: administered systemically, the drug may cause nausea, headache and dizziness; there may also be diarrhoea. In the eye, the drug may cause red coloration for a few hours, or temporary drooping of the upper eyelid.

Related article: OPILON.

T

thyroxine sodium is a preparation of one of the natural thyroid HORMONES. It is used therapeutically to make up a hormonal deficiency on a regular maintenance basis, and to treat associated symptoms (myxoedema). It may also be used in the treatment of goitre and of thyroid cancer. Administration is oral in the form of tablets.

✚ warning: thyroxine sodium should not be administered to patients with cardiovascular disease or angina pectoris (heart pain), or impaired secretion by the adrenal glands. It has a delayed action; repeated doses are cumulative in effect.

▲ side-effects: there may be an increase in the heart rate, heartbeat irregularities and angina; some patients experience headache, muscle cramp, flushing, and sweating; there may also be diarrhoea. Dramatic weight loss occurs in some patients.

Related article: ELTROXIN.

Thyrotropar (*Armour*) is a proprietary form of the HORMONE thyroid-stimulating hormone (TSH), available only on prescription. Derived from oxen, it is now used only rarely to stimulate thyroid activity and thus assist in the diagnosis of thyroid disorders. It is produced in the form of powder for reconstitution as a medium for injection.

✚/▲ warning/side-effects: *see* THYROTROPHIN.

thyrotrophin is the chemical name for the natural HORMONE thyroid-stimulating hormone (TSH). Derived from oxen, it is now used only rarely to stimulate thyroid activity and thus assist in the diagnosis of thyroid disorders. This growing unpopularity is because potentially severe allergic side-effects following the administration of thyrotrophin are relatively common, and because other diagnostic tests have become available. However, administration does still take place, by injection.

✚ warning: thyrotrophin should not be administered to patients with coronary thrombosis or insufficient secretion of hormones by the adrenal glands. It should be administered with caution to those with angina pectoris (heart pain), heart failure or insufficient secretion of hormones by the pituitary gland, or who are already taking corticosteroids.

▲ side-effects: there may be nausea and vomiting; the thyroid gland may swell (goitre). Some patients experience temporary low blood pressure (hypotension) or sensitivity reactions (such as urticaria).

Related article: THYROTROPAR.

tiaprofenic acid is a non-steroidal ANTI-INFLAMMATORY non-narcotic ANALGESIC used to treat pain and inflammation in rheumatic disease and other musculo-skeletal disorders. Administration is oral in the form of tablets or an infusion.

✚ warning: tiaprofenic acid should be administered with caution to patients with gastric ulcers, impaired kidney or liver function, or allergic disorders, or who are pregnant.

▲ side-effects: there may be nausea and gastrointestinal disturbance (to avoid which a patient may be advised to take the drug with food or milk), headache and ringing in the ears (tinnitus). Some patients experience sensitivity reactions (such as the symptoms of asthma). Fluid retention and/or blood disorders may occur.
Related article: SURGAM.

Ticar (*Beecham*) is a proprietary ANTIBIOTIC, available only on prescription, used to treat serious infections such as septicaemia and peritonitis, in addition to infections of the respiratory tract or urinary tract. It may also be used to prevent infection in wounds. Produced in the form of a powder for reconstitution as a medium for injection, and in infusion bottles, Ticar is a preparation of the penicillin ticarcillin sodium.

✚/▲ warning/side-effects: *see* TICARCILLIN.

ticarcillin is an ANTIBIOTIC, one of the penicillins, used to treat serious infections such as septicaemia and peritonitis, in addition to infections of the respiratory tract or of the urinary tract. It may also be used to prevent infection in wounds. Administration is by injection or infusion.

✚ warning: ticarcillin should not be administered to patients known to be allergic to penicillins; it should be administered with caution to those with impaired kidney function.

▲ side-effects: there may be sensitivity reactions ranging from a minor rash to urticaria and joint pains, and (occasionally) to high temperature or anaphylactic shock. High doses may in any case cause convulsions.
Related articles: TICAR; TIMENTIN.

Tiempe (*DDSA Pharmaceuticals*) is a proprietary ANTIBACTERIAL, available only on prescription, used primarily to treat infections of the urinary or respiratory tracts, and especially bronchitis. Produced in the form of tablets (in two strengths), it is a preparation of the SULPHONAMIDE-like antibacterial agent trimethoprim.

✚/▲ warning/side-effects: *see* TRIMETHOPRIM.

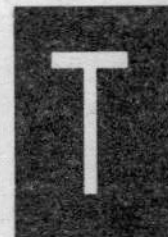

Tigason (*Roche*) is a proprietary preparation of the drug etretinate, available only on prescription, administered orally to treat severe, resistant or complicated psoriasis or certain hereditary disorders that harden and thicken the skin. It is used generally only under specialist supervision in hospitals, and is produced in the form of capsules.

✚/▲ warning/side-effects: *see* ETRETINATE.

Tilade (*Fisons*) is a proprietary preparation of the drug nedocromil sodium, available only on prescription, used to prevent recurrent attacks of asthma. It is not capable of

treating an acute attack, but is particularly effective in forestalling attacks in patients whose asthma corresponds to allergy, and especially when administered before exercise. Dosage should be adjusted to the requirements of each individual patient (and should be administered regularly whether symptoms are present or not). It is produced in the form of an inhalant in an aerosol that emits metered doses, and is not recommended for children.
✚/▲ warning/side-effects: *see* NEDOCROMIL.

Timentin (*Beecham*) is a proprietary ANTIBIOTIC, available only on prescription, used to treat severe infections in patients whose immune systems are undermined by disease or drugs. (Patients with such conditions are generally in hospital.) Produced in the form of a powder for reconstitution as a medium for injection, Timentin is a compound preparation of the catalytic additive CLAVULANIC ACID with the penicillin ticarcillin.
✚/▲ warning/side-effects: *see* TICARCILLIN.

Timodine (*Lloyd-Hamol, Reckitt & Colman*) is a proprietary CORTICOSTEROID cream, available only on prescription, used for topical application on mild skin inflammation, especially where there is a yeast infection (such as candidiasis or thrush). It is a compound preparation that contains the steroid hydrocortisone, the ANTIFUNGAL drug nystatin, the ANTISEPTIC BENZALKONIUM CHLORIDE and the antifoaming agent DIMETHICONE.
✚/▲ warning/side-effects: *see* HYDROCORTISONE; NYSTATIN.

timolol maleate is a BETA-BLOCKER used as an ANTIHYPERTENSIVE to treat high blood pressure or angina pectoris (heart pain), and to prevent recurrent heart attacks or attacks of migraine. Like many other beta-blockers, the drug is also used to reduce the formation of aqueous humour in the eye and so relieve intra-ocular pressure in the treatment of glaucoma. Administration is thus oral in the form of tablets or capsules, and topical in the form of eye-drops.
✚ warning: timolol maleate should not be administered to patients with asthma, bradycardia (slow heartbeat) or partial heart block; it should be administered with caution to those with congestive heart failure, impaired liver or kidney function, who are diabetic, or who are pregnant or lactating. Withdrawal of treatment should be gradual.
▲ side-effects: there may be gastrointestinal disturbances, slow heart rate and cold fingertips and toes, and symptoms much like asthma.
Related articles: BETIM; BLOCADREN; TIMOPTOL.

Timoped (*Reckitt & Colman*) is a proprietary non-prescription cream for topical application to fungal skin infections (such as athlete's foot). Intended to be massaged into the affected area and allowed to dry to a white powder, the cream is a preparation of the ANTIFUNGAL drug TOLNAFTATE with the ANTISEPTIC TRICLOSAN.

Timoptol (*Merck, Sharp & Dohme*) is a proprietary BETA-BLOCKER used in the form of eye-drops to reduce the formation of aqueous humour in the eye and so relieve intra-ocular pressure in the treatment of glaucoma.

Available only on prescription, and produced in its own metered-dosage unit, it is a preparation of timolol maleate.
✚/▲ warning/side-effects: *see* TIMOLOL MALEATE.

Tinaderm-M (*Kirby-Warrick*) is a proprietary non-prescription cream for topical application to fungal infections of the skin and nails. Intended to be applied two or three times a day, the cream is a preparation of the ANTIFUNGAL drugs TOLNAFTATE and nystatin.
✚/▲ warning/side-effects: *see* NYSTATIN.

Tineafax (*Wellcome*) is a proprietary non-prescription ointment for topical application to fungal skin infections (such as athlete's foot). It is a preparation of two ANTIFUNGAL zinc salts. A powdered form containing zinc salt is also available for use as a dusting-powder in a puffer pack, and is intended to prevent fungal skin infection.

tinidazole is a powerful ANTIBACTERIAL compound drug, effective against infection by various types of micro-organism, particularly in the lower intestines and the vagina, but also effective in the treatment of ulcerative gingivitis. Administration is oral in the form of tablets, or by intravenous infusion.
✚ warning: tinidazole should be administered with caution to patients with impaired liver function, or who are pregnant or lactating. On no account should alcohol be consumed during treatment (for even a small amount can cause severe reaction).
▲ side-effects: there may be nausea and vomiting, with gastrointestinal disturbance; drowsiness and headache may occur. Less commonly, there may be a rash, discoloration of the urine, tingling or numbness of the extremities and a reduction in white cells in the blood. High doses in susceptible patients may bring on epilepsy-like seizures.
Related article: FASIGYN.

Tinset (*Janssen*) is a proprietary non-prescription ANTIHISTAMINE used in oral administration to treat allergic conditions such as hay fever and urticaria. Produced in the form of tablets, it is a preparation of the modern antihistamine oxatomide. It is not recommended for children aged under 5 years.
✚/▲ warning/side-effects: *see* OXATOMIDE.

Tisept (*Schering*) is a DISINFECTANT used mainly for surgical procedures in obstetrics or in dressing wounds and burns. Produced in sachets and in bottles, it is a compound solution of the two ANTISEPTICS CHLORHEXIDINE gluconate and CETRIMIDE.

titanium dioxide paste is a non-proprietary formulation that combines the mild astringent titanium dioxide with a number of other mineral salts (including ZINC OXIDE) and water, forming a paste that is effective as a barrier preparation for topical application on the skin. There, it protects not only against infection and dirt, but also against ultraviolet radiation (providing what is known as a sunscreen).

Titralac (*Riker*) is a proprietary non-prescription calcium supplement used to make up body deficiency of the mineral, particularly following kidney failure. It is a preparation of

CALCIUM CARBONATE and is produced in the form of tablets.
✚ warning: Titralac should not be taken by patients already being treated with TETRACYCLINE antibiotics.

Tixylix (*May & Baker*) is a proprietary non-prescription compound cough linctus that is not available from the National Health Service. Produced in the form of a syrup for dilution (the potency of the syrup once dilute is retained for 14 days), Tixylix is a preparation of the OPIATE ANTITUSSIVE pholcodine citrate and the ANTIHISTAMINE promethazine hydrochloride.
✚/▲ warning/side-effects: *see* PHOLCODINE; PROMETHAZINE HYDROCHLORIDE.

T

Tobralex (*Alcon*) is a proprietary preparation of the ANTIBACTERIAL drug tobramycin, available only on prescription, used in the form of eye-drops to treat bacterial infections of the eye.
✚/▲ warning/side-effects: *see* TOBRAMYCIN.

tobramycin is an ANTIBIOTIC, one of the aminoglycosides, effective against many forms of bacteria and against some other micro-organisms. However, it is not absorbed from the intestine (except in the case of local infection or liver failure) and so is administered by injection when treating systemic disease. It is also produced in the form of eye-drops to treat bacterial infections of the eye.
✚ warning: tobramycin should not be administered to patients who are pregnant, or who are already taking drugs that affect the neural system. It should be administered with caution to those with parkinsonism or impaired kidney function. Prolonged or high dosage can cause deafness; regular blood counts are essential in such cases.
▲ side-effects: treatment must be discontinued if there are any signs of deafness. There may be dysfunction of the kidneys.
Related articles: NEBCIN; TOBRALEX.

tocainide hydrochloride is an ANTIARRHYTHMIC drug that is an analogue of the local ANAESTHETIC LIGNOCAINE. Its use, however, is associated with an unacceptably high level of blood disorders, for which reason it is now restricted to life-threatening emergencies in patients who do not respond to other forms of therapy. Administration is oral in the form of tablets, or by injection.
✚ warning: tocainide hydrochloride should not be administered to patients whose natural heart pacemaker (the sino-atrial node) is dysfunctioning, or who are in the process of undergoing a heart attack. It should be administered with extreme caution to patients with severely impaired liver or kidney function or from heart failure, or who are pregnant. Regular and frequent blood counts are essential.
▲ side-effects: there may be nausea, vomiting and gastrointestinal disturbance; tremor, dizziness and loss of sensation are not uncommon, and may lead to convulsions. Injection sometimes results in low blood pressure and slow heart rate.
Related article: TONOCARD.

tocopherol is a general name for a group of substances known collectively as VITAMIN E (and chemically classed as tocopherols and tocotrienols). They have anti-oxidant properties, and are

thought to maintain the structure of cell membranes by preventing the oxidation of their fatty acid constituents. It is also possible that vitamin E has some significance in fertility. Vitamin E deficiency may lead to a form of anaemia through the rupture of red blood cells. Good food sources include eggs, vegetable oils, wheat germ and green vegetables. The form of tocopherol most used in therapy to make up vitamin deficiency is alpha tocopheryl acetate. Administration is oral in the form of tablets or capsules.
Related articles: EPHYNAL; VITA-E.

tocopheryl acetate, or alpha tocopheryl acetate, is one of the forms of tocopherol (VITAMIN E) most used in vitamin replacement therapy.
see TOCOPHEROL.

Tofranil (*Geigy*) is a proprietary ANTIDEPRESSANT drug, available only on prescription, used to treat depressive illness particularly in patients who are withdrawn and apathetic. It may also be used to treat nocturnal bedwetting by children (aged over 7 years). Produced in the form of tablets (in two strengths) and as a syrup for dilution (the potency of the syrup once diluted is retained for 14 days), Tofranil is a preparation of imipramine hydrochloride. Treatment may be prolonged.
✚/▲ warning/side-effects: *see* IMIPRAMINE.

Tolanase (*Upjohn*) is a proprietary form of the SULPHONYLUREA tolazamide, available only on prescription, used to treat adult-onset diabetes mellitus. It works by augmenting what remains of insulin production in the pancreas, and is produced in the form of tablets (in two strengths).
✚/▲ warning/side-effects: *see* TOLAZAMIDE.

tolazamide is a drug used to treat adult-onset diabetes mellitus, one of the SULPHONYLUREAS, which works by augmenting whatever remains of the capacity of the pancreas still to produce insulin (as opposed to compensating for its absence). Administration is oral in the form of tablets.
✚ warning: tolazamide should not be administered to patients with liver or kidney damage, with endocrine disorders, or who are under stress; who are pregnant or lactating; or who are already taking corticosteroids or oral contraceptives, oral anticoagulants, or aspirin or antibiotics.
▲ side-effects: there may be some sensitivity reactions (such as a rash).
Related article: TOLANASE.

tolbutamide is a drug used to treat adult-onset diabetes mellitus, one of the SULPHONYLUREAS, which works by augmenting whatever remains of the capacity of the pancreas still to produce insulin (as opposed to compensating for its absence). Administration is oral in the form of tablets.
✚ warning: tolbutamide should not be administered to patients with liver or kidney damage, with endocrine disorders, or who are under stress; who are pregnant or lactating; or who are already taking corticosteroids or oral contraceptives, oral anticoagulants, or aspirin or antibiotics.
▲ side-effects: there may be some sensitivity reactions (such as a skin rash).

Related articles: GLYCONON; PRAMIDEX; RASTINON.

Tolectin (*Ortho-Cilag*) is a proprietary preparation of the non-steroidal drug tolmetrin which has ANTI-INFLAMMATORY non-narcotic ANALGESIC properties. Available only on prescription, it is used to treat the pain of rheumatic disease and other musculo-skeletal disorders (including bone fusion). It is produced in the form of capsules in two strengths.
✚/▲ warning/side-effects: *see* TOLMETIN.

Tolerzide (*Bristol-Myers*) is a proprietary ANTIHYPERTENSIVE drug, available only on prescription, used to treat mild to moderate high blood pressure (hypertension). Produced in the form of tablets, it is a compound preparation of the BETA-BLOCKER sotalol hydrochloride together with the THIAZIDE DIURETIC hydrochlorothiazide. It is not recommended for children.
✚/▲ warning/side-effects: *see* HYDROCHLOROTHIAZIDE; SOTALOL HYDROCHLORIDE.

tolmetin is a non-steroidal drug with ANTI-INFLAMMATORY and ANALGESIC properties used to treat the pain of rheumatic disease and other musculo-skeletal disorders. Administration is oral in the form of capsules.
✚ warning: tolmetin should be administered with caution to patients with gastric ulcers, impaired kidney or liver function, bleeding disorders, cardio-vascular disease or allergic disorders, or who are pregnant.
▲ side-effects: there may be nausea and gastrointestinal disturbance (to avoid which a patient might be advised to take the drug with food or milk), headache and ringing in the ears (tinnitus). Some patients experience sensitivity reactions (such as the symptoms of asthma). Fluid retention and/or blood disorders may occur.
Related article: TOLECTIN.

tolnaftate is a mild, synthetic, ANTIFUNGAL drug used principally in the topical treatment of infections by the Tinea species known as ringworm (such as athlete's foot). Administration is in the form of a cream, a powder or a solution. Rarely, sensitivity reactions occur.
Related article: TIMOPED; TINADERM-N.

tolu linctus is a non-proprietary formulation that is a cough linctus for children. Its various constituents (including citric acid and GLYCEROL) are mixed in with a syrup derived from tolu balsam (itself obtained from the bark of the South American tolu tree) which has very mild ANTISEPTIC and EXPECTORANT action.

Tonivitan (*Medo*) is a proprietary multivitamin supplement, available on prescription only to private patients, used to treat overall VITAMIN deficiency. Produced in the form of capsules, it contains RETINOL (vitamin A), THIAMINE (vitamin B_1), NICOTINIC ACID (of the B complex), ASCORBIC ACID (vitamin C), CALCIFEROL (vitamin D) and a dried preparation of yeast.

Tonivitan A & D (*Medo*) is a proprietary non-prescription VITAMIN-and-mineral compound that is not available from the National Health Service. Used as a general tonic, and produced in the form of a syrup, it contains RETINOL (vitamin A), CALCIFEROL (vitamin D), IRON, CALCIUM, manganese, phosphorus, and copper.

Tonivitan B (*Medo*) is a proprietary non-prescription VITAMIN-and-mineral compound that is not available from the National Health Service. Used as a general tonic, and produced in the form of a syrup, it contains THIAMINE (vitamin B_1), RIBOFLAVINE (vitamin B_2), PYRIDOXINE (vitamin B_6), NICOTINAMIDE (of the B complex), calcium, manganese and phosphorus.

Tonocard (*Astra*) is a proprietary form of the ANTI-ARRHYTHMIC drug tocainide hydrochloride, available only on prescription. Its use, however, is associated with an unacceptably high level of blood disorders, for which reason it is now restricted to life-threatening emergencies immediately following a heart attack in patients who do not respond to other forms of therapy. It is produced in the form of tablets (in two strengths) and in vials for injection.
✚/▲ warning/side-effects: *see* TOCAINIDE HYDROCHLORIDE.

Topal (*Concept*) is a proprietary non-prescription ANTACID used to treat heartburn, severe indigestion, and the symptoms of hiatus hernia. Produced in the form of tablets for chewing between meals and at bedtime, Topal is a compound preparation that includes ALUMINIUM HYDROXIDE and MAGNESIUM CARBONATE.

Topiclens (*Smith & Nephew*) is a proprietary non-prescription preparation of mild saline solution (0.9%) that can be used either as an eye-wash or eye lubricant, or as a cleansing lotion for minor wounds and burns.
see SODIUM CHLORIDE.

Topicycline (*Norwich Eaton*) is a proprietary ANTIBIOTIC, available only on prescription, used to treat acne. Produced in the form of a solution for topical application, it is a preparation of the TETRACYCLINE tetracycline hydrochloride, and is not recommended for children.
✚/▲ warning/side-effects: *see* TETRACYCLINE.

Topilar (*Syntex*) is a proprietary CORTICOSTEROID cream, available only on prescription, used in topical application to treat serious non-infective skin inflammation (such as psoriasis and certain forms of dermatitis). Produced as a water-miscible cream and an ointment for dilution with paraffin (the potency of the ointment once diluted is retained for 14 days), Topilar is a preparation of fluclorolone acetonide.
✚/▲ warning/side-effects: *see* FLUCLOROLONE ACETONIDE.

Torecan (*Sandoz*) is a proprietary ANTI-EMETIC drug, available only on prescription, used to relieve nausea and vomiting that may be caused by the vertigo associated with infections of the middle or inner ear, or by therapy with cytotoxic drugs in the treatment of cancer. Produced in the form of tablets, as anal suppositories, and in ampoules for injection, Torecan is a preparation of thiethylperazine.
✚/▲ warning/side-effects: *see* THIETHYLPERAZINE.

Tracrium (*Calmic*) is a proprietary SKELETAL MUSCLE RELAXANT, available only on prescription, used mainly under general anaesthesia during surgery. Produced in ampoules for injection, Tracrium is a preparation of atracurium besylate.

✚ warning: *see* ATRACURIUM BESYLATE.

Tramil (*Whitehall Laboratories*) is a proprietary non-prescription compound ANALGESIC containing the active constituents paracetamol and caffeine.
✚/▲ warning/side-effects: *see* CAFFEINE; PARACETAMOL.

Trancopal (*Winthrop*) is a proprietary ANXIOLYTIC drug that also has the properties of a SKELETAL MUSCLE RELAXANT. Available only on prescription, it is used principally in the short-term treatment of insomnia, and produced in the form of tablets containing the TRANQUILLIZER chlormezanone. It is not recommended for children.
✚/▲ warning/side-effects: *see* CHLORMEZANONE.

Trancoprin (*Winthrop*) is a proprietary compound ANALGESIC and MUSCLE RELAXANT, available on prescription only to private patients. It is used to treat headache and the pain of menstruation problems, and also to relieve the pain of muscle spasm. Produced in the form of tablets, Trancoprin is a preparation of aspirin together with the ANXIOLYTIC muscle relaxant chlormezanone.
✚/▲ warning/side-effects: *see* ASPIRIN; CHLORMEZANONE.

Trandate (*Duncan, Flockhart*) is a proprietary ANTIHYPERTENSIVE drug, available only on prescription, used to treat all forms of high blood pressure (including those caused by heart disease, by pregnancy or by surgery). Produced in the form of tablets (in four strengths), and in ampoules for injection, Trandate is a preparation of the BETA-BLOCKER labetalol hydrochloride.
✚/▲ warning/side-effects: *see* LABETALOL HYDROCHLORIDE.

tranexamic acid is a HAEMOSTATIC drug used to stem the flow of blood in such circumstances as dental extraction in a haemophiliac patient, or following surgical removal of the prostate gland, or continual menstrual flow (menorrhagia). It works by inhibiting the action of one of the blood's natural anticoagulant factors. Administration is oral in the form of tablets or a dilute syrup, or by injection.
✚ warning: tranexamic acid should not be administered to patients who are known to have any form of thrombosis; it should be administered with caution to those with impaired kidney function or severe urinary disorders. Prolonged treatment requires regular ophthalmic checks and monitoring of liver function.
▲ side-effects: there may be nausea and vomiting, with diarrhoea; injection may cause temporary giddiness.
Related article: CYKLOKAPRON.

***tranquillizers** are drugs that calm and soothe, and relieve anxiety. Many also cause some degree of sedation. They are often classified in two groups, major tranquillizers and minor. The major tranquillizers are used primarily to treat severe mental disorders – the psychoses (including schizophrenia and mania) – not only to relieve patients of their own private fears and terrors, but also to control violent behavioural disturbances that present a danger to the patients themselves and to those who look after them. The minor tranquillizers may also be used to treat mental disorders, such as neuroses, but are more commonly used in short-term therapies to treat anxiety and nervous tension.

Best known and most used major tranquillizers include the PHENOTHIAZINES (such as CHLORPROMAZINE, THIORIDAZINE and PROCHLORPERAZINE) and such drugs as HALOPERIDOL, FLUSPIRILENE and FLUPENTHIXOL. Best known and most used minor tranquillizers include the BENZODIAZEPINES (such as DIAZEPAM and CHLORDIAZEPOXIDE) and such drugs as MEPROBAMATE. Prolonged treatment with some minor tranquillizers can lead to dependence (addiction).

Transiderm-Nitro (*Ciba*) is a proprietary VASODILATOR, available only on prescription, used to prevent recurrent attacks of angina pectoris (heart pain). Produced in the form of dressings to be applied to the chest wall so that the drug is slowly absorbed through the skin, and presented in packs of 5 or 10 dressings, Transiderm-Nitro is a preparation of glyceryl trinitrate.
✚/▲ warning/side-effects: *see* GLYCERYL TRINITRATE.

Translet (*Franklin*) is a proprietary non-prescription perfumed barrier cream for use in protecting, freshening and sanitizing the area of skin around a stoma (an outlet on the skin surface following the surgical curtailment of the intestines).

Translet Plus (*Franklin*) is a proprietary non-prescription deodorant for use in the appliance (bag) attached to a stoma (an outlet on the skin surface following the surgical curtailment of the intestines). There are two versions: Translet Plus One is intended for men; Translet Plus Two for women.

Transvasin (*Lloyds*) is a proprietary non-prescription cream for topical application which, when applied to the skin, produces an irritation of the sensory nerve endings that offsets the pain of underlying muscle or joint disorders (counter-irritant). Active constituents include the local anaesthetic BENZOCAINE and salts of NICOTINIC ACID and SALICYLIC ACID.

Tranxene (*Boehringer Ingelheim*) is a proprietary ANXIOLYTIC drug, available only on prescription, used principally in the short-term treatment of anxiety. Produced in the form of capsules (in two strengths), it is a preparation of the TRANQUILLIZER clorazepate dipotassium. It is not recommended for children.
✚/▲ warning/side-effects: *see* CLORAZEPATE DIPOTASSIUM.

tranylcypromine is an ANTIDEPRESSANT drug, an MAO INHIBITOR that also has some stimulant effect and is therefore less used than most in the treatment of depressive illness. Administration is oral in the form of tablets.
✚ warning: tranylcypromine should not be administered to patients with heart or liver disease, circulatory disorders, abnormal secretion of hormones by the adrenal glands, epilepsy, or overactivity of the thyroid gland (hyperthyroidism), or who are children. It should be administered with caution to those who are elderly or debilitated. Treatment requires a strict dietary regime (that includes the avoidance of meat or yeast extracts, cheese, and alcohol) and the avoidance also of virtually all other forms of medication. Withdrawal of treatment must be gradual.
▲ side-effects: concentration and

speed of thought and movement are usually affected; there may also be dizziness, especially when rising from sitting or lying down (because of low blood pressure), and insomnia, muscular weakness and dry mouth. Some patients experience headache, which implies that treatment should be withdrawn.
Related article: PARNATE.

Trasicor (*Ciba*) is a proprietary ANTIHYPERTENSIVE drug, available only on prescription, used to treat high blood pressure, heartbeat irregularities, angina pectoris (heart pain), and the effects of an excess of thyroid hormones in the bloodstream (thyrotoxicosis). Produced in the form of tablets, and in ampoules for injection, Trasicor is a preparation of the BETA-BLOCKER oxprenolol hydrochloride.
✚/▲ warning/side-effects: *see* OXPRENOLOL.

Trasidrex (*Ciba*) is a proprietary compound ANTIHYPERTENSIVE drug, available only on prescription, used to treat high blood pressure, heartbeat irregularities, angina pectoris (heart pain), and an excess of thyroid hormones in the bloodstream (thyrotoxicosis). Produced in the form of sustained-release tablets, Trasidrex is a preparation of the BETA-BLOCKER oxprenolol hydrochloride with the THIAZIDE DIURETIC cyclopenthiazide.
✚/▲ warning/side-effects: *see* CYCLOPENTHIAZIDE; OXPRENOLOL.

Trasylol (*Bayer*) is a proprietary preparation of the enzyme aprotinin, available only on prescription, used in the treatment of acute inflammation of the pancreas, or to prevent such inflammation following abdominal surgery. It is produced in ampoules for injection.
▲ side-effects: *see* APROTININ.

Travamulsion (*Travenol*) is a proprietary nutritional supplement for administration via intravenous infusion in patients for whom feeding via the alimentary tract is not possible. It is a compound emulsion of protein in the form of soya bean oil with glycerol and a phosphate extract from egg, and is produced in two strengths (under the names Travamulsion 10% and Travamulsion 20%).

Travasept (*Travenol*) is a proprietary non-prescription DISINFECTANT for use in cleaning wounds and burns. Produced in sachets of solution (not for further dilution), Travasept is a compound preparation of the antiseptics CETRIMIDE and CHLORHEXIDINE acetate (in two strengths, under the trade names Travasept 30 and Travasept 100).

Travogyn (*Schering*) is a proprietary ANTIFUNGAL drug, available only on prescription, used in the treatment of fungal or fungal-and-bacterial infections of the vagina or the ano-genital area. Produced in the form of a cream for topical application, and as vaginal tablets (pessaries), it is a preparation of isoconazole nitrate.
▲ side-effects: *see* ISOCONAZOLE.

trazodone hydrochloride is an ANTIDEPRESSANT drug used to treat depressive illness, particularly in cases where some degree of sedation is called for. Administration is oral in the form of capsules or a liquid.
✚ warning: trazodone hydrochloride should be administered with caution to

patients who have serious heart complaints or have recently had a heart attack, or to those who have manic episodes. It should be administered with caution to those with epilepsy, diabetes, impaired liver function, heartbeat irregularities, thyroid disorders, glaucoma, or urinary retention; who are pregnant; or who are mentally unstable. Withdrawal of treatment should be gradual.

▲ side-effects: concentration and speed of thought and movement may be affected. There may be an increased or decreased heart rate, sweating and tremor; constipation and difficulty in urinating; blurred vision and drowsiness; and weight changes, weakness and vomiting.

Related article: MOLIPAXIN.

Tremonil (*Sandoz*) is a proprietary drug used to treat the tremor of parkinsonism, of drug-induced states, or simply of old age (*see* ANTIPARKINSONISM). Available only on prescription, and produced in the form of tablets, it is a preparation of methixene hydrochloride.

✚/▲ warning/side-effects: *see* METHIXENE HYDROCHLORIDE.

Trental (*Hoechst*) is a proprietary VASODILATOR that principally affects the blood vessels of the limbs and is used to treat circulatory disorders of the hands and feet. Available only on prescription, and produced in the form of tablets and in ampoules for injection, Trental is a preparation of oxpentifylline.

✚/▲ warning/side-effects: *see* OXPENTIFYLLINE.

treosulfan is a CYTOTOXIC drug used specifically in the treatment of cancer of the ovary. It works by interfering with the DNA of new-forming cells, so preventing normal cell replication. Administration is oral in the form of capsules, or by injection. (The identically named proprietary form of the drug is manufactured by Leo.)

✚ warning: prolonged use may cause sterility in men and an early menopause in women; in both sexes it may lead to permanent bone-marrow damage. Prolonged treatment has also been associated with the incidence of leukaemia following simultaneous irradiation treatment. Blood count monitoring is essential. Dosage should be the minimum still to be effective.

▲ side-effects: there is commonly nausea and vomiting; there may also be (temporary) hair loss. The blood-cell-producing capacity of the bone-marrow is impaired.

tretinoin is a derivative of RETINOL (vitamin A) that is used mostly in topical application to treat acne. Rather astringent, it tends to cause a redness of the skin following several days' treatment. Administration is in the form of a cream, gel or lotion.

✚ warning: tretinoin should not be applied to broken skin or to conditions such as eczema. It should be kept away from the eyes, mouth and mucous membranes, and should not be used in combination with other peeling agents (keratolytics) or with sun-ray lamps.

▲ side-effects: there may be irritation. Prolonged treatment brings out first a redness, and may then go on to change pigmentation in the skin. Rarely, there is sensitivity to light.

Related article: RETIN-A.

TRH (*Roche*) is a proprietary preparation of the natural HORMONE thyrotrophin-releasing hormone (TRH, or protirelin) used primarily in diagnosing thryoid function in patients who suffer from overactivity of the thyroid gland (hyperthyroidism). It is produced in the form of tablets and in ampoules for injection.
✚/▲ warning/side-effects: *see* PROTIRELIN.

Tri-Adcortyl (*Squibb*) is a proprietary preparation for topical application in the treatment of severe non-infective skin inflammation (such as eczema), especially in cases that have not responded to less powerful therapies. Available only on prescription, and produced in the form of a cream and an ointment, it is a compound of the CORTICOSTEROID triamcinolone acetonide together with the ANTIFUNGAL drug nystatin, and the ANTIBIOTICS GRAMICIDIN and NEOMYCIN. A form of the ointment prepared especially for the topical treatment of infection of the outer ear is also available (under the name Tri-Adcortyl Otic).
✚/▲ warning/side-effects: *see* NYSTATIN; TRIAMCINOLONE ACETONIDE.

triamcinolone is a synthetic CORTICOSTEROID used to suppress the symptoms of inflammation, especially when caused by allergic disorders. It is administered in the form of tablets, or by injection, to relieve such conditions as hay fever or asthma.
✚ warning: triamcinolone should not be administered to patients who suffer from psoriasis; it should be administered with caution to the elderly (in whom overdosage can cause osteoporosis, "brittle bones"). In children, administration may lead to stunting of growth. Prolonged use may cause muscular weakness. As with all corticosteroids, triamcinolone treats only inflammatory symptoms; an undetected and potentially serious infection may have its effects masked by the drug until it is well established.
▲ side-effects: treatment of susceptible patients may engender a euphoria – or a state of confusion or depression. Rarely, there is peptic ulcer.
Related article: LEDERCORT.

triamcinolone acetonide is a synthetic CORTICOSTEROID used to suppress the symptoms of inflammation, especially when caused by allergic disorders. It is administered sometimes as a systemic medication (in the form of an injection) to relieve such conditions as hay fever or asthma but, more commonly, is instead applied by local injection to treat skin inflammations or such conditions as rheumatoid arthritis and bursitis. Several proprietary preparations are in the form of a cream for topical application, mostly in the treatment of severe non-infective skin inflammations such as eczema, but one or two are for treating inflammations in the mouth.
✚ warning: triamcinolone acetonide should not be administered to patients with psoriasis; it should be administered with caution to the elderly (in whom overdosage can cause osteoporosis, "brittle bones"). In children, systemic administration may lead to stunting of growth. Prolonged

use may cause muscular weakness, and in any case should be avoided. As with all corticosteroids, triamcinolone acetonide treats only inflammatory symptoms; an undetected and potentially serious infection may have its effects masked by the drug until it is well established.

▲ side-effects: systemic treatment of susceptible patients may engender a euphoria – or a state of confusion or depression. Rarely, there is peptic ulcer.
Related articles: ADCORTYL; AUDICORT; AUREOCORT; KENALOG; LEDERCORT; NYSTADERMAL; SILDERM; TRI-ADCORTYL.

triamcinolone hexacetonide is a synthetic CORTICOSTEROID used to suppress the symptoms of inflammation. It is administered by local injection to treat skin inflammation or such conditions as rheumatoid arthritis and bursitis.

✚ warning: triamcinolone hexacetonide should not be administered to patients with psoriasis; it should be administered with caution to the elderly (in whom overdosage can cause osteoporosis, "brittle bones"). In children, administration may lead to stunting of growth. Prolonged use may cause muscular weakness, and in any case should be avoided. As with all corticosteroids, triamcinolone hexacetonide treats only inflammatory symptoms; an undetected and potentially serious infection may have its effects masked by the drug until it is well established.

▲ side-effects: systemic treatment of susceptible patients may engender a euphoria – or a state of confusion or depression. Rarely, there is peptic ulcer.
Related article: LEDERSPAN.

Triamco (*Norton*) is a proprietary compound DIURETIC, available only on prescription, used for general diuresis. Produced in the form of tablets, it is a combination of the THIAZIDE diuretic hydrochlorothiazide together with a complementary potassium-sparing diuretic triamterene.

✚/▲ warning/side-effects: *see* HYDROCHLOROTHIAZIDE; TRIAMTERENE.

triamterene is a DIURETIC that does not deplete the body's reserves of potassium; although it is sometimes used by itself in the treatment of fluid retention in the tissues (oedema), it is therefore more commonly used in combination with diuretics that do promote the excretion of potassium, particularly the THIAZIDES. Singly, administration is oral in the form of capsules.

✚ warning: triamterene should not be administered to patients with kidney failure or high levels of potassium in the blood; it should be administered with caution to those with diabetes or cirrhosis of the liver, or who are pregnant. Regular monitoring of blood levels of urea and potassium is essential.

▲ side-effects: there may be gastrointestinal disturbance and dry mouth; some patients come out in a rash. The urine may be discoloured (and even fluorescent).
Related articles: DYAZIDE; DYTAC; DYTIDE; FRUSENE; KALSPARE; TRIAMCO.

triazolam is a short-acting

HYPNOTIC drug, a derivative of the BENZODIAZEPINES, used as a TRANQUILLIZER to treat insomnia (particularly in the elderly). Administration is oral in the form of tablets.

✚ warning: triazolam should be administered with caution to patients with lung disease or depressed breathing, or who are pregnant or lactating. Susceptible patients may experience psychological changes.

▲ side-effects: concentration and speed of thought and movement are affected. There may also be drowsiness, dry mouth, and dizziness. Prolonged use may eventually result in tolerance, and finally dependence.
Related article: HALCION.

T

Tribiotic (*Riker*) is a proprietary ANTIBIOTIC, available only on prescription, used as a spray in topical application to infections of the skin. Produced in aerosol units, it is a compound preparation of three antibiotics: NEOMYCIN sulphate, POLYMYXIN B sulphate and bacitracin zinc.

trichloroethylene is an inhalant general ANAESTHETIC with powerful ANALGESIC properties used primarily in combination with nitrous oxide-oxygen mixtures, but it also has rather poor MUSCLE RELAXANT properties. It is normally administered only after anaesthesia has been initially induced with some other agent.

✚ warning: trichloroethylene is not suitable for induction of anaesthesia; moreover, administration of the drug should be discontinued some time before the end of surgery because the recovery rate from the drug afterwards is comparatively slow.

▲ side-effects: side-effects are rare (in fact the drug helps stabilize several body functions, such as blood pressure). But the respiratory rate may increase, and post-operative vomiting is not uncommon. It may decrease the function of the liver and kidneys.
Related article: TRILENE.

triclofos sodium is a derivative of the soluble SEDATIVE chloral, used as a HYPNOTIC to treat insomnia. Administration is oral in the form of an elixir: the liquid is less irritant to the stomach lining than chloral hydrate.

✚ warning: triclofos sodium should not be administered to patients with severe heart disease, or severe impairment of kidney or liver function. It should be administered with caution to those with lung disease, particularly if there is depressed breathing, who are elderly or debilitated, or who are pregnant or lactating. The consumption of alcohol enhances the hypnotic effect of the drug. Withdrawal of treatment should be gradual. Prolonged use may lead to tolerance and dependence (addiction).

▲ side-effects: concentration and speed of thought and movement are affected. There is commonly drowsiness, dry mouth and gastric irritation; there may also be sensitivity reactions (such as a rash) and, in the elderly, a mild state of confusion.

triclosan is a mildly ANTIBIOTIC DISINFECTANT for topical application to the skin. It is sometimes used to treat staphylococcal infection, but it is primarily used to prevent the spread of infection within hospitals or households. It should be kept away from the eyes. *Related articles:* ATLAS DERMALEX; MANUSEPT; STER-ZAC; TIMOPED.

tricyclic drugs are one of the two main classes of ANTIDEPRESSANT, and often have SEDATIVE and TRANQUILLIZER effects. Chemically, they are dibenzazipine or debenzocycloheptone derivatives. Examples include AMYTRIPTYLINE and LOFEPRAMINE.

Tridesilon (*Lagap*) is a proprietary CORTICOSTEROID preparation, available only on prescription, used in topical application to treat severe non-infective skin inflammation (such as eczema), especially when therapy with less powerful corticosteroids has failed. Produced in the form of a water-miscible cream and a paraffin-based ointment, Tridesilon's major active constituent is the steroid desonide.

✚/▲ warning/side-effects: *see* DESONIDE.

Tridil (*American Hospital Supply*) is a proprietary VASODILATOR, available only on prescription, used to treat angina pectoris (heart pain) or to prevent recurrent attacks. Produced in ampoules for injection, or in polyethylene infusion sets, Tridil is a preparation of the NITRATE glyceryl trinitrate.

✚/▲ warning/side-effects: *see* GLYCERYL TRINITRATE.

trientine dihydrochloride is an unusual drug used in the treatment of the rare congenital defect in metabolism that causes a potentially dangerous accumulation of copper in the body (Wilson's disease). Ordinarily this defect is readily remedied through the use of PENICILLAMINE – but some patients are unable to tolerate that drug, and so trientine dihydrochloride is then used instead. Administration is oral in the form of capsules.

✚ warning: trientine dihydrochloride should be administered with caution to patients who are pregnant.

▲ side-effects: there may be nausea. Skin conditions that arise as a sensitivity reaction to initial treatment with penicillamine may require independent treatment to resolve them.

trifluoperazine is a powerful ANTIPSYCHOTIC drug used to treat and tranquillize psychosis (such as schizophrenia), in which it is particularly suitable for treating forms of behavioural disturbance. The drug may additionally be used to treat severe anxiety in the short term. In low dosages the drug is also sometimes used as an ANTI-EMETIC in the treatment of nausea and vomiting caused by underlying disease or by drug therapies. Administration is oral in the form of tablets, capsules, sustained-release capsules, and a liquid, or by injection.

✚ warning: trifluoperazine should not be administered to patients who suffer from reduction in the bone-marrow's capacity to produce blood cells, or from certain types of glaucoma. It should be administered only with caution to those with heart or vascular disease, kidney or liver disease, or parkinsonism; or who are pregnant or lactating; or who are children.

▲ side-effects: concentration and speed of thought and movement are affected. There may be restlessness, insomnia

T

and nightmares; rashes and jaundice may occur; and there may be dry mouth, slight gastrointestinal disturbance, and blurred vision. Some patients experience muscle weakness.
Related article: STELAZINE.

trifluperidol is a powerful ANTIPSYCHOTIC drug used to treat and tranquillize psychosis (such as schizophrenia), in which it is particularly suitable for treating forms of manic behavioural disturbance. Administration is oral in the form of tablets.

✚ warning: trifluperidol should not be administered to patients who suffer from reduction in the bone-marrow's capacity to produce blood cells, or from certain types of glaucoma. It should be administered only with caution to those with heart or vascular disease, kidney or liver disease, or parkinsonism; or who are pregnant or lactating.

▲ side-effects: concentration and speed of thought and movement are affected. There may be restlessness, insomnia and nightmares; rashes and jaundice may occur; and there may be dry mouth, gastrointestinal disturbance, difficulty in urinating, and blurred vision. Some patients experience muscle weakness or spasm. Rarely, there is weight loss.
Related article: TRIPERIDOL.

Trifyba (*Labaz*) is a proprietary non-prescription LAXATIVE that is not available from the National Health Service. A bulking agent – which works by increasing the overall mass of faeces within the rectum, so stimulating bowel movement – Trifyba is produced in the form of sachets of powder for mixing with food and liquids, and consists of wheat fibre (BRAN).

triiodothyronine is a natural thyroid HORMONE, administered therapuetically in the form of liothyronine sodium to make up a hormonal deficiency (hypothyroidism) and to treat associated symptoms (myxoedema). It may also be used in the treatment of goitre and of thyroid cancer.
see LIOTHYRONINE SODIUM.

Trilene (*ICI*) is a proprietary preparation of the inhalant general ANAESTHETIC trichlorethylase, which has good ANALGESIC properties and weak MUSCLE RELAXANT actions. It is used in combination with other anaesthetics to provide general anaesthesia, and is produced in the form of a liquid in a gas canister, for administration through a vaporizer.

✚/▲ warning/side-effects: *see* TRICHLOROETHYLENE.

Trilisate (*Napp*) is a proprietary non-prescription non-narcotic ANALGESIC used to treat pain and inflammation in rheumatic disease and other musculo-skeletal disorders. Produced in the form of tablets, it is a compound preparation of the natural body substance choline and SALICYLIC ACID.

✚/▲ warning/side-effects: *see* CHOLINE MAGNESIUM TRISALICYLATE.

trilostane is an unusual drug that inhibits the production of corticosteroids by the adrenal glands. It is thus used to treat conditions that result from the excessive secretion of corticosteroids into the bloodstream (such as Cushing's syndrome). Administration is oral in the form of capsules.

T

✚ warning: trilostane should not be administered to patients who are pregnant or who are using hormonal contraceptive methods; it should be administered with caution to those with impaired liver or kidney function. Monitoring of blood levels of corticosteroids and electrolytes is essential.
▲ side-effects: side-effects are rare, but following high dosage may include nausea, flushing and a running nose.
Related article: MODRENAL.

Triludan (*Merrell*) is a proprietary non-prescription ANTIHISTAMINE used to treat the symptoms of allergic disorders such as hay fever and urticaria. Produced in the form of tablets and as a suspension for dilution (the potency of the suspension once dilute is retained for 14 days), it is a preparation of terfenadine.
✚/▲ warning/side-effects: *see* TERFENADINE.

trimeprazine tartrate is an ANTIHISTAMINE that has additional SEDATIVE properties. It is used to treat the symptoms of allergic disorders (particularly rashes and itching), as a premedication prior to surgery, and sometimes even as an ANTI-EMETIC.
Administration is oral in the form of tablets or as a dilute syrup.
✚ warning: trimeprazine tartrate should be administered with caution to patients with epilepsy, glaucoma, liver disease or enlargement of the prostate gland. During treatment, alcohol consumption must be avoided.
▲ side-effects: there may be headache, drowsiness and dry mouth. Some patients experience sensitivity reactions on the skin.
Related article: VALLERGAN.

trimetaphan camsylate is a drug that reduces blood pressure (technically, it is a hypotensive drug with a ganglion-blocking action that reduces sympathetic vascular tone). Short-acting, it is used primarily during neurosurgery and vascular surgery. The advantage of its use is that, once the patient's individual response to the drug has been gauged, its hypotensive effect is highly controllable. Administration is by injection.
✚ warning: trimetaphan camsylate should be administered with caution to patients with heart disease or severe arteriosclerosis; it should be administered with caution to those with diabetes, Addison's disease, or any degenerative disease of the brain, or whose liver or kidney function is impaired.
▲ side-effects: there is an increase in the heart rate, and depression of respiration; the pupils of the eyes are dilated.
Related article: ARFONAD.

trimethoprim is an ANTIMICROBIAL agent similar in action to the sulphonamides, used to treat and to prevent the spread of many forms of bacterial infection but particularly those of the urinary and respiratory tracts. It is peculiarly effective in combination with a sulphonamide drug, for the combined effect is greater than twice the individual effect of either partner. This is the basis of the medicinal compound co-trimoxazole (which forms the active constituent of many proprietary preparations). Administration of trimethoprim is oral in the form of tablets or a dilute suspension, or by injection.

✚ warning: trimethoprim should not be administered to newborn babies, or to patients who are pregnant, or who have severely impaired kidney function. Dosage should be reduced for patients with poor kidney function. Prolonged therapy requires frequent blood counts.

▲ side-effects: there may be nausea, vomiting and gastrointestinal disturbances; rashes may break out, with itching (pruritus).

Related articles: IPRAL; MONOTRIM; SYRAPRIM; TIEMPE; TRIMOGAL; TRIMOPAN.

see also CO-TRIMOXAZOLE.

trimipramine is an ANTIDEPRESSANT drug used to treat depressive illness, especially in cases where sedation is advantageous to the patient. Administration of trimipramine is oral in the form of capsules or tablets.

✚ warning: trimipramine should not be administered to patients with heart disease or psychosis; it should be administered with caution to those with epilepsy, diabetes, liver or thyroid disease, glaucoma, or urinary retention, or who are pregnant or lactating. Withdrawal of treatment must be gradual.

▲ side-effects: concentration and speed of thought and movement are commonly affected; there may also be dry mouth and blurred vision, difficulty in urinating, a rash, sweating, and irregular heartbeat. Some patients experience a behavioural disturbance, a state of confusion, and/or a loss of libido. Rarely, there are also blood disorders or tingling in the hands and feet.

Related article: SURMONTIL.

Trimogal (*Lagap*) is a proprietary ANTIMICROBIAL, available only on prescription, used to treat and to prevent the spread of many forms of bacterial infection but particularly those of the urinary and respiratory tracts. Produced in the form of tablets (in two strengths), it is a preparation of the SULPHONAMIDE-like drug trimethoprim.

✚/▲ warning/side-effects: *see* TRIMETHOPRIM.

Trimopan (*Berk*) is a proprietary ANTIMICROBIAL agent, available only on prescription, used to treat and to prevent the spread of many forms of bacterial infection but particularly those of the urinary and respiratory tracts. Produced in the form of tablets (in two strengths), and as a sugar-free suspension for dilution (the potency of the suspension once dilute is retained for 14 days), it is a preparation of the SULPHONAMIDE-like drug trimethoprim.

✚/▲ warning/side-effects: *see* TRIMETHOPRIM.

Trimovate (*Glaxo*) is a proprietary CORTICOSTEROID and ANTIBIOTIC preparation, available only on prescription, used in topical application to treat severe skin inflammation, especially when therapy with less powerful corticosteroids has failed. Produced in the form of a water-miscible cream and a paraffin-based ointment, Trimovate's major active constituents are the steroid clobetasone butyrate, the ANTIFUNGAL drug nystatin, and the TETRACYCLINE antibiotic chlortetracycline hydrochloride.

✚/▲ warning/side-effects: *see* CHLORTETRACYCLINE; CLOBETASONE BUTYRATE; NYSTATIN.

TriNordiol (*Wyeth*) is a

proprietary ORAL CONTRACEPTIVE, available only on prescription, that combines the OESTROGEN ethinyloestradiol with the PROGESTOGEN levonorgestrel. It is produced in a packet of 63 tablets, made in three differing ratios of the two constituents, corresponding to three complete menstrual cycles of 21 days plus 7 days without.

✚/▲ warning/side-effects: *see* ETHINYLOESTRADIOL; LEVONORGESTREL.

Tri-Novum (*Ortho-Cilag*) is a proprietary ORAL CONTRACEPTIVE, available only on prescription, that combines the OESTROGEN ethinyloestradiol with the PROGESTOGEN norethisterone. It is produced in a packet of 63 tablets, made in three differing ratios of the two constituents, corresponding to three complete menstrual cycles of 21 days plus 7 days without.

✚/▲ warning/side-effects: *see* ETHINYLOESTRADIOL; NORETHISTERONE.

Triogesic (*Beecham*) is a proprietary non-prescription nasal DECONGESTANT that is not available from the National Health Service. Unlike many decongestants, however, it is produced in the form of tablets and as a sugar-free elixir for dilution (the potency of the elixir once dilute is retained for 14 days). Both forms are preparations of the non-narcotic ANALGESIC paracetamol in combination with the SYMPATHOMIMETIC phenylpropanolamine hydrochloride.

✚/▲ warning/side-effects: *see* PARACETAMOL; PHENYLPROPANOLAMINE HYDROCHLORIDE.

Triominic (*Beecham*) is a proprietary non-prescription nasal DECONGESTANT that is not available from the National Health Service. Unlike many decongestants, however, it is produced in the form of tablets and as a sugar-free syrup for dilution (the potency of the syrup once dilute is retained for 14 days). Both forms are preparations of the ANTIHISTAMINE pheniramine maleate in combination with the SYMPATHOMIMETIC phenylpropanolamine hydrochloride.

✚/▲ warning/side-effects: *see* PHENIRAMINE MALEATE; PHENYLPROPANOLAMINE HYDROCHLORIDE.

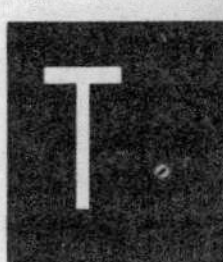

Triosorbon (*Merck*) is a proprietary non-prescription dietary supplement for patients who are severely undernourished (as with anorexia nervosa) or who have serious problems with the internal absorption of food (as following gastrectomy). It consists of a gluten-, sucrose- and galactose-free, lactose-low powder that contains protein, carbohydrates, fats, vitamins and minerals. It is not suitable for children aged under 5 years.

Triperidol (*Lagap*) is a proprietary ANTIPSYCHOTIC drug, available only on prescription, used to treat and tranquillize psychosis (such as schizophrenia), in which it is particularly suitable for treating forms of manic behavioural disturbance. Produced in the form of tablets (in two strengths), Triperidol is a preparation of trifluperidol.

✚/▲ warning/side-effects: *see* TRIFLUPERIDOL.

Triplopen (*Glaxo*) is a proprietary ANTIBIOTIC used in the treatment or prevention of many forms of bacterial infection. Produced in the form of powder for reconstitution as a medium for injection, it is a compound preparation of three penicillin-type antibiotics: benzylpenicillin sodium, procaine penicillin and benethamine penicillin.

✚/▲ warning/side-effects: *see* BENETHAMINE PENICILLIN; BENZYLPENICILLIN; PROCAINE PENICILLIN.

tripotassium dicitrato-bismuthate is a drug which assists in the healing of gastric and duodenal ulcers. It is thought to work by creating a protective coating over the ulcer under which healing can take place. Administration is oral in the form of tablets or an elixir – food and drink should be avoided for some time before and after treatment.
Related articles: DE-NOL; DE-NOLTAB.

T

triprolidine is an ANTIHISTAMINE used to treat the symptoms of allergic disorders such as hay fever and urticaria. A long-acting drug, its effect may last for more than 12 hours. Administration (in the form of triprolidine hydrochloride) is oral as tablets, sustained-release tablets, and a dilute elixir.

✚ warning: triprolidine should be administered with caution to patients with epilepsy, glaucoma, liver disease or enlargement of the prostate gland. During treatment, alcohol consumption must be avoided.

▲ side-effects: there may be headache, drowsiness and dry mouth. Some patients experience sensitivity reactions on the skin.
Related articles: ACTIDIL; PRO-ACTIDIL.

Triptafen (*Allen & Hanburys*) is a proprietary compound ANTIDEPRESSANT, available only on prescription, used to treat depressive illness particularly in cases in which there is also anxiety. Produced in the form of tablets (in two strengths, the weaker under the name Triptafen-M), it is a combination of amitriptyline hydrochloride with the PHENOTHIAZINE perphenazine. It is not recommended for children.

✚/▲ warning/side-effects: *see* AMITRIPTYLINE; PERPHENAZINE.

Trisequens (*Novo*) is a proprietary hormonal supplement, available only on prescription, used in HORMONE replacement therapy for women during and following the menopause. It contains both the OESTROGENS oestradiol and oestriol, together with the PROGESTOGEN norethisterone acetate, and is produced in a calendar pack of 28 tablets corresponding to one complete menstrual cycle.

✚/▲ warning/side-effects: *see* NORETHISTERONE; OESTRADIOL; OESTRIOL.

trisodium edetate is a CHELATING AGENT that absorbs calcium. It is thus used primarily to treat conditions in which there is excessive calcium in the bloodstream (hypercalcaemia), but may also be used in the form of eye-drops (in dilute solution) to treat calcification of the cornea or lime burns of the eyeball. In the case of hypercalcaemia, administration is in the form of slow intravenous infusion.

✚ warning: trisodium edetate should not be administered to patients with impaired kidney function; it should be administered with caution to those who suffer from tuberculosis. Regular blood counts to check calcium levels are essential during treatment.

▲ side-effects: administration by slow intravenous infusion may cause pain in the limb in which the infusion is given. There may be nausea, diarrhoea and cramps. Overdosage may lead to kidney damage.
Related article: LIMCLAIR.

Tritamyl (*Procea*) is the name of a brand of gluten-free starch-based self-raising flour with which bread (and other delicacies) can be made for patients who cannot tolerate dietary gluten (as with coeliac disease and other amino acid deficiencies). A low-protein version is also available (under the name Tritamyl PK).

Trivax (*Wellcome*) is a proprietary preparation of the triple vaccine diphtheria-pertussis-tetanus (DPT) vaccine, consisting of a combination of the toxoids (antibodies produced in response to the toxins) of the diphtheria and tetanus bacteria with pertussis vaccine. It is produced in ampoules for injection.
see DIPHTHERIA-PERTUSSIS-TETANUS (DPT) VACCINE.

Trivax-AD (*Wellcome*) is a proprietary preparation of the triple vaccine diphtheria-pertussis-tetanus (DPT) vaccine, consisting of a combination of the toxoids (antibodies produced in response to the toxins) of the diphtheria and tetanus bacteria with pertussis vaccine, all adsorbed on to a mineral carrier (in the form of aluminium hydroxide). It is produced in ampoules for injection.
see DIPHTHERIA-PERTUSSIS-TETANUS (DPT) VACCINE.

Trobicin (*Upjohn*) is a proprietary ANTIBIOTIC, available only on prescription, used specifically in the treatment of the sexually transmitted disease gonorrhoea in patients who are allergic to penicillins, or in cases resistant to penicillins. Produced in the form of a powder for reconstitution as a medium for injection, it is a preparation of spectinomycin.

✚/▲ warning/side-effects: *see* SPECTINOMYCIN.

tropicamide is a short-acting ANTICHOLINERGIC drug used (in mild solution) to dilate the pupil of the eye for ophthalmic examination. Administration is in the form of eye-drops.

✚ warning: tropicamide should not be administered to patients with certain forms of glaucoma, or who are known to have soft lenses.

▲ side-effects: vision is blurred or otherwise disturbed. Overdosage may lead to increased heart rate and to behavioural changes in susceptible patients.
Related articles: MINIMS; MYDRIACYL.

Tropium (*DDSA Pharmaceuticals*) is a proprietary ANXIOLYTIC drug, available on prescription only to private patients, used to treat anxiety or to assist in the treatment of acute alcohol withdrawal symptoms. Produced in the form of capsules (in two strengths) and tablets (in three strengths), Tropium is a preparation of the BENZODIAZEPINE chlordiazepoxide.

✚/▲ warning/side-effects: *see* CHLORDIAZEPOXIDE.

Trufree (*Cantassium*) is a proprietary brand of gluten-free flours which are used in baking for patients who cannot tolerate gluten (as in the case of coeliac disease and other amino acid deficiency conditions).

trypsin is an enzyme secreted by the pancreas in the process of digestion. It may be administered therapeutically either to assist digestion locally, or – more commonly – to treat inflammation, bruising or swelling of the soft tissues. In this it is supposed to work by removing coagulated blood and cellular debris. Administration is usually by injection.

✚ warning: trypsin should not be administered to a patient who is already taking anticoagulant drugs.

▲ side-effects: there may be nausea and vomiting, with diarrhoea. Rarely, there are sensitivity reactions.

T

Tryptizol (*Morson*) is a proprietary ANTIDEPRESSANT drug, available only on prescription, used in the treatment of depressive illness and especially in cases where its additional SEDATIVE properties may be advantageous to the patients or to those that care for them. However, the drug is additionally used to prevent bedwetting at night in youngsters. Produced in the form of tablets (in three strengths), as sustained-release capsules, as a sugar-free liquid for dilution (the potency of the liquid once dilute is retained for 14 days), and in vials for injection, Tryptizol is a preparation of amitryptiline hydrochloride.

✚/▲ warning/side-effects: *see* AMITRYPTILINE.

tryptophan is an amino acid present in an ordinary diet, from which the natural body substance serotonin is derived. Serotonin is much like histamine in its role in inflammation, but even more importantly, deficiency of serotonin (specifically in the brain) is thought to contribute to depression. Therapeutic administration of tryptophan, singly or in combination with ANTIDEPRESSANT drugs, is therefore aimed mainly at treating depressive illness. The response to treatment with tryptophan by itself is slow, taking at least 4 weeks for genuine improvement to occur. Administration is oral in the form of tablets or in solution.

✚ warning: tryptophan should not be administered to patients known to have defective metabolism of tryptophan in the diet, or who have disease of the bladder.

▲ side-effects: concentration and speed of thought and movement may initially be affected; with drowsiness, there may also be nausea and/or a headache.
Related articles: OPTIMAX; PACITRON.

TSH, or thyroid-stimulating hormone, is also known as thyrotrophin.
see THYROTROPHIN.

Tubarine Miscible (*Calmic*) is a proprietary preparation of the SKELETAL MUSCLE RELAXANT tubocurarine chloride, used under general anaesthesia for medium- or long-duration paralysis. Available only on prescription, it is produced in ampoules for injection.

✚/▲ warning/side-effects: *see* TUBOCURARINE.

tubocurarine is a SKELETAL MUSCLE RELAXANT used primarily (in the form of tubocurarine chloride) under general anaesthesia for medium- or long-duration paralysis. It is the paralytic factor in the well-known South American poison curare. Apart from its use in surgical operations, the drug may also be used occasionally to treat the spasm associated with tetanus or with some mental disorders. Administration is ordinarily by injection.

✚ warning: following injection, a rash may appear on the chest and neck, due to the release of histamine. Onset of the paralysis may be accompanied by hypotension.

▲ side-effects: effects begin some 3 to 5 minutes after injection, and last for about 30 minutes. *Related articles:* JEXIN; TUBARINE MISCIBLE.

tub/vac/BCG, dried, is an abbreviation for the freeze-dried version of BCG VACCINE (against tuberculosis).
see BCG VACCINE.

tub/vac/BCG, perc, is an abbreviation for the live version of BCG vaccine (against tuberculosis) for percutaneous administration by multiple puncture with a suitable instrument.
see BCG VACCINE.

Tuinal (*Lilly*) is a proprietary HYPNOTIC, a BARBITURATE on the controlled drugs list, and used to treat intractable insomnia. Produced in the form of capsules, it is a preparation of amylobarbitone sodium. It is not recommended for children.

✚/▲ warning/side-effects: *see* AMYLOBARBITONE.

Tums (*Beecham Health Care*) are proprietary non-prescription ANTACID tablets containing calcium carbonate.

✚/▲ warning/side-effects: *see* CALCIUM CARBONATE.

Tunes (*Mars*) are proprietary non-prescription sweets formulated for the relief of cold symptoms. Tunes contain GLUCOSE syrup, citric acid, MENTHOL, balsam of tolu, camphor and thyme.

turpentine liniment is a non-proprietary formulation of turpentine oil, camphor and soap all in solution, for gentle massage into the skin as a topical treatment for underlying muscular or rheumatic pain. It stimulates the sensory nerve endings in the skin and so offsets the underlying ache (as a COUNTER-IRRITANT).

Two's Company (*Family Planning Sales*) is a proprietary non-prescription SPERMICIDAL preparation for use in combination with one of the barrier methods of contraception (such as a condom). Produced in the form of vaginal inserts (pessaries), Two's Company's active constituent is an alcohol ester.

tyloxapol is a MUCOLYTIC drug, used via a nebuliser to reduce the viscosity of sputum and thus facilitate expectoration (coughing up sputum) mostly in conditions such as asthma and bronchitis. It is now used rather seldom, although there are no contra-indications and side-effects are rare (constituted by the occasional high temperature).

typhoid vaccine is a suspension of dead typhoid bacteria, administered by deep subcutaneous or intramuscular injection. Full protection is, however, not guaranteed, and travellers at risk are advised not to eat prepared but uncooked food or to drink untreated water. Dosage is normally repeated after 4 to 6 weeks – unless reactions have been severe. Some reaction is to be expected: swelling, pain and tenderness occur after a couple of hours, followed by high temperature and malaise, possibly with a headache.

typhus vaccine is not normally available in the United Kingdom, although there are small stocks that can be used if necessary. It consists of inactivated Rickettsia organisms grown in the yolk-sacs of hens' eggs. The organisms are carried by body lice, but hygienic conditions in any part of the world, even where the disease is endemic, are usually enough for protection.

Tyrozets (*Merck, Sharp & Dohme*) is a proprietary non-prescription brand of ANTISEPTIC lozenges used to sanitize and relieve pain in the mouth and throat. They contain the local ANAESTHETIC benzocaine together with the ANTIBACTERIAL compound tyrothricin.

✚/▲ warning/side-effects: *see* BENZOCAINE.

T

Ubretid (*Berk*) is a proprietary preparation used mainly to stimulate bladder or intestinal activity; it may also form part of treatment for serious skeletal muscular disease. Available only on prescription, Ubretid is produced in the form of tablets or ampules for injection, and contains distigmine bromide.
✚/▲ warning/side-effects: *see* DISTIGMINE BROMIDE.

Ukidan (*Serono*) is a proprietary FIBRINOLYTIC drug available only on prescription, containing urokinase. Produced as a powder for reconstitution, it is used in intravenous infusions to treat various forms of thrombosis.
✚/▲ warning/side-effects: *see* UROKINASE.

Ultrabase (*Schering*) is a proprietary water-miscible cream used as a skin emollient (softener and soother) and as a medium for various other skin preparations. Available without prescription, it contains liquid paraffin, stearyl alcohol and white soft paraffin.

Ultradil Plain (*Schering*) is a proprietary CORTICOSTEROID preparation, available only on prescription, in the form of either a water-miscible cream or a more oily ointment. Its active constituents are fluocortolone hexanoate and fluocortolone pivalate, which are effective in treating inflammatory skin conditions such as eczema and psoriasis. In made-up dilute form, either version retains its potency for 14 days.
✚/▲ warning/side-effects: *see* FLUOCORTOLONE.

Ultralanum Plain (*Schering*) is a proprietary CORTICOSTEROID preparation, available only on prescription, in the form of either a water-miscible cream or a more oily ointment. Its active constituents are fluocortolone hexanoate and fluocortolone pivalate at higher concentrations than present in ULTRADIL PLAIN. Ultralanum is also used to treat inflammatory skin conditions, and in made-up dilute form also retains its potency for 14 days.
✚/▲ warning/side-effects: *see* FLUOCORTOLONE.

Ultraproct (*Schering*) is a proprietary CORTICOSTEROID-ANTIHISTAMINE compound with local ANAESTHETIC properties. Available only on prescription, it is made up of fluocortolone hexanoate and fluocortolone pivalate, with the local anaesthetic cinchocaine and the antihistamine chemizole undeconate. Produced in the form of ointment and anal suppositories, Ultraproct is prescribed to treat piles (haemorrhoids), anal fissure and infection of the anal region.
✚ warning: ultraproct is not suitable as treatment for children or for women during pregnancy. Prolonged use should be avoided.
▲ side-effects: *see* FLUOCORTOLONE.

Ultratard, MC (*Novo*) is a proprietary preparation of insulin zinc suspension, available in ampoules for injection by diabetics according to individual requirements.
✚/▲ warning/side-effects: *see* INSULIN.

Unguentum Merck (*Merck*) is a proprietary, non-prescription skin emollient (softener and soother) and barrier ointment, also used as a medium for other skin preparations. Because it contains similar proportions of fats and water it is particularly stable; its principal constituent is white soft paraffin. One of the safest of all ointments, its complex formula includes no known allergen.

Uniflu Plus Gregovite C (*Unigreg*) is a proprietary combination of two drugs issued as separate tablets to be taken simultaneously to treat the symptoms of colds and influenza. Uniflu is an ANTITUSSIVE and ANTIHISTAMINE that also has some ANALGESIC properties. Because Uniflu contains the OPIATE codeine, however, the combination is not available on a National Health Service prescription; other principal constituents of Uniflu include paracetamol and caffeine. Gregovite C is a form of ASCORBIC ACID (vitamin C).
✚/▲ warning/side-effects: *see* CAFFEINE; CODEINE PHOSPHATE; PARACETAMOL.

Unigesic (*Unimed*) is a proprietary compound ANALGESIC, not available on a National Health Service prescription, that principally consists of a mixture of paracetamol and caffeine.
✚/▲ warning/side-effects: *see* CAFFEINE; PARACETAMOL.

Unigest (*Unigreg*) is a proprietary ANTACID, not available on a National Health Service prescription, that principally consists of aluminium hydroxide (its active ingredient) and dimethicone (an antifoaming agent).
✚/▲ warning/side-effects: *see* ALUMINIUM HYDROXIDE.

Unihep (*Leo*) is a proprietary preparation of the ANTICOAGULANT heparin sodium in a mode suitable for injection. Available only on prescription, Unihep is used to treat various forms of thrombosis.
✚/▲ warning/side-effects: *see* HEPARIN.

Unimycin (*Unigreg*) is a proprietary ANTIBIOTIC, available only on prescription, containing oxytetracycline hydrochloride; it is administered in the form of capsules, and is effective against a wide range of infections and infestations.
✚/▲ warning/side-effects: *see* OXYTETRACYCLINE.

Uniparin (*CP Pharmaceuticals*) is a proprietary preparation of the ANTICOAGULANT heparin sodium in a mode suitable for subcutaneous injection. Available only on prescription, Uniparin is used to treat various forms of thrombosis.
✚/▲ warning/side-effects: *see* HEPARIN.

Uniparin Calcium (*CP Pharmaceuticals*) is a proprietary preparation of the ANTICOAGULANT heparin calcium in a mode suitable for subcutaneous injection. Available only on prescription, Uniparin Calcium is used to treat various forms of thrombosis.
✚/▲ warning/side-effects: *see* HEPARIN.

Uniphyllin Continus (*Napp*) is a proprietary, non-prescription BRONCHODILATOR consisting of tablets containing theophylline. It is used to treat respiratory difficulties caused by bronchial infection, asthma and emphysema, and by cardiac deficiency. There is a half-strength children's version – Uniphyllin Paediatric Continus – although even this is not advised for children aged under 12 months.
✚/▲ warning/side-effects: *see* THEOPHYLLINE.

Uniroid (*Unigreg*) is a proprietary steroid compound, available only on prescription, which has

ANTIBIOTIC and local ANAESTHETIC properties. Produced as both ointment and anal suppositories, its main constituents are cinchocaine hydrochloride, hydrocortisone, neomycin sulphate and polymyxin B sulphate. Uniroid is prescribed to treat piles (haemorrhoids), anal fissure and inflammation of the anal region.
✚ warning: uniroid is unsuitable as treatment for children or for women during pregnancy. Prolonged use should be avoided.
▲ side-effects: *see* CINCHOCAINE; HYDROCORTISONE; NEOMYCIN; POLYMIXIN B.

Unisept (*Schering*) is a proprietary, non-prescription DISINFECTANT and wound cleanser that is available in sachets: each sachet contains chlorhexidine gluconate in very dilute solution.
✚/▲ warning/side-effects: *see* CHLORHEXIDINE.

Unisomnia (*Unigreg*) is a proprietary form of the BENZODIAZEPINE nitrazepam. A powerful and long-acting HYPNOTIC produced in the form of tablets, Unisomnia is available only by prescription for private patients.
✚/▲ warning/side-effects: *see* NITRAZEPAM.

Urantoin (*DDSA Pharmaceuticals*) is a proprietary form of the antimicrobial drug nitrofurantoin, used specifically to treat infections of the urinary tract. Produced as tablets, Urantoin is available only on prescription.
✚/▲ warning/side-effects: *see* NITROFURANTOIN.

Ureaphil (*Abbott*) is a proprietary, powdered form of the DIURETIC body-substance urea. Available only on prescription, it is used in solution for intravenous infusion in cases of cerebral oedema (accumulation of fluid in the brain) or to test renal function.
✚ warning: urea should not be administered to patients with cerebral haemorrhage, kidney or liver failure, or any wound or injury that might cause the spread of body fluids from vessels into the tissues, or to those who are dehydrated.

Uriben (*RP Drugs*) is a proprietary ANTIBACTERIAL agent, available only on prescription, in the form of a syrupy suspension of nalidixic acid. Used in solution to treat gastrointestinal infections and infections of the urinary tract, once made up its potency is retained for 14 days.
✚/▲ warning/side-effects: *see* NALIDIXIC ACID.

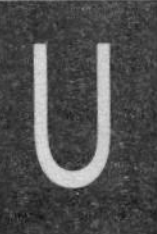

Urisal (*Winthrop*) is a proprietary preparation, available only on prescription, in the form of sachets of soluble granules of sodium citrate. In solution, the granules treat cystitis and other relatively mild infections of the urinary tract.
✚/▲ warning/side-effects: *see* SODIUM CITRATE.

Urispas (*Syntex*) is a proprietary ANTIPASMODIC, available only on prescription, consisting of tablets containing flavoxate hydrochloride. Urispas is used to treat urinary incontinence and associated difficulties (dysuria).
✚/▲ warning/side-effects: *see* FLAVOXATE HYDROCHLORIDE.

Urizide (*DDSA Pharmaceuticals*) is a proprietary DIURETIC, available only on prescription, consisting of tablets containing bendrofluazide. Urizide is prescribed to treat the accumulation of fluid in the

tissues (oedema) or high blood pressure (hypertension).
✚/▲ warning/side-effects: *see* BENDROFLUAZIDE.

urofollitrophin is a form of follicle-stimulating hormone (FSH) found in, and processed from, human menopausal urine. *see* FSH.
Related article: METRODIN.

urokinase is a FIBRINOLYTIC found in, and processed from, human male urine. It is valuable in the treatment of thrombosis, and particularly of blood clots in the eye; administration is by infusion in a medium of saline solution.
✚ warning: urokinase should not be administered to patients who have recently suffered haemorrhage (as for example during surgery), or to pregnant women. If for any reason bleeding occurs, further treatment to stem the flow will be required.
▲ side-effects: there may be fever, haemorrhage, and allergic reactions.
Related article: UKIDAN.

U

Uromide (*Consolidated*) is a proprietary SULPHONAMIDE, available only on prescription, in the form of tablets containing sulphaurea and phenazopyridine hydrochloride. Uromide is used to treat infections of the urinary tract, and apart from its ANTIBACTERIAL properties also has soothing and alkalinizing effects.
✚/▲ warning/side-effects: *see* PHENAZOPYRIDINE; SULPHAUREA.

Uromitexan (*Boehringer Ingelheim*) is a proprietary form of the drug MESNA, used to combat the toxicity of CYTOTOXIC drugs by reacting with their metabolites in the urinary tract. Available only on prescription, Uromitexan is produced as ampoules for injection.

Uro-Tainer (*CliniMed*) is the proprietary name for a selection of solutions designed to wash and maintain a latex or silicone catheter replacing or assisting part of the urinary tract. Solutions – available without prescription in the form of sachets – include CHLORHEXIDINE 0.02%; saline [sodium chloride] 0.9%; mandelic acid 1%; and some proprietary compounds.

ursodeoxycholic acid is a drug taken orally to dissolve small, light, cholesterol gallstones. X-ray monitoring of treatment is also required to supervise progress. The course may last up to two years, and treatment must be continued for at least three months after stones have been dissolved.
✚ warning: ursodeoxycholic acid is not suitable for patients with larger, radio-opaque gallstones; nor for those who suffer from chronic liver disease, intestinal inflammation or an inoperative gall bladder; nor for pregnant women.
▲ side-effects: there may be pruritus (itching) and minor dysfunctioning of the liver. Diarrhoea is rare.
Related articles: DESTOLIT; URSOFALK.

Ursofalk (*Thames*) is a proprietary form of the drug ursodeoxycholic acid, available only on prescription, in the form of capsules.
✚/▲ warning/side-effects: *see* URSODEOXYCHOLIC ACID.

Uticillin (*Beecham*) is a proprietary ANTIBACTERIAL drug, available only on prescription, in the form of tablets containing

carfecillin sodium. The tablets are prescribed to treat infections of the urinary tract.
✚/▲ warning/side-effects: *see* CARFECILLIN SODIUM.

Utovlan (*Syntex*) is a proprietary PROGESTOGEN (ovulation-suppressing sex HORMONE), available only on prescription, in the form of tablets containing norethisterone. It is used to treat uterine bleeding, abnormally heavy menstruation, and other menstrual problems, and may additionally be used as an effective contraceptive preparation.
✚/▲ warning/side-effects: *see* NORETHISTERONE.

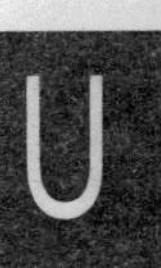

***vaccines** confer active immunity against specific diseases: that is, they cause a patient's own body to create a defence (in the form of antibodies against the disease). Most are administered in the form of a suspension of dead viruses (as in flu vaccine) or bacteria (as in typhoid vaccine), or of live but attenuated viruses (as in rubella vaccine) or bacteria (as in BCG vaccine against tuberculosis). A third type is a suspension containing extracts of the toxins emitted by the invading organism that also cause the formation of antibodies (as in tetanus vaccine). Vaccines that incorporate dead micro-organisms generally require a series of administrations (most often three) to build up a sufficient supply in the body of antibodies; booster shots may thereafter be necessary at regular intervals to reinforce immunity. Vaccines that incorporate live micro-organisms may confer immunity with a single dose, because the organisms multiply within the body, although some vaccines still require 3 administrations (as in oral poliomyelitis vaccine).
✚ warning: vaccination should not be administered to patients who have a febrile illness or any form of infection. Vaccines containing live material should not be administered routinely to patients who are pregnant, or who are known to have an immunodeficiency disorder.
▲ side-effects: side-effects range from little or no reaction to severe discomfort, high temperature and pain.

Vaginyl (*DDSA Pharmaceuticals*) is a proprietary preparation with ANTIPROTOZOAL and ANTIBACTERIAL actions, available only on prescription, in the form of tablets containing the antimicrobial drug metronidazole. It is prescribed to treat bacterial infections of the intestines (causing dysentery) and of the vagina.
✚/▲ warning/side-effects: *see* METRONIDAZOLE.

Valium (*Roche*) is a proprietary form of the powerful BENZODIAZEPINE diazepam, useful both as an AXIOLYTIC or minor TRANQUILLIZER and also as a SKELETAL MUSCLE RELAXANT. Available only on prescription, it is produced as anal suppositories and in ampoules for injection (available on National Health Service prescription), and as capsules, tablets and syrup (available only to private patients). It is prescribed mainly to treat anxiety.
✚/▲ warning/side-effects: *see* DIAZEPAM.

Vallergan (*May & Baker*) is a proprietary ANTIHISTAMINE, available only on prescription, consisting of trimeprazine tartrate in the form either of tablets or of syrup for dilution (the syrup once diluted retains potency for 14 days). Vallergan is prescribed to treat various types of allergic reaction, particularly those which include itching skin. It has SEDATIVE effects as with most antihistamines.
✚/▲ warning/side-effects: *see* TRIMEPRAZINE TARTRATE.

Valoid (*Calmic*) is a proprietary form of ANTIHISTAMINE prescribed to treat vomiting, motion sickness and loss of the sense of balance (labyrinthitis). It comes in two forms: tablets, containing cyclizine hydrochloride and available without prescription; and ampoules for injection, containing cyclizine lactate and available only on prescription.

✚/▲ warning/side-effects: *see* ANTIHISTAMINE; CYCLIZINE.

Vamin (*KabiVitrum*) is the name of a selection of proprietary infusion fluids for the intravenous nutrition of a patient in whom feeding via the alimentary tract is not possible. All contain amino acids and provide energy, some in the form of glucose, others in the form of various electrolytes.

Vancocin (*Lilly*) is the name of a selection of proprietary forms of the ANTIBACTERIAL ANTIBIOTIC vancomycin hydrochloride. Available only on prescription, there are capsules (produced under the name Matrigel) and powdered forms for use in solution orally and as injections.
✚/▲ warning/side-effects: *see* VANCOMYCIN.

vancomycin is an ANTIBACTERIAL ANTIBIOTIC most commonly administered orally to treat certain forms of colitis, but also used in intravenous infusion to treat endocarditis and other serious infections. Because incautious use may have deleterious effects on the organs of the ear, on the kidney, and on the tissues at the site of injection, blood counts and tests on liver and kidney functions are necessary during treatment.
✚ warning: vancomycin should not be administered to patients with impaired kidney function or who are deaf; or to patients in whom there is a risk of the escape of body fluids from the vessels into the tissues.
▲ side-effects: infusion may cause high body temperature and a rash; incautious use may lead to ringing in the ears (tinnitus) and even to kidney disease.
Related article: VANCOCIN.

Vansil is a proprietary form of the ANTHELMINTIC drug OXAMNIQUINE, used specifically as an oral treatment for intestinal schistosomiasis (bilharziasis).

Variclene (*Dermal*) is a proprietary non-prescription ANTISEPTIC gel used to cleanse and soothe skin ulcers. Within an aqueous base its active constituents include lactic acid.

Varidase (*Lederle*) is a proprietary ANTISEPTIC, available only on prescription, in the form of a powdered enzymatic compound of streptokinase and streptodornase. Prescribed as treatment to cleanse and soothe skin ulcers, the combination of enzymes also helps to slough off surrounding lesioned skin.
✚/▲ warning/side-effects: *see* STREPTOKINASE.

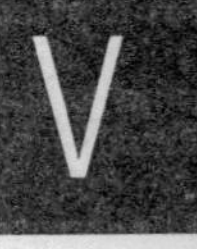

Varihesive (*Squibb*) is a proprietary non-prescription dressing compound for use in treating leg ulcers. Constituents are CARMELLOSE SODIUM, GELATIN, pectin and polyisobutylene.

var/vac is an abbreviation for variola vaccine.
see SMALLPOX VACCINE.

Vascardin (*Nicholas*) is a proprietary VASODILATOR used in treatment for angina pectoris (heart pain) and for cardiac arrhythmia, and is available without prescription. It consists of tablets containing isosorbide dinitrate (two strengths are available), and should not be used by patients who have high blood pressure, those who are undergoing other drug treatments, or by children.
✚/▲ warning/side-effects: *see* ISOSORBIDE DINITRATE.

Vasculit (*Boehringer Ingelheim*) is

a proprietary form of the VASODILATOR bamethan sulphate, used to treat circulation problems in the extremities and the attendant neural effects. Available without prescription, Vasculit is produced in the form of tablets.

✚/▲ warning/side-effects: *see* BAMETHAN SULPHATE.

Vasocon A (*CooperVision*) is a proprietary form of ANTIHISTAMINE eye-drops, available only on prescription, used to treat acute allergic conjunctivitis. Its active constituents are antazoline phosphate and naphazoline hydrochloride.

✚/▲ warning/side-effects: *see* ANTAZOLINE.

V

***vasoconstrictors** cause a narrowing of the blood vessels, and thus a reduction in the rate of blood flow and an increase in blood pressure. They are used to increase blood pressure in circulatory disorders, in cases of shock, or in cases where pressure has fallen during lengthy or complex surgery. Different vasoconstrictors work in different ways: vasoconstrictors that have a marked or local effect on mucous membranes, for example, may be used to relieve nasal congestion. Some are used to prolong the effects of local anaesthetics. Best known and most used vasoconstrictors include PHENYLEPHRINE, XYLOMETAZOLINE and METHOXAMINE.

***vasodilators** cause a widening of the blood vessels, causing changes in blood flow and a reduction in blood pressure. They are used to reduce blood pressure mainly in the treatment of heart failure or angina pectoris (heart pain), to improve the circulation in the brain or in the limbs, or simply to treat high blood pressure (hypertension). Different vasodilators work in different ways: short-acting nitrates, for example, work by both expanding the blood vessels of the heart and reducing the flow of blood back to the heart in the veins; in order to prolong the effect, some nitrates are administered in the form of tablets to be held under the tongue, or in the form of an aerosol spray for repeated doses. Best known and most used vasodilators include GLYCERYL TRINITRATE, ISOSORBIDE DINITRATE, DIAZOXIDE, NIFEDIPINE, CINNARIZINE, THYMOXAMINE and CO-DERGACRINE.

Vasogen (*Pharmax*) is a proprietary non-prescription barrier cream, used to soothe and dress nappy rash, bedsores, and rashes in excretory areas. Active constituents are CALAMINE, DIMETHICONE and ZINC OXIDE.

vasopressin is a natural body HORMONE secreted by the posterior lobe of the pituitary gland; it is known also as antidiuretic hormone, or ADH. In therapy, vasopressin – a VASOCONSTRICTOR – is used mostly to treat pituitary-originated diabetes insipidus. There are two main forms: DESMOPRESSIN and LYPRESSIN; TERLIPRESSIN is another derivative. Preparations include nose-drops, nasal spray, injections and solutions for infusion. Treatment must not be prolonged, and should be carefully and regularly monitored to avoid overdosage.

✚ warning: doses should be adjusted to individual response, to balance water levels in the body. Treatment with vasopressin is not advisable for patients with asthma, epilepsy or migraine, and should not be administered to patients with chronic kidney disease or disease of the blood vessels.

▲ side-effects: potential side-effects include hypersensitivity reactions, constriction of coronary arteries (possibly leading to angina pectoris), nausea, cramps and an overpowering urge to defecate. *Related article:* PITRESSIN.

Vasoxine (*Calmic*) is a proprietary SYMPATHOMIMETIC VASOCONSTRICTOR, available only on prescription, most often used to raise blood pressure in a patient under general anaesthesia. It is a preparation of methoxamine hydrochloride in ampoules for injection.

✚/▲ warning/side-effects: *see* METHOXAMINE HYDROCHLORIDE.

V-Cil-K (*Lilly*) is a proprietary preparation of the penicillin-type ANTIBIOTIC phenoxymethylpenicillin, used mainly to treat infections of the head and throat, and some skin conditions; it is also used to reduce high body temperature. Available only on prescription, it is produced in the form of capsules, tablets (in two strengths), a syrup for dilution, and a children's syrup (in two strengths) for dilution (the potency of the diluted syrups is retained for 7 days).

✚/▲ warning/side-effects: *see* PHENOXYMETHYLPENICILLIN.

vecuronium bromide is a relatively recently derived SKELETAL MUSCLE RELAXANT, of the type known as non-depolarizing or competitive. Administration is by injection, commonly under general anaesthetic during surgery.

✚ warning: patients treated with vecuronium bromide must have their respiration controlled and monitored until the drug has been inactivated or antagonized. The effect of repeated large doses is cumulative. *Related article:* NORCURON.

Veganin (*Warner*) is a proprietary non-prescription compound ANALGESIC that is not available from the National Health Service, consisting of tablets that contain aspirin, codeine phosphate and paracetamol.

✚/▲ warning/side-effects: *see* ASPIRIN; CODEINE PHOSPHATE; PARACETAMOL.

Veil (*Blake*) is a proprietary (non-prescription) series of camouflage creams in eleven shades designed for use in masking scars and other skin disfigurements. They may be obtained on prescription if the skin disfigurement is the result of surgery or is giving rise to emotional disturbance in the patient.

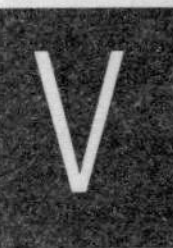

Velbe (*Lilly*) is a proprietary form of the CYTOTOXIC drug vinblastine sulphate, produced in the form of the powdered sulphate together with an ampoule of diluent. Available only on prescription, Velbe is used to treat cancer particularly lymphomas, Hodgkin's disease, and some neoplasms.

✚/▲ warning/side-effects: *see* VINBLASTINE SULPHATE.

Velosef (*Squibb*) is a proprietary form of the CEPHALOSPORIN ANTIBIOTIC cephradine, available only on prescription, as capsules (in two strengths), a syrup (for dilution) or a powdered form for use in solution as injections. The potency of the syrup once diluted is retained for 7 days.

✚/▲ warning/side-effects: *see* CEPHRADINE.

Velosulin (*Nordisk Wellcome*) is a proprietary form of insulin, derived from pigs and highly purified, for use in treating and maintaining diabetic patients. It is produced in the form of ampoules for injection.
✚/▲ warning/side-effects: *see* INSULIN.
Related article: HUMAN VELOSULIN.

Venos (*Beecham Health Care*) is a proprietary non-prescription cough mixture produced in the form of an ANTITUSSIVE formula and as an EXPECTORANT. The active constituents of the antitussive is the cough suppressant noscapine, and the expectorant contains guaiphensin, aniseed oil, capiscum and camphor.
✚/▲ warning/side-effects: *see* NOSCAPINE.

Ventide (*Allen & Hanburys*) is a proprietary CORTICOSTEROID compound, available only on prescription, used to treat the symptoms of asthma and chronic bronchitis. It is produced in the form of an aerosol inhalant containing the steroid beclomethasone dipropionate with the BRONCHODILATOR salbutamol.
✚/▲ warning/side-effects: *see* BECLOMETHASONE DIPROPIONATE; SALBUTAMOL.

Ventolin (*Allen & Hanburys*) is a proprietary form of the selective BETA-RECEPTOR STIMULANT salbutamol, used as a BRONCHODILATOR in patients with asthma and other breathing problems. Available only on prescription, Ventolin appears in many forms: as tablets (in three strengths, one form under the name Spandets), as sugar-free syrup (for dilution; potency once diluted is retained for 28 days), as ampoules for injection (in two strengths), as infusion fluid (after dilution), as aerosol inhalant, as ampoules for nebulization spray, and as a solution (for further dilution). In every case, patients should not exceed the prescribed or stated dose, and should follow the manufacturer's directions closely.
✚/▲ warning/side-effects: *see* SALBUTAMOL.

Vepesid (*Bristol-Myers*) is a proprietary form of the CYTOTOXIC drug etoposide, produced in the form either of capsules (in two strengths) or of ampoules for injection (after dilution). Available only on prescription, Vepesid is used to treat cancer, particularly lymphoma or carcinoma of the bronchus or testicle. Caution must be used in handling: Vepesid may dissolve certain types of filter.
✚/▲ warning/side-effects: *see* ETOPOSIDE.

Veractil (*May & Baker*) is a proprietary form of the ANTIPSYCHOTIC drug methotrimeprazine maleate (used primarily to treat schizophrenia and other psychoses). Available only on prescription, and not recommended for young or elderly patients, Veractil is produced in the form of tablets.
✚/▲ warning/side-effects: *see* METHOTRIMEPRAZINE.

Veracur (*Typharm*) is a proprietary non-prescription gel made from a 1.5% formaldehyde solution in a water-miscible base and used to treat warts, especially verrucas (plantar warts).
✚/▲ warning/side-effects: *see* FORMALDEHYDE.

verapamil hydrochloride is a

CALCIUM ANTAGONIST ANTIARRHYTHMIC drug used to treat heartbeat irregularities, high blood pressure (hypertension) and angina pectoris (heart pain). It is most commonly administered orally at first, although thereafter ampoules for injection or infusion are also available.

✚ warning: verapamil hydrochloride should not be administered to patients already taking beta-blockers, or who have heart block or heart failure, or to those with bradycardia (slow heartbeat).

▲ side-effects: potential side-effects include nausea, vomiting and constipation; infusion may result in low blood pressure. Very rarely there is liver damage.
Related articles: BERKATENS; CORDILOX; SECURON.

Verdiviton (*Squibb*) is a proprietary non-prescription MULTIVITAMIN elixir that is not available from the National Health Service. It contains THIAMINE (vitamin B_1), RIBOFLAVINE (vitamin B_2), PYRIDOXINE (vitamin B_6), CYANOCOBALAMIN (vitamin B_{12}), NICOTINAMIDE (of the vitamin B complex) and various mineral salts.

Veripaque (*Sterling Research*) is a proprietary non-prescription form of enema administered rectally to promote bowel movement. Containing oxyphenisatin, it is produced as powder for reconstitution in solution, and is commonly used in hospitals in combination with a barium sulphate enema or before colonic surgery.

✚ warning: careful monitoring should accompany treatment of patients with irritable or inflamed colons. Reduced dosage is recommended for elderly or infirm patients. Prolonged use as a laxative is inadvisable.

▲ side-effects: mild cramps, sweating and nausea may occur, in which case the dosage should be reduced.

Verkade (*G F Dietary Supplies*) is the name of a proprietary non-prescription brand of gluten-free biscuits, produced for patients who suffer from coeliac disease and other forms of gluten sensitivity.

Vermox (*Janssen*) is a proprietary ANTHELMINTIC drug, available only on prescription, used to treat infestation by pinworms (threadworms) and similar intestinal parasites. Comprising mebendazole, Vermox is produced in two forms: as tablets and in suspension.

✚/▲ warning/side-effects: *see* MEBENDAZOLE.

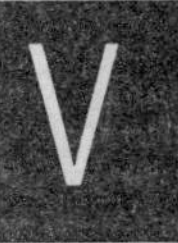

Verrugon (*Pickles*) is a proprietary non-prescription ointment consisting of salicylic acid in a paraffin base, used to treat warts and remove hard, dead skin.

✚ warning: *see* SALICYLIC ACID.

Vertigon (*Smith, Kline & French*) is a proprietary ANTI-EMETIC, available only on prescription, used to relieve symptoms of nausea caused by the vertigo and loss of balance experienced in infections of the inner and middle ears, or as a result of the administration of CYTOTOXIC drugs in the treatment of cancer. It is produced as spansules (soluble capsules) containing the major TRANQUILLIZER prochlorperazine (in two strengths).

✚/▲ warning/side-effects: *see* PROCHLORPERAZINE.

Verucasep (*Galen*) is a proprietary non-prescription gel containing the KERATOLYTIC glutaraldehyde, used to treat warts and remove hard, dead skin.
✚ warning: *see* GLUTARALDEHYDE.

Vibramycin (*Pfizer*) is a proprietary form of the TETRACYCLINE ANTIBIOTIC doxycycline, available only on prescription, as capsules (in two strengths), a sugar-free syrup (for dilution) or – under the separate name Vibramycin-D – soluble (dispersible) tablets. Vibramycin is prescribed to treat many serious bacterial and microbial infections.
✚/▲ warning/side-effects: *see* DOXYCYCLINE.

V

Vibrocil (*Zyma*) is a proprietary anti-infective nasal preparation, available only on prescription, produced in the form of a nasal spray, nose-drops, and a gel. All contain DIMETHINDENE MALEATE, NEOMYCIN sulphate and PHENYLEPHRINE, have ANTIHISTAMINE, ANTIBIOTIC and nasal DECONGESTANT properties, and are used to treat sinusitis and hay fever.

Vicks Coldcare (*Richardson-Vicks*) is a proprietary non-prescription cold relief preparation in the form of capsules, which contain paracetamol, the ANTITUSSIVE dextromethorphan and the DECONGESTANT phenylpropanolamine.
✚/▲ warning/side-effects: *see* DEXTROMETHORPHAN; PARACETAMOL; PHENYLPROPANOLOMINE.

vidarabine is an ANTIVIRAL drug used to treat serious infections by herpes viruses (such as chickenpox and shingles) in patients whose immune systems are already suppressed by other drugs. Administration is by intravenous infusion.
✚ warning: careful monitoring of blood count and kidney function is required: dosage should be balanced at an optimum. Treatment with vidarabine is not suitable for pregnant or lactating women.
▲ side-effects: there may be nausea and vomiting, diarrhoea and/or anorexia; a tremor may become apparent, with dizziness or a state of confusion; in the blood, white cells and platelets may decrease.
Related article: VIRA-A.

Vi-Daylin (*Abbott*) is a proprietary non-prescription MULTIVITAMIN syrup that is not available from the National Health Service. It contains RETINOL (vitamin A), THIAMINE (vitamin B_1), RIBOFLAVINE (vitamin B_2), PYRIDOXINE (vitamin B_3), NICOTINAMIDE (of the vitamin B complex), ASCORBIC ACID (vitamin C) and ERGOCALCIFEROL (vitamin D).

Videne (*Riker*) is a proprietary non-prescription skin disinfectant and cleanser containing povidone-iodine. Much used in hospitals, several forms are available: a water-based solution, a detergent-based surgical scrub, a tincture in methylated spirit (for washing skin preparatory to surgery), and dusting powder (for direct application to minor wounds).
✚/▲ warning/side-effects: *see* POVIDONE-IODINE.

Vidopen (*Berk*) is a proprietary form of the broad-spectrum PENICILLIN called ampicillin, available only on prescription. A powerful ANTIBIOTIC used mainly

to treat infections of the respiratory passages, the middle ear and the urinary tract, it is also effective against gonorrhoea. Vidopen is produced as capsules (in two strengths) and as a syrup (in two strengths, for dilution); the potency of the syrup once diluted is retained for 7 days.
✚/▲ warning/side-effects: *see* AMPICILLIN.

Vigranon B (*Wallace*) is a proprietary non-prescription compound of B complex VITAMINS that is not available from the National Health Service. Produced in the form of a syrup, it contains THIAMINE (vitamin B_1), RIBOFLAVINE (vitamin B_2), PYRIDOXINE (vitamin B_6), NICOTINAMIDE and PANTOTHENIC ACID (panthenol).

Villescon (*Boehringer Ingelheim*) is a proprietary compound containing the weak stimulant prolintane with VITAMIN supplements; it is used to treat debility or fatigue. Available on prescription only to private patients, it is produced in the form of tablets or an elixir.
✚/▲ warning/side-effects: *see* PROLINTANE.

viloxazine is an ANTIDEPRESSANT drug that has less of a sedative effect than many. Used to treat depression, dosage must be carefully monitored to remain at an optimum for each individual patient.
✚ warning: the sedative effect, though mild, may affect a patient's ability to operate controls on machinery or vehicles. Viloxazine should not be administered to patients who have had recent heart attacks or heart failure, who have a psychosis, who have liver damage or glaucoma, or who are pregnant. Age is also relevant: elderly patients should receive a reduced dosage.
▲ side-effects: there may be drowsiness, nausea and vomiting, and sweating; a weight change may become apparent.
Related article: VIVALAN.

vinblastine sulphate is a CYTOTOXIC drug, one of the VINCA ALKALOIDS. Available in its proprietary forms only on prescription, its ability to halt the process of cell reproduction means that it is used to treat cancer, particularly Hodgkin's disease, lymphoma and some neoplasms. But treatment with vinblastine sulphate may cause unpleasant side-effects, and even handling the material may cause problems: it is an irritant to tissue.
✚ warning: the use of vinblastine sulphate must be closely monitored in relation to each individual patient's tolerance of the toxicity of the drug.
▲ side-effects: as part of chemotherapy for cancer, its inevitable toxicity may produce unpleasant side-effects. These range from nausea and vomiting, depression of the bone-marrow's ability to produce red blood cells, and hair loss, to loss of sensation at the extremities, abdominal bloating and serious constipation.
Related article: VELBE.

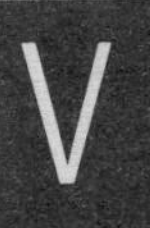

vinca alkaloids are a type of CYTOTOXIC drug; they work by halting the process of cell reproduction and are thus used to treat cancer, especially leukaemia, lymphoma and some sarcomas. But their toxicity inevitably causes some serious side-effects, in particular some

loss of neural function at the extremities, and such symptoms may become so severe as to oblige a reduction in dosage.
Related articles: ELDISINE; ONCOVIN; VELBE; VINBLASTINE SULPHATE; VINCRISTINE SULPHATE; VINDESINE SULPHATE.

vincristine sulphate is a CYTOTOXIC drug, one of the VINCA ALKALOIDS. Available in its proprietary forms only on prescription, its ability to halt the process of cell reproduction means that it is used to treat cancer, particularly acute leukaemia, Hodgkin's disease and other lymphomas. But treatment with vincristine sulphate may cause unpleasant side-effects, and even handling the material may cause problems: it is an irritant to tissue.
✚ warning: the use of vincristine sulphate must be closely monitored in relation to each individual patient's tolerance of the toxicity of the drug.
▲ side-effects: as part of chemotherapy for cancer, its inevitable toxicity may produce unpleasant side-effects. These range from nausea and vomiting, constipation and hair loss, to loss of sensation at the extremities, neural failure and abdominal bloating.
Related article: ONCOVIN.

vindesine sulphate is a CYTOTOXIC drug, derived from one of the VINCA ALKALOIDS. Available in its proprietary form (which also contains MANNITOL) only on prescription, its ability to halt the process of cell reproduction means that it is used to treat cancer, particularly leukaemia, lymphoma and some sarcomas. But treatment with vindesine sulphate may cause unpleasant side-effects, and even handling the material may cause problems: it is an irritant to tissue.
✚ warning: the use of vindesine sulphate must be closely monitored in relation to each individual patient's tolerance of the toxicity of the drug.
▲ side-effects: as part of chemotherapy for cancer, its inevitable toxicity may produce unpleasant side-effects. These range from nausea and vomiting, constipation and hair loss, to loss of sensation at the extremities, neural failure and abdominal bloating.
Related article: ELDISINE.

Vioform-Hydrocortisone (*Ciba*) is a proprietary ANTBACTERIAL, ANTIFUNGAL steroid compound preparation of hydrocortisone and CLIOQUINOL used to treat inflammatory skin disorders when infection is not the cause of the inflammation. It is produced as a water-based cream (for further dilution) and a more oily white soft paraffin-based ointment (also for dilution); the potency of either form in dilution is retained for 14 days.
✚/▲ warning/side-effects: *see* HYDROCORTISONE.

Vira-A (*Parke-Davis*) is a proprietary ANTIVIRAL drug, available only on prescription, used to treat herpes infections. It is produced in two forms: as a concentrated fluid for dilution before intravenous infusion or injection, and as an eye ointment. In both cases the active constituent is vidarabine.
✚/▲ warning/side-effects: *see* VIDARABINE.

Virormone (*Paines & Byrne*) is a proprietary form of the male sex HORMONE testosterone (in the form of testosterone propionate),

V

available only on prescription, and used primarily in hormone replacement therapy. Virormone is produced in ampoules for injection (in three strengths) and (under the trade name Virormone-Oral) in the form of tablets (in three strengths).
✚/▲ warning/side-effects: *see* TESTOSTERONE.

Visclair (*Sinclair*) is a proprietary non-prescription MUCOLYTIC that is not available from the National Health Service. Used to reduce the viscosity of sputum and thus facilitate expectoration in patients with asthma or bronchitis, Visclair tablets contain METHYLCYSTEINE hydrochloride. They are not recommended for children aged under 5 years.

Viscopaste PB7 (*Smith & Nephew*) is a proprietary non-prescription form of bandaging impregnated with ZINC paste. This kind of bandaging is used to treat and dress wounds and ulcers (and further bandaging is required to keep it in place).

Vi-Siblin (*Parke-Davis*) is a proprietary form of the type of laxative known as a bulking agent, which works by increasing the overall mass of faeces within the rectum, so stimulating bowel movement. In the case of Vi-Siblin, the agent involved is ispaghula husk, presented in the form of brown granules for swallowing with water.
✚/▲ warning/side-effects: *see* ISPAGHULA HUSK.

Viskaldix (*Sandoz*) is a proprietary ANTIHYPERTENSIVE combination of the drugs pindolol and clopamide, used to treat and control moderately high blood pressure. Available only on prescription, Viskaldix is produced as tablets. It is not recommended for children.
✚/▲ warning/side-effects: *see* CLOPAMIDE; PINDOLOL.

Visken (*Sandoz*) is a proprietary form of the BETA-BLOCKER drug pindolol, used as an ANTIHYPERTENSIVE in the treatment of high blood pressure, and to treat angina pectoris. Available only on prescription, Visken is produced as tablets in either of two strengths. It is not recommended for children.
✚/▲ warning/side-effects: *see* PINDOLOL.

Vista-Methasone (*Daniel*) is a proprietary ANTI-INFLAMMATORY steroid drug, available only on prescription, in the form of drops to treat inflammation in the ear, eye or nose. Used solely where infection is not the cause of the inflammation, its active constituent is betamethasone sodium phosphate. A second version – called Vista-Methasone N – additionally contains NEOMYCIN sulphate.
✚/▲ warning/side-effects: *see* BETAMETHASONE SODIUM PHOSPHATE.

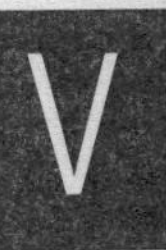

Vita-E (*Bioglan*) is a proprietary non-prescription form of vitamin E (TOCOPHEROL) supplements. Vita-E Gels are capsules containing alpha tocopheryl acetate, and are produced in three strengths; Vita-E Gelucaps also contain alpha tocopheryl acetate but are chewy tablets; Vita-E Succinate is in the form of tablets containing alpha tocopheryl succinate. There is also Vita-E Ointment, a paraffin-based ointment containing alpha tocopheryl acetate, for treating bedsores and similar conditions.

vitamin A is another term for retinol.
see RETINOL.

vitamin B is the collective term for a number of water-soluble vitamins found particularly in dairy products, cereals and liver. *see* CYANOCOBALAMIN; FOLIC ACID; NICOTINAMIDE; NICOTINIC ACID; PANTOTHENIC ACID; PYRIDOXINE; RIBOFLAVINE; THIAMINE.

vitamin C is another term for ascorbic acid. *see* ASCORBIC ACID.

vitamin D is another term for calciferol; it occurs naturally in plants (ergocalciferol) and through the action of sunlight on the skin (cholecalciferol). *see* CHOLECALCIFEROL; ERGOCALCIFEROL.

vitamin E is a group of chemically-related oxidant compounds consisting of tocopherols and tocotrienols. Their main effect is thought to be to increase the stability of cell membranes. Good food sources are dairy products, vegetable oils and cereals; deficiency is rare. *Related article:* VITA-E.

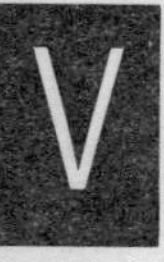

vitamin K is a fat-soluble vitamin that occurs naturally in plants (phytomenadione) and in animals (menaquinone) and derived in the diet from fresh green vegetables, fruit and egg-yolk. It is essential to the process of blood clotting. Deficiency of the vitamin is very rare. *see* PHYTOMENADIONE.

vitamins are substances required in small quantities for healthy growth, development and metabolism; lack of any one vitamin causes a specific deficiency disorder. Because they cannot usually be synthesized by the body, vitamins have to be absorbed or ingested from external sources – generally these are food substances.

Vitavel (*Bencard*) is a proprietary non-prescription sugar-free multivitamin elixir that is not available from the National Health Service. It contains THIAMINE (vitamin B_1), RIBOFLAVINE (vitamin B_2), NICOTINAMIDE (of the vitamin B complex), ASCORBIC ACID (vitamin C) and ERGOCALCIFEROL (vitamin D), and is used after dilution. The potency of the diluted elixir is retained for 30 days.

Vitlipid (*KabiVitrum*) is a proprietary form of liquid VITAMIN supplement for intravenous infusion into patients who cannot be adequately fed via the alimentary canal. An emulsion intended to be combined with a lipid-based intravenous infusion, Vitlipid is a compound of RETINOL (vitamin A), ERGOCALCIFEROL (vitamin D) and PHYTOMENADIONE (vitamin K). It is produced in two strengths: one for adults, the other for children.

Vivalan (*ICI*) is a proprietary ANTIDEPRESSANT drug, available only on prescription, consisting of tablets containing viloxazine hydrochloride.
✚/▲ warning/side-effects: *see* VILOXAZINE.

Vivonex (*Norwich Eaton*) is a proprietary form of nutritional compound, available only on prescription, for patients who are undernourished (such as with anorexia nervosa) or who have severe problems in digestion (such as following gastrectomy). There are two versions: both contain amino acids, glucose solids, fats, vitamins and minerals, and are produced in sachets of powder for dilution. Administration is oral or by tube.
✚ warning: Vivonex is not suitable as the sole source of

nutrition for children aged under 5 years.

Volital (*LAB*) is a proprietary form of the weak STIMULANT pemoline, used to treat debility, lassitude or fatigue. Available only on prescription, it is produced as tablets. It is not recommended for children aged under 6 years.
✚/▲ warning/side-effects: *see* PEMOLINE.

Voltarol (*Geigy*) is a proprietary, non-steroid, ANTI-INFLAMMATORY non-narcotic ANALGESIC, available only on prescription, used to treat arthritic and rheumatic pain and other musculo-skeletal disorders. Its active constituent is diclofenac sodium, and it is produced in the form of tablets (in either of two strengths, plus a sustained-release version called Voltarol Retard), ampoules for injection, and anal suppositories (in either of two strengths). Voltarol should not be administered to patients with a peptic ulcer or asthma, who are known to be allergic to aspirin, or who are pregnant or lactating.
✚/▲ warning/side-effects: *see* DICLOFENAC SODIUM.

Volumatic (*Allen & Hanburys*) is a large-volume inhaler device for use with the bronchodilators BECLOFORTE, BECOTIDE, VENTIDE and VENTOLIN, all of which rely on the corticosteroid BECLOMETHASONE DIPROPIONATE and/or the sympathomimetic SALBUTAMOL.

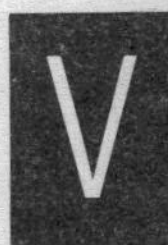

Wallachol (*Wallace*) is a proprietary non-prescription compound primarily of B complex VITAMINS that is not available from the National Health Service. Produced in the form of tablets and a syrup, Wallachol contains THIAMINE (vitamin B_1), RIBOFLAVINE (vitamin B_2), PYRIDOXINE (vitamin B_6), CYANOCOBALAMIN (vitamin B_{12}), NICOTINAMIDE and other metabolic constituents.

warfarin is an orally administered ANTICOAGULANT, used primarily to treat patients who suffer from deep-vein thrombosis or from transient attacks of ischaemia (restriction of the blood supply) in the brain. It may also be used following surgery to replace a heart valve, although – as with all anticoagulants – it should not be administered when there is any risk of haemorrhage. The anticoagulant effect may take up to 48 hours to develop. There are two proprietary forms, both produced as tablets in several strengths.

✚ warning: warfarin (in the form of warfarin sodium) should not be administered to patients with kidney or liver disease, seriously high blood pressure (hypertension), bacterial endocarditis or a peptic ulcer; who are regularly taking anabolic steroids, aspirin, barbiturates or phytomenadione (vitamin K) supplements; who are using oral contraceptives; or who are in the first three months or last two months of pregnancy.

▲ side-effects: internal haemorrhaging may occur; monitoring is required.
Related article: MAREVAN.

Waxsol (*Norgine*) is a proprietary non-prescription form of ear-drops designed to soften and dissolve ear-wax (cerumen), and commonly prescribed for use at home two nights consecutively before syringing of the ears in a doctor's surgery. Its solvent constituent is DIOCTYL SODIUM SULPHOSUCCINATE (also called docusate sodium).

✚ warning: Waxsol should not be used if there is inflammation in the ear, or where there is any chance that the eardrum has been perforated.

Welldorm (*Smith & Nephew*) is a proprietary HYPNOTIC and SEDATIVE, available only on prescription, used to treat insomnia. Produced as tablets and as an elixir for dilution (the potency of the dilute elixir is retained for 14 days), Welldorm's active constituent is dichloralphenazone, a derivative of CHLORAL HYDRATE.

✚/▲ warning/side-effects: *see* DICHLORALPHENAZONE.

Wellferon (*Wellcome*) is a proprietary preparation of interferon (in the form of alfa interferon), available only on prescription, and used mainly to treat leukaemia. Administration is by injection. As with virtually all anticancer drugs, some fairly severe side-effects are inevitable.

✚/▲ warning/side-effects: *see* INTERFERONS.

white liniment is a non-proprietary compound liniment which, massaged into the skin, produces an irritation that offsets the pain of underlying muscle or joint ailments. Its main constituent is water, but it also contains ammonia solution, AMMONIUM CHLORIDE, oleic acid and turpentine oil in various proportions.

✚ warning: avoid broken or inflamed skin surfaces.

Whitfield's ointment is a common name for the non-proprietary compound benzoic acid ointment, used most commonly to treat patches of the fungal infection ringworm.
see BENZOIC ACID OINTMENT.

wool alcohols ointment is a non-proprietary skin emollient (softener and soother) made up of wool alcohols (a water-in-oil emulsifying agent) together with various forms of paraffin.

Wyeth Standard Enteral Feed (*Wyeth*) is a proprietary non- prescription form of nutritional compound for patients who are undernourished (such as with anorexia nervosa) or who have severe problems in digestion (such as following gastrectomy). The Enteral Feed provides a virtually complete diet, containing protein, carbohydrate, fat, vitamins and minerals; it is also gluten-free. Produced in the form of a liquid, its administration is oral or by tube.
✚ warning: Wyeth Standard Enteral Feed is not suitable as the sole source of nutrition for children aged under 5 years, and not suitable at all for children aged under 12 months.

Wysoy (*Wyeth*) is a proprietary non-prescription form of nutritional compound for patients who in one way or another are unable to tolerate cow's milk. Produced in the form of powder, for reconstitution, Wysoy provides a virtually complete diet, containing protein, carbohydrate, fat, vitamins, minerals and trace elements; it is – naturally – free of milk protein and lactose, but it is also gluten-free.

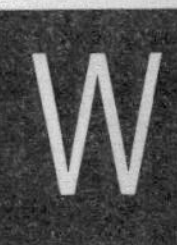

Xanax (*Upjohn*) is a proprietary ANXIOLYTIC, available on prescription only to private patients. It is produced in the form of tablets (in two strengths) containing the BENZODIAZEPINE alprazolam, and is used to treat short-term anxiety and anxiety accompanying depression.
✚/▲ warning/side-effects: *see* ALPRAZOLAM.

xanthine-oxidase inhibitor is a type of drug that interferes with the breakdown of nucleic acids, the process by which the purines adenine and guanine (constituents of DNA) are broken down, resulting in the formation of uric acid. The most widely used xanthine-oxidase inhibitor is ALLOPURINOL (which is prescribed particularly in the long-term treatment of gout – a condition caused by an excess of uric acid and its salts).
✚ warning: xanthine-oxidase inhibitors should not be used when a high level of uric acid in the bloodstream has led to acute inflammation; treatment at this time may exacerbate the effect of the inflammation (and anti-inflammatory drugs should be used first).

xipamide is a DIURETIC drug, similar to the THIAZIDES, used mainly to relieve the accumulation of fluids in the tissues (oedema) due to heart failure, and in lower dosages or in combination to relieve high blood pressure (hypertension). Administration is oral (in the form of proprietary tablets) early in the day (so that the diuretic effect does not inhibit sleep).
✚ warning: treatment with xipamide may cause abnormally low levels of potassium in the bloodstream (hypokalaemia), and may accordingly require the provision of potassium supplements. The drug may also aggravate the conditions of gout and diabetes. Xipamide should not be used on patients with kidney failure or cirrhosis of the liver. Caution should be exercised in treating patients with impaired functioning of the kidneys or the liver, or who are pregnant or lactating.
▲ side-effects: there may be minor gastrointestinal disturbances; mild dizziness, allergies, and/or thirst may be experienced.
Related article: DIUREXAN.

X-Prep (*Napp*) is a proprietary non-prescription form of the stimulant LAXATIVE senna, used particularly in hospitals and clinics for bowel evacuation before X-ray examination. Produced as a liquid, X-Prep should be taken by the patient on the afternoon of the day before the X-ray session.
✚/▲ warning/side-effects: *see* SENNA.

Xylocaine (*Astra*) is a series of proprietary preparations of the local ANAESTHETIC lignocaine, mostly available only on prescription. In the form of anhydrous lignocaine hydrochloride, Xylocaine is produced in ampoules for injection, in various strengths, with and without ADRENALINE (which increases duration of effect). Cartridges of this form of Xylocaine are also available for use in dental surgery, as are (non-prescription) tubes or syringes of Xylocaine Gel (with and without CHLORHEXIDINE gluconate). In addition, there is (non-prescription) Xylocaine Viscous solution and Xylocaine 4% Topical solution for local use on skin or mucous membranes. Containing lignocaine – as

opposed to the hydrochloride – there is (non-prescription) Xylocaine Ointment and Xylocaine Spray (with cetylpyridinium chloride).
✚/▲ warning/side-effects: *see* LIGNOCAINE.

Xylocard (*Astra*) is a proprietary ANTIARRHYTHMIC drug, available only on prescription, used to treat irregularities in the heartbeat, especially after a heart attack. Produced in the form of pre-loaded hypodermics for injection and as pre-loaded syringes for intravenous infusion (following dilution), Xylocard's active constituent is anhydrous lignocaine hydrochloride (also used as a local ANAESTHETIC).
✚/▲ warning/side-effects: *see* LIGNOCAINE.

Xylodase (*Astra*) is a proprietary, non-prescription, local ANAESTHETIC cream, intended for use on the mucous membranes of the mouth. Its major active constituent is lignocaine, but it also contains HYALURONIDASE (a "spreading" factor).
✚/▲ warning/side-effects: *see* LIGNOCAINE.

xylometazoline hydrochloride is a VASOCONSTRICTOR. As nose-drops it is available in two strengths; there is also a proprietary nasal spray.
✚ warning: prolonged use is to be avoided. In combination with certain other drugs, xylometazoline hydrochloride may cause extremely high blood pressure.
▲ side-effects: there may be local irritation. Increasing tolerance in the body corresponds to diminishing effect of the drug.
Related articles: OTRIVINE; OTRIVINE-ANTISTIN; RYNACROM.

Xyloproct (*Astra*) is a proprietary compound, available only on prescription, used to treat, dress and soothe various painful conditions of the anus and rectum. It is produced both as water-miscible ointment and as anal suppositories. The active constituents of Xyloproct are HYDROCORTISONE acetate (a CORTICOSTEROID), LIGNOCAINE (a local ANAESTHETIC), ALUMINIUM ACETATE and ZINC OXIDE (both mild astringents).

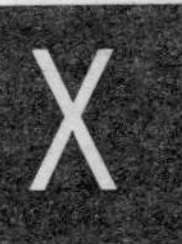

Xylotox (*Astra*) is a proprietary dental local ANAESTHETIC, available only on prescription, containing lignocaine hydrochloride and ADRENALINE (the latter to add duration to the effect). It is produced in cartridges for easy attachment to a dentist's hypodermic.
✚/▲ warning/side-effects: *see* LIGNOCAINE.

yellow fever vaccine consists of a protein suspension containing live but attenuated yellow fever viruses (cultured in chick embryos). Immunity may last for a good deal longer than the official ten years. The disease remains relatively well established in parts of tropical Africa and northern South America.
✚ warning: vaccination should not be administered to patients with an impaired immune response; who are sensitive to eggs; who are pregnant; or who are aged under 9 months.
▲ side-effects: reactions are rare.
Related articles: ARILVAX; YEL/VAC.

yel/vac is an abbreviation for yellow fever vaccine.
see YELLOW FEVER VACCINE.

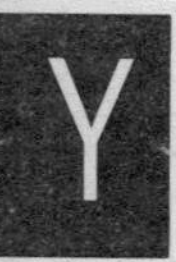

Yomesan (*Bayer*) is a proprietary, non-prescription form of the ANTHELMINTIC drug niclosamide, used to treat infestation by tapeworms; it is produced as chewy yellow tablets. Careful monitoring of the infestation is required, together with reassuring counselling of the patient.
✚ warning: consumption of alcohol should be avoided during treatment.
▲ side-effects: *see* NICLOSAMIDE.

Yutopar (*Duphar*) is a proprietary form of the BETA-RECEPTOR STIMULANT ritodrine hydrochloride, available only on prescription, used initially as an emergency measure to halt premature labour, and thereafter as a holding dosage until full term is attained (if there are no apparent fetal complications) or until preparations have been rapidly made for a premature delivery (if fetal complications are apparent). Yutopar is produced both in the form of ampoules for injection and as tablets.
✚/▲ warning/side-effects: *see* RITODRINE HYDROCHLORIDE.

Zaditen (*Sandoz*) is a proprietary drug, available only on prescription, intended to reduce the incidence of asthmatic attacks, or to treat allergic rhinitis or conjunctivitis. It is produced in the form of capsules, tablets, and an elixir for dilution. (The potency of the dilute elixir is retained for 14 days.) Zaditen's active constituent is ketotifen (in the form of the fumarate), which may take several weeks of treatment to achieve its full effect in the body.
✚ warning: consumption of alcohol should be avoided during treatment. Zaditen should not be administered to children aged under 2 years.
▲ side-effects: *see* KETOTIFEN.

Zadstat (*Lederle*) is a proprietary ANTIBACTERIAL and ANTIPROTOZOAL drug, available only on prescription, used to treat infections by anaerobic bacteria, amoebae and protozoa, particularly infections of the rectum, colon and vagina. It may also be used to treat ulcerative infections of the gums. Produced in the form of tablets, suppositories (in either of two strengths), and in a Minipack for intravenous infusion, Zadstat is a preparation of the drug metronidazole.
✚/▲ warning/side-effects: *see* METRONIDAZOLE.

Zagreb antivenom (*Regent*) is a proprietary antidote to the poison injected by an adder. The systemic effects of an adder's bite are rarely serious enough to warrant the use of the antivenom (which has to be diluted with saline solution), but severely low blood pressure, heart arrhythmia or extensive swelling of the bitten limb are indications that more than cleaning, dressing and immobilization is required. Antivenoms for other snakes' poisons are available from the National Poisons Information Centre in London, and the Walton Hospital in Liverpool.

Zantac (*Glaxo*) is a proprietary form of the anti-ulcer drug ranitidine hydrochloride, available only on prescription, used to reduce the acidity of stomach juices in the presence of a non- expanding gastric or duodenal ulcer, or following gastric surgery. It is produced in the form of tablets (in either of two strengths), soluble (dispersible) tablets, or ampoules for injection. Treatment is not recommended for children aged under 8 years.
✚/▲ warning/side-effects: *see* RANITIDINE.

Zarontin (*Parke-Davis*) is a proprietary form of the ANTI-EPILEPTIC drug ethosuximide, available only on prescription, used to treat and suppress petit mal ("absence") seizures – the mild form of epilepsy. Available in the form of capsules and an elixir for dilution – the potency of the dilute elixir is retained for 14 days – monitoring of seizures following the initiation of treatment with Zarontin should establish an optimum treatment level.
✚/▲ warning/side-effects: *see* ETHOSUXIMIDE.

ZeaSORB (*Stiefel*) is a proprietary non-prescription dusting powder, used to dry and soothe skin in folds or on surfaces where friction may occur. Active constituents include CHLOROXYLENOL (a DISINFECTANT cleanser).

Zinacef (*Glaxo*) is a proprietary broad-spectrum ANTIBIOTIC, available only on prescription, used to treat bacterial infections

and to retain asepsis during surgery. Produced in the form of powder for reconstitution as a medium for injections, Zinacef is a preparation of the CEPHALOSPORIN cefuroxime.
✚/▲ warning/side-effects: *see* CEFUROXIME.

Zinamide (*Merck, Sharp & Dohme*) is a proprietary ANTITUBERCULAR drug, available only on prescription, consisting of tablets containing pyrazinamide. Usually prescribed in combination with other antitubercular drugs, it is not recommended for children.
✚/▲ warning/side-effects: *see* PYRAZINAMIDE.

zinc is a trace element, necessary in tiny quantities in a daily diet. Deficiency demanding the administration of zinc supplements is rare, however, but occurs with inadequate diet, in cases of malabsorption of ingested food, and where trauma causes loss of zinc from the blood. Conversely, zinc supplements cause some uncomfortable side-effects such as dyspepsia.
Related articles: ZINC OXIDE; ZINC SULPHATE.

zinc oxide is a mild ASTRINGENT used primarily to treat skin disorders such as nappy rash, urinary rash and eczema. It is available (without prescription) in any of a number of compound forms – as a water-based cream (with arachis oil, oleic acid and wool fat; or with ichthammol and wool fat); as an ointment, and as an ointment with castor oil; as dusting powder (with starch and talc); as a paste (with starch and white soft paraffin; or with starch and salicylic acid – Lassar's paste), sometimes in impregnated bandages.
Related article: ZINC PASTE.

zinc paste is a non-proprietary compound made up of ZINC OXIDE, starch and white soft paraffin, which is slightly ASTRINGENT and is used as a base to which other active constituents can be added, especially within impregnated bandages. Of all such pastes (compounded to treat and protect the lesions of skin diseases such as eczema and psoriasis), zinc paste is the standard type.

zinc sulphate is one form in which zinc supplements can be administered in order to make up a ZINC deficiency in the body. There are several proprietary preparations, all different in form although all oral in administration. In solution, zinc sulphate is also used as an astringent and wound cleanser, in eye-drops (with or without ADRENALINE), and as an occasional EMETIC.
✚ warning: zinc sulphate should not be administered in combination with tetracycline antibiotics.
▲ side-effects: there may be abdominal pain or mild gastrointestinal upsets.
Related articles: SOLVAZINC; ZINCFRIN; ZINCOMED; Z SPAN.

Zincaband (*Seton*) is a proprietary non-prescription form of impregnated bandaging, impregnated with gelatinous ZINC PASTE and used to treat eczema, varicose veins and skin ulcers. (Further bandaging is required to hold it in place.)

Zincfrin (*Alcon*) is a proprietary non-prescription form of eye-drops containing ZINC SULPHATE and PHENYLEPHRINE, used to treat eyes that are watering too freely, and for mild conjunctivitis.

Zincomed (*Medo*) is a proprietary non-prescription form of ZINC

supplement, used to treat zinc deficiency in the body. It is produced in the form of capsules containing zinc sulphate.
✚/▲ warning/side-effects: *see* ZINC SULPHATE.

Zonulysin (*Henleys*) is a proprietary form of an enzyme preparation used to dissolve the ligament that suspends the lens of the eye within the eyeball (the zonule of Zinn) in order to facilitate the surgical removal of a lens that has become opaque through cataract. Available only on prescription, Zonulysin is produced as a powder for reconstitution as an injection; the fluid – in which the active constituent is alpha-chymotrypsin – is injected behind the iris a minute or so before the lens is removed, and affects no other part of the eye.

Zovirax (*Wellcome*) is a proprietary form of the ANTIVIRAL drug acyclovir, available only on prescription, used to treat infection by herpes simplex and herpes zoster organisms. It is available in the form of tablets (in either of two strengths), a suspension (for dilution with syrup or sorbitol; the potency of the dilute suspension is retained for 28 days), and a powder for reconstitution as an intravenous infusion. To treat one form of herpes simplex, there is also an eye ointment; urogenital forms of herpes are treated by a water-based cream. Treatment by any of these preparations is required at least 4 times a day.
✚/▲ warning/side-effects: *see* ACYCLOVIR.

Z Span (*Smith, Kline & French*) is a proprietary non-prescription form of ZINC supplement, used to treat zinc deficiency in the body. Produced in the form of spansules (slow-release capsules) containing zinc sulphate monohydrate, Z Span is not recommended for children aged under 12 months.
✚/▲ warning/side-effects: *see* ZINC SULPHATE.

zuclopenthixol is an ANTIPSYCHOTIC drug, one of the thioxanthenes, used to treat and restrain psychotic patients, particularly the more aggressive or agitated schizophrenic ones. It is administered in the form of tablets (as zuclopenthixol dihydrochloride) or injection (as zuclopenthixol decanoate).
✚ warning: zuclopenthixol should not be administered to patients with heart disease, respiratory disease, epilepsy, parkinsonism, severe arteriosclerosis or acute infection; who are in a withdrawn or apathetic state; who are pregnant or lactating; who have impaired functioning of the liver or kidneys; whose prostate gland is enlarged; who are old and infirm (especially in very hot or cold weather); or who are children. Withdrawal of treatment must be gradual.
▲ side-effects: there may be involuntary (reflex) movements, hypothermia, drowsiness, lethargy, insomnia and depression; low blood pressure and heartbeat irregularities; allergic symptoms; and/or dry mouth, constipation, blurred vision, rashes and difficulties in urinating. Prolonged high dosage may cause eventual eye defects and pigmentation of the skin.
Related article: CLOPIXOL.

Zyloric (*Calmic*) is a proprietary form of the XANTHINE-OXIDASE INHIBITOR allopurinol, used to treat high levels of uric acid in

the bloodstream (which may otherwise cause gout). Available only on prescription, Zyloric is produced for oral administration in the form of tablets.
✚/▲ warning/side-effects: *see* ALLOPURINOL.

Zymafluor (*Zyma*) is a proprietary non-prescription form of fluoride supplement for administration in areas where the water supply is not fluoridated, especially to growing children. Produced in the form of tablets (in either of two strengths, to correspond with local water fluoridation levels), Zymafluor's active constituent is SODIUM FLUORIDE.

Z

Glossary

abscess Pus-filled cavity surrounded by inflamed tissue.

acute disorder Condition that occurs suddenly and usually severely, but is brief.

addiction Physical or psychological dependence on a substance such as a drug.

adenoids Lymphatic tissue located at the rear of the nasal cavity. The adenoids are relatively large in children, and usually shrink in adulthood.

adhesion Union of normally separate surfaces by fibrous tissue. The term may also refer to the formation of scar tissue as part of the normal healing process.

adrenal gland Small endocrine gland situated above the kidney. It consists of two parts: the outer cortex and the inner medulla. The adrenal cortex releases corticosteroid hormones, and the medulla releases adrenaline and noradrenaline.

airways Tubular passages through which air passes into and out of the lungs.

alkaloids Diverse group of chemical substances – including morphine and quinine – that are derived from plants; many are physiologically active.

alveoli Tiny air-sacs in the lungs where oxygen from inhaled air is transferred to the blood and carbon dioxide is removed from the blood.

amino acid One of a group of more than twenty organic compounds, which are the chemical building blocks of all proteins. The human body can synthesize many of them, but eight that are essential for health can only be obtained in the diet.

anaemia Deficiency of haemoglobin (the oxygen-carrying substance in red blood cells). There are several possible causes, including lack of red blood cells, iron deficiency and a deficiency of vitamin B_{12}.

aneurysm Abnormal swelling of an artery, commonly caused by weakness in the wall.

angina pectoris Chest pain that is caused by the heart muscle receiving too little oxygen, commonly as a result of coronary artery disease. The pain typically spreads to the neck or left arm. Angina pectoris is often referred to simply as angina.

antibody Specific protein produced by the immune system in order to defend the body against a substance which it regards as alien and therefore potentially dangerous.

antigen Substance that stimulates the formation of antibodies. Examples include bacteria, bacterial toxins, transplanted organs, and various substances that cause allergic reactions (such as plant pollens).
anxiety Feeling of fear and dread about a real or imagined threat.
appendix Small tube-like extension that is attached to the caecum of the large intestine. Inflammation of the appendix is called appendicitis.
arrhythmia Deviation from the normal rhythm of the heart.
artery Blood vessel that carries blood under pressure from the heart to the rest of the body.
astringent Substance that causes tissues to contract. Because astringents constrict blood vessels, they are sometimes used to reduce bleeding from minor abrasions.
autoimmune disease Condition in which the immune system produces antibodies that act against the body's own tissues.
autonomic nervous system Part of the nervous system that controls involuntary bodily functions, such as sweating, the heartbeat, glandular secretions and the function of smooth muscle. It has two divisions: the sympathetic and the parasympathetic nervous systems.
bacteria Single-celled micro-organisms, many of which are harmless, but some of which cause disease.
benign Non-cancerous tumour, which does not invade or destroy surrounding tissue or spread through the body. It may also be used to describe any condition that is harmless.
bile Digestive secretion that emulsifies fats. It is a product of the breakdown of red blood cells by the liver. It is stored in the gall bladder, and enters the duodenum (small intestine) through the bile duct.
biopsy Removal of a small amount of living tissue for laboratory examination.
bladder Organ that holds fluid, such as the gall bladder or the urinary bladder. The term used on its own usually refers to the urinary bladder.
blood clot Mass of coagulated blood.
blood count Laboratory investigation used to measure the quantity of certain constituents of blood, such as red blood cells.
blood pressure Pressure of the blood in major arteries, usually measured in the arm using a sphygmomanometer.
blood vessels Tubes in which the blood circulates throughout the body (that is, the arteries, veins and capillaries).
bronchus Main airway from the trachea (windpipe) to the bronchioles.
bronchiole Small airway in the lung that carries air from the bronchi to the alveoli.
bruising Discoloration in or under the skin, caused by leakage of blood into the tissues.
caecum First part of the large intestine, into which digested food passes from the small intestine.
calcification Deposition of calcium salts into the tissues. Calcification can be the result of a number of normal or abnormal conditions.
cancer Any malignant growth of tissue, which may invade or destroy surrounding tissue and spread throughout the body.
capillaries Microscopically small blood vessels that are involved in the supply of nutrients (including oxygen) to, and the removal of wastes from, the tissues of the body.
carbohydrates Large group of compounds, which includes sugars and starches, an important source of energy.
cardiac Relating to the heart.

cardiovascular Relating to the heart and blood vessels.
central nervous system Brain and spinal cord.
cholera Acute bacterial infection of the small intestine that causes severe vomiting and diarrhoea, which may lead to dangerous dehydration.
chronic disorder Condition that is long-term or of long duration. Chronic diseases often have a gradual onset and involve slow changes. The term does not imply anything about the severity of the disease.
circulatory system Another term for the cardiovascular system.
clotting Process by which blood coagulates and then solidifies to form a blood clot (thrombus), often in response to tissue damage.
coagulation Another term for clotting.
colic Fluctuating abdominal pain, which typically recurs after a period of seconds or minutes, in a way that is often described as wave-like.
colon Another term for the large intestine.
congenital Something present from birth; often used to describe a psychological disorder or physical defect.
conjunctiva Mucous membrane covering the front of the eyeball and the inside of the eyelids.
cornea Transparent, curved and tough covering of the iris and the pupil.
coronary Referring to the blood vessels that supply the heart. In common usage it may refer to a heart attack.
dehydration Lack of fluid in the tissues and blood.
dependence Usually applied to a person's need for a drug. Physical dependence means that withdrawal symptoms (such as sweating, vomiting or even epilepsy) will occur if a particular substance that is being taken is discontinued too quickly. Psychological dependence means that a person requires a substance in order to maintain contentment or a feeling of well-being, even though the absence of that substance would have no significant physical effect.
diabetes mellitus Disorder caused by a deficiency of the hormone insulin, which is produced by the pancreas. This condition has widespread effects because of the failure of sugar absorption by the tissues. Diabetes mellitus is often referred to simply as diabetes, although there are other conditions known as diabetes – such as diabetes indsipidus, which is a rare deficiency of the hormone vasopressin.
digestive system Series of organs through which food and drink pass, in which nutrients are absorbed and from which waste products are excreted. The digestive tract consists of the mouth, oesophagus, stomach, small intestine (duodenum, jejunum, ileum), and large intestine (caecum, colon, rectum and anus). The liver, gall bladder and pancreas are also important parts of the digestive system.
dilate Widen, open up or expand a hollow organ (such as a blood vessel), a cavity or the pupil of the eye.
diuretic Substance that increases the output of urine by the kidneys.
electrolyte Solution that produces ions. The term is also commonly used when talking about the concentration of ions themselves.
embolism Obstruction of a blood vessel by a material (usually by a blood clot) that is carried by the bloodstream from one part of the body to another. The consequences depend on where the clot finally lodges and on its size.
emollient Substance that softens and soothes. The term is usually used for substances applied to the skin.

endocrine system System composed of glands that secrete hormones directly into the bloodstream, by which means they can exert various effects on other organs. The endocrine glands include the adrenals, ovaries, pancreas, pituitary, testicles and thyroid.

enema Fluid that is passed into the rectum through the anus by means of a tube, for diagnostic or therapeutic purposes.

enzyme Biological substance that acts like a catalyst to enable a specific biochemical reaction to occur (or to occur faster than it would otherwise) in the body.

epithelium Thin layer of cells covering external and internal body surfaces.

extremities Limbs.

faeces Solid or semisolid waste that is excreted through the anus.

fascia Sheet of fibrous tissue surrounding a muscle or lying between the skin and underlying tissue.

fats Substances – correctly called lipids – containing chemicals known as fatty acids. They play an important role in the body's metabolism, and also form part of the structure of cells and certain organs. In the body, excess carbohydrate or protein is converted to fat for storage.

fever Symptom of a body temperature that is higher than normal.

fibre Indigestible, non-nutritious element in food, that is nevertheless important in the diet because it provides the substance that the muscles of the intestines need to push food through the digestive tract. Dietary fibre is also known as roughage.

fibroid Benign tumour of the womb.

glaucoma Disease involving increased pressure in the fluids within the eyeball. If untreated, glaucoma can lead to blindness.

fissure Cleft or break in a mucous membrane or skin surface.

gallbladder Small, sac-like organ lying under the liver. Its main function is to store bile produced by the liver, and to secrete the bile into the small intestine when food leaves the stomach.

gangrene Death and decay of a tissue resulting from loss of the local blood supply.

gastrointestinal system Series of organs through which food passes in the digestive system.

gland Organ or tissue that produces and secretes fluid.

glucose Simple sugar that circulates in the blood and is used for energy by the tissues of the body.

gluten Protein in wheat and rye, which must be avoided by anyone suffering from coeliac disease.

haemoglobin Pigmented substance in red blood cells that carries oxygen from the lungs to the tissues.

haemorrhage Internal or external bleeding.

hangover Unpleasant symptoms produced after taking excessive alcohol or certain other drugs.

host Animal or plant that has a parasite living on, or within, it.

hypercalcaemia Abnormally high concentration of calcium in the blood.

hypersensivity Exaggerated response to a specific stimulus. The term usually applies to an allergic response or some other hypersensitivity of the immune system.

hypothalamus Small part of the brain connected with the pituitary gland. The hypothalamus is important in regulating various functions, including body temperature, hunger and thirst.

immune system Body's natural defence system against infection. The white blood cells and the lymphatic system are the principal elements of the immune system.

immunity Resistance to infection.

immunization Production of immunity by artificial means.

incubation period Time between being exposed to or "catching" an infection, and actually developing the symptoms of the illness.

infection Disease caused by the invasion of the tissues by organisms such as bacteria, viruses or fungi.

inflammation Tenderness, swelling and redness in part of the body, often caused by injury or infection.

infusion Introduction of a fluid into a vein.

injection Forcing a fluid into the body by way of a needle.

inoculation Act of producing immunization, for example by injecting a vaccine.

intestinal tract Another term for the gastrointestinal system.

intestine Long, tube-like structure between the stomach and the anus, through which food or faeces pass. Also known as the bowel.

ion Atom or molecule with an electrical charge. Dissolved substances take the form of ions, thus common salt (sodium chloride) will take the form of positively-charged sodium ions and negatively-charged chlorine ions.

iris Coloured membrane in the eye that dilates and contracts to regulate the amount of light falling on the retina.

jaundice Unnatural yellow appearance of the skin and the whites of the eyes that is caused by the presence in the blood of bilirubin (a waste product from the liver normally excreted in bile).

larynx Organ at the top of the windpipe (trachea), also known as the voice box.

lesion Abnormality of a tissue.

lower respiratory tract That part of the respiratory system consisting of the bronchi and the lungs.

lymphatic system System of channels and valve-like nodes that conveys fluid from the tissues of the body back into the bloodstream. It is an important part of the immune system.

malignant Harmful. It is a term usually used to describe a cancerous growth, but it can also be applied to a number of other conditions.

membrane Very thin boundary. The term may be used to describe the boundary of a single cell, a thin piece of tissue covering an organ or the lining of a cavity.

metabolism Complete set of all chemical reactions and physical changes in the body.

mucus Viscous fluid secreted by mucous membranes.

mucous membrane Lining of certain parts of the body (such as the mouth, the nose and the intestine) that secretes mucus.

nausea Unpleasant feeling that one is about to vomit.

nebulizer Device for converting a liquid into a fine mist for inhalation.

neuritis Inflammation of a nerve.

neurosis Severe mental illness in which the patient nevertheless retains contact with reality.

neurotransmitter Chemical "messenger" substance secreted by nerve cells.

oedema Swelling of a tissue.

oesophagus Gullet, joining the mouth to the stomach.

oral Relating to the mouth.

ovary Female reproductive organ that produces an ovum in each menstrual cycle. The two ovaries also secrete hormones.
pacemaker Electrical device that can trigger the heartbeat. The natural pacemaker in the heart is called the sinus or sinoatrial node.
palpitations Irregular or regular "fluttering" of the heart, powerful enough to be noticed by the person suffering from them.
pancreas Organ in the abdomen that secretes the hormone insulin into the blood and digestive juices into the digestive tract.
parasympathetic nervous system Part of the autonomic nervous system. Its effects generally oppose those of the sympathetic nervous system.
perforation Hole or opening, usually the result of disease.
peripheral nervous system System of motor and sensory nerves emerging from the spinal cord, supplying all the organs of the body.
peripheral vascular system System of arteries and veins, excluding the largest vessels.
peristalsis Involuntary, wave-like muscular contractions of smooth muscle that propel substances along hollow organs (such as the intestine).
phobia Unreasonable fear.
pituitary gland Small gland in the brain that secretes hormones controlling growth and the functioning of other endocrine glands.
plasma Liquid part of the blood, which contains minerals, proteins and salts.
platelets Very small particles found in the blood. Their main function is in blood clotting.
prolapse Part or all of an organ slipping downwards from its normal position because of poor structural support.
prophylaxis Prevention.
psychosis Severe mental illness with varying symptoms (which may include hallucination) in which the patient loses contact with reality.
pulmonary Relating to the lungs.
pus Yellow or green viscous fluid consisting of dead white blood cells and bacteria. It is a product of the body's reaction to infection.
rectum Last segment of the large intestine, through which the products of digestion pass.
red blood cell Type of cell that circulates in the blood and contains the oxygen-carrying pigment haemoglobin. Red blood cells are also known as erythrocytes.
renal Relating to the kidneys.
renal dialysis Method of artificially performing certain of the kidney's excretory functions.
retina Light-sensitive lining at the back of the eye.
schizophrenia Form of psychosis characterized by a number of symptoms, which may include auditory hallucinations and the disintegration of thought processes and personality.
septicaemia Infection of the blood.
sympathetic nervous system Part of the autonomic nervous system. It is involved in the type of responses that occur when coping with an emergency, and its effects are generally opposed to those of the parasympathetic nervous system.
septic Infected.
serum Part of the blood that remains after the cells have formed a clot.
shock Inability of the cardiovascular system to supply the body with an

adequate amount of blood. The term is often used to describe an emotional reaction, so a distinction is made between emotional and physiological shock; the latter is far more serious and can be life-threatening, although extreme cases of emotional shock can also produce a physiological reaction.

spastic/spasticity Weakness associated with increased reflex activity, caused by a defect in the central nervous system.

spleen Organ in the abdomen involved in the regulation of blood cells and the immune response.

sputum Phlegm, or secretions from the lungs.

stroke Interruption of the blood flow to part of the brain.

syndrome Specific set of physical signs and/or symptoms.

systemic Affecting or relating to the whole of the body, or a complete body system.

thyroid gland Endocrine gland that is found in the neck, which secretes hormones, some of which have important regulatory functions for the entire body.

tissue Group of cells with similar functions.

tolerance Decrease in the body's normal reaction to a drug. Tolerance is sometimes linked with dependence.

tonic Any medicine that is given to increase vigour and vitality.

tonsils Mass of lymphatic tissue on either side of the back of the mouth.

topical Indicating a medicine that is directly applied to the affected area.

toxin Poison (such as those produced by certain bacteria).

trachea Medical name for the windpipe, the airway from the larynx to the bronchial tubes.

tumour Abnormal growth of tissue in the body, which can be either benign or malignant.

ulceration Breach in the lining of a tissue (such as the skin or a mucous membrane). Ulceration of certain tissues may lead to perforation.

upper respiratory tract Airways leading into the lungs (i.e. the mouth, nose, throat and windpipe).

urinary bladder Distensible reservoir that collects urine from the kidneys before excretion.

urinary tract System involved in the production and removal of urine from the body. The kidneys produce urine and the bladder stores it. The ureters and urethra are the tubes through which urine passes.

vein Blood vessel that returns blood from the tissues to the heart.

virus Minute particle that can reproduce within living cells, causing disease. There are few medicines that can cure such diseases (an example of one being the common cold), but vaccines may aid the body's own immune system in dealing with the infection.

white blood cell Type of cell that is usually carried by the blood and lymphatic system, the major functions of which are involved with the body's immune system. There are many varieties of white blood cell. They are also known as leukocytes.

Chart of Common Disorders

This chart provides rapid access to the alphabetical listing of drugs and drug types in terms of various common disorders and the types of drug often used to treat them. However, it is not a guide to treatment. In all cases of illness, a professional medical practitioner should be consulted before any drug is taken. (Words in SMALL CAPITALS appear as headings in the alphabetical listing.)

COMMON DISORDERS	DRUG TYPE COMMONLY USED
Aches, mild pain	
Headache, period pains, joint and muscle ache, toothache, and other mild local pain	ANALGESICS

It is very important that a medical practitioner is consulted about any ache or pain that persists or grows worse.

COMMON DISORDERS	DRUG TYPE COMMONLY USED
Allergies	
General	ANTIHISTAMINES
Small skin reactions, such as rashes and insect bites	ANTIHISTAMINES; and other various proprietary ANTI-INFLAMMATORY preparations
Itching	Various soothing lotions and creams
Babies' problems	
Teething	ANALGESICS; various topical preparations containing analgesic or local ANAESTHETIC agents
Fungal infections (such as thrush)	ANTIFUNGALS
Nappy rash	Various soothing creams and lotions

Diarrhoea, vomiting	In infants these should not treated with drugs. Dilute glucose solutions with mineral additives are sometimes used to replace lost fluids and minerals

Cold, cough, fever, sore throat

Headache, fever, aching muscles	ANALGESICS
Sore throat	Various medicated throat lozenges and syrups
Nasal congestion	DECONGESTANTS
Cough	ANTITUSSIVES; EXPECTORANTS

Medicated inhalations and various proprietary mixtures are also available.

Gastrointestinal problems

Acid or irritated stomach, hiatus hernia, mild ulcer symptoms	ANTACIDS
Nausea, travel sickness	ANTI-EMETICS
Diarrhoea	ANTIDIARRHOEALS
Constipation	LAXATIVES
Haemorrhoids (piles)	Various antihaemorrhoid creams and suppositories

Skin problems (see also allergies)

Burns, cuts and grazes	ANTISEPTICS
Fungal infection (such as athlete's foot)	ANTIFUNGALS
Boils	ANTISEPTICS
Head and body lice	Various lotions or shampoos are available
Acne	ANTISEPTICS; KERATOLYTICS
Dandruff	Various medicated shampoos
Dermatitis	ANTIHISTAMINES; hormonal preparations

Home Medicine Cabinet

A typical home medicine cabinet contains a number of over-the-counter preparations used to treat common disorders, such as those in the chart above; it also has a number of other items that may be useful in first aid. It is recommended that anyone preparing a complete home medicine cabinet should consult his or her family doctor for advice about specific products that may suit their needs, but a basic home first aid kit might contain the following:

antiseptic cream or lotion
analgesics
mild saline eyewash
travel sickness tablets
antihistamines
soothing lotions
antacids
cough and cold remedies
mild laxatives
smelling salts
bandages (wide and narrow)
adhesive plasters
absorbent gauze dressings
tissues for cleansing
cotton wool
safety pins
scissors

Warnings

- All medicines should be kept well out of the reach of children.
- Prescribed drugs should not be kept in a first aid cabinet in case they are used by someone to whom they were not prescribed.
- Courses of drugs prescribed by a doctor should always be completed, so usually there will not be any drugs left over. If there are, however, when the course is finished they should be disposed of by flushing them down the toilet, so that there is no risk of them being found and used incorrectly – for example by children thinking they are sweets.
- Never use drugs that have been prescribed to another person.
- Most drugs have a limited lifespan; this is usually marked on the container. Do not use drugs after their expiry date.